The Family Nurse Practitioner

The Family Nurse Practitioner

Clinical Case Studies

SECOND EDITION

Edited by

Leslie Neal-Boylan, PhD, APRN, CRRN, FAAN, FARN

Mansfield Kaseman Health Clinic
Rockville, MD, USA

WILEY Blackwell

This edition first published 2021
© 2021 John Wiley & Sons Ltd

Edition History
John Wiley & Sons, Inc. (1e, 2011)

Registered Office(s)
John Wiley & Sons, Inc., 111 River Street, Hoboken, NJ 07030, USA
John Wiley & Sons Ltd, The Atrium, Southern Gate, Chichester, West Sussex, PO19 8SQ, UK

Editorial Office
9600 Garsington Road, Oxford, OX4 2DQ, UK

For details of our global editorial offices, customer services, and more information about Wiley products visit us at www.wiley.com.

Wiley also publishes its books in a variety of electronic formats and by print-on-demand. Some content that appears in standard print versions of this book may not be available in other formats.

Library of Congress Cataloging-in-Publication Data
Names: Neal-Boylan, Leslie, editor.
Title: The family nurse practitioner : clinical case studies / [edited by]
    Leslie Neal-Boylan.
Other titles: Clinical case studies for the family nurse practitioner. |
    Case studies in nursing.
Description: Second edition. | Hoboken, NJ : Wiley-Blackwell, 2021. |
    Series: Case studies in nursing | Preceded by Clinical case studies for
    the family nurse practitioner / [edited by] Leslie Neal-Boylan. 2011. |
    Includes bibliographical references and index.
Identifiers: LCCN 2020026509 (print) | LCCN 2020026510 (ebook) |
    ISBN 9781119603191 (paperback) | ISBN 9781119603214 (adobe pdf) |
    ISBN 9781119603221 (epub)
Subjects: MESH: Family Nurse Practitioners | Family Nursing | Primary Care
    Nursing | Case Reports
Classification: LCC RT82.8 (print) | LCC RT82.8 (ebook) | NLM WY 128 |
    DDC 610.7306/92–dc23
LC record available at https://lccn.loc.gov/2020026509
LC ebook record available at https://lccn.loc.gov/2020026510

Cover Design: Wiley
Cover Image: © Arthur Tilley/Getty Images

Set in 10/12pt PalatinoLTStd by SPi Global, Pondicherry, India

10 9 8 7 6 5 4 3 2 1

Contents

Contributors

EDITOR

Leslie Neal-Boylan, PhD, APRN, CRRN, FAAN, FARN
Mansfield Kaseman Health Clinic
Rockville, MD, USA

CONTRIBUTORS

Ivy M. Alexander, PhD, APRN, ANP-BC, FAANP, FAAN
Professor and Director, Adult-Gerontology Primary Care Track
Coordinator, Clinical Scholarship
School of Nursing
University of Connecticut
Storrs, CT, USA

Nancy Cantey Banasiak, DNP, PPCNP-BC, APRN
Associate Professor
Yale University School of Nursing
New Haven, CT, USA

Vera Borkowski, MSN, APRN, FNP-C
Family Nurse Practitioner
Child and Family Agency of Southeastern CT
New London, CT, USA

Suellen Breakey, PhD, RN
Associate Professor
School of Nursing
MGH Institute of Health Professions
Boston, MA, USA

Amy Bruno, PhD, RN, ANP-BC
Term Lecturer
School of Nursing
MGH Institute of Health Professions
Boston, MA, USA

Adult Nurse Practitioner
Galileo Health
New York, NY, USA

Jessica Chan, MSN, APRN, PPCNP-BC
Coordinator of Medical Services
Child and Family Agency of Southeastern CT
New London, CT, USA

Karen M. Flaherty, MSN, MEd, APRN-BC, CBCN
Instructor, Academic Support Counselor
School of Nursing
MGH Institute of Health Professions
Boston, MA, USA

Betsy Gaffney, MSN, APRN, FNP-BC
Family Nurse Practitioner
Child and Family Agency of Southeastern CT
New London, CT, USA

Anna Goddard, PhD, APRN, CPNP-PC
Assistant Professor
College of Nursing
Sacred Heart University
Fairfield, CT, USA

Pediatric Nurse Practitioner
Child and Family Agency of Southeastern CT
New London, CT, USA

Clara Gona, PhD, FNP-BC, RN
Assistant Professors
School of Nursing
MGH Institute of Health Professions
Boston, MA, USA

Allison Grady, MSN, APNP
Clinical Instructor
College of Nursing
University of Wisconsin–Milwaukee
Milwaukee, WI, USA

Pediatric Nurse Practitioner
Medical College of Wisconsin/Children's Wisconsin Clinics
Milwaukee, WI, USA

Millie Hepburn, PhD, RN, SCRN, ACNS-BC
Assistant Professor
Quinnipiac University
Hamden, CT, USA

Rebecca Hill, DNP, RN, FNP-C, CNE
Assistant Professor
School of Nursing
MGH Institute of Health Professions
Boston, MA, USA

Family Nurse Practitioner
Family Doctors, LLC
Swampscott, MA, USA

Erin Janicek, LCSW
Senior Director of Clinical Services
Child and Family Agency of Southeastern CT
New London, CT, USA

Sara Ann Jakub, MA, SYC, LPC
Director of Clinical Services for School-Based Health Centers
Director of Quality Assurance
Child and Family Agency of Southeastern CT
New London, CT, USA

Annette Jakubisin-Konicki, PhD, ANP-BC, FNP-BC, FAANP
Associate Professor
Director, Family Nurse Practitioner Primary Care Track
School of Nursing
University of Connecticut
Storrs, CT, USA

Erin Janicek, LCSW
Senior Director of Clinical Services
Child and Family Agency of Southeastern CT
New London, CT, USA

Susan M. Jussaume, MSN, APRN, FNP-BC, AHN-BC
Instructor and Family Nurse Practitioner
School of Nursing
MGH Institute of Health Professions
Boston, MA, USA

Andrew Konesky, MSN, APRN
Pediatric Nurse Practitioner
Child and Family Agency of Southeastern CT
New London, CT, USA

Jason R. Lucey, DNP, FNP-BC
Assistant Professor
Family Track Co-Coordinator
School of Nursing
MGH Institute of Health Professions
Boston, MA, USA

Antonia C. Makosky, DNP, MPH, ANP-BC, ANP
Assistant Professor
Adult-Gerontology Primary Care Track Co-Coordinator
School of Nursing
MGH Institute of Health Professions
Boston, MA, USA

Mikki Meadows-Oliver, PhD, RN, FAAN
Associate Professor
School of Nursing
Quinnipiac University
Hamden, CT, USA

Sheila L. Molony, PhD, APRN, GNP-BC, FGSA, FAAN
Professor of Nursing
Quinnipiac University
Hamden, CT, USA

Patrice K. Nicholas, DNSc, DHL (Hon), MPH, MS, RN, NP-C, FAAN
Distinguished Teaching Professor and Director
Center for Climate Change, Climate Justice, and Health
School of Nursing
MGH Institute of Health Professions
Boston, MA, USA

Meredith Scannell, PhD, MSN, MPH, CNM, CEN, SANE-A
Clinical Research Nurse and Emergency Nurse
Brigham and Women's Hospital
Boston, MA, USA

Sara Smoller, RN, MSN, ANP-BC
Assistant Professor
School of Nursing
MGH Institute of Health Professions
Boston, MA

Adult Nurse Practitioner
Family Doctors, LLC
Swampscott, MA, USA

Sheila Swales, MS, RN, PMHNP-BC
Instructor
School of Nursing
MGH Institute of Health Professions
Boston, MA, USA

Nancy M. Terres, PhD, RN
Associate Professor of Nursing
School of Nursing
MGH Institute of Health Professions
Boston, MA, USA

Preface

The purpose of this book is to help clinicians and students better understand how to diagnose and manage typical (and some atypical) patient cases. While the focus is on the nurse practitioner role, this book will be useful to other patient care providers, such as physicians and physician's assistants. The contributing authors have worked hard to update cases from the first edition of this book to better reflect patient-centered language and advances in care. We have developed several new cases, such as one on climate change, to assist clinicians with scenarios that were not as predominant as they are today.

We have presented a variety of patients in these cases with regard to age, gender identity, socioeconomic status, family status, and other considerations. However, please don't hesitate to alter these demographics to tailor the cases for your specific needs.

The contributing authors in this book are all subject matter experts. They have written these cases from real life. Consequently, the cases do not result in cookie-cutter solutions. Critical thinking questions encourage the reader to think carefully about the case as presented and about potential resolutions to the case given variations that occur in real life. These cases should be used to jump-start conversations among students, faculty, and clinicians regarding possible treatment options depending on the individual patient. All cases include the most current research and guidelines for treatment.

The cases are presented chronologically from pediatric to adolescent to adult and older adult. Cases in women's health and men's health have their own separate chapters. Mental health cases are now in a separate chapter.

For this second edition we moved the case resolutions to the end of the book. The best use of the book is to read and analyze the case, alter the demographics of the patient to view the case from multiple perspectives, and then review and discuss the resolutions. Keep in mind that there is typically more than one way to treat a patient and patients should always be diagnosed and treated on an individual basis, so there is often more than one possible resolution to a case. We have only included one resolution per case in this book.

Acknowledgments

I am so grateful to the readers of the first edition of this book. Thank you for using it. I hope you will find this second edition even more helpful. Many thanks to the contributing authors of this second edition. Several rejoined me from the first edition and others are new to this edition. All were easy to work with and are consummate professionals and excellent clinicians.

Thanks to all the patients and colleagues who've taught me so much throughout the years. Clinical practice and nursing education are my great passions and I'm grateful for all I learn every day.

Finally, thank you to Edward and Natalie Rotkoff, Kevin Boylan, Paul Neal, Corinne Neal, Andrew Neal, and Bonnie Brown.

Introduction

By Leslie Neal-Boylan, PhD, APRN, CRRN, FAAN, FARN

Family practice is not simply the practice of caring for individuals across the lifespan. Contrary to the perceptions of many students who enter the world of family practice, it is not simply to care for people "from womb to tomb." Practice that is guided by that philosophy risks missing so much, not only regarding the individual patient's own health but the family dynamics and the tangible and intangible aspects of the family that impact the individual patient. If the "family" aspect of family practice is ignored or neglected, then the clinician is simply caring for individuals as any clinician would and cannot really style themselves as a family practice clinician regardless of title or certification.

To practice as a family practice clinician, it is important to have a basic understanding first about what is meant by "family" and then how the family is integrated into the plan of care and ultimately often becomes the "patient." In previous work about home health clinicians, this author found that home health clinicians care for the "patient entity," which is defined as all those who impact or potentially impact the patient's health. In family practice, the clinician also cares for and, at the very least, considers the patient entity when developing and pursuing a plan of care for an individual who seeks health care.

The meaning of "family" has undergone significant societal change. Consequently, it is important that the clinician not make assumptions about who is "family" and who is not. It is important to ask the patient who they consider their family. As I write this, society, both nationally and globally, is undergoing the crisis brought on by the coronavirus. Aside from the medical implications, the virus is already having an impact on how people interact with each other. We are required to practice "social distancing," which requires us to maintain our relationships, whether personal or professional, in other ways besides close proximity or touching. Neighbors are calling to check in on the elderly, especially those who don't have family nearby, and older adults are checking on the young parents in their neighborhoods who are working from home while trying to manage children who are unable to attend school due to the pandemic. What is the definition of family during a crisis like this? How will we keep each other from becoming socially isolated?

Crises like these imply a new definition of family. Technology allows us to keep in contact despite the prohibition on being physically within six feet of another human being. A crisis like this reminds us how vulnerable we are as human beings, not only to disease but to loneliness and despair. Knowing that others care about us takes on even greater significance. We are reminded that "family," however we define it, is crucial to our survival.

As clinicians, we are just as vulnerable but have the advantage of a vast store of medical knowledge. As laypersons disseminate misconceptions about how to prevent and treat the virus, nurse practitioners and our health professions colleagues are stepping up to make sure the public has accurate health care information.

Our care of individuals and families does not just take place in the clinic or health care setting. It occurs via every encounter we have with the people in our communities and across cyberspace. The coronavirus crisis illustrates that while we have better means of communication than in years past, we are also vulnerable to more misinformation.

The cases in this book were chosen in an attempt to illustrate mostly typical (and some atypical) cases that occur in family practice. Remembering the impact "family" has on our physical and mental health and that the patient is part of a subsystem within the larger family system can help the reader see that the patient's illness or condition not only impacts the patient but potentially has a ripple effect on many others both within and outside of the family system.

Abbreviations and Acronyms

AAA: Abdominal aortic aneurysm
AACE: American Association of Clinical Endocrinologists
AAP: American Academy of Pediatrics
ABG: Arterial blood gas
ABI: Ankle brachial index
ACC: American College of Cardiology
ACIP: Advisory Committee on Immunization Practices
ACL: Anterior cruciate ligament
ACS: Acute coronary syndrome
ADHD: Attention-deficit hyperactive disorder
ad lib: At liberty or whenever the patient wants to do something
AGS: American Geriatrics Society
AHA: American Heart Association
AMI: Acute myocardial infarction or heart attack
ANA: Anti-nuclear antibody
AP: Anterior-posterior
APA: American Psychiatric Association
Apgar: The score given to newborns at 1 minute and 5 minutes after birth. The newborn is scored on activity (muscle tone), pulse, grimace (reflex irritability), appearance (skin color), and respirations.
AS: Active surveillance
BD: Blastomycoses dermatitidis
BDI: Beck Depression Inventory
BMI: Body mass index
BMP: Basic metabolic panel
BP: Blood pressure
BS: Bowel sounds
BUN: Blood urea nitrogen
CAD: Coronary artery disease
CAM: Complementary and alternative medicine *or* Confusion Assessment Method
CBC: Complete blood count, with or without diff (differential)
CBT: Cognitive behavioral therapy
CCB: Calcium channel blocker
CCRC: Continuing care retirement community
CKD: Chronic kidney disease
CLI: Critical limb ischemia

CLIA:	Clinical Laboratory Improvement Amendment
CMP:	Complete metabolic panel
CMT:	Cervical motion tenderness
COC:	Combined oral contraceptive pill
COPD:	Chronic obstructive pulmonary disease
COWS:	Clinical Opiate Withdrawal Scale
CRP:	C-reactive protein
C-SSRS:	Columbia–Suicide Severity Rating Scale
CT:	Computed tomography
CTA:	Clear to auscultation
CVA:	Cerebrovascular accident
CXR:	Chest X-ray
D&C:	Dilatation and curettage
DASH:	Dietary Approaches to Stop Hypertension
DDVAP:	Desmopressin acetate vasopressin
DEA:	Drug Enforcement Agency
DFA:	Direct fluorescent antibody (testing)
DMARD:	Disease-modifying antirheumatic drug
DMPA:	Depo-Provera
DoD:	Department of Defense
DOE:	Dyspnea on exertion
DRE:	Digital rectal examination
DVT/PE:	Deep vein thrombosis/pulmonary embolism
DXA:	Dual-energy absorptiometry
EBV:	Epstein-Barr virus
ECG:	Electrocardiogram
ED:	Emergency department
EEG:	Electroencephalogram
ELISA:	Enzyme-linked immunosorbent assay
EM:	Erythema migrans
EMA:	Endomysial antibody
EMDR:	Eye movement desensitization and reprocessing
ENT:	Ear, nose, and throat
EOB:	Explanation of benefits
EOM:	Extraocular movement
EPT:	Expedited partner therapy
ESPGN:	European Society for Pediatric Gastroenterology, Hepatology, and Nutrition
ESR:	Erythrocyte sedimentation rate
ETOH:	Alcohol (drinking kind)
FBG:	Fasting blood glucose
FBS:	Fasting blood sugar
FIT:	Fecal immunochemical test
FM:	Fibromyalgia
FROM:	Full range of motion
FTT:	Failure to thrive
GABHS:	Group A beta-hemolytic streptococci
GAD:	Glutamic acid decarboxylase
GC/CHL:	Gonorrhea/chlamydia
GCA:	Giant cell arteritis
GCS:	Glasgow Coma Scale
GDMT:	Guideline-directed medical therapy
GDS:	Geriatric Depression Scale

GERD:	Gastroesophageal reflux disease
GFR:	Glomerular filtration rate
GI:	Gastrointestinal
GINA:	Global Initiative for Asthma
HA1c:	Hemoglobin A1c
HCV:	Hepatitis C virus
HPV:	Human papilloma virus
HR:	Heart rate
HRI:	Heat-related illness
HSDD:	Hypoactive sexual desire disorder
HSM:	Hepatosplenomegaly
HSV:	Herpes simplex virus
HT:	Hormone therapy
HTN:	Hypertension
HZO:	Herpes zoster opthalmica
IBD:	Inflammatory bowel disease
IBS:	Irritable bowel syndrome
IgA:	Immunoglobulin A
IgE:	Immunoglobulin E
ITP:	Idiopathic thrombocytopenic purpura
IUC:	Intrauterine contraception
IUD:	Intrauterine device
KOH:	Potassium hydroxide
KUB:	Kidneys, ureters, and bladder
LARC:	Long-acting reversible contraceptives
LDH:	Lactic acid dehydrogenase
LEAP:	Learning Early About Peanut
LFT:	Liver function test
LLSB:	Left lower sternal border
LMP:	Last menstrual period
LNMP:	Last normal menstrual period
LR:	Light reflex
LRI:	Lower respiratory infections
LROM:	Limited range of motion
MCI:	Mild cognitive impairment
MCP:	Metacarpal phalangeal (joint)
MCV:	Mean corpuscular volume
MDD:	Major depressive disorder
MDI:	Metered dose inhaler
MGF:	Maternal grandfather
MGM:	Maternal grandmother
MI:	Myocardial infarction *or* motivational interviewing
MMSE:	Mini-Mental State Examination
MoCA:	Montreal Cognitive Assessment
MRI:	Magnetic resonance imaging
MRSA:	Methicillin-resistant *Staphylococcus aureus*
MSSA:	Methicillin-susceptible *Staphylococcus aureus*
MSU:	Monosodium urate
MTP:	Metatarsophalangeal (joint)
MVI:	Multiple vitamin
NAAT:	Nucleic acid amplification test
NAD:	No apparent distress

NAPNAP:	National Association of Pediatric Nurse Practitioners
NARES:	Nonallergic rhinitis with eosinophilia syndrome
NIAAA:	National Institute of Alcohol Abuse and Alcoholism
NICU:	Neonatal intensive care unit
NIDA:	National Institute on Drug Abuse
NKDA:	No known drug allergies
NKFA:	No known food allergies
NOF:	National Osteoporosis Foundation
NP:	Nurse practitioner
NPH:	Normal pressure hydrocephalus
NSAID:	Nonsteroidal anti-inflammatory drug
NSTEMI:	Non-ST elevation myocardial infarction
NSVD:	Normal spontaneous vaginal delivery
NT/ND:	Nontender/nondistended
OA:	Osteoarthritis
O2 sat:	Oxygen saturation
OCP:	Oral contraceptive pill
ODD:	Oppositional defiant disorder
OGTT:	Oral glucose tolerance test
OP:	Osteoporosis
OSA:	Obstructive sleep apnea
OTC:	Over-the-counter (medication)
OUD:	Opioid use disorder
PAD:	Peripheral artery disease
PCOS:	Polycystic ovarian syndrome
PCR:	Polymerase chain reaction
PDA:	Patent ductus arteriosus
PE:	Pulmonary embolism
PEG:	Polyethylene glycol
PEP:	Post-exposure prophylaxis
PERRLA:	Pupils equal, round, reactive to light and accommodation
PGF:	Paternal grandfather
PGM:	Paternal grandmother
PH/G:	Pubic hair/gonads
PHN:	Postherpetic neuralgia
PHQ:	Patient Health Questionnaire
PID:	Pelvic inflammatory disease
PIP:	Proximal interphalangeal (joint)
PLP:	Phantom limb pain
PMDD:	Premenstrual dysphoric disorder
PMR:	Polymyalgia rheumatica
PMS:	Premenstrual syndrome
PNE:	Primary nocturnal enuresis
PPD:	Postpartum depression
PPI:	Proton pump inhibitor
PRN:	As needed
PSI:	Pneumonia Severity Index
PTSD:	Post-traumatic stress disorder
PVD:	Peripheral vascular disease
QD:	Once daily
RAI:	Radionucleotide uptake scan with iodine
RED-S:	Relative energy deficiency in sports

REM:	Rapid eye movement
RICE:	Rest, ice, compression, and elevation
ROS:	Review of systems
RR:	Respiratory rate
RRR:	Regular rate and rhythm
RSV:	Respiratory syncytial virus
RUQ:	Right upper quadrant
SAFE-T:	Suicide Assessment Five-Step Evaluation and Triage
SAMHSA:	Substance Abuse and Mental Health Services Administration
SANE:	Sexual assault nurse examiner
SART:	Sexual assault response team
SBHC:	School-based health center
SBIRT:	Screening, Brief Intervention, and Referral for Treatment
SEM:	Systolic ejection murmur
SERM:	Selective estrogen receptor modulator
SGA:	Small for gestational age
SIB:	Self-injurious behavior
SJS:	Stevens-Johnson Syndrome
SLE:	Systemic lupus erythematosus
SM:	Stroke mimic
SNRI:	Serotonin norepinephrine reuptake inhibitor
SSP:	Syringe services program
SSRI:	Selective serotonin reuptake inhibitor
STI:	Sexually transmitted infection
SUD:	Substance use disorder
SWS:	Slow-wave sleep
TANF:	Temporary Assistance for Needy Families
TBI:	Traumatic brain injury *or* toe brachial index
TBSA:	Total body surface area
TCA:	Tricyclic antidepressant
TEN:	Toxic epidermal necrosis
TENS:	Transcutaneous electrical nerve stimulation
TM:	Tympanic membrane
TPO:	Antithydroperoxidase antibody
TRAb:	Thyrotropin receptor antibody
TRUS:	Transrectal ultrasound
TSH:	Thyroid-stimulating hormone
tTG:	Tissue transglutaminase
TTN:	Transient tachypnea of the newborn
TTP:	Tenderness to palpation
ULT:	Urate-lowering therapy
URI:	Upper respiratory infection
USPSTF:	U.S. Preventive Services Task Force
UTI:	Urinary tract infection
VA:	Veterans Administration
VCF:	Vertebral compression fracture
VCUG:	Voiding cystourethrography
VDRL:	Venereal disease research laboratory
VZV:	Varicella zoster virus
WBC:	White blood cell
WHI:	Women's Health Initiative
WIC:	Women, Infants, and Children Supplemental Nutrition Program

Section 1

The Neonate

Case 1.1 Cardiovascular Screening Exam

By Mikki Meadows-Oliver, PhD, RN, FAAN

SUBJECTIVE

Justin, a 10-day-old male, presents in the primary care office for a weight check. He is accompanied by his parents. His mother is concerned about his feeding habits. She believes that he takes awhile to drink his formula—longer than his siblings did; she also thinks that he sweats more than they did, even when he doesn't feel warm.

Birth history: Significant for a 36-week gestation. His birth weight was 2600 grams. Because of his premature birth, Justin required hospitalization for the first week of life in the Neonatal Intensive Care Unit (NICU). During his stay in the NICU, he was noted to feed without problems, maintain his temperature without assistance, and gain weight. His weight at discharge from the hospital 3 days ago was 2400 grams. Because of his premature birth status and his decreased weight, the family was told to follow up with their primary care provider in 3 days.

In the office today, his weight is 2490 grams. Further questioning about Justin's birth history reveals that the mother's pregnancy was normal. She had no infections, falls, or known exposures to environmental hazards. She did not drink alcohol, take prescription medication (other than prenatal vitamins), use tobacco products, or use illicit drugs. During labor, she experienced a failure to progress, which resulted in her having a cesarean birth. The baby's Apgar scores were 8 at 1 minute and 9 at 5 minutes.

Social history: Justin was born to a single, 29-year-old mother. His father is involved but does not reside in the household. Justin lives in an apartment with his mother and two other siblings (ages 2 and 4 years). The maternal grandmother (MGM) lives nearby and is able to help Justin's mother provide care. The family receives several governmental subsidies such as the Women, Infants, and Children (WIC) Supplemental Nutrition Program, Temporary Assistance for Needy Families (TANF), and Medicaid. Educationally, Justin's mother has a high school diploma. She works in a local retail store. Justin's father works in a manufacturing plant. The family has no pets. The MGM smokes but does not smoke in the home.

Diet: Breastfeeding ad lib with supplementation of a milk-based formula.

Elimination: 6–8 wet diapers daily with 3–4 yellow, seedy bowel movements.

Sleep: Sleeps between feedings.

The Family Nurse Practitioner: Clinical Case Studies, Second Edition. Edited by Leslie Neal-Boylan.
© 2021 John Wiley & Sons Ltd. Published 2021 by John Wiley & Sons Ltd.

Family medical history: PGF (age 54): diabetes mellitus, heart attack at age 50; PGM (age 53): healthy; MGF: deceased from stroke at age 47; MGM (age 54): asthma; mother (age 29): asthma; father (age 31): healthy; Sibling #1 (age 4): asthma; Sibling #2 (age 2): heart murmur.

Medications: Currently taking no prescription, herbal, or OTC medications.

Allergies: No known allergies to food, medications, or environment.

OBJECTIVE

Vital signs: Weight: 2490 grams; length: 44 centimeters; temperature: 37°C (rectal).

General: Alert, well-nourished, well-hydrated baby.

Skin: Clear with no lesions noted; no cyanosis of lips, nails, or skin; no diaphoresis noted; skin turgor with elastic recoil.

Head: Normocephalic; anterior fontanel open and flat (2 cm × 3 cm); posterior fontanel open and flat (1 cm × 1 cm).

Eyes: Red reflex present bilaterally; pupils equal, round, and reactive to light; no discharge noted.

Ears: Pinnae normal; tympanic membranes gray bilaterally with positive light reflex.

Nose: Both nostrils patent; no discharge.

Oropharynx: Mucous membranes moist; no teeth present; no lesions.

Neck: Supple; no nodes.

Respiratory: RR = 28; clear in all lobes; no adventitious sounds noted; no retractions; no deformities of the thoracic cage noted.

Cardiac/Peripheral vascular: HR = 120; thrill noted in pulmonic area; continuous, systolic, grade 3 heart murmur noted on exam in the pulmonic area of the chest with both the bell and diaphragm; no radiation of the murmur to the back or axilla; brachial and femoral pulses present and 2+ bilaterally.

Abdomen/Gastrointestinal: Soft, nontender, nondistended, no evidence of hepatosplenomegaly. Umbilical cord is in place with no signs and symptoms of infection.

Genitourinary: Normal male; testes descended bilaterally; circumcision healing well.

Back: Spine straight.

Extremities: Full range of motion of all extremities; warm and well perfused; capillary refill <2 seconds. Negative hip click.

Neurologic: Good suck and cry; good tone in all extremities; positive Moro, rooting, plantar, palmar, and Babinski reflexes.

CRITICAL THINKING

Which diagnostic or imaging studies should be considered to assist with or confirm the diagnosis?
___Chest X-ray (CXR)
___Echocardiogram
___Electrocardiogram

What is the most likely differential diagnosis and why?

___Patent ductus arteriosus

___Venous hum

___Atrioventricular malformation

What is the plan of treatment, and what should be the plan for follow-up care?

Are there any referrals needed?

Does this patient's psychosocial history influence how you might treat her?

What if this baby were a girl?

What if this baby had been born full term?

What if this baby had been born at a higher altitude?

Are there any standardized guidelines that should be used to assess or treat this case?

Case 1.2 Pulmonary Screening Exam

By Mikki Meadows-Oliver, PhD, RN, FAAN

SUBJECTIVE

Cassidy, a 12-hour-old female, was born at home via planned home birth. She was brought into the office for an initial health maintenance visit. On initial examination, she was found to have rapid breathing when the office nurse weighed her. Cassidy is accompanied by both parents. There are no parental concerns.

Birth history: Cassidy is the product of a 40-week gestation. She was delivered vaginally at home by a certified nurse midwife. During the pregnancy, Cassidy's mother had no falls, infections, or known exposures to environmental hazards. She did not drink alcohol, take prescription medication (other than prenatal vitamins), use tobacco products, or use illicit drugs. The total labor duration was 2 hours. Cassidy's birth weight was 3380 g and her Apgar scores were 9 at 1 minute and 9 at 5 minutes.

Social history: Cassidy was born to a 37-year-old mother. Cassidy is the second child and has a 3-year-old sibling. She lives at home with both parents and her older sibling. The family employs an au pair who also resides in the home. Both parents are college educated. The mother works as a research assistant, and the father works as an accountant. There are no pets or smokers in the home.

Diet: Breastfeeding ad lib, but mother feels that Cassidy is having problems latching on. Colostrum is present. Milk has not come in yet.

Elimination: Urinated at birth, and has had 3 wet diapers since that time. Passed meconium at 10 hours of age.

Sleep: Sleeps between feedings.

Family medical history: PGF (age 67): sarcoidosis; PGM (age 63): healthy; MGF (age 64): Type 2 diabetes; MGM (age 64): history of MI at age 63; mother (age 37): healthy; father (age 42): healthy; Sibling #1 (age 3): healthy; history of bronchiolitis.

Medications: Currently taking no prescription, herbal, or over-the-counter medications.

Allergies: No known allergies to food, medications, or environment.

OBJECTIVE

Vital signs: Weight in the office today is 3360 g; length: 48 cm; temperature: 37.2°C (rectal); pulse oximeter reading: 95% on room air.

General: Alert, active baby.

Skin: Clear with no lesions noted; no cyanosis of skin, lips, or nails; no diaphoresis noted; skin turgor intact.

Head: Molding present; anterior fontanel open and flat (2 cm × 2 cm); posterior fontanel open and flat (1 cm × 1 cm).

Eyes: Red reflex present bilaterally; pupils equal, round, and reactive to light; no discharge noted.

Ears: Pinnae normal; tympanic membranes gray bilaterally with positive light reflex.

Nose: Both nostrils patent; no discharge; mild nasal flaring.

Oropharynx: Mucous membranes moist; no teeth present; no lesions.

Neck: Supple; no nodes.

Respiratory: RR = 68; crackles present in lower lung fields bilaterally; mild intercostal retractions; no grunting. No deformities of the thoracic cage noted.

Cardiac/Peripheral vascular: HR = 120; regular rhythm; no murmur noted; brachial and femoral pulses present and 2+ bilaterally.

Abdomen/Gastrointestinal: Soft, nontender, nondistended, no evidence of hepatosplenomegaly. Umbilical cord is in place with no signs and symptoms of infection.

Genitourinary: Normal female genitalia.

Back: Spine straight.

Extremities: Full range of motion of all extremities; warm and well-perfused; capillary refill <2 seconds; negative hip click.

Neurologic: Good suck and cry; good tone in all extremities; positive Moro, rooting, gag, plantar, palmar, and Babinski reflexes.

CRITICAL THINKING

Which diagnostic or imaging studies should be considered to assist with or confirm the diagnosis?
___Chest radiograph
___Arterial blood gas (ABG)
___Pulmonary function tests

What is the most likely differential diagnosis and why?
___Transient tachypnea of the newborn
___Pneumonia
___Neonatal sepsis

What is the plan of treatment, referral, and follow-up care?

Are there any demographic characteristics that would affect this case?

What if the patient lived in a rural, isolated setting?

Are there any standardized guidelines that should be used to assess or treat this case?

Case 1.3 Skin Screening Exam

By Mikki Meadows-Oliver, PhD, RN, FAAN

SUBJECTIVE

Siobhan is a 4-day-old infant in the office with her mother for an initial visit and weight check. Her mother states that Siobhan has a rash on her chest and arms that has been intermittent for the past 2 days. There do not seem to be any triggers for the rash. Siobhan's mother has washed all of the baby's clothes in a hypoallergenic cleanser only and has not used any moisturizers on the skin since the baby was discharged from the hospital. The rash also appears when Siobhan is clad in only a diaper. The rash does not appear to cause discomfort for Siobhan. Siobhan's mother has not found anything that makes the rash better or worse.

Birth history: Siobhan is the product of a 40-week gestation. Her birth weight was 3600 g. Further questioning about Siobhan's birth history reveals that the mother's pregnancy was normal. She had no infections, falls, or known exposures to environmental hazards. She did not use alcohol, take prescription medication (other than prenatal vitamins), use tobacco products, or use illicit drugs. During labor, Siobhan's mother received a narcotic analgesic 1 hour prior to birth. Siobhan was delivered via spontaneous vaginal delivery and her Apgar scores were 7 at 1 minute and 9 at 5 minutes.

Social history: Siobhan was born to a single, 18-year-old mother. Siobhan's father is involved but does not reside in the household. Siobhan lives in a 2-bedroom apartment with her mother and maternal grandmother (MGM). The MGM is able to help Siobhan's mother provide care. Siobhan's mother receives several governmental subsidies such as the Women, Infants, and Children (WIC) Supplemental Nutrition Program, Temporary Assistance for Needy Families (TANF), and Medicaid. Educationally, Siobhan's mother is completing coursework for her high school diploma. Siobhan's father is also a high school student. There are no smokers in the home. The family has a dog.

Diet: Siobhan is being fed a milk-based formula—2 oz every 3–4 hours.

Elimination: 6–8 wet diapers daily with 3–4 yellow, seedy bowel movements.

Sleep: Sleeps between feedings.

Family medical history: PGF (age 40): asthma; PGM (age 38): obesity, high cholesterol, hypertension; MGF (age 36): sickle cell trait; MGM (age 34): bipolar disorder; mother (age 18): sickle cell trait; father (age 17): eczema.

The Family Nurse Practitioner: Clinical Case Studies, Second Edition. Edited by Leslie Neal-Boylan.
© 2021 John Wiley & Sons Ltd. Published 2021 by John Wiley & Sons Ltd.

Medications: Currently taking no prescription, herbal, or over-the-counter medications.

Allergies: No known allergies to food, medications, or environment.

OBJECTIVE

Vital signs: Weight: 3690 g; length: 44 cm; temperature: 36.8°C (rectal).

General: Alert, well-nourished, well-hydrated baby.

Skin: Scattered 1-cm, yellow-white papules on an erythematous base on the trunk, upper arms, and thighs; lesions are nontender to touch; lanugo over shoulders; no cyanosis of lips, nails, or skin; no diaphoresis noted; good skin turgor.

Head: Normocephalic; anterior fontanel open and flat (0.3 cm × 3 cm); posterior fontanel open and flat (0.5 cm × 0.5 cm).

Eyes: Red reflex present bilaterally; pupils equal, round, and reactive to light; no discharge noted.

Ears: Pinnae normal; tympanic membranes gray bilaterally with positive light reflex.

Nose: Both nostrils patent; no discharge.

Oropharynx: Mucous membranes moist; no teeth present; no lesions.

Neck: Supple; no nodes.

Respiratory: RR = 28; clear in all lobes; no adventitious sounds noted; no retractions; no deformities of the thoracic cage noted.

Cardiac/Peripheral vascular: HR = 120; regular rhythm; no murmur noted; brachial and femoral pulses present and 2+ bilaterally.

Abdomen/Gastrointestinal: Soft, nontender, nondistended, no evidence of hepatosplenomegaly. Umbilical cord is in place without signs and symptoms of infection.

Genitourinary: Normal male; testes descended bilaterally; circumcision healing well.

Back: Spine straight.

Extremities: Full range of motion of all extremities; warm and well-perfused; capillary refill <2 seconds; negative hip click.

Neurologic: Good suck and cry; good tone in all extremities; positive Moro, rooting, plantar, palmar, and Babinski reflexes.

CRITICAL THINKING

Which diagnostic or imaging studies should be considered to assist with or confirm the diagnosis?
___Skin biopsy
___Peripheral blood smear
___Bacterial/viral culture from the lesion

What is the most likely differential diagnosis and why?
___Milia
___Erythema toxicum
___Herpes simplex virus

What is the plan of treatment?

Does the patient's psychosocial history impact how you might treat her?

Are any referrals needed?

Are there any demographic characteristics that would affect this case?

Are there any standardized guidelines that should be used to assess or treat this case?

Case 1.4 Oxygenation

By Mikki Meadows-Oliver, PhD, RN, FAAN

SUBJECTIVE

Matthew, a 27-day-old infant, arrives at the office with complaints of "breathing fast" and conges-tion since yesterday. He is accompanied by both parents. He has had no fever. At home, his rectal temperature was 37.2 degrees this morning. The parents tried using a humidifier to alleviate the symptoms, but they do not feel that this helped. They also used a bulb syringe with nasal saline to help relieve nasal congestion. Matthew has had several visitors at his home during the first few weeks of his life, including small children who attend day-care centers. His mother thinks that some of those visitors may have had cold symptoms, although she tried to keep anyone who seemed sick away from Matthew.

Diet: Normally breastfeeding every 2–3 hours; occasionally supplementing with a milk-based formula. Since yesterday, intake has decreased.

Elimination: 4–6 wet diapers since yesterday, which is decreased from his normal urine output. 2–3 bowel movements.

Sleep: Normally sleeps approximately 5 hours at night with several naps throughout the day. However, since yesterday, Matthew's sleep has been interrupted.

Medications: Currently taking no prescription, herbal, or over-the-counter medications.

Allergies: No known allergies to food, medications, or environment.

Birth history: Matthew was the product of a 39-week gestation. He was delivered via planned cesarean section. Matthew's mother had no falls or known exposures to environmental hazards. She has a history of chlamydia during the pregnancy at 36 weeks' gestation. She was treated with antibiotics. The only other prescription medications taken during the pregnancy were prenatal vitamins. She did not use tobacco products or use illicit drugs. She stated that she drank an occa-sional glass of wine during the third trimester. Matthew's birth weight was 3250 g, and his Apgar scores were 9 at 1 minute and 9 at 5 minutes.

Social history: Matthew was born to a 32-year-old mother. He lives at home with both parents. Neither parent has any other children. The mother works as a secretary, and the father works in construction. Matthew's father is a smoker. The family has 2 cats.

The Family Nurse Practitioner: Clinical Case Studies, Second Edition. Edited by Leslie Neal-Boylan.
© 2021 John Wiley & Sons Ltd. Published 2021 by John Wiley & Sons Ltd.

Family medical history: PGF (age 65): Type 2 diabetes mellitus; PGM (age 64): breast cancer at age 55; MGF (age 60): asthma; MGM (age 64): healthy; mother (age 32): asthma; father (age 32): seasonal allergies.

OBJECTIVE

Vital signs: Weight: 4050 grams; length: 48 cm; temperature: 37.2°C (rectal); pulse oximeter reading: 91% on room air.

General: Alert, well-hydrated, well-nourished baby in mild respiratory distress.

Skin: Clear with no lesions noted; no cyanosis of skin, lips, or nails; no diaphoresis noted; good skin turgor.

Head: Normocephalic; anterior fontanelle open and flat (2 cm × 2 cm); posterior fontanelle open and flat (0.5 cm × 0.5 cm).

Eyes: Red reflex present bilaterally; pupils equal, round, and reactive to light; no discharge noted.

Ears: Pinnae normal; tympanic membranes gray bilaterally with positive light reflex.

Nose: Both nostrils congested; cloudy discharge present in nares; mild nasal flaring.

Oropharynx: Mucous membranes moist; no teeth present; no lesions.

Neck: Supple; no nodes.

Respiratory: RR = 42; expiratory wheezing present in all lobes; intercostal retractions present; no grunting; no deformities of the thoracic cage noted.

Cardiac/Peripheral vascular: HR = 120; regular rhythm; no murmur noted; brachial and femoral pulses present and 2+ bilaterally.

Abdomen/Gastrointestinal: Soft, nontender, nondistended, no evidence of hepatosplenomegaly.

Genitourinary: Normal male genitalia; testes descended bilaterally.

Back: Spine straight.

Extremities: Full range of motion of all extremities; warm and well-perfused; capillary refill <2 seconds; negative hip click.

Neurologic: Good suck and cry; good tone in all extremities; positive Moro, rooting, plantar, palmar, and Babinski reflexes.

CRITICAL THINKING

Which diagnostic or imaging studies should be considered to assist with or confirm the diagnosis?
___Chest radiograph (anterior-posterior [AP] and lateral views)
___Nasopharyngeal swab to detect respiratory syncytial virus (RSV)
___Complete blood count

What is the most likely differential diagnosis and why?

___Bronchiolitis

___Upper respiratory infection (URI)

___Chlamydial pneumonia

What is the plan of treatment, referral, and follow-up care?

What demographic characteristics might affect this case?

Does the patient's psychosocial history impact how you might treat him?

What if the patient lived in a rural, isolated setting?

Case 1.5 Nutrition and Weight

By Mikki Meadows-Oliver, PhD, RN, FAAN

SUBJECTIVE

Anita is a 2-week-old Hispanic female in for her well-child check. She is accompanied by her 15-year-old mother. The family speaks only Spanish. A Spanish-speaking interpreter is used for the visit. Anita's mother is concerned that Anita spits up a lot after eating. The mother states that the vomit is not projectile. The mother is worried that, since the baby is vomiting so much, she is not getting enough food. Therefore, the mother has been feeding Anita even more formula. Also, Anita's mother is worried that she will run out of formula since the baby takes so much.

Diet: Formula feeding: 5 oz every 2–3 hours.

Elimination: 6 wet diapers and 3 bowel movements since yesterday.

Sleep: Sleeps approximately 4 hours at night with several naps throughout the day.

Medications: Currently taking no prescription, herbal, or over-the-counter medications.

Allergies: No known allergies to food, medications, environment.

Birth history: Anita was the product of a 38-week gestation. She was delivered via spontaneous vaginal delivery. Anita's mother had no falls, infections, or known exposures to environmental hazards. The only prescription medications taken during the pregnancy were prenatal vitamins. She did not use alcohol, tobacco products, or illicit drugs during the pregnancy. Anita's birth weight was 3250 g and her Apgar scores were 8 at 1 minute and 9 at 5 minutes. Her discharge weight was 3180 g.

Social history: Anita lives at home with her teenage mother and her maternal grandmother (MGM), who emigrated from Mexico. The father of the baby is involved. Neither parent has any other children. Both parents are students at a local high school. The family has a dog.

Family medical history: PGF (age 37): high blood pressure; PGM (age 33): thyroid problems; MGF (age 35): health history unknown; MGM (age 30): healthy; mother (age 15): healthy; father (age 15): healthy.

The Family Nurse Practitioner: Clinical Case Studies, Second Edition. Edited by Leslie Neal-Boylan.
© 2021 John Wiley & Sons Ltd. Published 2021 by John Wiley & Sons Ltd.

OBJECTIVE

Vital signs: Weight: 4050 g; length: 48 cm; temperature: 37.3°C (rectal).

General: Alert, well-developed baby.

Skin: Clear with no lesions noted; no cyanosis of skin, lips, or nails; no diaphoresis noted; good skin turgor.

Head: Normocephalic; anterior fontanel is open and flat (3 cm × 2 cm); posterior fontanel is open and flat (1.0 cm × 0.5 cm).

Eyes: Red reflex present bilaterally; pupils equal, round, and reactive to light; no discharge noted.

Ears: Pinnae normal; tympanic membranes gray bilaterally with positive light reflex.

Nose: Both nostrils congested; cloudy discharge present in nares; mild nasal flaring.

Oropharynx: Mucous membranes moist; no teeth present; no lesions.

Neck: Supple; no nodes.

Respiratory: RR = 24; lungs with clear breath sounds in all lobes; no retractions present; no grunting; no deformities of the thoracic cage noted.

Cardiac/Peripheral vascular: HR = 120; regular rhythm; no murmur noted; brachial and femoral pulses present and 2+ bilaterally.

Abdomen/Gastrointestinal: Soft, nontender, nondistended, no evidence of hepatosplenomegaly.

Genitourinary: Normal female genitalia.

Back: Spine straight.

Extremities: Full range of motion of all extremities; warm and well-perfused; capillary refill <2 seconds; negative hip click.

Neurologic: Good suck and cry; good tone in all extremities; positive Moro, rooting, plantar, palmar, and Babinski reflexes.

CRITICAL THINKING

Which diagnostic or imaging studies should be considered to assist with or confirm the diagnosis?
___Upper gastrointestinal (GI) imaging series
___Manometry to assess esophageal motility and lower esophageal sphincter function
___Complete blood count

What is the most likely differential diagnosis and why?
___Overfeeding
___Gastroesophageal reflux disease
___Gastroenteritis

What is the plan of treatment and follow-up care?

Does the patient's psychosocial history impact how you might treat this case?

What demographic characteristics might affect this case?

Are there any standardized guidelines that should be used to assess or treat this case?

Section 2

The Infant

Case 2.1 Nutrition and Weight

By Mikki Meadows-Oliver, PhD, RN, FAAN

SUBJECTIVE

Neil, a 12-month-old infant, presents to the office for a well-baby visit. He is accompanied by his mother, Kayla. Kayla states that Neil has been healthy since his last well-baby visit at 9 months of age. He has had no visits to the urgent care clinic or to the emergency room in the interim. Kayla is concerned that Neil's appetite has diminished. She states that he is not eating as much lately as he had been.

Diet: Neil's nutrition history reveals that he has successfully transitioned to a diet with whole milk. He drinks five 8-oz bottles of whole milk daily. Neil is a "picky eater." He rarely eats foods that are offered to him and, instead, prefers to drink from the bottle. He is not currently taking any multivitamins.

Elimination: Kayla states that Neil has 4–6 wet diapers daily. He does not have any diarrhea but does have occasional constipation that is relieved with prune juice.

Sleep: Neil sleeps 13 hours nightly but does not take any naps during the day. He does not have any problems falling asleep or staying asleep. His nighttime bedtime routine includes a bath and bedtime story read to him by Kayla.

Developmental: Neil is able to walk while holding onto furniture. He can also stand unassisted for about 5 seconds. Neil says "dada" and "mama" and has words for bottle and milk.

Birth history: Neil was the product of a 37-week gestation. He was delivered vaginally with the assistance of a vacuum. During the pregnancy, Kayla had no falls or infections. She did not drink alcohol, take over-the-counter or prescription medications (other than prenatal vitamins), use tobacco products, or use illicit drugs. Neil's birth weight was 3000 g, and his Apgar scores were 8 at 1 minute and 9 at 5 minutes. Past medical history reveals that Neil has had 3 episodes of acute otitis media since birth. He has had no injuries or illnesses requiring visits to the emergency department.

Social history: Neil was born to a 20-year-old mother. He has a 2-month-old younger sibling. He lives at home with his mother and his paternal grandmother. Neil's father is currently incarcerated.

The Family Nurse Practitioner: Clinical Case Studies, Second Edition. Edited by Leslie Neal-Boylan.
© 2021 John Wiley & Sons Ltd. Published 2021 by John Wiley & Sons Ltd.

Neil's mother does not currently work outside the home. The family receives a rent subsidy from Section 8 and a food subsidy from the Women, Infants, and Children (WIC) program and food stamps.

The family also receives monthly cash assistance from the Temporary Aid to Needy Families (TANF) program. The family has no pets and there are no smokers in the home.

Family medical history: Neil's mother has no health problems. His father is 32 years old and has no history of chronic medical conditions. His maternal grandmother has a history of breast cancer. His maternal grandfather has high blood pressure. His paternal grandmother (48 years of age) is healthy with no health problems. The health history of his paternal grandfather is unknown.

Neil is not currently taking any over-the-counter, prescription, or herbal medications. He has no known allergies to food, medications, or the environment. He is up to date on required immunizations.

OBJECTIVE

Neil's vital signs were taken in the office. His weight is 6.4 kg, and his length is 66 cm. His temperature is within the normal range at 36.8°C (temporal). When observing Neil's general appearance, he is alert, active, and playful. He appears well hydrated and well nourished.

Skin: Clear of lesions; no cyanosis of his skin, lips, or nails; no diaphoresis noted. Neil has good skin turgor on examination.

HEENT: Neil's head is normocephalic. His anterior fontanel is open and flat (0.5 cm × 0.5 cm). Red reflex is present bilaterally; and his pupils are equal, round, and reactive to light. There is no discharge noted. Pinnae are normal, and the tympanic membranes are gray bilaterally with positive light reflexes. Bony landmarks are visible, and there is no fluid noted behind the tympanic membrane. Both nostrils are patent. There is no nasal discharge, and there is no nasal flaring. Neil's mucous membranes are noted to be moist when examining his oropharynx. He has 8 teeth present, with white spots present on both upper central incisors. There are no lesions present in the oral cavity.

Neck: Supple and able to move in all directions without resistance; shotty nodes present in the posterior cervical region.

Respiratory: Respiratory rate is 20 breaths per minute, and his lungs are clear to auscultation in all lobes. There is good air entry, and no retractions or grunting are noted on examination. No deformities of the thoracic cage noted.

Cardiovascular: Heart rate is 106 beats per minute with a regular rhythm. There is no murmur noted upon auscultation; brachial and femoral pulses are present and 2+ bilaterally.

Abdomen: Normoactive bowel sounds are present throughout; soft and nontender. There is no evidence of hepatosplenomegaly.

Genitourinary: Normal male genitalia. Neil is circumcised and his testes are descended bilaterally.

Neuromusculoskeletal: Good tone in all extremities; full range of motion in all extremities. His extremities are warm and well perfused. Capillary refill is less than 2 seconds, and his spine is straight.

CRITICAL THINKING

Which laboratory tests should be ordered as part of a 12-month, well-child visit?

Other than "well child," what additional diagnoses should be considered for Neil?

What is the plan of treatment, referral, and follow-up care?

Does this patient's psychosocial history affect how you might treat this case?

What if the patient lived in a rural setting?

Are there any demographic characteristics that might affect this case?

Are there any standardized guidelines that should be used to assess or treat this case?

Case 2.2 Breastfeeding

By Mikki Meadows-Oliver, PhD, RN, FAAN

SUBJECTIVE

Julio, a 9-month-old male, presents to the office for a well-baby visit. He is accompanied by his mother, Lupita. Lupita is Spanish speaking, so a medical interpreter is used for the visit. Lupita has no concerns and states that Julio has been healthy since his last well-child visit at 6 months of age. He has had no visits to the urgent care clinic or to the emergency room in the interim.

Diet: Julio's nutrition history reveals that he is still being breastfed but that he is also being supplemented with a low-iron, milk-based formula. Lupita states that she gives Julio low-iron formula because formula that is not low-iron makes him constipated. He eats a diet of regular food that the family eats. He eats fruits and vegetables daily. Lupita introduced finely chopped meats into Julio's diet last week, and he has tolerated the addition well. Julio also enjoys Cheerios®, which he is able to grasp and bring to his mouth without assistance. He is not currently taking any multivitamins.

Elimination: Lupita states that Julio has 4–6 wet diapers daily and voids easily with a straight urine stream. He does not have any diarrhea or constipation since beginning the low-iron formula.

Sleep: Julio is sleeping 10 hours at night and takes one 2-hour nap daily. He does not have any problems falling asleep or staying asleep. At night, he has a bedtime routine that includes a bath and bedtime story read to him by an older sibling.

Development: Julio is crawling and pulling up to stand. He makes lots of vocalizations and is saying "da-da," although Lupita is not sure if he is just making sounds or referring to his father when he says "da-da." Julio has a beginning pincer grasp that allows him to eat small items such as Cheerios®.

Birth history: Julio is the product of a 40-week gestation. He was delivered vaginally without complications. During the pregnancy, his mother had no falls or infections. Lupita did not drink alcohol, take over-the-counter or prescription medications (other than prenatal vitamins), use tobacco products, or use illicit drugs. Julio's birth weight was 3500 g, and his Apgar scores were 9 at 1 minute and 9 at 5 minutes. Past medical history reveals that he was hospitalized at 4 months of age for bronchiolitis. He has had no episodes of wheezing since that time.

The Family Nurse Practitioner: Clinical Case Studies, Second Edition. Edited by Leslie Neal-Boylan.
© 2021 John Wiley & Sons Ltd. Published 2021 by John Wiley & Sons Ltd.

Social history: Julio was born to a 31-year-old mother. He has 2 older siblings (7 and 9 years old). He lives at home with both parents and his maternal grandfather. The family is from Ecuador.

His mother works as a housekeeper, and his father works in construction. The family has a pet bird. There are no smokers in the home.

Family medical history: Julio's mother has asthma and seasonal allergies. His 33-year-old father is healthy and has no history of chronic medical conditions. Julio's maternal grandmother died at age 55 years from a myocardial infarction. His maternal grandfather has a history of Type 2 diabetes mellitus and obesity. His paternal grandparents are both deceased; both died in a motor vehicle accident several years ago.

Julio is not currently taking any over-the-counter, prescription, or herbal medications. He has no known allergies to food, medications, or the environment. He is up to date on required immunizations.

OBJECTIVE

Julio's vital signs were taken in the office today. His weight is 6.0 kg, and his length is 64 cm. Julio's temperature is within the normal range at 37°C (temporal). When observing his general appearance, he is alert, active, and playful. He appears well hydrated and well nourished.

Skin: His skin is clear of lesions. There is no cyanosis of his skin, lips, or nails. There was no diaphoresis noted. Julio has good skin turgor on examination.

HEENT: Julio's head is normocephalic. His anterior fontanel is open and flat (0.5 cm × 0.5 cm). Red reflexes are present bilaterally and pupils are equal, round, and reactive to light. There is no discharge noted. Pinnae are normal; tympanic membranes are gray bilaterally with positive light reflexes. Bony landmarks are visible, and there is no fluid noted behind the tympanic membrane. Both nostrils are patent. There is no nasal discharge, and there is no nasal flaring. Julio's mucous membranes are noted to be moist when examining his oropharynx. He has 2 teeth present without evidence of caries. There are no lesions present in the oral cavity.

Neck: Supple and able to move in all directions without resistance. There is no cervical lymphadenopathy.

Respiratory: Respiratory rate is 22 breaths per minute and his lungs are clear to auscultation in all lobes. There is good air entry, and no retractions or grunting are noted on examination. No deformities of the thoracic cage are noted.

Cardiovascular: Heart rate is 102 beats per minute with a regular rhythm. There is no murmur noted upon auscultation; brachial and femoral pulses are present and 2+ bilaterally.

Abdomen: Normoactive bowel sounds are present throughout; soft and nontender. There is no evidence of hepatosplenomegaly.

Genitourinary: Genitourinary examination reveals normal male genitalia. Julio is uncircumcised, and his testes are descended bilaterally.

Neuromusculoskeletal: Good tone in all extremities; full range of motion of all extremities. His extremities are warm and well perfused. Capillary refill is less than 2 seconds, and his spine is straight.

CRITICAL THINKING

Which laboratory or diagnostic imaging tests should be ordered as part of a 9-month, well-child visit?

___CBC

___Lead screening test

___Liver function tests

___Cholesterol level

___Baseline chest radiograph

What is the most likely differential diagnosis and why?

___Iron deficiency anemia

___Constipation

___Other

What is the plan of treatment, referral, and follow-up care?

Does this patient's psychosocial history affect how you might treat this case?

What if the patient lived in a rural setting?

Are there any demographic characteristics that might affect this case?

Are there any standardized guidelines that should be used to assess or treat this case?

Case 2.3 Growth and Development

By Mikki Meadows-Oliver, PhD, RN, FAAN

SUBJECTIVE

Kilah, a 9-month-old infant, presents to the office for a well-baby visit. She is accompanied by her foster mother, Angela. Angela states that Kilah has been in her care for the past 7 months. Kilah is the first infant that Angela has cared for. According to Angela, Kilah has been healthy since her last well-child visit at 6 months of age. She has had no visits to the urgent care clinic or to the emergency room in the interim. Angela is concerned that Kilah appears thin.

Diet: Kilah's nutrition history reveals that she drinks three 8-oz bottles of milk-based formula daily. Kilah also eats 1 jar of stage 1 baby food twice daily. She is not currently taking any multivitamins.

Elimination: Angela states that Kilah has 4–6 wet diapers daily. She does not have any diarrhea or constipation.

Sleeps: Kilah sleeps 10 hours nightly and takes 2 naps daily. Angela states that Kilah does not have any problems falling asleep or staying asleep. The family does not currently have a bedtime routine for Kilah.

Birth history: Angela does not know any of the details of Kilah's birth history or family history.

Past medical history: Kilah has been healthy since being placed in Angela's care. Since placement, Kilah has had no injuries or illnesses requiring visits to the emergency department. Developmentally, Kilah is able to crawl. She is able to pick up small objects such as Cheerios® using only her thumb and forefinger. Kilah makes many sounds and is beginning to say "dada."

Social history: Kilah lives at home with her foster mother, Angela. Angela does not currently work outside the home. The family receives a rent subsidy from Section 8, food subsidies from the Women, Infants, and Children (WIC) program, and food stamps. The family also receives monthly cash assistance from the Temporary Aid to Needy Families (TANF) program. The family has no pets, and there are no smokers in the home.

Medications: Kilah is not currently taking any over-the-counter, prescription, or herbal medications.

Allergies: Kilah has no known allergies to food, medications, or the environment. She is up to date on required immunizations.

The Family Nurse Practitioner: Clinical Case Studies, Second Edition. Edited by Leslie Neal-Boylan.
© 2021 John Wiley & Sons Ltd. Published 2021 by John Wiley & Sons Ltd.

OBJECTIVE

General: Appears thin but alert, active, and playful.

Vital signs: Weight in the office today is 6.4 kg and her length is 66 centimeters. Kilah's temperature is within the normal range at 36.8°C (temporal). Kilah's weight has not changed since her last well child visit.

Skin: She appears well hydrated, and her skin was clear of lesions. There is no cyanosis of her skin, lips, or nails. There was no diaphoresis noted. Kilah has good skin turgor on examination.

HEENT: Kilah's head is normocephalic. Her anterior fontanel is open and flat (0.5 cm × 0.5 cm). Red reflexes are present bilaterally; and pupils are equal, round, and reactive to light. There is no discharge noted. Pinnae are normal; the tympanic membranes were gray bilaterally with positive light reflexes. Bony landmarks are visible and there was no fluid noted behind the tympanic membrane. Both nostrils are patent. There is no nasal discharge, and there is no nasal flaring. Kilah's mucous membranes are noted to be moist when examining her oropharynx. She has 2 teeth present—lower central incisors. There are no lesions present on the teeth or in the oral cavity.

Neck: Supple and able to move in all directions without resistance. There are no lymph nodes present in the neck area.

Respiratory: Rate is 22 breaths per minute, and her lungs are clear to auscultation in all lobes. There is good air entry, and no retractions or grunting are noted on examination. There are no deformities of the thoracic cage noted.

Cardiovascular: Heart rate is 110 beats per minute with a regular rhythm. There is no murmur noted upon auscultation; brachial and femoral pulses are present and 2+ bilaterally.

Abdomen: Normoactive bowel sounds are present throughout; soft and nontender. There is no evidence of hepatosplenomegaly.

Genitourinary: Genitourinary examination reveals normal female genitalia.

Neuromusculoskeletal: Good tone in all extremities. She has full range of motion in all extremities and her extremities are warm and well perfused. Capillary refill is less than 2 seconds, and her spine is straight.

CRITICAL THINKING

Which diagnostic or imaging studies should be considered to assist with or confirm the diagnosis?
___CBC count
___Urinalysis
___Urine culture
___Electrolytes, including creatinine and BUN
___Liver function tests, including total protein and albumin
___Barium swallow
___Chest radiograph

What is the most likely differential diagnosis and why?

___Organic failure to thrive (FTT)

___Nonorganic FTT (FTT)

___Constitutional growth delay

___Fetal alcohol spectrum disorder

What is the plan of treatment, referral, and follow-up care?

Does this patient's psychosocial history affect how you might treat this case?

What if the patient lived in a rural setting?

Are there any demographic characteristics that might affect this case?

Are there any standardized guidelines that should be used to assess or treat this case?

Case 2.4 Heart Murmur

By Mikki Meadows-Oliver, PhD, RN, FAAN

SUBJECTIVE

Jonathan, a 12-month-old infant, presents to the primary care office for a well-child visit. He is accompanied by his parents. His mother is concerned that Jonathan is eating less than usual but says that he is drinking his normal amount. His activity level has not changed.

Birth history: Jonathan was born at 39 weeks' gestation. His birth weight was 3200 g. There were no complications during the labor or delivery. The mother had no infections, falls, or known exposures to environmental hazards. She did not drink alcohol, take prescription medication (other than prenatal vitamins), use tobacco products, or use illicit drugs. The immediate neonatal period was unremarkable. Jonathan was discharged at 2 days of age to home with his mother.

The social history reveals that Jonathan was born to a 23-year-old single mother. His father is involved but does not reside in the household. Jonathan lives in an apartment with his mother and 19-year-old cousin. The maternal grandmother (MGM) lives in the neighborhood and is able to help Jonathan's mother with child care. The family receives assistance from governmental subsidies such as the Women, Infants, and Children supplemental nutrition program (WIC), Temporary Assistance for Needy Families (TANF), and Medicaid. Educationally, both Jonathan's mother and father have high school diplomas. She works at a fast-food restaurant. Jonathan's father works as a construction worker. The family has no pets. There are no smokers in the home.

Diet: Jonathan eats a balanced diet of table foods. He still breastfeeds but is transitioning to whole milk. He takes a daily multivitamin.

Elimination: 4–6 wet diapers daily with 1 bowel movement.

Sleep: Takes one 2-hour nap daily and sleeps 12 hours at night.

Family medical history: PGF (age 54): healthy; PGM (age 53): diabetes mellitus; MGF (age 46): high blood pressure; MGM (age 44): asthma; mother (age 23): asthma; father (age 32): healthy.

Medications: Currently taking no prescription, herbal, or over-the-counter medications.

Immunizations: Up to date.

Allergies: No known allergies to food, medications, or environment.

The Family Nurse Practitioner: Clinical Case Studies, Second Edition. Edited by Leslie Neal-Boylan.
© 2021 John Wiley & Sons Ltd. Published 2021 by John Wiley & Sons Ltd.

OBJECTIVE

Vital signs: Weight: 10 kg; length: 84 cm; temperature: 37°C (axillary).

General: Alert; well nourished; well hydrated; interactive.

Skin: Clear with no lesions noted; no cyanosis of lips, nails, or skin; no diaphoresis noted; good skin turgor.

Head: Normocephalic; anterior fontanel is open and flat (1 cm × 1 cm).

Eyes: Red reflexes present bilaterally; pupils equal, round, and reactive to light; no discharge noted.

Ears: Pinnae normal; tympanic membranes gray bilaterally with positive light reflex.

Nose: Both nostrils are patent; no discharge.

Oropharynx: Mucous membranes are moist; no teeth are present; no lesions.

Neck: Supple; no nodes.

Respiratory: RR = 24; clear in all lobes; no adventitious sounds noted; no retractions; no deformities of the thoracic cage noted.

Cardiac/Peripheral vascular: HR = 120; vibratory, systolic, grade 2 heart murmur noted on exam at the lower left sternal border area of the chest with both the bell and diaphragm; heard best in the supine position; no heaves or thrills noted; no radiation of the murmur to the back or axilla; brachial and femoral pulses present and 2+ bilaterally.

Abdomen/Gastrointestinal: Soft, nontender, nondistended, no evidence of hepatosplenomegaly.

Genitourinary: Normal circumcised male genitalia; testes descended bilaterally.

Back: Spine straight.

Ext: Full range of motion of all extremities; warm and well perfused; capillary refill < 2 seconds.

Neurologic: Good strength and tone.

CRITICAL THINKING

Which diagnostic or imaging studies should be considered to assist with or confirm the diagnosis?
___Chest radiograph
___Echocardiogram
___Electrocardiogram

What is the most likely differential diagnosis and why?
___Patent ductus arteriosus (PDA)
___Ventricular septal defect (VSD)
___Still's murmur

What is the plan of treatment, referral, and follow-up care?

Are there any referrals needed?

Does the patient's psychosocial history impact how you might treat him?

What if this baby were a girl?

What if this baby were 6 months old?

Are there any standardized guidelines that should used to assess or treat this case?

Case 2.5 Cough

By Mikki Meadows-Oliver, PhD, RN, FAAN

SUBJECTIVE

Katelynn, a 7-month-old infant, presents to the office with complaints of cough for 2 days and "breathing heavy" since this morning. Katelynn is accompanied by both parents. She has had a fever for 2 days. Her maximum temperature at home was 101°F (rectal). She also has a runny nose. Her mother has tried an over-the-counter cough medicine without much relief. Katelynn's mother has not found much that helps the symptoms; but she notices that, when Katelynn cries, the breathing sounds get worse. Katelynn attends day care and her mother states that many of the kids there have coughs and runny noses. Katelynn's mother also has had cold symptoms for nearly 5 days.

Birth history: Katelynn was the product of a 40-week gestation. She was delivered vaginally without complications. During the pregnancy, Katelynn's mother had no falls, infections, or known exposures to environmental hazards. She did not drink alcohol, take over-the-counter or prescription medication (other than prenatal vitamins), use tobacco products, or use illicit drugs. Katelynn's birth weight was 3300 g and her Apgar scores were 9 at 1 minute and 9 at 5 minutes.

Social history: Katelynn was born to a 31-year-old mother. Katelynn has a 2-year-old sibling. She lives at home with both parents and her older sibling. Both parents have high school diplomas. The mother works as an administrative assistant, and the father works as a maintenance worker. There are no pets or smokers in the home.

Diet: Decreased solid and liquid intake since yesterday.

Elimination: Decreased urine output; no diarrhea or constipation.

Sleep: Sleep is interrupted by coughing.

Family medical history: Paternal grandfather (PGF) (age 60): history of prostate cancer; paternal grandmother (PGM) (age 59): healthy; maternal grandfather (MGF) (age 61): Type 2 diabetes mellitus, high cholesterol, high blood pressure; maternal grandmother (MGM) (age 61): asthma; mother (age 31): asthma; father (age 30): healthy; sibling (age 2): healthy; history of bronchiolitis.

Medications: Currently taking no prescription or herbal medications. Taking a children's over-the-counter cough suppressant.

The Family Nurse Practitioner: Clinical Case Studies, Second Edition. Edited by Leslie Neal-Boylan.
© 2021 John Wiley & Sons Ltd. Published 2021 by John Wiley & Sons Ltd.

Immunizations: Up to date.

Allergies: No known allergies to food, medications, or environment.

OBJECTIVE

Vital signs: Weight: 7.1 kg; length: 65 cm; temperature: 37.9°C (rectal); pulse oximeter reading: 95% on room air.

General: Alert, active, well-hydrated, interactive baby.

Skin: Clear with no lesions noted; no cyanosis of skin, lips, or nails; no diaphoresis noted; good skin turgor.

Head: Normocephalic; anterior fontanel is open and flat (1.5 cm × 1.5 cm).

Eyes: Red reflexes present bilaterally; pupils equal, round, and reactive to light; no discharge noted.

Ears: Pinnae normal; tympanic membranes gray bilaterally with positive light reflex.

Nose: Both nostrils patent; no discharge; mild nasal flaring.

Oropharynx: Mucous membranes moist; no teeth present; no lesions.

Neck: Supple; no nodes.

Respiratory: RR = 32; barking cough noted; inspiratory stridor with activity; no intercostal, supra-sternal, or subcostal retractions; no grunting; no deformities of the thoracic cage noted.

Cardiac/Peripheral vascular: HR = 120; regular rhythm; no murmur noted; brachial and femoral pulses present and 2+ bilaterally.

Abdomen/Gastrointestinal: Soft, nontender, nondistended, no evidence of hepatosplenomegaly.

Genitourinary: Normal female genitalia.

Back: Spine straight.

Extremities: Full range of motion of all extremities; warm and well perfused; capillary refill < 2 seconds.

Neurologic: Good tone in all extremities.

CRITICAL THINKING

Which diagnostic or imaging studies should be considered to assist with or confirm the diagnosis?
___Chest X-ray (CXR)
___Arterial blood gas (ABG)
___Complete blood count (CBC)

What is the most likely differential diagnosis and why?
___Croup (laryngotracheobronchitis)
___Bronchiolitis
___Epiglottitis

What is the plan of treatment, referral, and follow-up care?

Are there any demographic characteristics that would affect this case?

What if the patient lived in a rural, isolated setting?

Case 2.6 Diarrhea

By Mikki Meadows-Oliver, PhD, RN, FAAN

SUBJECTIVE

David, an 11-month-old infant, presents to the office with complaints of watery diarrhea for 1 day. David is accompanied by his mother. In addition to the diarrhea, he has had vomiting for 1 day and a fever for 2 days. His maximum temperature at home was 102°F (rectal). David has not vomited today, although the fever continues and the diarrhea seems to be getting worse. He has had at least 10 diapers with diarrhea since yesterday. David's mother is unsure of his urine output because each diaper is so full of stool. No blood or mucus has been noted in the stool. His mother believes that a rash is starting on his buttocks due to the diarrhea. She knows that another child in the day care center had diarrhea a few days ago. No one at home has any similar symptoms.

Yesterday, David completed a course of amoxicillin for otitis media. David's mother states that earlier in the week she began to introduce whole milk into his diet and that she also gave him Indian take-out food with a strong curry flavor. She is concerned that one of these factors may have caused or contributed to David's diarrhea. Further review of systems reveals that David has had decreased solid food and soy formula intake since yesterday and that he has been sleeping more than usual.

Birth history: David is the product of a 41-week gestation. He was delivered vaginally without complications. During the pregnancy, his mother had no falls or infections. She was in a car accident when she was 6 months pregnant and had to receive an X-ray of her right wrist. There was no break in the wrist, and she was told to take Tylenol for pain. David's mother did not drink alcohol, take prescription medication (other than prenatal vitamins), use tobacco products, or use illicit drugs. His birth weight was 3480 g, and his Apgar scores were 7 at 1 minute and 8 at 5 minutes.

Social history: David was born to a 39-year-old mother. He is an only child. He lives at home with his mother. She works as a psychologist with her own private practice. David's father is not involved. There are no pets or smokers in the home.

Family medical history: The health history of David's father and the paternal grandparents is unknown. David's mother is positive for Crohn disease. His maternal grandmother has a history of Type 2 diabetes, and the maternal grandfather has a history of prostate cancer.

David is currently taking no prescription or herbal medications. His mother gave him an over-the-counter antiemetic, Emetrol®, to help reduce nausea and vomiting. She has not given him any

The Family Nurse Practitioner: Clinical Case Studies, Second Edition. Edited by Leslie Neal-Boylan.
© 2021 John Wiley & Sons Ltd. Published 2021 by John Wiley & Sons Ltd.

antidiarrheal agents. David has no known allergies to food, medications, or the environment. He is up to date for required vaccinations, but he did not receive a rotavirus vaccination due to a recall of the vaccination.

OBJECTIVE

David's vital signs were taken in the office today. His weight is 6.8 kg, and his length is 69 cm. David's temperature is elevated at 38°C (rectal). When observing David's general appearance, he is alert and consolable by his mother when crying.

Skin: The skin on David's buttocks is mildly erythematous. There is no cyanosis of his skin, lips, or nails. There is no diaphoresis noted. David has good skin turgor on examination.

HEENT: David's head is normocephalic. His anterior fontanel is open and flat (0.5 cm × 0.5 cm). Upon examination of David's eyes, his red reflexes are present bilaterally and his pupils are equal, round, and reactive to light. There is no discharge noted, and tears are present when crying. David's external ear reveals that the pinnae are normal. On otoscopic examination, the tympanic membranes are pink bilaterally with positive light reflex. Bony landmarks are visible, and there is no fluid noted behind the tympanic membrane. Both nostrils are patent. There is no nasal discharge, and there is no nasal flaring. David's mucous membranes are noted to be moist when examining his oropharynx. He has 4 teeth present without evidence of caries. There are no lesions present in the oral cavity.

Neck: David's neck is supple and able to move in all directions without resistance. There is no cervical lymphadenopathy.

Respirations: Respiratory rate is 28 breaths per minute, and lungs are clear to auscultation in all lobes. There is good air entry, and no retractions or grunting are noted on examination. No deformities of the thoracic cage are noted.

Cardiovascular: Heart rate is 110 beats per minute with a regular rhythm. There is no murmur noted upon auscultation. Brachial and femoral pulses are present and 2+ bilaterally.

Abdomen: Hyperactive bowel sounds are present throughout. David has diffuse tenderness on abdominal palpation. His abdomen is mildly distended; there is no evidence of hepatosplenomegaly.

Genitourinary: Genitourinary examination revealed normal male genitalia. David is circumcised, and his testes are descended bilaterally.

Neuromusculoskeletal: David was noted to have good tone in all extremities. He has full range of motion of all extremities. His extremities are warm and well perfused. Capillary refill is less than 2 seconds. David's spine is straight.

CRITICAL THINKING

Which laboratory or imaging studies should be considered to assist with or confirm the diagnosis?
___Complete blood count (CBC)
___Stool culture
___Electrolyte levels
___Hydrogen breath test
___Lactose tolerance test

What is the most likely differential diagnosis and why?

What is the plan of treatment, referral, and follow-up care?

Are there any demographic factors that should be considered?

Are there any standardized guidelines that should be used to assess or treat this case?

Case 2.7 Fall from Height

By Mikki Meadows-Oliver, PhD, RN, FAAN

SUBJECTIVE

Victor, a 2-month-old infant, presents in the office for an examination after he fell off the changing table. He is accompanied by his mother, Amy. Amy states that she was preparing to change Victor's diaper, and she placed him on the changing table. She then realized that she had forgotten to bring the diaper wipes to the changing table. When she turned around to retrieve the wipes, Victor rolled off the table and onto the floor. Amy states that Victor cried immediately after falling. She did not notice any bleeding after the fall but she did notice bruising on the left side of Victor's head, which prompted her to bring him in to the office. The injury occurred approximately 1 hour ago. Since that time, Victor has not had anything to eat or drink. He has not had any wet diapers. Amy stated that she did not let Victor sleep after his head injury.

Diet: Normally, Victor takes six 4-oz bottles of soy-based formula daily. He has not yet started any solids.

Elimination: Amy states that Victor normally has 6–8 wet diapers daily. He has 2 bowel movements daily. Amy denies that Victor has diarrhea or constipation.

Sleep: Victor normally sleeps 2–3 hours at a time between feedings. He has one 5-hour stretch of sleep during the night.

Birth history: Victor is the product of a 40-week gestation. He was born via spontaneous vaginal delivery. During the pregnancy, Amy had no falls or infections. She did not drink alcohol, take over-the-counter or prescription medications (other than prenatal vitamins), use tobacco products, or use illicit drugs. His birth weight was 3280 g, and his Apgar scores were 9 at 1 minute and 9 at 5 minutes. Since birth, he has had no other injuries or illnesses.

Social history: Victor was born to an 18-year-old mother. He lives at home with his mother and his maternal grandmother. Victor's father is not involved in his care. His mother does not currently work outside the home but plans to return to work at a local fast-food restaurant soon. She is looking for child care. The family receives a rent subsidy from Section 8, food subsidies from the Women, Infants, and Children (WIC) program, and food stamps. The family also receives monthly cash assistance from the Temporary Aid to Needy Families (TANF) program. The family has no pets, and there are no smokers in the home.

Family medical history: Victor's mother has no health problems. His father is 17 years old and has no history of chronic medical conditions. His maternal grandmother (38 years of age) has a history of high blood pressure. His maternal grandfather (39 years of age) also has high blood pressure. His paternal grandmother (48 years of age) is healthy with no health problems, and his paternal grandfather's health history is unknown.

Medications: Victor is not currently taking any over-the-counter, prescription, or herbal medications. He has no known allergies to food, medications, or the environment. He has not yet received any recommended immunizations other than the hepatitis B vaccination received at 1 day of age.

OBJECTIVE

Victor's vital signs are taken, and his weight in the office today is 5.24 kg. His temperature is within the normal range at 37.1°C (rectal). He is alert, active, and playful. He appears well hydrated and well nourished.

Skin: His skin shows a 1.5 cm × 1.0 cm area of ecchymosis over the left forehead. The area appears mildly tender to touch. There is no cyanosis of his skin, lips, or nails. There is no diaphoresis noted, and he has good skin turgor on examination.

HEENT: Normocephalic with no swelling of the scalp. His anterior fontanel is open and flat (2 cm × 2 cm). Victor's red reflexes are present bilaterally; and his pupils are equal, round, and reactive to light. He is able to fix and follow the examination past midline. There is no ocular discharge noted. The external ear reveals that the pinnae are normal. On otoscopic examination, the tympanic membranes are gray bilaterally with positive light reflexes. Bony landmarks are visible, and there is no fluid noted behind the tympanic membrane. Both nostrils are patent. There are no nasal discharge and no nasal flaring. Victor's mucous membranes are noted to be moist when examining his oropharynx. He has no teeth, and there are no lesions present in the oral cavity.

Neck: Victor's neck is supple and able to move in all directions without resistance. He has no cervical lymphadenopathy.

Respiratory: Respiratory rate is 24 breaths per minute, and lungs are clear to auscultation in all lobes. There is good air entry, and no retractions or grunting are noted on examination. No deformities of the thoracic cage are noted.

Cardiovascular: Heart rate is 116 beats per minute with a regular rhythm. There is no murmur noted upon auscultation. When palpating, brachial and femoral pulses are present and 2+ bilaterally.

Abdomen: Normoactive bowel sounds are present throughout; soft and nontender. There is no evidence of hepatosplenomegaly.

Genitourinary: Normal male genitalia. Victor is uncircumcised and his testes are descended bilaterally.

Neuromusculoskeletal: Good tone in all extremities; full range of motion in all extremities. His extremities are warm and well perfused. Capillary refill is less than 2 seconds, and his spine is straight.

CRITICAL THINKING

Which laboratory tests should be ordered as part of a workup after a fall from height?

What is the most likely differential diagnosis and why?

What is the plan of treatment, referral, and follow-up care?

Does this patient's psychosocial history affect how you might treat this case?

What if the patient lived in a rural setting?

Are there any demographic characteristics that might affect this case?

Section 3

The Toddler/Preschool Child

Case 3.1 Earache

By Mikki Meadows-Oliver, PhD, RN, FAAN

SUBJECTIVE

Janice, a 3-year-old preschool child, presents to the office with a complaint of left ear pain for 2 days. She is accompanied by her mother, Marsha. She has had an intermittent fever and her maximum temperature at home was 101°F (axillary). The pain is worse sometimes when she is lying down. The pain is occasionally relieved with the use of over-the-counter pain relievers. Janice has had no vomiting or diarrhea. She has had a slight runny nose, but no cough.

Diet: Janice's nutrition history reveals that she has a balanced diet with enough dairy, protein, fruits, and vegetables. Her appetite has decreased over the past 2 days since the ear pain began.

Elimination: She is voiding well with no complaints of dysuria.

Sleep: Janice sleeps approximately 10 hours at night and takes one 1-hour nap at her preschool. She usually has no problems falling or staying asleep but since the ear pain has started, her sleep has been interrupted.

Past medical history: Janice was born via vaginal delivery at 40 weeks' gestation. Since being discharged at 2 days of age, she has had no emergency department (ED) visits or hospitalizations. Janice has had 2 episodes of otitis media that were cleared with antibiotics. She has had no injuries or illnesses since that time. Janice passed her developmental screening at her last well-child visit. She currently attends preschool and is doing well, according to Marsha. She has no chronic illnesses and is currently taking no medications.

Social history: Janice lives at home with both parents. Her mother works as a teacher, and her father is a commercial fisherman. The family has a pet cat. Janice's father smokes, but not in the home.

Family medical history: Janice's mother (31 years old) and father (30 years old) are healthy and have no history of chronic medical conditions. Her maternal grandmother (age 52 years) has a history of lupus. Her maternal grandfather (54 years of age) has a history of prostate cancer (in remission). Janice's paternal grandfather (age 59 years) has a history of hypertension. Her paternal grandmother (53 years of age) has a history of asthma.

Medications: Janice is currently taking no prescription or herbal medications. She has been taking over-the-counter pain relievers/antipyretics to relieve symptoms associated with ear pain. Janice

The Family Nurse Practitioner: Clinical Case Studies, Second Edition. Edited by Leslie Neal-Boylan.
© 2021 John Wiley & Sons Ltd. Published 2021 by John Wiley & Sons Ltd.

has an allergy to penicillin. She gets hives when she takes penicillin. Janice has no known allergies to food or the environment. She is up to date on required immunizations.

OBJECTIVE

Janice's vital signs are taken, and her weight in the office today is 14 kg. Her temperature is slightly elevated at 38°C (temporal). Janice is alert and quiet, sitting in her mother's lap. She appears well hydrated and well nourished.

Skin: Her skin is clear of lesions and warm to touch. There is no cyanosis of her skin, lips, or nails. There is no diaphoresis noted. Janice has good skin turgor on examination.

HEENT: Janice's head is normocephalic. Her red reflexes are present bilaterally; and her pupils are equal, round, and reactive to light. There is no ocular discharge noted. Janice's external ear reveals that the pinnae are normal, and there is no tenderness to touch on the external ear. On otoscopic examination, the right tympanic membrane (TM) is gray, in normal position, with positive light reflexes. Bony landmarks are visible, and there is no fluid noted behind the TM. The left TM is erythematous and bulging with purulent fluid visible behind the TM. The TM is opaque with no light reflex or bony landmarks present. Both nostrils are patent. There is no nasal discharge, and there is no nasal flaring. Janice's mucous membranes are noted to be moist. She has 20 teeth present without evidence of caries. There are no lesions present in the oral cavity.

Neck: Janice's neck is supple and able to move in all directions without resistance. There are shotty anterior cervical nodes present on the left side of the neck. There is no erythema or tenderness of the nodes.

Respiratory: Janice's respiratory rate is 26 breaths per minute and her lungs are clear to auscultation in all lobes. There is good air entry, and no retractions or grunting are noted on examination. No deformities of the thoracic cage are noted.

Cardiovascular: Janice's heart rate is 102 beats per minute with a regular rhythm. There is no murmur noted upon auscultation.

Abdomen: Normoactive bowel sounds are present throughout. Janice's abdomen is soft and non-tender. There is no evidence of hepatosplenomegaly.

Genitourinary: Genitourinary examination reveals normal female genitalia.

Neuromusculoskeletal: Janice is noted to have good tone in all extremities. She has full range of motion of all extremities. Her extremities are warm and well perfused. Capillary refill is less than 2 seconds, and her spine is straight.

CRITICAL THINKING

Are there laboratory tests or diagnostic imaging studies that should be ordered as part of a workup for ear pain?

What is the most likely differential diagnosis and why?

What is the plan of treatment, referral, and follow-up care?

Does this patient's psychosocial history affect how you might treat this case?

What if the patient lived in a rural setting?

Are there any demographic characteristics that might affect this case?

Case 3.2 Bedwetting

By Mikki Meadows-Oliver, PhD, RN, FAAN

SUBJECTIVE

Four-year-old Javier presents to the office with his mother, Carol, with a complaint of bedwetting. Carol states that Javier consistently wets the bed each night although he remains dry throughout the day. According to his mother, Javier has never been dry at night but has been toilet-trained during the daytime for 2 years. Carol is frustrated with this behavior because she is frequently washing bedsheets and having to buy new mattresses. She has a 5-year-old daughter who achieved daytime and nighttime dryness by the age of 3 years old. Carol said that Javier's father is also frustrated with the bedwetting and will sometime spank Javier when he wets the bed. Carol says that her 5-year-old daughter teases Javier and calls him names such as "pee-pee boy." She says that she has already tried strategies such as limiting his liquid intake 2 hours before bed and waking him to urinate before she goes to bed. Carol states that often, when she goes to wake Javier before going to bed herself, he has already wet the bed. She does not know what to do now and has come to the office today because she would like assistance in resolving this issue. Javier has no other symptoms of illness.

Diet: Javier's nutrition history reveals that he has a balanced diet with enough dairy, protein, fruits, and vegetables. He does not appear to eat or drink large amounts.

Elimination: He is voiding well (normal amounts) with no complaints of dysuria. Javier does have occasional constipation that is relieved with an over-the-counter laxative.

Sleep: Javier sleeps 11 hours at night and has no trouble falling or staying asleep.

Past medical history: Born via cesarean section at 38 weeks' gestation. This was a repeat C-section for Carol. Since being discharged at 4 days of age, Javier has had no hospitalizations. Javier had 4 teeth removed at 2 years of age, under general anesthesia, due to early childhood caries. He had an emergency department (ED) visit at 3 years of age for a broken arm after he fell from the jungle gym at day care. Javier passed his developmental screening at his last well-child visit. He currently attends preschool and is doing well. He has no chronic illnesses and is taking no medications.

The Family Nurse Practitioner: Clinical Case Studies, Second Edition. Edited by Leslie Neal-Boylan.
© 2021 John Wiley & Sons Ltd. Published 2021 by John Wiley & Sons Ltd.

Social history: Javier lives at home with both parents and a 5-year-old sibling. His mother works as a store clerk, and his father is a school custodian. The family has no pets. There are no smokers in the home.

Family medical history: Javier's mother (26 years old) and father (26 years old) are healthy and have no history of chronic medical conditions. His mother has sickle cell trait. His maternal grandmother (48 years old) has a history of heart disease. His maternal grandfather (50 years old) has a history of liver disease. Javier's paternal grandfather (51 years old) has a history of vertigo. His paternal grandmother (50 years old) has a history of high cholesterol.

Medications: Javier is currently taking no over-the-counter, prescription, or herbal medications. He has no known allergies to medication, food, or the environment. He is up to date for required immunizations.

OBJECTIVE

Javier's vital signs are taken, and his weight in the office is 20 kg. His temperature is within the normal range at 36.7°C (temporal). When observing Javier's general appearance, he is alert, pleasant, and interactive. He appears well hydrated and well nourished.

Skin: Javier's skin is clear of lesions. There is no cyanosis of his skin, lips, or nails. There is no diaphoresis noted, and Javier has good skin turgor on examination.

HEENT: Javier's head is normocephalic. His red reflexes are present bilaterally; and his pupils are equal, round, and reactive to light. There is no ocular discharge noted. Javier's external ear reveals that the pinnae are normal and that there is no tenderness to touch on the external ear. On otoscopic examination, the tympanic membranes are gray bilaterally, in normal position with positive light reflexes. Bony landmarks are visible, and there is no fluid noted behind the tympanic membranes. Both nostrils are patent. There is no nasal discharge, and there is no nasal flaring. Javier's mucous membranes are noted to be moist. He has 16 teeth present. There are no lesions present in the oral cavity.

Neck: Javier's neck is supple and able to move in all directions without resistance. There is no cervical lymphadenopathy present.

Respiratory: Javier's respiratory rate is 20 breaths per minute, and his lungs are clear to auscultation in all lobes. There is good air entry, and no retractions or grunting are noted on examination. No deformities of the thoracic cage are noted.

Cardiovascular: Javier's heart rate is 96 beats per minute with a regular rhythm. There is no murmur noted upon auscultation.

Abdomen: Normoactive bowel sounds are present throughout, and Javier's abdomen is soft and nontender. Javier has shotty nodes present in his inguinal area bilaterally. These nodes are mobile, nontender, and nonerythematous. There is no evidence of hepatosplenomegaly.

Genitourinary: Normal circumcised male genitalia without erythema or lesions. His testes are descended bilaterally.

Neuromusculoskeletal: Good tone and full range of motion in all extremities; extremities are warm and well perfused. Capillary refill is less than 2 seconds, and his spine is straight.

CRITICAL THINKING

What laboratory tests or diagnostic imaging studies should be ordered as part of a workup for bedwetting?

What is the most likely differential diagnosis and why?

What is the plan of treatment, referral, and follow-up care?

Does this patient's psychosocial history affect how you might treat this case?

What if the patient lived in a rural setting?

Are there any demographic characteristics that might affect this case?

Case 3.3 Burn

By Mikki Meadows-Oliver, PhD, RN, FAAN

SUBJECTIVE

Two-year-old Faye presents to the office with her mother, Kellie, with a complaint of a burn to the right hand. Kellie states that she was curling her hair in the bathroom when her telephone rang. She left the bathroom to retrieve the telephone. While she was answering the telephone, Faye entered the bathroom and pulled on the curling iron cord that was hanging down below. The incident was unwitnessed, but Kellie heard Faye scream. She ran to the bathroom to find both Faye and the curling iron on the floor. She then noticed that Faye's right hand was red and swollen. She immediately brought her in to the office. Faye has no symptoms of illness.

Diet: Faye's nutrition history reveals that she has a balanced diet with enough dairy, protein, fruits, and vegetables. She has not eaten since she burned her hand.

Elimination: She is voiding well with no complaints of dysuria. She is not yet toilet-trained.

Sleep: Faye sleeps 10 hours at night and has no trouble falling or staying asleep. She takes one 2-hour nap during the day.

Past medical history: Faye was born via vaginal delivery at 37 weeks' gestation. Since being discharged at 2 days of age, she has had no hospitalizations. She had an emergency department (ED) visit 3 months ago for ingestion of cigarette butts. Faye passed her developmental screening at her last well-child visit. She currently attends an in-home day care while her mother is working. Faye has no chronic illnesses and is currently taking no medications.

Social history: Faye lives at home with her 18-year-old mother, 6-month-old sibling, and maternal grandmother. Her father is not involved. Faye's mother works as a nurse's aide in a long-term care facility. The family has 2 cats. There are no smokers in the home.

Family medical history: Faye's mother (18 years old) and father (19 years old) are healthy and have no history of chronic medical conditions. Kellie did have high blood pressure with both pregnancies but the condition resolved after she delivered her children. Her maternal grandmother (age 34 years) has thalassemia trait. Her maternal grandfather (35 years old) is healthy with no chronic illnesses. The health history of Faye's paternal grandfather is unknown. Her paternal grandmother (40 years old) has a history of obesity and high blood pressure.

The Family Nurse Practitioner: Clinical Case Studies, Second Edition. Edited by Leslie Neal-Boylan.
© 2021 John Wiley & Sons Ltd. Published 2021 by John Wiley & Sons Ltd.

Medications: Faye is not currently taking any over-the-counter, prescription, or herbal medications. She has no known allergies to medication, food, or the environment. She is up to date on required immunizations, although her mother declines the flu vaccine yearly.

OBJECTIVE

Faye's vital signs are taken, and her weight in the office is 14 kg. Her temperature is within the normal range at 37.2°C (temporal). She is alert, crying at times, but consolable. She appears well hydrated and well nourished.

Skin: The skin on the palm of her right hand is erythematous and beginning to blister. The affected area is painful to touch. The rest of her skin is without lesions. There is no cyanosis of her skin, lips, or nails. There is no diaphoresis noted, and Faye has good skin turgor on examination.

HEENT: Faye's head is normocephalic. Her red reflexes are present bilaterally; and her pupils are equal, round, and reactive to light. There is no ocular discharge noted. Faye's external ear reveals that the pinnae are normal, and there is no tenderness to touch on the external ear. On otoscopic examination, the tympanic membranes are gray bilaterally and in normal position with positive light reflexes. Bony landmarks are visible, and there is no fluid noted behind the tympanic membranes. Both nostrils are patent. There is no nasal discharge and no nasal flaring. Faye's mucous membranes are noted to be moist. She has 20 teeth present. There are no lesions present in the oral cavity.

Neck: Faye's neck is supple and able to move in all directions without resistance. There is no cervical lymphadenopathy present.

Respiratory: Her respiratory rate is 28 breaths per minute, and her lungs are clear to auscultation in all lobes. There is good air entry, and no retractions or grunting are noted on examination. No deformities of the thoracic cage are noted.

Cardiovascular: Faye's heart rate is 106 beats per minute with a regular rhythm. There is no murmur noted upon auscultation.

Abdomen: Normoactive bowel sounds are present throughout and Faye's abdomen is soft and nontender. There is no evidence of hepatosplenomegaly.

Genitourinary: Normal female genitalia without erythema or lesions.

Neuromusculoskeletal: Good tone and full range of motion in all extremities. Her extremities are warm and well perfused. Capillary refill is less than 2 seconds, and her spine is straight.

CRITICAL THINKING

Are there any laboratory tests or diagnostic imaging studies that should be ordered as part of a workup for a burn?

What additional diagnoses should be considered for a pediatric patient with a burn?

What is the plan of treatment, referral, and follow-up care?

Does this patient's psychosocial history affect how you might treat this case?

What if the patient lived in a rural setting?

Are there any demographic characteristics that might affect this case?

Are there any standardized guidelines that should be used to assess or treat this case?

Case 3.4 Toothache

By Mikki Meadows-Oliver, PhD, RN, FAAN

SUBJECTIVE

Five-year-old Lamont presents to the office with his father, Allen, with a complaint of a toothache. Allen states that Lamont woke in the middle of the night, crying, stating that his tooth (on the back, left side of his mouth) hurt. Allen gave Lamont an over-the-counter pain reliever to help with the pain. The pain reliever helped, and Lamont went back to sleep. However, when Lamont awakened this morning, he was again complaining of a toothache, and Allen decided to bring him in for a visit. Allen states that he thinks that Lamont had a fever. The family does not have a thermometer, but Lamont's forehead felt hot. Lamont has no cough, runny nose, vomiting, or diarrhea.

Diet: Lamont's nutrition history reveals that he has a balanced diet with enough dairy, protein, fruits, and vegetables. He also ingests quite a bit of junk food, including chips and cookies. Allen admits that Lamont sometimes drinks juice and soda from a baby bottle.

Elimination: Lamont is voiding well with no complaints of dysuria. He has 1 bowel movement daily and denies constipation or diarrhea.

Sleep: Lamont sleeps approximately 10 hours at night and has no trouble falling asleep or staying asleep.

Past medical history: Lamont was born via vaginal birth in Senegal. His birth was a home birth attended by a local midwife. The exact number of weeks' gestation is unknown, but Lamont's parents state that his was a full-term birth. Lamont has had no injuries or illnesses requiring visits to the emergency department. He passed his developmental screening at his last well-child visit. He currently attends kindergarten and is doing well.

   He has no chronic illnesses and is currently taking no medications.

Social history: Lamont lives at home with both parents and his 1-year-old sibling. The family has been in the United States for 2 years. They are in the United States so that Lamont's father can study biology at a local university. His mother is currently not working because her visa does not allow her to work. The family has no pets. There are no smokers in the home.

The Family Nurse Practitioner: Clinical Case Studies, Second Edition. Edited by Leslie Neal-Boylan.
© 2021 John Wiley & Sons Ltd. Published 2021 by John Wiley & Sons Ltd.

Family medical history: Lamont's mother (26 years old) and father (30 years old) both have sickle cell trait, but neither has a history of chronic medical conditions. Lamont's 1-year-old sister also has sickle cell trait. His maternal grandmother (46 years old) has a history of hepatitis. His maternal grandfather (50 years old) has a history of tuberculosis (successfully treated before Lamont was born). Lamont's paternal grandfather (51 years old) has no known history of health problems. His paternal grandmother (50 years old) has a history of malaria.

Medications: Lamont is not currently taking any over-the-counter, prescription, or herbal medications. He has no known allergies to medication, food, or the environment. He is up to date on required immunizations.

OBJECTIVE

Lamont's vital signs are taken, and his weight in the office is 24 kg. His temperature is 37.5°C (temporal). He is alert, cooperative, and interactive. He appears well hydrated and well nourished.

Skin: His skin is clear of lesions. There is no cyanosis of his skin, lips, or nails. There is no diaphoresis noted, and Lamont has good skin turgor on examination.

HEENT: Lamont is normocephalic. Red reflexes are present bilaterally; and his pupils are equal, round, and reactive to light. There is no ocular discharge noted. Lamont's external ear reveals that the pinnae are normal and that there is no tenderness to touch on the external ear. On otoscopic examination, the tympanic membranes are gray bilaterally, in normal position with positive light reflexes. Bony landmarks are visible, and there is no fluid noted behind the tympanic membranes. Both nostrils are patent. There is no nasal discharge, and there is no nasal flaring. Lamont's mucous membranes are noted to be moist when examining his oropharynx. He has 20 teeth present. Both premolars on the lower, left side are noted to have visible caries. The gingival area surrounding those 2 teeth is erythematous and edematous. The area is tender to touch. There are no other lesions present in the oral cavity.

Neck: Supple and able to move in all directions without resistance. There is a 1-cm diameter left, anterior cervical node present. The node is nonerythematous, mobile, and mildly tender to touch.

Respiratory: Respiratory rate is 20 breaths per minute, and lungs are clear to auscultation in all lobes. There is good air entry, and no retractions or grunting are noted on examination. No deformities of the thoracic cage are noted.

Cardiovascular: Heart rate is 92 beats per minute with a regular rhythm. There is no murmur noted upon auscultation.

Abdomen: Normoactive bowel sounds throughout; soft and nontender. No evidence of hepatosplenomegaly.

Genitourinary: Normal uncircumcised male genitalia without erythema or lesions. His testes are descended bilaterally.

Neuromuscular: Good tone and full range of motion in all extremities, warm, and well-perfused. Capillary refill is less than 2 seconds, and his spine is straight.

CRITICAL THINKING

Which diagnostic or imaging studies should be considered to assist with or confirm the diagnosis?

___Complete blood count

___Erythrocyte sedimentation test

___Dental X-ray

What are the most likely differential diagnoses and why?

___Gingivitis

___Dental caries

___Periodontitis

What is the plan of treatment, referral, and follow-up care?

Does this patient's psychosocial history affect how you might treat this case?

What if the patient lived in a rural setting?

Are there any demographic characteristics that might affect this case?

Are there any standardized guidelines that should be used to assess or treat this case?

Case 3.5 Abdominal Pain

By Mikki Meadows-Oliver, PhD, RN, FAAN

SUBJECTIVE

Four-year-old Jennifer presents to the office with a complaint of abdominal pain for 2 days. She is accompanied by her mother, Anat. Anat states that Jennifer's pain is intermittent and is mainly on the left side of her abdomen. She states that the pain is sometimes worse after eating and that the pain is sometimes relieved by passing gas. Jennifer is unable to describe the quality of the pain, but Anat states that Jennifer will sometimes "double over" in pain. Jennifer has had no vomiting or diarrhea. She has had no cough or runny nose.

Diet: Jennifer's nutrition history reveals that she eats bananas and rice almost daily. She drinks 4–5 cups of whole milk daily.

Elimination: She is voiding well with no complaints of dysuria. Jennifer has 2–3 bowel movements per week. Anat is unsure of the amount or consistency, since she rarely accompanies Jennifer into the bathroom.

Sleep: Jennifer sleeps approximately 10 hours at night. She has no problems falling asleep or staying asleep. Her sleep has not been interrupted by her abdominal pain.

Past medical history: Jennifer was born via cesarean section at 37 weeks' gestation. Since being discharged at 4 days of age, she has had no emergency department visits or hospitalizations. Jennifer had bronchiolitis at 6 months of age but has had no injuries or illnesses since that time. Jennifer passed her developmental screening at her last well-child visit. She currently attends pre-kindergarten and is doing well, according to Anat. She has no chronic illnesses and is not currently taking any medications.

Social history: Jennifer lives at home with both parents and a 2-year-old sibling. Her mother works as a nurse, and her father is a firefighter. The family has a pet chihuahua. There are no smokers in the home.

Family medical history: Jennifer's mother (29 years old) and father (29 years old) are healthy and have no history of chronic medical conditions. Her 2-year-old sibling is healthy as well. Her maternal grandmother (52 years old) has a history of Crohn's disease. Her maternal grandfather (54 years old) has a history of asthma. Jennifer's paternal grandfather passed away at 47 years of

The Family Nurse Practitioner: Clinical Case Studies, Second Edition. Edited by Leslie Neal-Boylan.
© 2021 John Wiley & Sons Ltd. Published 2021 by John Wiley & Sons Ltd.

age from stomach cancer. Her paternal grandmother (53 years old) has a history of obesity and Type 2 diabetes.

Medications: Jennifer is currently taking no over-the-counter, prescription, or herbal medications. She has no known allergies to medications, food, or the environment. She is up to date on required immunizations.

OBJECTIVE

Jennifer's vital signs are taken, and her weight in the office today is 27 kg. Her temperature is 37°C (temporal). She is alert, cooperative, and interactive. She appears well hydrated and well nourished.

Skin: Her skin is clear of lesions. There is no cyanosis of her skin, lips, or nails. There is no diaphoresis noted. Jennifer has good skin turgor on examination.

HEENT: Jennifer's head is normocephalic. Red reflexes are present bilaterally; and pupils are equal, round, and reactive to light. There is no ocular discharge noted. Julia's external ear reveals that the pinnae are normal and that there is no tenderness to touch on the external ear. On otoscopic examination, the tympanic membranes are gray bilaterally and in normal position with positive light reflexes. Bony landmarks are visible, and there is no fluid noted behind the tympanic membranes. Both nostrils are patent. There is scant nasal discharge, and there is no nasal flaring. Jennifer's mucous membranes are noted to be moist when examining her oropharynx. She has 20 teeth present without evidence of caries. There are no lesions present in the oral cavity.

Neck: Supple and able to move in all directions without resistance; no cervical lymphadenopathy.

Respiratory: Respiratory rate is 24 breaths per minute, and lungs are clear to auscultation in all lobes. There is good air entry, and no retractions or grunting are noted on examination. No deformities of the thoracic cage are noted.

Cardiovascular: Heart rate is 104 beats per minute with a regular rhythm. There is no murmur noted upon auscultation.

Abdomen: Normoactive bowel sounds are present throughout; abdomen is soft and mildly tender in the lower left quadrant. There is no evidence of hepatosplenomegaly.

Genitourinary: Normal female genitalia.

Neuromusculoskeletal: Good tone in all extremities; full range of motion of all extremities. Extremities are warm and well perfused. Capillary refill is <2 seconds, and spine is straight.

CRITICAL THINKING

Are there laboratory tests or diagnostic imaging studies that should be ordered as part of a workup for abdominal pain?
___Stool test for occult blood
___Anorectal manometry
___Digital rectal exam
___Abdominal radiograph
___Blood test for celiac disease

___Erythrocyte sedimentation rate (ESR)
___Barium enema
___Total colonic motility studies
___Thyroid function test
___Stool culture
___Endoscopy/Colonoscopy

What is the most likely differential diagnosis and why?
___Functional dyspepsia
___Functional constipation
___Irritable bowel syndrome
___Cyclic vomiting syndrome
___Abdominal migraine
___Functional abdominal pain syndrome
___Gastrointestinal infection
___Hirschsprung disease
___Intussusception
___Celiac disease
___Crohn's disease
___Dietary intolerances

What is the plan of treatment, referral, and follow-up care?

Does this patient's psychosocial history affect how you might treat this case?

What if the patient lived in a rural setting?

Are there any demographic characteristics that might affect this case?

Case 3.6 Lesion on Penis

By Mikki Meadows-Oliver, PhD, RN, FAAN

SUBJECTIVE

Two-year-old Lydell presents to the office with his mother and maternal grandmother with a complaint of a red area on his penis. Lydell's mother, Stacy, states that when she was changing his diaper 2 days ago, she noticed that Lydell's foreskin was red. She states that she has been putting a diaper rash cream on the area but that it has not helped to relieve the redness. She feels that the area of redness is getting larger and that the area is now painful. Lydell has no fever, cough, runny nose, vomiting, or diarrhea.

Diet: Lydell's nutrition history reveals that he has a balanced diet with enough dairy, protein, fruits, and vegetables. His appetite is good and has not changed in the past 2 days.

Elimination: Lydell is voiding well, but Stacy thinks that he may have some pain when he urinates. She states that diaper changes seem to cause him pain when she cleans the area of redness with the baby wipes. He has 1 bowel movement daily, and Stacy denies that he has constipation or diarrhea.

Sleep: Lydell sleeps approximately 11 hours at night and takes one nap daily. He has no trouble falling asleep or staying asleep.

Past medical history: Lydell was born at 40 weeks' gestation via vaginal delivery with vacuum assist. Since birth, Lydell has been healthy and has had no injuries or illnesses requiring visits to the emergency department. Lydell passed his developmental screening at his last well-child visit. He does not currently attend a day care or preschool program. He has no chronic illnesses and is currently taking no medications.

Social history: Lydell lives at home with his mother and maternal grandmother. Lydell's father is involved but does not reside in the home. His mother is currently not working outside of the home. The family has a cat. There are no smokers in the home.

Family medical history: Lydell's mother (21 years old) has a history of having leukemia as child. She is followed periodically by an oncologist. Lydell's father (23 years old) has a history of asthma. Lydell's maternal grandmother (age 39 years) has a history of multiple sclerosis. His maternal grandfather (40 years old) has a history of Type I diabetes. Lydell's paternal grandfather (41 years

The Family Nurse Practitioner: Clinical Case Studies, Second Edition. Edited by Leslie Neal-Boylan.
© 2021 John Wiley & Sons Ltd. Published 2021 by John Wiley & Sons Ltd.

old) has no known history of health problems. His paternal grandmother (40 years old) has a history of asthma.

Medications: Lydell is not currently taking any over-the-counter, prescription, or herbal medications. His mother does apply diaper rash cream to the genital area during diaper changes. Lydell has no known allergies to medication, food, or the environment. He is up to date on required immunizations.

OBJECTIVE

Lydell's vital signs are taken, and his weight in the office is 17 kg. His temperature is 37.0°C (temporal). He is alert, playful, and interactive. When crying, he is easily consolable. He appears well hydrated and well nourished. There is no cyanosis of his skin, lips, or nails. There is no diaphoresis noted, and Lydell has good skin turgor on examination.

HEENT: Lydell's head is normocephalic. His red reflexes are present bilaterally; and his pupils are equal, round, and reactive to light. There is no ocular discharge noted. Lydell's external ear reveals that the pinnae are normal, and there is no tenderness to touch on the external ear. On otoscopic examination, the tympanic membranes are gray bilaterally, in normal position with positive light reflexes. Bony landmarks are visible, and there is no fluid noted behind the tympanic membranes. Both nostrils are patent. There is no nasal discharge, and there is no nasal flaring. Lydell's mucous membranes are noted to be moist. He has 18 teeth present. There are no visible caries or other lesions present in the oral cavity.

Neck: Lydell's neck is supple and able to move in all directions without resistance. There is no cervical lymphadenopathy noted.

Respiratory: Lydell's respiratory rate is 24 breaths per minute, and his lungs are clear to auscultation in all lobes. There is good air entry, and no retractions or grunting are noted on examination. No deformities of the thoracic cage are noted.

Cardiovascular: Lydell's heart rate is 96 beats per minute with a regular rhythm. There is no murmur noted upon auscultation.

Abdomen: Normoactive bowel sounds are present throughout, and Lydell's abdomen is soft and nontender. There is no evidence of hepatosplenomegaly.

Genitourinary: Uncircumcised male genitalia with erythema and mild edema on the foreskin. The affected area is mildly tender to touch. A portion of the glans is visible; and there is no discharge, erythema, or swelling noted. His testes are descended bilaterally. There is no erythema or edema of the scrotum. He has shotty lymph nodes present in the inguinal area.

Neuromuscular: Good tone and full range of motion in all extremities; extremities are warm and well perfused. Capillary refill is less than 2 seconds, and his spine is straight.

CRITICAL THINKING

Which diagnostic or imaging studies should be considered to assist with or confirm the diagnosis?
___Bacterial culture
___Gram stain
___Microscopic examination

___Potassium hydroxide (KOH)
___Urinalysis

What is the most likely differential diagnosis and why?
___Balanitis
___Phimosis
___Paraphimosis
___Balanoposthitis

What is the plan of treatment, referral, and follow-up care?

Does this patient's psychosocial history affect how you might treat this case?

What if the patient lived in a rural setting?

Are there any demographic characteristics that might affect this case?

Case 4.1 Rash without Fever

By Mikki Meadows-Oliver, PhD, RN, FAAN

SUBJECTIVE

A 4-year-old female, Abigail, comes to the clinic for evaluation of a rash. She is accompanied to the visit by her mother. According to her mother, Abigail first developed a small, red papule between her nose and her upper lip a few days prior to the appointment today. Her mother thinks that she might have scratched or picked at that area. A few more papules appeared that became fluid-filled vesicles for a brief amount of time. The fragile roofs of these vesicles quickly sloughed off. The newly eroded skin developed overlying honey-colored crusts. The patient complains that the rash is sometimes pruritic, so she has been scratching the area. Abigail's mother feels that the rash is spreading due to Abigail's manipulation of the area. Abigail has been afebrile and has maintained a normal appetite and activity level by report.

Diet: Adequate and varied.

Elimination: Voids every 3–4 hours. Normal bowel movements daily.

Past medical history: Abigail is a healthy 4-year-old with no significant medical history. She does not have any chronic medical problems and has not had surgery.

Family history: One of Abigail's cousins has a similar rash on her arm. Otherwise noncontributory.

Social history: Abigail and her mother live in a 4-bedroom duplex with her 2 siblings, a grandmother, a grandfather, an aunt, an uncle, and 3 cousins. There are no pets in the home. Abigail's mother works part-time doing housekeeping for a nearby hotel. She reports that she earns minimum wage. Abigail's father has not been in contact with the family since before she was born.

Medications: Abigail does not take any medications regularly. Her mother has not given her any oral medications to treat this problem. Her mother did apply some over-the-counter 1% hydrocortisone cream to the area but does not feel that it helped.

Allergies: Abigail is not allergic to any medications. There are no suspected allergies to soaps, detergents, foods, or other environmental factors.

The Family Nurse Practitioner: Clinical Case Studies, Second Edition. Edited by Leslie Neal-Boylan.
© 2021 John Wiley & Sons Ltd. Published 2021 by John Wiley & Sons Ltd.

OBJECTIVE

General: Alert, well-nourished female in no apparent distress. She appears nontoxic and is coloring pictures calmly during the exam.

Vital signs: Heart rate: 96; respiratory rate: 16; temperature: 98.8°F; height: 40 inches; weight: 42 lbs (19 kg).

HEENT: Moist mucous membranes without ulcerations; nares patent bilaterally without drainage. Conjunctivae clear without erythema or discharge.

Lymphatic: No cervical, supraclavicular, or occipital lymphadenopathy.

Cardiovascular: Regular heart rate and rhythm; no murmur.

Respiratory: Regular respiratory rate with clear and equal air movement bilaterally.

Skin: Mildly erythematous, confluent plaque of eroded skin inferior to nares and superior to upper lip. Honey-colored crusts overlying the affected area.

CRITICAL THINKING

Which diagnostic or imaging studies should be considered to assist with or confirm the diagnosis?
___Bacterial culture
___Bacterial culture of the nares
___Examination of Tzanck smear
___Fluorescent antibody testing of smears
___Fungal culture
___Gram stain
___Potassium hydroxide (KOH) examination
___Viral culture

What is the most likely differential diagnosis and why?
___Atopic dermatitis
___Herpes simplex virus (HSV)
___Impetigo

What is the treatment plan?

What would the appropriate treatment plan for this diagnosis be if the patient were febrile and/or showing other signs of systemic illness?

What is the plan for follow-up care?

Are any referrals needed?

Should the patient stay out of school and/or day care during treatment? If so, for how long?

What, if anything, should be recommended to unaffected household members?

Case 4.2 Rash with Fever

By Mikki Meadows-Oliver, PhD, RN, FAAN

Seven-year-old Aubrey presents to the office with a complaint of a rash for 2 days. She is accompanied by her mother, Jessica. Aubrey has also had a mildly runny nose and cough for 3 days. She has had a low-grade fever, and her maximum temperature at home was 37.9°C (oral). Aubrey has had no vomiting or diarrhea.

Diet: Normally has a balanced diet with enough dairy, protein, fruits, and vegetables. There has been no change in appetite since her symptoms began.

Elimination: Voiding well with no complaints of dysuria.

Sleep: Sleeps approximately 9 hours at night and has no problems falling asleep or staying asleep.

Past medical history: Aubrey was born via cesarean section at 38 weeks' gestation for a breech presentation. Since being discharged home at 4 days of age, she has had no hospitalizations. Aubrey had an emergency department visit at 5 years of age for sutures to her head after she fell and struck her head on the corner of a table. She has had no injuries or illnesses since that time

Family history: Aubrey's mother (34 years old) has a history of migraine headaches. Her father (30 years old) is healthy and has no history of chronic medical conditions. Her 5-year-old sibling has Type 1 diabetes. Her maternal grandmother (68 years old) has Type 2 diabetes. Her maternal grandfather (68 years old) has a history of chronic obstructive pulmonary disease (COPD). Aubrey's paternal grandfather (58 years old) has a history of skin cancer. Her paternal grandmother (53 years old) has hypertension.

Social history: Aubrey currently attends elementary school. She is in the second grade and is doing well, according to her mother. Aubrey lives at home with her parents and her 5-year-old sibling. Her father is a graduate student, and her mother is an accountant. The family has a pet rabbit.

Medications: Aubrey is not currently taking any over-the-counter, prescription, or herbal medications. Aubrey has no known allergies to food, medications, or the environment. At her last well-child check, her mother refused the annual flu shot and the second varicella vaccination because Aubrey had a cold. The family did not return to the office to receive these 2 vaccines.

The Family Nurse Practitioner: Clinical Case Studies, Second Edition. Edited by Leslie Neal-Boylan.
© 2021 John Wiley & Sons Ltd. Published 2021 by John Wiley & Sons Ltd.

OBJECTIVE

General: Aubrey is alert, active, and cooperative. She appears well hydrated and well nourished.

Vital signs: Weight in the office today is 33 kg. Her temperature is slightly elevated at 37.9° Celsius (oral).

Skin: A predominantly maculopapular rash is noted on her back and chest. Two vesicles are noted on the upper right side of her chest. There is no rash noted elsewhere in her body. There is no cyanosis of her skin, lips, or nails. There is no diaphoresis noted. Skin has elastic recoil.

HEENT: Normocephalic; red reflexes are present bilaterally; and her pupils were equal, round, and reactive to light. There is no ocular discharge noted. Aubrey's external ear reveals that the pinnae are normal and that there is no tenderness to touch on the external ear. On otoscopic examination, both tympanic membranes are gray, in normal position, with positive light reflexes. Bony landmarks are visible, and there is no fluid noted behind the tympanic membranes. Both nostrils are patent. There is no nasal discharge, and there is no nasal flaring. Aubrey's mucous membranes are noted to be moist when examining her oropharynx. There is no inflammation of her tonsils, and there are no oral lesions noted.

Neck: Supple and able to move in all directions without resistance. There is no cervical lymphadenopathy noted.

Respiratory: Rate is 20 breaths per minute, and lungs are clear to auscultation in all lobes. There is good air entry, and no retractions or grunting are noted on examination. No deformities of the thoracic cage are noted.

Cardiac: Heart rate is 102 beats per minute with a regular rhythm. There is no murmur noted upon auscultation.

Abdomen: Normoactive bowel sounds are present throughout; soft and nontender. No evidence of hepatosplenomegaly.

Genitourinary: Normal prepubertal female genitalia.

Neuromusculoskeletal: Good tone and full range of motion of all extremities; extremities are warm and well perfused. Capillary refill is less than 2 seconds. Spine is straight.

CRITICAL THINKING

Which diagnostic or imaging studies should be considered to assist with or confirm the diagnosis?
___Tzanck smear
___Viral culture
___Direct fluorescent antigen testing
___Varicella polymerase chain reaction
___Potassium hydroxide (KOH) smear
___Throat culture for group A beta-hemolytic streptococci (GABHS)
___Nasal swab for influenza

What is the most likely differential diagnosis and why?
___Varicella zoster virus (breakthrough)
___Herpes zoster
___Scarlet fever
___Viral exanthem
___Lyme disease
___Tinea corporis

What is the plan of treatment, referral, and follow-up care?

Does this patient's psychosocial history affect how you might treat this case?

What if the patient lived in a rural setting?

Are there any demographic characteristics that might affect this case?

By Andrew Konesky, MSN, APRN

SUBJECTIVE

Will, a 12-year-old male, was referred to the school-based health center (SBHC) at the request of his mother for a red right eye, noticed this morning upon awakening. Will reports waking up this morning with his right eyelid "stuck together like glue." He reports washing his face and eyes with warm water, allowing him to open his eye. He noticed his eye was "a little red," but did not report any pain or itch. He has had to wipe his eye a few times since washing his face, as "yellow stuff keeps coming out." Will reports wearing glasses daily and has never worn contact lenses. He is experiencing no visual disturbances and denies blurriness and double vision. Will's mother was contacted by the SBHC to provide confirmation of history and further details. His mother denies sick contacts at home, but Will's cousin, whose house he slept at over the weekend, was given "eye drops" last week by his primary care provider.

Birth history: Will was born full term. His birth weight was 8 lbs 5 oz and birth length was 20 in.

Past medical history: Will has seasonal allergies, which are exacerbated every fall, that are well controlled on daily allergy medication. He has myopia and has been wearing glasses since age 6. He had an appendectomy 2 years ago when he was 10 years old. He has multiple visits to the SBHC for acute, unrelated presentations. He has no further significant history, hospitalizations, or surgeries.

Social history: Will lives with his mother, father, and older sister in a single-family house. Will is in the seventh grade and plays on the school lacrosse team. He wants to one day be a professional lacrosse player. He is also the team manager for the town's local hockey team, and enjoys art and music in his spare time. Will has multiple friends at school and a few close friendships.

Diet: Will eats 3 meals a day and reports a normal appetite. He consumes a varied diet of fruits, vegetables, dairy products, and protein sources.

Elimination: Denies difficulty going to the bathroom. Reports regular bowel patterns.

Sleep: Sleeps an average of 8 hours per night. Denies nighttime awakenings, snoring, and restlessness.

Family medical history: Will's family history is positive for heart disease on his father's side; his father had a myocardial infarction several years ago. His father may have high blood pressure,

---

The Family Nurse Practitioner: Clinical Case Studies, Second Edition. Edited by Leslie Neal-Boylan.
© 2021 John Wiley & Sons Ltd. Published 2021 by John Wiley & Sons Ltd.

but he is not sure. Will denies family history of cancer and or diabetes. His paternal and maternal grandparents are alive and well. He is unsure of his grandparent's medical history.

Medications: 10 mg Zyrtec daily, Naphcon allergy eye drops as needed, daily multivitamin.

Allergies: Seasonal. No medication allergies reported. No food allergies reported.

OBJECTIVE

General: Male presenting in no acute distress, well hydrated, conversational and appropriate with provider.

Vital signs: Height: 68 in; weight: 135 lbs; BMI: 20.5; BP: 116/70; HR: 75; RR: 16.

Skin: Skin is clear with no rashes noted. Small scar is noted at right lower abdominal quadrant s/p appendectomy. Skin is warm and dry.

HEENT: On examination, right eye is mildly injected, with thick, yellow discharge draining from inner canthus. Dried, yellow crusting is noted across lower lid. Upon cleansing the canthus, discharge reappears spontaneously throughout duration of exam. Pupils are equal and round, reactive to light, with accommodation showing normal pupillary reflex. Visual acuity is 20/20 on Snellen test with corrective lenses. Red reflex is noted and optic discs are without hemorrhage.

Head is normocephalic and atraumatic. Tympanic membranes are clear, intact, with landmarks and cone of light visualized, bilaterally. Nasal turbinates are pale, swollen, and with mild clear discharge. Nasal septum is vertically aligned with no report of pain or discomfort upon palpation of frontal and maxillary sinuses. Oral pharynx is clear with no erythema noted. Tonsils +2 of 4 with no exudate or erythema. Posterior pharynx has minimal post nasal drainage and mild cobbling.

Neck: Supple with full range of motion in all directions. No cervical lymphadenopathy.

Cardiovascular: Regular rate and rhythm. S1/S2 auscultated with no murmur, clicks, rubs, gallops. Equal +2 carotid and radial pulse bilaterally.

Respiratory: Clear to auscultation. No wheezes, rhonchi, rales noted. Good air exchange.

Abdomen: Soft, nontender, nondistended, normal active bowel sounds in all 4 quadrants.

Genitourinary: Deferred.

Neurologic: Alert and oriented. Cranial nerves grossly intact. Good eye contact. Gait normal. Uvula rises midline and symmetrically.

CRITICAL THINKING

What are the top three differential diagnoses in this case and why?

What are the diagnostic tests required in this case and why?

What is the plan of treatment?

Are there any standardized guidelines that should be used to treat this case? If so, what are they?

What are the plans for follow-up care and referral?

Are there any special examination and or treatment considerations that may affect this case?

Case 4.4 Sore Throat

By Mikki Meadows-Oliver, PhD, RN, FAAN

SUBJECTIVE

Eight-year-old Suzanna presents to the office with a complaint of a sore throat for 2 days. She is accompanied by her mother, Mikayla. Suzanna has had an intermittent fever and her maximum temperature at home was 101°F (oral). Suzanna complains that she has pain when she swallows. She also complains of a headache. Both the throat pain and headache are relieved slightly with the use of over-the-counter pain relievers. Suzanna has had no vomiting or diarrhea. She has had no runny nose or cough. She denies drooling or difficulty breathing.

Diet: Suzanna's nutrition history reveals that she normally has a balanced diet with enough dairy, protein, fruits, and vegetables. Her appetite has decreased over the past 2 days since the throat pain began.

Elimination: She is voiding well with no complaints of dysuria.

Sleep: Suzanna usually sleeps approximately 9 hours at night. She usually has no problems falling or staying asleep but since the throat pain has started, her sleep has been interrupted.

Past medical history: Suzanna was born via vaginal delivery at 38 weeks' gestation. Since being discharged at 2 days of age, she has had no hospitalizations. Suzanna had an emergency department visit at 4 years of age for a broken clavicle that she sustained after falling from the jungle gym at preschool. She has had no injuries or illnesses since that time.

Family history: Suzanna's mother (28 years old) has a history of hyperthyroidism. Her father (30 years old) is healthy and has no history of chronic medical conditions. Her maternal grandmother (56 years old) has emphysema. Her maternal grandfather (57 years old) has a history of asthma. Suzanna's paternal grandfather (58 years old) has a history of hypertension. Her paternal grandmother (53 years old) has multiple sclerosis.

Social history: Suzanna currently attends elementary school. She is in the third grade and is doing well, according to Mikayla. Suzanna lives at home with her mother, who works as an office manager, and her father, Joe, who is a professional carpenter. The family has a pet fish. Suzanna attends an after-school program.

The Family Nurse Practitioner: Clinical Case Studies, Second Edition. Edited by Leslie Neal-Boylan.
© 2021 John Wiley & Sons Ltd. Published 2021 by John Wiley & Sons Ltd.

Medications: Suzanna is currently taking no prescription or herbal medications. She has been taking over-the-counter pain relievers/antipyretics to relieve symptoms associated with her throat pain.

Allergies: Suzanna has no known allergies to food, medications, or the environment. She is up to date on required immunizations.

OBJECTIVE

General: Alert, quiet, and cooperative; appears well hydrated and well nourished.

Vital signs: Weight in the office today is 36 kg; temperature is slightly elevated at 38.4°C (oral).

Skin: Clear of lesions and warm to touch. There was no cyanosis of her skin, lips, or nails. There was no diaphoresis noted; skin with elastic recoil.

HEENT: Normocephalic; red reflexes are present bilaterally; and pupils are equal, round, and reactive to light. There is no ocular discharge noted. External ear reveals that the pinnae are normal and that there is no tenderness to touch on the external ear. On otoscopic examination, both tympanic membranes are gray, in normal position, with positive light reflexes. Bony landmarks are visible, and there is no fluid noted behind the tympanic membranes. Both nostrils are patent. There is no nasal discharge and no nasal flaring. Samantha's mucous membranes are noted to be moist when examining her oropharynx. Both tonsils are erythematous and inflamed. There are exudates present bilaterally, as well as palatal petechiae.

Neck: Supple and able to move in all directions without resistance; tender anterior cervical nodes present on both sides of the neck; no erythema of the nodes.

Respiratory: Respiratory rate was 28 breaths per minute, and her lungs are clear to auscultation in all lobes. There is good air entry, and no retractions or grunting are noted on examination. No deformities of the thoracic cage are noted.

Cardiac: Heart rate was 112 beats per minute with a regular rhythm. There is no murmur noted upon auscultation.

Abdomen: Normoactive bowel sounds were present throughout; soft and nontender; no evidence of hepatosplenomegaly.

Genitourinary: Normal prepubertal female genitalia.

Neuromusculoskeletal: Good tone in all extremities; full range of motion of all extremities; extremities warm and well-perfused. Capillary refill is less than 2 seconds. Her spine is straight.

CRITICAL THINKING

Which diagnostic or imaging studies should be considered to assist with or confirm the diagnosis?
___Throat culture
___Rapid strep test
___Complete blood count (CBC)
___Monospot
___Liver function tests (LFTs)

What is the most likely differential diagnosis and why?
___Viral pharyngitis
___Bacterial pharyngitis
___Fungal pharyngitis
___Peritonsillar abscess
___Group A beta-hemolytic streptococci (GABHS)

What is the plan for treatment, referral, and follow-up care?

Does this patient's psychosocial history affect how you might treat this case?

What if the patient lived in a rural setting?

Are there any demographic characteristics that might affect this case?

Case 4.5 Disruptive Behavior

By Mikki Meadows-Oliver, PhD, RN, FAAN

SUBJECTIVE

This mother presents with 6-year-old Jason with concerns about his increasingly disruptive behavior at home. She reports that Jason has always been a difficult child to manage, often is irritable, angers easily, and resists any changes in routine. He argues constantly with his 8-year-old sister about simple activities. He grabs her toys, interferes with her play, and has begun to be more physically aggressive with her. Jason argues with his mother and grandmother when any limits are put on his behavior. He is uncooperative regarding the simplest of requests like coming to the table for meals, turning off his video games, or staying in the yard. Jason has had a few good relationships with children in the neighborhood. His mother has attempted to discipline Jason through a variety of methods, such as talking, screaming, time out, losing TV and video game time, and occasional spankings. His mother reports that no methods work. She is exhausted by the attention she spends on his behavior and is frustrated facing discipline issues every day from breakfast to bedtime. She is confused because her daughter has never demonstrated these types of issues, and she used basically the same parenting strategies with her daughter as she did with Jason. His mother has not spoken with Jason's first-grade teacher to see if similar behaviors are occurring in school.

Diet: Jason has been a healthy child. He had some initial feeding issues as an infant with excessive irritability causing multiple formula changes. Since then he has had no food allergies or intolerances and eats a fairly well-balanced diet with the exception of excessive juice consumption.

Elimination: No difficulties.

Sleep: Jason has had difficulty establishing nighttime sleep patterns. He continues to have difficulty with sleep onset, wakes frequently, and goes into his mother's bed.

Past medical history: Jason was the second child born to a 27-year-old mother by vaginal delivery after an uneventful full-term pregnancy. He weighed 7 lbs 9 oz and had no problems in the newborn nursery (no temperature instability, no jaundice, and no respiratory issues). He was discharged home with his mother on cow's-milk formula at 48 hours of age. Jason experienced a head injury with a loss of consciousness at the age of 3 years. His head CT was normal, but he was admitted to the pediatric unit for overnight observation. He has not had any obvious sequelae from this incident. Jason has had no respiratory, cardiac, neurologic, or allergic problems.

The Family Nurse Practitioner: Clinical Case Studies, Second Edition. Edited by Leslie Neal-Boylan.
© 2021 John Wiley & Sons Ltd. Published 2021 by John Wiley & Sons Ltd.

Family history: Jason's mother has history of Hashimoto thyroiditis and depression and is medicated for both of these conditions. She is fairly adherent to her medication regime. She was an average student, graduated from high school, and works as a cashier. Jason's 33-year-old father has a history of substance abuse, depression, and hypertension. He was incarcerated briefly for selling drugs and now declines all medications. He did not complete high school, has a history of delinquency and attention problems, and currently works intermittently in construction. The maternal grandparents both have well-controlled hypertension and hypercholesterolemia. The paternal grandparents' histories are unknown to the father since he has not had contact with them in 15 years. Jason's sister is healthy and doing average schoolwork.

Social history: Jason's mom is single and lives on the second floor of a 1940s 2-family house with the maternal grandparents on the first floor. Jason's household consists of his mother, an 8-year-old sister, 2 dogs, and several cats. His mother and the children have frequent contact with the father, but he is not a regular part of the household. Both parents smoke while with the children. Jason attended day care full-time until school entry but now returns home to the care of his grandparents after school. Toward the end of his time in day care, his mom reports that she had received a few calls about Jason's behavior, specifically some difficulties participating in group activities and following directions.

Medications: Takes no medications.

OBJECTIVE

General: Alert, active, responsive to most requests with good articulation, some fidgeting with instruments.

Vital signs: Height: 46 inches (115 cm); weight: 45 lbs (20.9 kg); heart rate: 92; respiratory rate: 18; blood pressure: 98/62.

HEENT: Normocephalic; PERRL full EOMs, normal convergence, normal discs; gray TMs with good light reflexes and landmarks. Nose is normal, midline septum, boggy turbinates. Throat reveals large tonsils, no erythema, and uvula midline.

Neck: Supple; full range of motion; thyroid not palpable; no lymphadenopathy.

Cardiac: Regular rate and rhythm; S1/S2; no murmur; pulses full and equal.

Respiratory: Clear breath sounds throughout.

Abdomen: Soft, no mass, no hepatosplenomegaly.

Genitourinary: Normal male, circumcised, testes descended ×2.

Musculoskeletal: Full range of motion for all extremities; symmetric movement.

Neurologic: Normal tone, strength, coordination, reflexes and cranial nerves II-XII grossly intact.

Skin: Clear, dry patches on elbows and knees.

CRITICAL THINKING

Which diagnostic or imaging studies should be considered to assist with or confirm the diagnosis?
___CBC
___Thyroid studies

___Lead screening
___Vision screening
___Hearing screening
___Vanderbilt ADHD screening for school and parent
___Learning disability evaluation
___Pediatric Symptom Checklist

What is the most likely differential diagnosis and why?
___Normal active behavior of early childhood
___Hearing impairment
___Attention-deficit hyperactive disorder (ADHD)
___Learning disability
___Oppositional defiant disorder (ODD)
___Conduct disorder
___Depression

What is the plan of treatment?

What is the plan for follow-up care?

Are there any demographic factors that might affect this case?

NOTE: The author would like to acknowledge Patricia Ryan-Krause, MSN, APRN, who co-authored this case in the first edition of this book.

Case 4.6 Cough and Difficulty Breathing

By Nancy Cantey Banasiak, DNP, PPCNP-BC, APRN

SUBJECTIVE

Emily is a 6-year-old female who presents to the clinic with her mother. She presents with complaints of cough and difficulty breathing. Two days prior, Emily developed a nonproductive cough that is worse at night, clear rhinorrhea, and a fever with a maximum temperature of 102°F. The mother has treated the fever with Tylenol 320 mg every 4 hours, as needed, when the temperature was greater than 101°F. Her mother also complains that "when she gets a cold, it lasts longer than normal."

Birth history: Emily was born full term weighing 3200 g by normal spontaneous vaginal delivery (NSVD). Pregnancy and delivery were uncomplicated with Apgar scores of 8 (1 minute) and 9 (5 minutes).

Social history: Emily is a 6-year-old female in the first grade who lives with her mom, dad, and 2 siblings in a house in the city. They have 4 pets: 2 dogs, 1 cat, and 1 turtle. The parents work outside the home and have private health insurance. Emily and her siblings attend an after-school program until her mom picks them up after work. Emily attends regular medical and dental appointments, and they deny tobacco or alcohol use in the home. She plays soccer, ice hockey, and lacrosse.

Diet: Emily's appetite is fair with a fluid intake of 32 oz/day of juice/milk/water. She also reports normal eating habits without abdominal pain or diarrhea.

Elimination: Emily voided 4 times yesterday. No vomiting or diarrhea. Her mother complains that everyone in the house is sick with the same symptoms.

Sleep: Emily sleeps from 8 p.m. to 6 a.m. She coughs 1–2 times during the night.

Past medical history: Past medical history is positive for obstructive sleep apnea 4. Birth history was uneventful. Emily also has a history of bronchiolitis at 8 months of age, which did not require medication or hospitalization.

Family history: Mother (age 36): healthy, atopic dermatitis, seasonal allergies; father (age 35): healthy, asthma, seasonal allergies; sibling (age 4): healthy; sibling (age 2): healthy; maternal grandmother (age 80): hypertension, breast cancer, basal cell skin cancer; maternal grandfather

---

The Family Nurse Practitioner: Clinical Case Studies, Second Edition. Edited by Leslie Neal-Boylan.
© 2021 John Wiley & Sons Ltd. Published 2021 by John Wiley & Sons Ltd.

(age 81): hypertension, diabetes mellitus Type 2; paternal grandmother (age 76): hypertension, obesity; paternal grandfather (age 72): deceased, hypertension, stroke.

Medications: Emily is currently on no medications. Immunizations are up to date.

Allergies: Has no known allergies to medications, food, or the environment.

OBJECTIVE

General: Emily is alert, well hydrated, active, and cooperative.

Vital signs: Temperature 38°C, pulse 72, and respirations 28 per minute with a blood pressure of 100/52 in the left arm. The O2 saturation is 94%, and weight is 25 kg.

Skin: No lesions, rashes, or scars; and the patient is not cyanotic.

HEENT: Normocephalic with no evidence of trauma or lesions. Eyes show no signs of drainage; sclera white, with pink conjunctiva. Otoscopic examination reveals tympanic membranes gray bilaterally with positive light reflex and normal pinnae. The nose has clear rhinorrhea; no nasal polyps with pink turbinates. Examination of the throat shows a cobblestone appearance in the posterior pharynx, uvula midline, tonsils size 0/4 with no exudate or erythema, moist mucous membranes; and the trachea is midline.

Respiratory: Bilateral inspiratory and expiratory wheezing; mild intercostal retractions; mild shortness of breath; no rales, crackles, or nasal flaring.

Cardiovascular: No murmur; normal S1/S2; 2+ brachial and femoral pulses; no cyanosis, clubbing, or edema noted.

Lymphatic: There is no lymphadenopathy on examination.

Abdomen: Soft, nontender, nondistended; + bowel sounds; no hepatosplenomegaly during palpation.

Genitourinary: Normal female genitalia.

Neurological: Grossly intact.

CRITICAL THINKING

What diagnostic or imaging studies should be considered to assist with or confirm the diagnosis?
___Oxygen saturation
___Chest X-ray
___Nasal pharyngeal swab for direct fluorescent antibody (DFA)

What are the top differential diagnoses and why?

What is the most likely differential diagnosis and why?

What is the plan of treatment?

What is the plan for follow-up care?

Are any referrals needed at this time?

Are there any standardized guidelines that should be used to assess or treat this case?

Case 4.7 Left Arm Pain

By Mikki Meadows-Oliver, PhD, RN, FAAN

SUBJECTIVE

Jair, a 11-month-old infant, presents to the primary care office with a complaint of not using his left arm for one day. He is accompanied by his parents. His father states that Jair fell off the couch yesterday and he thinks that Jair may have landed on his left arm. The history provided by his mother is somewhat different. She states that Jair fell down two stairs while in a walker and hurt his left arm at that time.

Birth history: Jair was born at 35 weeks' gestation. His birth weight was 2200 g. There were no complications during the labor or delivery. The mother had no infections, falls, or known exposures to environmental hazards. She did not drink alcohol, take prescription medication (other than prenatal vitamins), use tobacco products, or use illicit drugs. Jair was discharged after 4 weeks in the neonatal intensive care unit to home with his mother.

The social history reveals that Jair was born to a adolescent single mother. His father, 18 years old, is involved but does not reside in the household. Jair lives in an apartment with his mother and 19-year-old cousin. The maternal grandmother (MGM) lives in the neighborhood and is able to help Jair's mother with child care. The family receives assistance from governmental subsidies such as the Women, Infants, and Children (WIC) supplemental nutrition program, Temporary Assistance for Needy Families (TANF), and Medicaid. Educationally, both Jair's mother and father have high school diplomas. She works at a fast-food restaurant. Joseph's father works as a construction worker. The family has no pets. There are no smokers in the home.

Diet: Jair eats a balanced diet of table foods. He is transitioning from formula to whole milk. He takes a daily multivitamin.

Elimination: 4–6 wet diapers daily with 1 bowel movement.

Sleep: Takes one 2-hour nap daily and sleeps 12 hours at night.

Family medical history: Paternal grandfather (age 54): healthy; paternal grandmother (age 53): hypertension; maternal grandfather (age 46): hypothyroidism; MGM (age 44): Type 2 diabetes; mother (age 18): asthma; father (age 18): healthy.

Medications: Currently taking no prescription, herbal, or over-the-counter medications.

Immunizations: Up to date.

Allergies: No known allergies to food, medications, or environment.

The Family Nurse Practitioner: Clinical Case Studies, Second Edition. Edited by Leslie Neal-Boylan.
© 2021 John Wiley & Sons Ltd. Published 2021 by John Wiley & Sons Ltd.

OBJECTIVE

Vital signs: Weight: 10 kg; length: 84 cm; temperature: 37°C (axillary).

General: Alert; well nourished; well hydrated; interactive.

Skin: Right side of forehead with ecchymosis and a 2 cm abrasion; no other lesions noted. No cyanosis of lips, nails, or skin; no diaphoresis noted; good skin turgor.

Head: Normocephalic; anterior fontanel is open and flat (1 cm × 1 cm).

Eyes: Red reflexes present bilaterally; pupils equal, round, and reactive to light; no discharge noted.

Ears: Pinnae normal; tympanic membranes gray bilaterally with positive light reflex.

Nose: Both nostrils are patent; no discharge.

Oropharynx: Mucous membranes are moist; 4 teeth are present; no lesions.

Neck: Supple; no nodes.

Respiratory: RR = 24; clear in all lobes; no adventitious sounds noted; no retractions; no deformities of the thoracic cage noted.

Cardiac/Peripheral vascular: HR = 100; regular rhythm. No murmur noted.

Abdomen/Gastrointestinal: Soft, nontender, nondistended, no evidence of hepatosplenomegaly.

Genitourinary: Normal circumcised male genitalia; testes descended bilaterally.

Back: Spine straight.

Ext/Musculoskeletal: Left arm with limited range of motion and tenderness to touch over left clavicle and left humerus. Both tender areas are slightly swollen and erythematous. Full range of motion of all other extremities; warm and well perfused; capillary refill < 3 seconds in all extremities.

Neurologic: Good strength and tone.

CRITICAL THINKING

Which diagnostic or imaging studies should be considered to assist with or confirm the diagnosis?
___Radiograph of left arm/clavicle
___CBC
___Metabolic panel

What is the most likely differential diagnosis and why?
___Fracture of left arm/clavicle to accidental fall
___Physical abuse
___Osteogenesis imperfecta

What is the plan for treatment, referral, and follow-up care?

Are there any referrals needed?

Does the patient's psychosocial history impact how you might treat him?

Case 4.8 Nightmares

By Mikki Meadows-Oliver, PhD, RN, FAAN

SUBJECTIVE

Six-year-old Daniel presents to the office with his mother, Donna, with complaints of frequent nightmares. Donna states that Daniel will be asleep and will suddenly sit upright with his eyes open and start to scream loudly. She says that Daniel looks terrified and that he sweats and breathes fast during these episodes. Donna says that while Daniel is screaming, she is unable to wake, console, or comfort him. The screaming episodes typically last about 5 minutes each and happen 3–4 times weekly. Donna states that after the screaming stops, Daniel returns to sleep and does not remember the screaming episodes when he awakens in the morning. Daniel does not have any problems falling asleep. He sleeps approximately 10 hours each night but does not have a set bedtime or a regular bedtime routine. He sleeps in his own bed and shares a room with his younger brother.

Diet: Balanced diet with sufficient sources of dairy, protein, fruits, and vegetables.

Elimination: Daniel is voiding well with no complaints of dysuria. He has 1 bowel movement daily and denies constipation or diarrhea.

Past medical history: Born via vaginal birth at 40 weeks' gestation. The mother's pregnancy was without problems. She had no infections, falls, or known exposures to environmental hazards. She did not drink alcohol, take prescription medication (other than prenatal vitamins), use tobacco products, or use illicit drugs. There were no problems for Daniel during his neonatal period. Since birth, he has had no injuries or illnesses requiring visits to the emergency department. He has no chronic illnesses.

Family history: Daniel's mother (27 years old) and father (26 years old) are both healthy and have no history of chronic medical conditions. His 3-year-old sibling also has no history of chronic medical conditions. His maternal grandmother (54 years old) has a history of asthma. His maternal grandfather (55 years old) has a history of high cholesterol. Daniel's paternal grandmother (52 years old) has a history of hypertension. His paternal grandfather (52 years old) has a history of hypertension and had a stroke at age 47 years.

Social history: Daniel lives at home with his mother, paternal grandmother, paternal uncle, and his younger brother (3 years old). His mother works as a restaurant waitress. Daniel's father is incarcerated. The family has no pets. There are no smokers in the home.

The Family Nurse Practitioner: Clinical Case Studies, Second Edition. Edited by Leslie Neal-Boylan.
© 2021 John Wiley & Sons Ltd. Published 2021 by John Wiley & Sons Ltd.

Medications: Daniel is not currently taking any over-the-counter, prescription, or herbal medications. He has no known allergies to medication, food, or the environment. He is up to date for required immunizations.

OBJECTIVE

General: Alert, cooperative, and active; appears well hydrated and well nourished.

Vital signs: Weight in the office was 28 kg. Temperature was 36.9°C (temporal).

HEENT: Normocephalic. Red reflexes are present bilaterally; and pupils are equal, round, and reactive to light. There is no ocular discharge noted; external ear reveals that the pinnae are normal and that there is no tenderness to touch on the external ear. On otoscopic examination, the tympanic membranes are gray bilaterally, in normal position, with positive light reflexes. Bony landmarks are visible, and there is no fluid noted behind the tympanic membranes. Both nostrils are patent. There is no nasal discharge and no nasal flaring. Daniel's mucous membranes were noted to be moist when examining his oropharynx. There is no evidence of visible caries or other lesions in the oral cavity.

Neck: Supple and able to move in all directions without resistance. There was no cervical lymphadenopathy present.

Skin: Clear of lesions; no cyanosis of his skin, lips, or nails; no diaphoresis noted; and there is elastic recoil.

Respiratory: Respiratory rate is 20 breaths per minute, and the lungs are clear to auscultation in all lobes. There is good air entry, and no retractions or grunting are noted on examination. No deformities of the thoracic cage are noted.

Cardiac: Heart rate is 102 beats per minute with a regular rhythm. There is no murmur noted upon auscultation.

Abdomen: Normoactive bowel sounds are present throughout. Soft and nontender. No evidence of hepatosplenomegaly.

Genitourinary: Normal circumcised male genitalia without erythema or lesions; testes are descended bilaterally.

Neuromusculoskeletal: Good tone and full range of motion in all extremities. Extremities are warm and well perfused. Capillary refill is less than 2 seconds. Spine is straight.

CRITICAL THINKING

Which diagnostic or imaging studies should be considered to assist with or confirm the diagnosis?
___EEG (electroencephalogram)
___Polysomnography
___MRI (magnetic resonance imaging)
___CT (computed tomography) scan
___Skull radiograph

What is the most likely differential diagnosis and why?
___Nightmares
___Nocturnal seizures
___Night terrors
___Sleepwalking (somnambulism)

What is the plan for treatment, referral, and follow-up care?

Does this patient's psychosocial history affect how you might treat this case?

What if the patient lived in a rural setting?

Are there any demographic characteristics that might affect this case?

NOTE: The author would like to acknowledge the contribution of Allison Grady, MSN, RN to this case in the first edition of this book.

Case 4.9 Gastrointestinal Complaint

By Allison Grady, MSN, APNP

SUBJECTIVE

Seven-year-old Katie presents with new onset gastrointestinal complaints. She has no significant past medical history and no known allergies. She was recently seen in her primary care provider's office for a well-child check. It was noted that her growth curve had plateaued for the past 2 years and she is now "falling off" her curve. Her mother describes Katie as a "classic picky eating toddler" who, in the past 2 years, has begun expanding list of acceptable foods. In the past several months, the mother has noticed that Katie has had increased incidences of diarrhea and abdominal pain. It has interfered in her ability to attend school and she is missing approximately 3 days per month due to symptoms. Her diarrhea is not accompanied by fever, upper respiratory infection (URI) symptoms, or vomiting. No one else in the house has experienced similar complaints.

Birth history: Katie was born at 38 weeks' gestation via spontaneous vaginal delivery. She weighed 7 lbs, 7 oz and required no NICU placement.

Social history: Katie is in second grade and lives with her mother and father. Katie does well in school and is easily able to name friends and her favorite subject. Katie has a 5-year-old sister, Madison. The family owns their own home in a suburb. They have 2 dogs.

Diet: Katie is described as a "reformed picky eater" by her mother. She eats steak and chicken for meat (refuses fish); flavored yogurt and cheese are her main sources of calcium; her favorite foods are turkey sandwiches, goldfish crackers, and pasta. Katie does not drink juice or soda. She has 3–5 servings of fruits or vegetables per day.

Elimination: Stools daily and these are described as soft and non-painful to pass. As noted by her mother, Katie has been experiencing greater frequency of diarrhea (1–3 times per week) which her mother describes as frequent, very loose, and malodorous. Katie urinates several times per day and denies any pain with urination. She has no history of urinary tract infection (UTI).

Sleep: Katie goes to bed at 8 p.m. and wakes up between 6:30 and 7 a.m. She generally sleeps through the night and sleeps alone in her own bed. Her mother reports that Katie has occasionally awakened during the night to stool.

Family history: Katie's mother reports a history of multiple miscarriages, and her father has a history of high cholesterol (on medication). Her maternal aunt has a history of celiac disease. Her

The Family Nurse Practitioner: Clinical Case Studies, Second Edition. Edited by Leslie Neal-Boylan.
© 2021 John Wiley & Sons Ltd. Published 2021 by John Wiley & Sons Ltd.

maternal grandmother has a history of colorectal cancer (deceased). Her paternal grandfather has Type 1 diabetes.

Medications: Katie takes a multivitamin daily.

Allergies: Katie has no known allergies.

OBJECTIVE

General: Katie is a 7-year-old feminine appearing child who presents in no acute distress. She is interactive and age-appropriate in her responses.

Vital signs: Heart rate is 90; respiratory rate is 14; blood pressure is 95/55, oxygen saturation is 100% on room air; pain is rated as a 0.

HEENT: Normocephalic; thick brown hair; eyes slightly sunken; tympanic membranes visible and with no evidence of effusion/infection; nostrils patent; trachea is midline. There is no evidence of enlarged thyroid.

Mouth: Mucous membranes with thick saliva. Mild enamel erosion on teeth. Dentition reveals mix of primary and secondary teeth.

Cardiac: Heart with regular rate and rhythm. There is no murmur noted.

Respiratory: Lungs are clear to auscultation bilaterally. There is equal air movement in all lobes.

Abdomen: Abdomen is soft, mildly tender to palpation. There is intermittent guarding in the right upper quadrant. Normoactive bowel sounds are present throughout. There are no masses or hepatosplenomegaly appreciated.

Genitourinary: Tanner stage 2 external female genitalia. There are no anal or rectal fissures, tags, or hemorrhoids.

Neuromusculoskeletal: Moves all 4 extremities equally with appropriate strength.

Neurologic: Alert and oriented to person, place, time, situation. Cranial nerves are grossly intact.

Psychological: Not visibly anxious or agitated.

CRITICAL THINKING

What are the three most likely differential diagnoses for this patient? What tests would help to confirm your suspicions?

What other information gathered through noninvasive methods would help to confirm the diagnosis?

What information from the family history helps to guide your differentials?

Once the diagnosis is established, what other multidisciplinary support would you offer the patient and family? What other medical specialties/subspecialties would you engage?

Case 4.10 Food Allergies

By Allison Grady, MSN, APNP

James is a 5-year-old male who presents to his pediatrician after being seen in the emergency room 2 days prior for hives and trouble breathing after eating a peanut butter and jelly sandwich. His mother reports that James has had peanut butter before and would occasionally cough but has never had any skin changes that she can remember and certainly never had trouble breathing. She wonders whether he was choking on the peanut butter instead of having an allergic reaction but concedes that he turned red and was gasping for breath. He was also found to have hives all over his back and trunk. "No one in our family has a peanut allergy and it's basically all that his older brother eats. It would be a real problem if we couldn't have it in the house." The provider explains to the mother that James recovered from his episode after receiving a dose of epinephrine, which would not have helped if he was choking, and hives are not caused by simply coughing. The provider asks if James has had any peanuts since the incident and mother says "no." James has also not had any further episodes of hives or respiratory distress since being discharged from the hospital. His mother grudgingly agrees that it probably *wasn't* choking, but asks "Are you *sure* that this was an allergy? Could we get him tested or something? What do we in the meantime?" She holds up the EpiPen that she was given at the hospital: "I don't want to carry this around all of the time and James isn't old enough to know how to use it."

Birth history: James was born via normal, spontaneous vaginal delivery at 42 weeks. He weighed 10 lbs, 1 oz. He did not spend any time in the neonatal intensive care unit (NICU) and was discharged to home with his mother at 2 days of life.

Social history: James lives with his mother, father, 8-year-old brother (Kevin), and 1-year-old sister (Kyla). James attends full-day kindergarten at a local public school. The family has 2 cats and a fish.

Diet: James is considered "overweight" by BMI, but is an active child with a lot of muscle. He plays soccer in the fall and baseball in the spring and summer. He has a total of 1 hour of recess per day at school. He eats a variety of foods, including grains, fruits, andvegetables, and his main protein sources are peanut butter and chicken. He drinks 8 oz of juice per day and about 12 oz of milk per day.

The Family Nurse Practitioner: Clinical Case Studies, Second Edition. Edited by Leslie Neal-Boylan.
© 2021 John Wiley & Sons Ltd. Published 2021 by John Wiley & Sons Ltd.

Elimination: James has no history of constipation and no history of urinary tract infection (UTI).

Sleep: James has an inconsistent bedtime routine, but generally goes to bed around 8 p.m. on school nights and wakes up at approximately 6 a.m. On the weekends, he is often up until 10 p.m. but still wakes up around 6 a.m.

Family medical history: James's father has lactose intolerance and James's mother has a history of eczema. Maternal grandmother: history of breast cancer (still living); paternal grandmother: hypertension (on medications); maternal grandfather: prostate cancer (still living) and Type 2 diabetes; paternal grandfather: deceased from heart attack at age 62; maternal aunt: history of celiac disease; paternal aunt: history of hypothyroid; paternal uncle: history of depression.

Medications: James does not take any medications.

Allergies: James has no known drug allergies but may have a peanut allergy.

OBJECTIVE

Vital signs: Heart rate is 110; respiratory rate is 13; oxygen saturation is 100% on room air; blood pressure is 98/62. Denies any pain.

General: Well-appearing 5-year-old child, appears masculine in dress and manner. He is in no distress.

HEENT: Normocephalic head with no appreciable lumps or bumps. Eyes demonstrate ability to fix and focus, pupils are equal, round, and reactive to light. Ears are set proportionately to head. Tympanic membranes are visible with no evidence of infection (no pus/fluid/erythema). Trachea is midline. Thyroid is appropriate in size. Mucous membranes are moist. Dentition demonstrates 1 loose tooth and 1 missing tooth. All primary teeth at this time.

Cardiovascular: Regular heart rate and rhythm. No rubs, murmurs, or gallops heard.

Respiratory: Lungs clear to auscultation in all fields. No wheezes, rhonchi, or rales.

Abdomen: Soft, nontender, nondistended. Normoactive bowel sounds are present in all four quadrants.

Gastrointestinal/Genitourinary: Deferred.

Neurological: Grossly intact. Demonstrates grossly normal hearing, vision, balance. No abnormal gait observed.

Musculoskeletal: All 4 extremities move equally with appropriate strength and range of motion.

Skin: Color is appropriate for race; no pallor. No rashes or hives noted. Patch of mild eczema on left lower extremity. Temperature and texture otherwise within normal limits.

CRITICAL THINKING

What are the top three differential diagnoses? What testing will confirm the diagnosis?

How should the provider educate the mother about the seriousness of anaphylaxis and the risk of it occurring again?

How can the provider help the school manage a child with food allergies?

If this family does not have insurance, what is the expected out-of-pocket expense for an EpiPen? Likely more than one will be needed, so how can a family navigate this barrier?

What is the essential information that all caregivers (not just parents) need to know when caring for James?

What advice should the mother be given regarding introduction of peanut-based products to the youngest child now that food allergies are known to be in the family?

Case 4.11 Obesity

By Mikki Meadows-Oliver, PhD, RN, FAAN

SUBJECTIVE

Tamika, a 12-year-old girl, came to the community health clinic with her mother, who had requested an urgent appointment to discuss a note from Tamika's physical education teacher with her nurse practitioner (NP). The note stated that Tamika was having difficulty keeping up with her classmates because she became short of breath when participating in activities. Tamika denies any other episodes of shortness of breath but reports that she occasionally has to stop and rest when climbing stairs. She has no persistent cough, wheeze, or seasonal allergies. She reports that she has not yet had a period.

Diet history: Tamika seldom eats breakfast at home and occasionally will eat cereal from the school breakfast. For lunch she likes pizza or macaroni and cheese but does not eat if these items are not on the school menu. She arrives at her grandmother's house around 3:30 p.m. and has a salty snack and a soda. She eats dinner with her father, either at home or at a local fast-food restaurant.

Sleep history: Tamika's mother notes that she snores loudly and sometimes awakens at night. She is currently not taking any medications.

Past medical history: Tamika was born after 36 weeks' gestation to a 39-year-old mother. She weighed 4 lb 14 oz; and, in addition to being preterm, she was small for gestational age. Her mother smoked ½ ppd. Her neonatal history was unremarkable, and she was discharged at 1 week of age weighing 5 lb 2 oz. She was formula fed.

Her past medical history is otherwise unremarkable except for treatment on 2 occasions for right otitis media at ages 1 and 5 and for day surgery at age 18 months to repair a bilateral inguinal hernia. There were no complications. She has no history of respiratory illness, asthma, or allergy.

Family history: Positive for Type 2 diabetes in Tamika's maternal grandmother. Her father is positive for cardiovascular disease and had a mild heart attack at age 48, has high blood pressure, and takes statins for elevated cholesterol. Her maternal grandfather died at age 42 from a heart attack and diabetes. Her paternal grandparents are reportedly alive and well and are living in Puerto Rico.

The Family Nurse Practitioner: Clinical Case Studies, Second Edition. Edited by Leslie Neal-Boylan.
© 2021 John Wiley & Sons Ltd. Published 2021 by John Wiley & Sons Ltd.

Social history: Tamika is in sixth grade. She is seldom absent and frequently makes the honor roll. She says she likes school but notes that she is shy and has few friends. She does not take part in any extracurricular activities and spends her after-school time helping her grandmother cook or watching TV. She likes to read. She denies ever using tobacco products, drugs, or alcohol. She admits to feeling sad and lonely at times but denies ever wanting to injure herself. She likes her parents but says they don't always understand her or have time to talk to her.

Tamika lives with both parents in a 2-bedroom, third-floor apartment near her school. Her father is employed as a laborer, and her mother works for a cleaning service 5 evenings a week. The family has a stable income. Tamika has 3 older siblings, ages 17, 19, and 21, living outside of the home. Her maternal grandmother lives nearby, and Tamika often goes to her home after school. Both parents were smokers previously but stopped 5 years ago. They moved to this area from Puerto Rico 20 years ago. Both speak fluent English.

OBJECTIVE

General: Tamika is a 12-year-old, Hispanic female who is neatly dressed and cooperative.

Vital signs: She is 5 feet tall and weighs 174 pounds. Her blood pressure is 116/70, pulse is 74, and respirations are 16 breaths/minute. Temperature is normal.

HEENT: PERRLA; EOMs intact. Oral pharynx is positive for 3+/4 tonsils, without lesions or exudate. No dental caries are noted.

Neck: Supple with full range of motion. No lymphadenopathy is present.

Respiratory: Her lungs are clear bilaterally with no wheezes, rales, or rhonchi.

Cardiac: Normal sinus rhythm with no murmur or irregular beats.

Chest: Breast buds are present bilaterally, with no tenderness or discharge.

Abdomen: Soft but protuberant with no masses or hepatosplenomegaly. Normal bowel sounds are heard in all 4 quadrants.

Neuromuscular: Back is straight with no curvature noted on forward bend. She has full range of motion in all extremities. Reflexes are normal.

Skin: Clear except for darkly pigmented areas on her neck.

CRITICAL THINKING

Which diagnostic or imaging studies should be considered to assist with or confirm the diagnosis?
___BMI
___Oral glucose tolerance test (OGGT)
___Insulin resistance
___Cholesterol screen
___Sleep study
___Psychosocial evaluation

What is the most likely differential diagnosis and why?
___Sleep apnea
___Obesity
___Insulin resistance
___Type 2 diabetes
___Exercise intolerance
___Psychosocial issues

Are any referrals needed at this time?

Can the school be of assistance?

What community resources are available to this family?

What type of nutrition support may aid this family?

NOTE: The author would like to acknowledge Elaine Gustafson, MSN, PNP, who co-authored this case in the first edition of this book.

Section 5

The Adolescent

Case 5.1 Drug Use

By Anna Goddard, PhD, APRN, CPNP-PC

SUBJECTIVE

Natalie is a 17 year-old female who presents to the school-based health center (SBHC) for the fourth time in 1 week with nonspecific complaints. Several teachers have reported Natalie falling asleep in class and "thinks she might be on drugs." Her grades have continued to decrease this semester from C averages to barely passing most of her classes. Natalie reports she is tired "all the time" even though she claims to sleep 8–10 hours a night. She reports frequently waking up and not being able to fall back asleep. She does not like school and states "I don't need anything I am learning in school." When offered the PHQ2 and CRAFFT to complete as part of routine screening, she refused to complete both of them. She is requesting to be sent home.

Past medical history: Natalie was hospitalized once as an infant with wheezing and bronchitis. She reports no primary care provider and receives care at minute clinics, emergency rooms, or urgent care when needed.

Family history: Natalie's mother has fibromyalgia, depression, and chronic headaches. Father's history is unknown.

Social history: Natalie lives in a single-parent household with her mother. No siblings live at home but she has half-siblings who are no longer living at home; one is incarcerated and one has unknown whereabouts. Natalie has previously had detention for marijuana possession and has been caught juuling in class. Her grade averages are Ds and Fs and she is not on-track to graduate this year. She admits to occasionally drinking with friends after school but has never blacked out and denies getting in the car while intoxicated. Natalie currently has a boyfriend but "it's nothing serious" and has also been involved with females.

Psychiatric: Natalie has no history of a known diagnosis of trauma, depression, anxiety, or substance use disorder.

Medications: Natalie has a previous prescription for Lexapro 10 mg but reports "it wasn't working" so she stopped taking it. The previous prescribing provider for Lexapro and age of treatment is unknown. She denies vitamins, supplements, or over-the-counter medications.

Allergies: Natalie has no known drug allergies (NKDA).

The Family Nurse Practitioner: Clinical Case Studies, Second Edition. Edited by Leslie Neal-Boylan.
© 2021 John Wiley & Sons Ltd. Published 2021 by John Wiley & Sons Ltd.

Review of systems: Natalie denies problems with weight gain or weight loss, fever, night sweats, or pain. She has no difficulty in hearing, runny nose, post-nasal drip, or ear pain. She denies history of cardiovascular issues, shortness of breath, night sweats, prolonged cough, wheezing, or gastro-intestinal issues.

OBJECTIVE

General: Natalie is dressed in leggings and an oversized sweatshirt with her hair in a ponytail, typical of adolescents.

Vital signs: Temperature: 98.8°F; heart rate: 70 beats per minute; BP: 118/60.

EENT: PERRLA, EOM intact, normal mucosa, no nasal discharge, swollen turbinates, tonsils 1+ with no exudate.

CV/Respiratory: Normal rate and rhythm. Lungs clear to auscultation with no wheezing and crackles.

Abdomen: Bowel sounds normal.

CRITICAL THINKING

What are the most likely differential diagnoses in this case and why?
__Substance use/abuse
__Alcohol use/abuse
__Depression
__School phobia
__Sleep problems
__Thyroid disorder

What are the top diagnostic tests required in this case and why?
__Toxicology screen
__Complete blood count (CBC) with differential
__Complete metabolic panel (CMP)
__Thyroid panel
__Suicide assessment

What are the concerns at this point?

What is the plan of treatment?

What are the plans for referral and follow-up care?

What health education should be provided to this patient?

Natalie asks, "Are you going to tell my mom about this?" How do you respond?

Does the patient's psychosocial history impact how you might treat her?

Can minors seek substance abuse counseling without parental consent?

Are there any standardized guidelines that should be used to treat this case? If so, what are they?

Case 5.2 Weight Loss

By Anna Goddard, PhD, APRN, CPNP-PC

SUBJECTIVE

Roseanne is a 15-year-old female who presents to the adolescent clinic with her mother for her annual wellness examination. Her mother reports she is "concerned with Roseanne's weight." Specifically she reports that Roseanne needs to "make weight for cheerleading competition." Roseanne is well-groomed, polite, and working on homework while the health care provider speaks to her mother. Her last physical examination was at the School-Based Health Center from a previous school she attended and was reported by her mother to be normal.

Past medical history: Roseanne has a history of a right ankle fracture from 2 years ago, treated with physical therapy and reported complete healing. Roseanne has also a history of right broken forearm and wrist injury from a previous cheerleading injury. She was hospitalized after both previous bone breaks, both requiring surgery. She reports no pain currently. Menarche occurred at age 13 and Roseanne reports that periods were monthly at first and then she started missing periods or having them sporadically. She is now on a triphasic birth control and reports she no longer gets her periods, which she likes because she is a competitive cheerleader and doesn't have to worry about her monthly menstruation while she is cheering.

Family history: Father is a Type 1 diabetic and has hypertension. Mother has history of anxiety and post-traumatic stress disorder (PTSD). Maternal and paternal grandparents are deceased. No siblings.

Social history: Roseanne lives in Dallas and moved to a new district with a "better cheerleading squad" in hopes of winning the district championship this year. Roseanne reports that she gets along well with her family and gets all As and A+s. She has friends at her new school and reports she enjoys cheerleading as "it is her life." Roseanne's mother reports that she has a chance for cheer-captain her senior year. Roseanne runs every day before school at 6 a.m. and then has cheerleading practice every day after school from 4:00–6:30 p.m. She competes and has football or basketball games almost every weekend. She studies and completes her homework from the time she gets home from cheerleading practice until 11 or sometimes 12 at night, when she then goes to bed.

Medications: Occasional ibuprofen for sore muscle aches and strains.

The Family Nurse Practitioner: Clinical Case Studies, Second Edition. Edited by Leslie Neal-Boylan.
© 2021 John Wiley & Sons Ltd. Published 2021 by John Wiley & Sons Ltd.

Allergies: NKDA; no allergies to foods or environment.

General: Denies fever, chills, or malaise. Denies restriction in food or decreased appetite.

Skin, hair, nails: No pigment changes, no current rashes although occasional tinea from tumbling on gymnastic mats; occasional bruises from cheerleading falls and acrobatics.

HEENT: Denies difficulty with hearing, sinus problems, runny nose, postnasal drip, tinnitus, mouth sores, teeth, ear pain, or sore throats. She reports "doesn't have time to be sick."

Cardiovascular: No history of irregular heartbeat, chest pains, swelling of feet or legs. No history of murmurs.

Respiratory: No shortness of breath, night sweats, prolonged cough or wheezing.

Gastrointestinal: No heartburn, constipation, diarrhea, constipation, nausea, vomiting, or blood in stools.

Genitourinary: Unremarkable.

Musculoskeletal: Occasional joint pain and aching muscles: relieved with Icy-Hot ointment, icing, and over-the-counter Motrin; occasional shoulder pain and joint swelling after competitions from certain tumbling and basket catches: treated by physical therapy and over-the-counter Motrin.

Hematologic: Does not "bruise easily" but does bruise from heavy athletics dance tumbling; no history of unknown swelling.

OBJECTIVE

General: Muscular teen dressed in athletic pants and tank top. Interactive and appropriate with provider and mother.

Vital signs: Height: 63 inches; weight: 100 lbs; BMI: 17.7 (6th percentile); BP: 92/61; HR: 52; RR: 16.

Skin: Bruising around both knees and shins; skin warm, dry, with sporadic mild acne covered by make-up.

HEENT: Normocephalic, +PERRLA, TMs gray and visible ossicles; intact, moist mucous membranes; nares patent; oropharynx clear.

Neck: No lymphadenopathy.

Cardiovascular: Regular rate and rhythm; no murmur; femoral pulses equal.

Respiratory: Lungs clear bilaterally.

Breast: Tanner IV symmetrical.

Abdomen: Flat, soft, nontender, muscular.

Genitourinary: Tanner stage IV.

Musculoskeletal: Full range of motion ×4 extremities; no pain or swelling, back straight; muscular.

Neurologic: Cranial nerves II–XII grossly intact, steady gait and balance; reflexes +2 and equal.

CRITICAL THINKING

What are the top differential diagnoses in this case and why?
___Eating disorder
___Excessive exercise
___Malnutrition
___Malabsorption
___Thyroid disorder
___Anxiety
___Female athlete triad

What are the diagnostic tests required in this case and why?
__Urine pregnancy test
___Glucose
___Urinalysis
___CBC with differential
___Thyroid panel
___Prolactin level
___Electrolytes

What are the concerns at this point?

Should Roseanne's mother be asked to leave the room at this time? Why or why not?

What is the plan of treatment?

What are the plans for referral and follow-up care?

What health education should be provided to this patient?

What demographic characteristics might affect this case?

Are there any standardized guidelines that should be used to treat this case? If so, what are they?

If this patient was male (instead of female), how would that change management and/or treatment?

SUBJECTIVE

Khaleesi is a 16-year-old who comes to the school-based health center (SBHC) after she just got her period in school. She is requesting a pad or tampon from SBHC because "I'm embarrassed . . . I soaked through my clothes." Khaleesi says she usually misses "about 1 or 2 days each month because of my period." While checking the patient into the electronic health system, it is noted her school absences are high. She reports she's gotten her period since age 11, every month, but once she got it twice in one month. She uses 6 pads or tampons on the heaviest days, but her period usually only lasts about 5 days. She says her cramps, "aren't too bad usually, but sometimes I will throw up when they are really bad." She reports "I think my mom gives me Advil some-times?," but she does not use medication every period, and "it only helps sometimes." Khaleesi denies any urinary frequency, urgency, dysuria, hematuria, vaginal discharge, pruritus, lesions, or lower abdominal pain other than "my normal cramps."

Past medical history: Tonsillectomy and adenoidectomy around age 8; seasonal allergies.

Family history: Khaleesi's mother and aunts with heavy periods.

Social history: Denies drug, alcohol, or vaping use. Denies any sexual activity (oral, anal, or vaginal) current or in past.

Medications: Zyrtec 10 mg only in springtime for allergies.

Allergies: NKDA, no food allergies.

OBJECTIVE

Vital signs: Height: 61 in; weight: 122 lbs; BP: 118/68; HR: 80; RR: 12; BMI: 23. Pain 5/10 on numeric scale, lower abdominal. Patient Health Questionnaire-2 = 0 negative screening.

General: Pleasant, well developed, well nourished, in no acute distress.

Respiratory: CTA bilaterally, no wheezes, rales, or rhonchi.

The Family Nurse Practitioner: Clinical Case Studies, Second Edition. Edited by Leslie Neal-Boylan.
© 2021 John Wiley & Sons Ltd. Published 2021 by John Wiley & Sons Ltd.

Cardiac: RRR, S1 S2 normal with no murmurs, rubs, or gallops.

Breast: Tanner V symmetrical.

Abdomen: Bowel sounds present, abdomen soft, nontender, nondistended with no hepatosplenomegaly.

Genitourinary: Pubic hair; Tanner V normal female; + menses.

CRITICAL THINKING

What is the most likely differential diagnosis and why?
___Dysmenorrhea
___Endometriosis
___Pelvic inflammatory disease (PID)
___Urinary tract infection (UTI)
___Appendicitis
___Pregnancy—threatened abortion
___Pregnancy—ectopic

Which diagnostic or imaging studies should be considered to assist with or confirm the diagnosis?
___Pelvic and transvaginal ultrasound
___CBC with differential
___CMP
___Urine pregnancy test
___Pelvic exam with cervical swab for GC/CT

What questions would you ask Khaleesi about her menstrual cycle?

What additional information/questions are needed?

What is the plan of treatment?

Are there other options?

Is it common for teen girls to miss school because of their periods?

When should she be seen for follow-up?

What health education should be provided to this patient?

Are there technologies available to assist this patient in her care?

Case 5.4 Missed Periods

By Vera Borkowski, MSN, APRN, FNP-C

SUBJECTIVE

Genevieve is a 17-year-old female who came to the clinic requesting a pregnancy test "because I haven't gotten my period and it is 3 weeks late." Genny reports that she normally gets her period every month and uses a period tracker, and is able to report her last period's exact start date 55 days ago. She reports that her last period was of normal duration and flow. She says she had multiple occurrences of unprotected sex with her boyfriend of the same age in the past month, and has not taken any pregnancy tests at home. Per her chart and report, Genny has not previously been screened for sexually transmitted infections (STIs). She states, "We lost our virginity to each other a few months ago, so I don't think he has any STIs." The clinician asks her if she wants to get pregnant and Genny states, "Not really, but my boyfriend doesn't like using condoms." Genny has not told her family she is sexually active, and is requesting that this visit be confidential. She is not on any type of birth control, "because I'm afraid if I ask, my mom will know I'm having sex."

Past medical history: Obesity.

Family history: No pertinent family history.

Social history: Denies substances, alcohol, or vaping use. Scores negative on PHQ-2 screening. Reports only vaginal intercourse in a monogamous relationship. 1 sexual partner.

Medications: None.

Allergies: NKDA

OBJECTIVE

Weight: 210 lbs; height: 65 in; BMI: 34.9; BP: 110/70; PHQ-2: 0 Negative.

General: Pleasant, well developed, obese, in no acute distress.

Respiratory: CTA bilaterally, no wheezes, rales, or rhonchi.

The Family Nurse Practitioner: Clinical Case Studies, Second Edition. Edited by Leslie Neal-Boylan.
© 2021 John Wiley & Sons Ltd. Published 2021 by John Wiley & Sons Ltd.

Cardiac: RRR, S1 S2 normal with no murmurs, rubs, or gallops.

Breast: Tanner V symmetrical.

Abdomen: Bowel sounds present, abdomen soft, nontender, nondistended, with no hepatospleno-megaly. Exam limited by adipose habitus.

Genitourinary: Pubic hair normal; Tanner V normal female; mucosa pale and pink, no lesions; no lymphadenopathy, discharge, or odor.

CRITICAL THINKING

Which diagnostic or imaging studies should be considered to assist with or confirm the diagnosis?
___Urine HCG
___HIV testing
___STI screening
___Pap smear
___Urine dipstick

Why is it important to ask Genny what she feels her boyfriend would want if she were pregnant?

What additional questions should Genny be asked?

If Genny is pregnant today, what are her options?

Should contraception be prescribed today?

What health education should be provided to this patient?

Are there technologies available to assist Genny in managing or understanding her menstruation?

Case 5.5 Birth Control Decision-Making

By Jessica Chan, MSN, APRN, PPCNP-BC

SUBJECTIVE

Lauren is a 17-year-old female who presents alone to the primary care office to discuss birth control options. She has been in a relationship with her boyfriend for 6 months and is currently sexually active with only him. She has a history of 1 partner prior to her current boyfriend. She reports using condoms always and never having unprotected intercourse. She has not discussed this with her mother yet, but does think she could be open about it. She has not had testing in the past for sexually transmitted infections (STIs), but would be interested and denies symptoms such as abnormal vaginal discharge, dysuria, pelvic pain, or any new rashes or lesions. She is due for her menses in 3 days. She generally has cramps the day before and the first day of her menses, and takes ibuprofen with good effect.

Past medical history: Lauren has a history of eczema and seasonal allergies.

Family history: Lauren's biological mother has a history of dysmenorrhea.

Social history: Lauren lives at home with her mother, father, and younger brother. She is in the 12th grade and plays tennis for fun. She reports having many good friends and denies substance use.

Medications: Lauren's medications include cetirizine (Zyrtec) 10 mg daily during allergy season and occasional triamcinolone cream for her eczema.

Allergies: NKDA.

OBJECTIVE

General: Well appearing, no acute distress

Vital signs: Weight: 145 lbs; height: 62 inches; BMI: 26.5; HR: 72; B/P: 116/74.

Cardiovascular: Regular rate and rhythm. S1/S2 normal.

Respiratory: Lungs clear to auscultation bilaterally.

The Family Nurse Practitioner: Clinical Case Studies, Second Edition. Edited by Leslie Neal-Boylan.
© 2021 John Wiley & Sons Ltd. Published 2021 by John Wiley & Sons Ltd.

Breast: Tanner V breast development noted. Not palpated at time of visit; at last annual physical exam had normal breast exam with no masses.

Gastrointestinal: Bowel sounds normoactive in all four quadrants. Soft, nontender, nondistended, with no hepatosplenomegaly.

Genitourinary: External exam with Tanner V pubic hair development noted and no lesions present.

CRITICAL THINKING

Given the information provided, what other questions would you ask?

What diagnostic or screening tests would you consider running on this patient?
___Urine pregnancy test
___Beta pregnancy test (serum hCG level)
___Urine gonorrhea and chlamydia (GC/CT)
___Serum HIV immunoassay and RT-PCR (viral load)
___Serum RPR (reactive plasma reagin) or VDRL (Venereal Disease Research laboratory) testing for syphilis
___Pelvic exam with wet mount
___Pap smear
___Complete blood count (CBC)
___Lipid panel (baseline cholesterol screening)

What are the concerns at this point?

What is the diagnosis at this point?

What types of contraceptives should be considered for Lauren?

How would each contraceptive option be initiated?

What are some common contraindications to contraceptives?

How should Lauren be counseled about side effects?

What are the plans for referral and follow-up care?

What other education should Lauren be provided with related to reproductive health?

If the patient chooses not to discuss her choice to seek out birth control options with her mother, how would you proceed?

Are there any standardized guidelines that should be used to treat this case? If so, what are they?

Case 5.6 Vaginal Discharge

By Betsy Gaffney, MSN, APRN, FNP-BC

SUBJECTIVE

Nora, an 18-year-old college student known to this family practice office, presents with a complaint of "some spotting since my last period and a vaginal discharge." Nora is home on a college break and states "I'm afraid I have an STD." She relates that she has "been healthy" while at school "except for this problem" and that she "did not feel comfortable going to the university health center." She denies any urinary burning or frequency. She denies any abdominal pain or pain with sex.

Past medical/surgical history: Negative with exception of tonsillectomy, age 7.

Medications: None.

Allergies: No known allergies.

Menstrual history: Menarche age 10 with regular 28-day cycle with 3–5 days of bleeding. Last menses 3 weeks ago with intermenstrual spotting 2 times since then.

Sexual history (obtained using the CDC's "5 P" approach):

- Partners: Nora's first sexual encounter was at age 16. She has had 4 encounters in the past 2 years with 2 different partners, with 2 encounters in the last 2 months.
- Prevention of pregnancy: Nora was prescribed a triphasic oral contraceptive at age 16 but says "I stopped taking it after a few months and haven't been on any since." Her partners "use condoms once in a while."
- Prevention of STIs: Limited to inconsistent condom use.
- Practices: Nora describes her encounters as limited to vaginal intercourse and "oral sex once in a while." She denies anal sex.
- Past history of STIs is negative.

The Family Nurse Practitioner: Clinical Case Studies, Second Edition. Edited by Leslie Neal-Boylan.
© 2021 John Wiley & Sons Ltd. Published 2021 by John Wiley & Sons Ltd.

OBJECTIVE

General: Anxious 18-year-old female in no acute distress. Well groomed with good hygiene. Cooperative.

Vital signs: Height: 5 ft 4 inches; weight: 112 lbs; BMI: 21.2; temperature: 97.8°F; B/P: 118/72; HR: 98.

Respiratory: Normal respiratory effort, CTA bilaterally.

Cardiac: Regular rate, rhythm. No murmurs, gallops.

Breasts: Tanner IV.

With Nora's consent a pelvic exam was done.

Pelvic/Genital exam: No vulvar or vaginal lesions. Mucoid, nonodorous discharge was noted and vaginal and endocervical swabs obtained. Cervix appeared inflamed but was nonfriable and there was no cervical motion tenderness (CMT). Discomfort but no tenderness on bimanual examination.

CRITICAL THINKING

Which diagnostic studies should be considered to assist with or confirm the diagnosis?
___Urine HCG
___Nucleic acid amplification test (NAAT) for chlamydia
___NAAT for gonorrhea
___Wet mount (saline, KOH prep of vaginal secretions) to rule out coexisting infection
___HIV-1 antibody testing
___Venereal Disease Research Laboratory (VDRL)

What is the most likely differential diagnosis and why?
___Chlamydia (*C. trachomatis*)
___Gonorrhea (*N. gonnorhoeae*)
___Bacterial vaginosis
___Trichomonas vaginalis
___Pregnancy
___HIV

What is the plan of treatment?

How should this patient be counseled regarding the prevention of STIs?

Is this patient at risk for HIV?

Should this patient be retested for cure after treatment?

Should this patient's partners be treated?

Case 5.7 Sexual Identity

By Betsy Gaffney, MSN, APRN, FNP-BC

SUBJECTIVE

Michelle, a 17-year-old Caucasian female, presents to a primary care practice where she has been a patient since 5 years of age. She is accompanied by her maternal aunt. Michelle is usually accompanied by her mother. She is up to date with her immunizations including HPV series. Her last visit was 10 months ago for strep pharyngitis. She was very quiet and less interactive at that visit but when asked if anything was bothering her said "just my throat."

Michelle tells you she is here today because she identifies "more as a boy," saying "I've felt this way for about 2 years but was afraid to tell anybody before. I'm not afraid now and have told my mother and my aunt. I'm tired of lying by not saying anything and want to do things differently. My mom said I should come and talk to you because we like and trust you." Michelle's aunt verifies this, saying, "My sister is still a little freaked out about this but wants what is best for Michelle. That's why she asked me to come with her today." Michelle's mom would also like her to have a physical check-up, since she hasn't been seen for almost a year. Michelle's aunt leaves the exam room to allow her privacy.

Past medical/surgical history: Michelle has a positive medical history for strep pharyngitis, which resolved with antibiotics. She has no chronic illnesses, surgery, or hospitalizations.

Menstrual history: She began menarche at age 11 with a regular 28-day cycle and moderate bleeding. She expresses a desire to "not have my period."

Family history: Maternal family history is positive for grandmother with COPD, grandfather with hypertension. Mother and 9-year-old sister have no health issues. Paternal history is unknown. Father has problems with substance abuse.

Social history: Michelle lives with her mother and younger sister in a rural, farming area. Her father is known but has little contact with the family. Michelle is a sophomore at the public high school. Her mother works full-time at a local manufacturing plant. Michelle has a close relationship with her mother and maternal aunt. She denies alcohol and tobacco use, does admit to "smoking weed once but I hated it." She denies depression but admits previous anxiety about her lifestyle choice. She reports her anxiety is "pretty much gone" since she has "come out" to her mother and aunt. She admits being attracted to other girls but denies any sexual experiences. She

The Family Nurse Practitioner: Clinical Case Studies, Second Edition. Edited by Leslie Neal-Boylan.
© 2021 John Wiley & Sons Ltd. Published 2021 by John Wiley & Sons Ltd.

has recently told a few other students about identifying as a boy, noting "it's hard to be different in this area."

Medications: No regular medications.

Allergies: Seasonal (spring) allergies. NKDA.

OBJECTIVE

General: Alert, pleasant adolescent; well groomed with good hygiene. Cooperative with good eye contact.

Vital signs: Height: 63.5 inches; weight: 112 pounds; BMI 19.5 (43rd percentile); B/P: 108/70; HR: 72; RR: 15.

Cardiac: RRR; S1-S2 normal; no murmur, rub, or gallop.

Respiratory: Normal respiratory effort; lungs clear to auscultation bilaterally.

Abdominal: Soft, nondistended, nontender, with positive bowel sounds x 4 quadrants.

Breasts: Tanner stage IV.

PHQ-9: Negative.

CRITICAL THINKING

What concerns should be addressed at this visit?
_____Sexual identity
_____Anxiety/Depression
_____Desire for amenorrhea

What case-specific questions should be asked addressing Michelle's desire for amenorrhea?

Are any referrals needed?

What complications exist related to the rural setting?

Are there implications for future medical care?

What psychosocial challenges present with "coming out"?

Case 5.8 Knee Pain

By Jessica Chan, MSN, APRN, PPCNP-BC

SUBJECTIVE

Peter is a 16-year-old male who presents to your pediatric primary care office with complaints of right knee pain and swelling for 1 week. He can bear weight on his leg with only mild discomfort. He lives in New York City, but reports that he spent the summer working as a camp counselor in Madison, Connecticut. He resides at the camp while working there and spends his days hiking and doing outdoor activities. He has also participated in summer soccer clinics but does not recall a specific injury, and has attributed his occasional muscle aches to his activity levels. Peter denies any current rashes, but does state that he had a lot of bug bites and poison ivy exposure during his time working as a camp counselor and has generally ignored the symptoms. He describes a few weeks of feeling more tired with intermittent headaches, but believes it's due to spending time in the sun and working with kids. He isn't sure whether he has had a fever. He also denies any pain or swelling in other joints. He did not go see the nurse on-site at the summer camp. He reports he is sleeping through the night and his appetite has been good with no recent weight loss.

Past medical history: Patient is a healthy 16-year-old male with no significant past medical history.

Family history: Maternal and paternal family history is unremarkable. Patient has 1 sibling, a sister, who is well. A maternal grandmother has rheumatoid arthritis, lupus, and hypertension.

Social history: Peter lives at home with his parents and younger sister. He has a pet dog that sleeps in his room. He is attending high school and in the 11th grade and is also an avid soccer player.

Medications: Daily multivitamin.

Allergies: Amoxicillin (hives, at age 2)

The Family Nurse Practitioner: Clinical Case Studies, Second Edition. Edited by Leslie Neal-Boylan.
© 2021 John Wiley & Sons Ltd. Published 2021 by John Wiley & Sons Ltd.

OBJECTIVE

Vital signs: Weight: 140 lbs; height: 68 inches; BMI: 21.3; temperature: 100.4°F; HR: 76; RR: 16; B/P: 108/72.

General: Alert, tired appearing but in no acute distress.

HEENT: Head is normocephalic and atraumatic. Scleras are clear. PERRLA bilaterally. Normal fundi exam bilaterally. Otoscopic exam reveals normal tympanic membranes with visible landmarks and appropriate light reflex. Nares are patent. Oropharynx is normal without erythema or exudate. Tongue is midline.

Skin: No rashes noted on exam. Skin is warm and dry.

Neck: No lymphadenopathy present. Full range of motion with no reported pain.

Respiratory: Lungs clear to auscultation bilaterally. No wheezes, rales, or rhonchi present.

Cardiovascular: Regular rate and rhythm. S1S2 normal. Pulses 2+ throughout.

Gastrointestinal: Abdomen soft, nontender, nondistended, with no masses or hepatosplenomegaly palpated. Bowel sounds normoactive in all 4 quadrants.

Neurological: Alert and oriented. Grossly normal. Sensation intact to lower extremities. Patellar and Achilles deep tendon reflexes 2+ bilaterally.

Musculoskeletal: Assessments of the joints, with a particular focus on those of his right lower extremity (hip and ankle) are normal with the exception of the right knee. Left lower extremity exam is normal, and there is obvious asymmetry between the two knees. To right lower extremity: minimal tenderness to the knee joint upon palpation. The knee feels warm to touch. Non-pitting edema is present. Further exam displays a positive "bulge" sign, evidence of fluid collection in the joint, as well as a negative McMurray test and negative anterior drawer sign test/Lachman test. The patella tracks normally. Range of motion of the right knee is limited due to swelling, with full extension but flexion limited to only 90°. No hypermobility is noted. Full strength (5/5) is noted to right lower extremity, and Peter's gait is normal with no limp at time of exam.

CRITICAL THINKING

Which diagnostic tests should be ordered in this case and why?
___Complete blood count (CBC)
___Comprehensive metabolic panel (CMP)
___Erythrocyte sedimentation rate (ESR)
___C-reactive protein (CRP)
___Rheumatoid factor
___Anti-nuclear antibody (ANA)
___Lactic acid dehydrogenase (LDH)
___Enzyme-linked immunosorbent assay with reflex Western blot (ELISA)
___X-ray
___Magnetic resonance imaging (MRI)
___Synovial fluid (cell counts, Gram stain, culture and sensitivity, PCR)

What is the most likely differential diagnosis and why?
___Infectious cause (septic arthritis, osteomyelitis, Lyme arthritis)
___Autoimmune diseases (juvenile idiopathic arthritis, systemic lupus erythematous)
___Trauma/Injury
___Malignancy (tumor secondary to osteosarcoma, lymphoma, neuroblastoma)

What is the plan of treatment?

What are the plans for referral and follow-up care?

What health education should be provided to this patient?

What demographic characteristics might affect this case?

Are there any standardized guidelines that should be used to treat this case? If so, what are they?

Is there any other information that would be helpful in determining a diagnosis?

If this patient were 6 years old, would it change how he would be tested and treated?

At what point would inpatient treatment be more appropriate than outpatient for this patient?

Case 6.1 Preconception Planning

By Sara Smoller, RN, MSN, ANP-BC

SUBJECTIVE

Delilah is a 28-year-old female who presents to discuss her plans to conceive. She is in a monogamous relationship with her husband. They are excited about the possibility of starting a family and want to do so in 6 months when her husband gets out of law school. Delilah wants to know what she should be doing to ensure that she is healthy and has a healthy pregnancy. She is worried she may have difficulty getting pregnant as her older sister had to go through in-vitro fertilization; she is wondering if she needs a referral to a fertility specialist. She has never been pregnant before. Her last Pap smear was 3 years ago and was normal. Her last menstrual period was 2 weeks ago. She reports regular menses.

Past medical history: G0P0; moderate persistent asthma, currently well controlled; appendectomy at age 21

Family history: Mother with Type 2 diabetes; father with bipolar depression (poorly managed)—she has minimal contact.

Social History: Delilah works as a flight attendant 7 days on, 7 days off. She engages in minimal physical activity other than being active/on her feet at work. She's been married for 2.5 years and feels safe at home. Her husband is in law school. Delilah drinks 1–2 glasses of wine per night and smokes "socially" about 5 cigarettes per week. She denies any marijuana or other drug use. Her sleeping habits are poor; when she is working she is flying between time zones and often is awake overnight. She states she averages about 5 hours of sleep per night. She drinks 3–4 cups of black coffee daily.

Medications: Fluticasone inhaler 220mcg 1 puff bid; albuterol inhaler 1–2 puffs q6h prn shortness of breath; Apri OCPs; Ibuprofen 200–400 mg prn headache

Allergies: NKDA

The Family Nurse Practitioner: Clinical Case Studies, Second Edition. Edited by Leslie Neal-Boylan.
© 2021 John Wiley & Sons Ltd. Published 2021 by John Wiley & Sons Ltd.

OBJECTIVE

Vital signs: Temperature 97.6°F (orally); BP 118/72; pulse 72 and regular. She is 5 ft 5 inches tall and 183 pounds.

General: Delilah is pleasant and cooperative and is sitting comfortably in the exam room.

Eyes: PERRL. No injection or icterus.

Mouth: No lesions or exudates.

Neck: Thyroid palpable without enlargement or nodules.

Cardiac: Regular rate and rhythm, no murmurs.

Lungs: Clear bilaterally.

Breasts: No lumps, masses, nipple discharge, or skin changes.

Abdomen: Soft, nontender, nondistended. No palpable masses or hepatosplenomegaly.

CRITICAL THINKING

What health recommendations should be made for Delilah in order to help her prepare for pregnancy?

What laboratory/diagnostic testing is recommended?

How Delilah's medication list be adjusted? Are any of the medications teratogenic? Are there any medications/vitamins or supplements she should start taking?

When should she stop her birth control pills?

How should she be counseled about seeing a fertility specialist? When would this be recommended?

Would anything be different if Delilah were 38 instead of 28?

Are any other referrals recommended?

Case 6.2 Bleeding in the First Trimester of Pregnancy

By Meredith Scannell, PhD, MSN, MPH, CNM, CEN, SANE-A

SUBJECTIVE

Tasha is a 44-year-old female who presents with a sudden onset of heavy vaginal bleeding. She reports that the bleeding started 2 days ago; it started slowly but progressed to heavy bleeding that required menstrual pads to be changed every 2–3 hours since awaking this morning. Tasha also reports significant cramping and pain in the lower abdomen. She describes having irregular menstrual cycles over the past year due to perimenopausal changes. Her last menstrual cycle was 2 months ago; it was light and lasted only 3–4 days. Tasha reports some occasional nausea over the past few weeks that occurs for short durations in the morning.

Past medical history: History of retinal detachments requiring surgical repair.

Menstrual history: Tasha began her menstrual cycle at the age of 14. Prior to beginning perimenopause, she had 28-day cycles lasting 5–6 days.

Obstetrical history: G4 T2 P0 A2 L3. Tasha had 2 full-term pregnancies. The first was a singleton at 38 weeks' gestation in which the delivery was an uncomplicated normal spontaneous vaginal birth. The second was a twin pregnancy at 37 weeks via uncomplicated Cesarean section. Tasha has also had 2 spontaneous miscarriages.

Family history: Tasha's mother has a history of tension headaches and transient ischemia attacks. Her father has a history of hypertension and myocardial infarction. Her sister has a history of systemic lupus erythematosus and infertility issues.

Social history: Tasha does not smoke; she drinks 4–5 times each week with 1–2 glasses of wine per setting. She reports occasionally drinking more than 6 drinks in a setting 1–2 times per year when there are celebratory occasions such as weddings. She is married and works as a funeral director. She has 1 teenage daughter who is in her senior year in college and two 19-year-old sons who started college in the fall. She has been married for 20 years to her high school sweetheart. She denies any concerns of domestic violence and reports feeling safe at home.

Sexual history: Tasha reports being in a mutually monogamous relationship with her husband. She engages in sexual activity 1–2 times per week and reports feeling satisfied with the level of sexual activity. She denies any use of condoms; she is not concerned about pregnancy because she is perimenopausal.

The Family Nurse Practitioner: Clinical Case Studies, Second Edition. Edited by Leslie Neal-Boylan.
© 2021 John Wiley & Sons Ltd. Published 2021 by John Wiley & Sons Ltd.

Genitourinary: Tasha denies any dysuria, frequency, or incontinence.

Medications: Tasha take no prescribed medication; over-the-counter medications include multi-vitamin QD, Vitamin D 200IU QD, fish oil 1,200 mg QD, ibuprofen 600 mg, as needed for pain.

Allergies: Shellfish (rash), IV contrast (rash), Reglan (difficulty breathing).

OBJECTIVE

General: Tasha appears in some distress and is guarding of her lower abdomen. She is neatly dressed; affect is appropriate for the situation.

Vital signs: BP: 110/52 (L) sitting; P: 90; RR: 18; temperature: 97.8°F; weight: 185 lbs; height: 5 ft 5 inches.

HEENT: Head: Nontender, without masses, hair with normal distribution. Eyes: Clear conjunctivae; PERRLA and intact. Ears: Clear external auditory canals, hearing normal. Mouth/throat: Light pink mucosa, dentition normal.

Skin: Pink, warm, no rashes, and no lesions.

Abdomen: Soft, nondistended, +tenderness lower abdomen above symphysis pubis, no rebound, no Turner sign, no Cullen sign.

Pelvic: Inguinal lymph nodes without swelling or tenderness; no adnexal masses, vaginal mucosa moist light pink. Uterus midline and globular. Cervical os dilated, with blood, no tissue observed. No cervical motion tenderness. Blood noted in the vaginal vault, no tissue noted.

CRITIAL THINKING

What is the most likely differential diagnosis in this case?
___Spontaneous inevitable abortion
___Ectopic pregnancy
___Cervicitis

Which diagnostic tests are required in this case and why?
___CBC with differential
___Blood type with Rhesus type and antibody screen
___Beta hCG
___Progesterone level
___Doppler fetal heart tones
___Transvaginal ultrasound
___Abdominal ultrasound

What are the concerns at this point?

What is the plan of treatment?

What are the plans for follow-up care?

Are there any standardized guidelines that should be used to treat this case? If so, what are they?

Case 6.3 Night Sweats

By Ivy M. Alexander, PhD, APRN, ANP-BC, FAANP, FAAN and
Annette Jakubisin-Konicki, PhD, ANP-BC, FNP-BC, FAANP

SUBJECTIVE

Susan is a 50-year-old Black female who presents for her annual physical with a complaint of hot flashes and night sweats. Susan reports that some of the night sweats are drenching. She is having difficulty sleeping and is finding it hard to function at work.

Susan says her symptoms have been present for about 4–8 months. They seem to be increasing in intensity and frequency. She says, "some days I think I am going crazy! I cannot sleep and I am so easily frustrated and tired all of the time." She expresses embarrassment about sweating at work and says that she sometimes has trouble remembering things and staying focused at work meetings.

Past medical history: No major chronic medical problems, + high blood pressure at the end of her second pregnancy (resolved with the birth), + seasonal allergies.

Surgical history: Tonsillectomy at age 6. Wisdom teeth excisions at age 20.

Family history: Mother: osteoporosis, mild depression; father: cardiovascular disease (CVD), hypertension, possibly diabetes mellitus; sister (3 years older): "terrible menopause symptoms," recently diagnosed with a thyroid problem; brother (2 years younger): hypertension; MGM: osteoporosis, depression; PGF: early CVD with myocardial infarction at age 50.

Social history: Susan lives with her husband of 19 years, their two daughters, and the family dog in a private home that they own. She is employed as an editor with a private press agency and enjoys her work. She reports feeling stressed at work lately due to difficulty remembering tasks and missing deadlines as a result. She reports that the most important recent life event was her daughter's graduation from high school. She is happy for her daughter as she was admitted to the university of her choice, but Susan is not looking forward to having her leave home in the fall. She describes her usual day as follows: awakes around 6 a.m., makes breakfast for herself and the family, showers and dresses for work, drives to work, and is at her desk by 8:30 a.m. She leaves work around 5:30 p.m. and drives home. She makes dinner most evenings and spends time in the evening assisting her younger daughter with homework and doing household chores. She starts getting ready for bed around 10 p.m. She reports walking the dog each day for about 1.5 miles, usually in the evening unless it is too hot.

The Family Nurse Practitioner: Clinical Case Studies, Second Edition. Edited by Leslie Neal-Boylan.
© 2021 John Wiley & Sons Ltd. Published 2021 by John Wiley & Sons Ltd.

Diet: Her 24-hour diet recall reveals a bagel with cream cheese and coffee (black) for breakfast, salad with cottage cheese for lunch, grilled fish with potatoes and salad for dinner, and no snacks. She reports that she eats out about once per week and enjoys dessert on occasion.

Substance use: Susan denies use of tobacco. She reports alcohol use as 1 glass of red wine most evenings. She denies use of recreational/illicit drugs.

Safety: She reports feeling safe at home with her husband and family. She had 1 partner long ago who threatened her physically, but she has had no contact with him for many years. Since then she has never been hit, slapped, kicked, or otherwise physically hurt by anyone. She denies ever being forced to have sexual activities when she did not want to. She uses a seatbelt and sunblock regularly and has working smoke detectors and carbon monoxide detectors at home. Her husband does have a hunting rifle, which is kept locked with the ammunition stored separately. She denies any concerns for her children or personal safety with regard to the rifle. She denies having any current concerns about HIV.

Medications: OTC antihistamines for allergies PRN; MVI daily; calcium (when she remembers); nasal spray for allergies PRN.

Allergies: NKDA, NKFA, +seasonal allergies.

General: Susan describes her overall health as "good, but getting weird lately." She reports a recent weight increase of about 4 lbs. She identifies her usual weight as 145 lbs. She reports fatigue and reduced energy since her hot flashes and poor sleep began. She denies any substantive premenstrual syndrome (PMS) symptoms. "I sometimes crave salty foods or chocolate, but it is not anything big." She denies symptoms of premenstrual dysphoric disorder (PMDD).

Mood: Susan reports her usual mood as "generally good, but I feel crabby when I don't sleep well." Recently she notes increased moodiness, especially after a night of poor sleep. She denies feeling nervous or anxious, but admits to feeling irritable and getting angry more easily than usual when she is tired and having more hot flashes. She says, "I feel depressed. I don't sleep well, and most of the things I used to enjoy doing irritate me now. I feel like I am going crazy." She denies anhedonia and with questioning says that she enjoys reading, eating out with her husband or friends, shopping with her daughters, and doing yoga classes. Susan denies eating disorders; she says, "sometimes I eat when I feel irritated, you know, comfort food like chips or chocolate; and it doesn't even make me feel better! But no, I don't think I have an eating disorder."

Cognitive: Susan describes difficulty with concentration and memory, especially at work after a night of particularly poor sleep or several nights of interrupted sleep. She denies problems with cognition, noting that she thinks clearly and can follow the conversation. Her issue is "with remembering what I said I would do. If I don't write it down, it is likely that it will not get done." She does use lists for shopping, puts appointments in a calendar, and carries a notebook to write down tasks when at work.

Systemic: Susan reports that she began having hot flashes about 8 months ago. They have been slowly and progressively getting worse. She does have night sweats as well; sometimes she has to change her pajamas and sheets. She describes the severity of the hot flashes as 4–10 on a 1–10 scale: "sometimes they are tolerable and I just feel hot; other times I am completely drenched with sweat." She reports having hot flashes during the day anywhere from 6 to 20 times. Her night sweats occur anywhere from 2 to 10 times nightly.

HEENT: Susan denies any problems with headaches, unless she forgets her morning coffee; and then, she says, "I get a headache around 2 p.m., but if I have a cup of coffee then it goes away. Of course then I don't sleep well." Susan reports minor changes in her vision over the past 3 years, requiring her to use reading glasses more and more often. She denies recent changes in hearing, smell, taste, or swallowing. She reports some increased dry eye symptoms and finds that she needs to use eye lubricating drops, especially when she is doing a lot of work on the computer. She has seasonal allergies and experiences sneezing, rhinorrhea, and itchy eyes year round and especially in the early fall.

Respiratory: Susan denies having any cough, wheeze, or shortness of breath in the recent past.

Cardiovascular: Susan denies chest pain, palpitations, dyspnea on exertion, peripheral edema, or a history of blood clots. She says that she has always had cold hands and feet: "Maybe it is Raynaud's. They get so cold and take a long time to warm up. I am okay if I remember to wear gloves and keep my feet warm."

Breast: Susan reports that she does do self-breast exams, usually each month right after her period. She has forgotten often this past year since she has been missing periods. She denies any concerns or recent breast changes. She denies any discharge, pain, or tingling. She breastfed each of her daughters.

Gastrointestinal: Susan reports occasional heartburn after a large or spicy meal that is relieved with Maalox. She denies persistent abdominal pain and reports daily regular bowel movements without constipation or recent changes in color, consistency, or pattern of stools. Specifically, she denies seeing any blood or experiencing fecal incontinence.

Genitourinary: Susan reports some urgency and occasional leakage of small amounts of urine, especially with coughing or laughing. She denies urinary frequency; history of recurrent urinary tract infections, pyelonephritis, or renal stones; and urine dribbling or outright incontinence. She says she does not have dysuria. She reports occasional nocturia of once or twice at night, but is unsure if this wakes her or if she is awake and then feels she needs to urinate before going back to sleep.

Gynecological: Susan reports no abnormal Pap smears or gynecological surgeries. She denies vaginal or vulvar discharge, itching, irritation, soreness, burning, abnormal bleeding, or lesions. She denies pelvic pain or rash. She reports some vaginal dryness, especially noticed with sexual activity.

Pregnancy history: Susan has been pregnant twice. She is P2, G2 with two healthy living daughters aged 15 and 18 years. She reports that she breastfed each daughter, the older one for 6 months and the younger one for 8 months.

Menstrual history: Susan reports that her last menstrual period was 6 weeks ago. She reports that the menses was typical and lasted for 6 days with 1–2 days of light flow, followed by 3 days of heavier flow, and then 1–2 days of light spotting. She experienced menarche at 13 years of age and after the first few years had pretty regular periods occurring every 28–30 days. Over the past year she has had some missed periods and some with flow that was lighter than her usual pattern. She had one period with light flow that continued for about 2 weeks.

Contraception: Susan reports that she used oral contraceptive pills for contraception in the past. She has not taken any type of hormone for contraception for the past 10 years because her husband had a vasectomy when they decided not to have any more children.

Sexual: Susan reports that she is sexually active with her husband. She is mostly satisfied but notes that it has become harder to get adequately lubricated and that it takes longer to achieve orgasm. She reports she has had 6 lifetime partners and has been monogamous with her husband for over 20 years. She reports that her desire/libido is satisfactory but is less strong than it was 1 year ago. She says that this is "a bummer. We have always had a good sex life and I miss wanting it like I used to." Her arousal is reported as satisfactory, but "it takes longer to get ready than it used to." She usually does achieve orgasm but "it takes longer than it used to and sometimes he is already finished and I am left feeling a bit frustrated." She denies dyspareunia. She reports their usual sexual practices include cuddling and kissing, then foreplay that includes genital manipulation, and then vaginal intercourse with penile penetration. They have used OTC lubricants recently, due to her dryness. She says she feels good and enjoys sex when it happens, but she doesn't initiate activity or wish for it like she used to. She reports their relationship quality as, "Oh, really good. When he finishes before me we laugh about it and talk it over. Sometimes he brings me to orgasm manually, but it can take a long time."

Musculoskeletal: Susan reports that she has noticed some vague joint and muscle pain over the past year. It seems better when she gets regular exercise and does not stop her from her usual activities.

Endocrine: Susan denies polydipsia, polyuria, polyphagia, and symptoms of diabetes mellitus type 2.

Skin/Hair: Susan denies noticing any recent skin changes or lesions of concern. She has noticed some increased acne around her mouth, skin dryness and wrinkles, and dry/thinning hair, especially on her head. She denies hirsutism or facial hair.

Hematologic: Susan denies any bleeding or bruising that doesn't correlate to a specific injury.

Neurologic: Susan reports some numbness and tingling if her hands or feet get too cold, but not otherwise. She denies fainting, dizziness (vertigo), feeling off balance, or having difficulty walking.

Sleep: Susan's usual bedtime routine includes nighttime washing and tooth brushing followed by reading or watching TV for about 30 minutes. She denies use of stimulants except for coffee each morning. She does wake every night with hot flashes/sweats. She is able to fall back to sleep but reports that it can take up to an hour depending on whether she needs to change her pajamas or sheets and how long it takes to feel cool again. She usually goes to bed around 10 p.m. and falls asleep around 10:30 p.m. She gets up for work around 6 a.m. most days. She reports that she usually does not feel refreshed when she wakes up.

OBJECTIVE

Vital signs: BP: 132/80 (L) sitting; P: 78; RR: 10; weight: 152 lbs; height: 5 ft 7 inches; BMI: 23.8.

General: Appears well; in no apparent distress; neatly dressed; appropriate affect.

HEENT: Head: Nontender; without masses; hair thinning slightly in some areas. Eyes: Clear conjunctivae; PERRLA intact; EOMI; fundi sharp optic discs; normal retinal arterioles; no A-V nicking. Ears: Clear external auditory canals; TMs + light reflex and landmarks visible; hearing grossly normal. Mouth/Throat: + normal mucosa, tongue, pharynx, and tonsils; dentition in good repair.

Neck: Supple, without lymphadenopathy. Thyroid nontender, without palpable masses or enlargement. Carotids without bruits.

Respiratory: Clear to auscultation and percussion, anterior and posterior; without wheezes, rales, or rhonchi.

Cardiac: RRR: normal S1 and S2 without murmurs, rubs, or gallops.

Breasts: Without masses, skin changes, or discharge bilaterally; no lymphadenopathy.

Abdomen: Soft, nondistended, nontender; + bowel sounds × 4 quadrants; without HSM, masses, or bruits.

Gynecological: Vaginal mucosa slightly dry, rugae present; uterus firm and anteverted, nontender, without palpable masses; adnexa nontender, without palpable masses bilaterally; no lesions noted.

Rectal: No lesions or masses noted; + external hemorrhoids; nontender; + normal sphincter tone.

Extremities: Without cyanosis, edema, or clubbing; +2 pulses bilaterally. + full range of motion throughout, nontender joints without crepitus.

Neurologic: CN II–XII grossly negative; 5/5 motor strength, gait even; DTRs 2+; Romberg negative.

CRITICAL THINKING

What are the top three differential diagnoses to consider for Susan and why?

Which diagnostic tests are required for managing Susan's condition and why?

What are the concerns at this point?

What is the plan of treatment options to be discussed with Susan?

What are the recommendations for referral and follow-up care?

What health education should be provided for Susan?

What if Susan also had diabetes or hypertension?

What if Susan were over age 65?

Does Susan's psychosocial history affect the management recommendations?

Are there any standardized guidelines that should be used when developing a management plan for Susan? If so, what are they?

Case **6.4** Pelvic Pain

By Meredith Scannell, PhD, MSN, MPH, CNM, CEN, SANE-A

SUBJECTIVE

Shanae is a 32-year-old female who presents with lower abdominal pain and fever. Fevers at home range between 99.4°F to a maximum of 101.7°F. She describes the lower abdominal pain as a constant dull ache, nonradiating, with a pain scale ranging from 5/10 to 8/10. The pain is worse with sexual intercourse. Shanae is taking acetaminophen 650 mg every 4 hours with minimal relief. She reports general malaise and that for the past 2 weeks she has been having heavy, purulent vaginal discharge. Three weeks ago, Shanae went to an urgent care clinic for dysuria. At that time, there was concern about a sexual transmitted infection and Shanae was treated for gonorrhea and chlamydia.

Past medical history: Polycystic ovarian syndrome, gonorrhea, herpes simplex virus type-2

Gynecologic history: Two abnormal Pap smears requiring repeat testing and cone biopsy with negative results.

Menstrual history: Menstrual cycles irregular between 28 and 35 days, lasting 5–7 days of heavy bleeding. LMP 1 week ago.

Family history: Mother with history of cervical cancer and died at the age of 38, father with alcohol and substance abuse, no other history known.

Sexual history: Shanae reports having a poor sexual relationship with her husband, from whom she is separated. She left her husband after finding out he was having extramarital relationships and has engaged in several sexual relationships of her own. She now reports current sexual activity as intercourse with only one partner. She and her partner use condoms on most occasions; however, there has been a few occasions when they did not use condoms. She is currently satisfied with her sexual partner with whom she engages in vaginal, oral, and rectal sexual intercourse.

Substance use: Shanae denies use of tobacco. She reports occasional alcohol use of 1–2 drinks per month. She reports daily or near daily smoking of marijuana and has used cocaine in the distant past, none recently.

The Family Nurse Practitioner: Clinical Case Studies, Second Edition. Edited by Leslie Neal-Boylan.
© 2021 John Wiley & Sons Ltd. Published 2021 by John Wiley & Sons Ltd.

Safety: Shanae reports feeling safe at home and in her current relationship. She says that the relationship with her husband was beginning to feel unsafe due to constant fighting. Since the separation, she has had no safety concerns and in the process of finalizing a divorce.

Medications: Ibuprofen 600 mg as needed, OCP (Yasmin) once daily.

Allergies: NKDA,

OBJECTIVE

General: Shanae is pleasant but appears in distress, guarding her abdomen.

Vital signs: Temperature: 100.4°F; BP: 100/52; HR: 110; respirations: 24.

Skin: Hot to touch, no lesions, no rashes.

Abdomen: Abdomen + bowel sounds, soft, nondistended. Positive suprapubic pain elicited upon palpation. No rebound tenderness, Turner sign, or Cullen sign.

Pelvic: Cervix midline, friable cervical OS; yellow discharge noted from the OS. Positive cervical motion tenderness. No lymphadenopathy and no adnexal masses.

Rectal: No lesions, no masses; normal sphincter tone.

CRITICAL THINKING

What is the most likely differential diagnosis in this case?
___Ectopic pregnancy
___Pyelonephritis
___Pelvic inflammatory disease

Which diagnostic tests are required in this case and why?
___CBC
___Nucleic acid amplification tests (NAAT)
___Beta hCG
___HIV
___Wet mount
___Treponema pallidum
___Transvaginal ultrasound

What is the plan of treatment?

What are the plans for follow-up care?

What health education should be provided to this patient?

Are there any standardized guidelines that should be used to treat this case? If so, what are they?

Case 6.5 Vaginal Itching

By Sara Smoller, RN, MSN, ANP-BC

SUBJECTIVE

Martha is a 24-year-old female who reports vaginal itching for 3 days. She says that she can barely focus on other things because of the itching. She also reports a copious, white vaginal discharge. Her last Pap smear was at age 22 and was negative. She has not received the HPV vaccine series. Martha denies previous episodes and states that she is otherwise healthy. She denies fever, chills, nausea, vomiting, or diarrhea. She is sexually active with both male and female partners since the age of 15. She states that recently she has been exclusively with females but has had 2 sexual partners in the past year. She states that she still feels somewhat confused about her sexual preferences. She admits to dyspareunia and burning with urination. She denies use of vaginal sprays, douches, or powders or the use of new soaps, detergent, or clothing. Her last menstrual period (LMP) was 3 weeks ago.

Past medical history: Recurrent strep pharyngitis—last episode 3 weeks ago.

Family history: Remarkable for diabetes mellitus and COPD.

Social history: Martha is a college graduate and still lives with her widowed mother. She feels safe and has a good relationship with her mother but has not disclosed her sexual preferences to her mother. Martha does worry about their financial status as she and her mother have low-paying jobs and do not have other financial support. They are currently renting their apartment from a friend. Martha does not smoke and denies substance use.

Medications: None currently. She completed a 10-day course of amoxicillin 1 week ago for strep pharyngitis.

Allergies: Seasonal in spring.

OBJECTIVE

Vital signs: Martha is afebrile. Her BP is 110/70. Pulse is 64 and regular. Respirations are 12 and unlabored. She is 5 ft 3 inches tall and weighs 120 lbs.

General: Martha is pleasant and cooperative but seems anxious about the visit.

The Family Nurse Practitioner: Clinical Case Studies, Second Edition. Edited by Leslie Neal-Boylan.
© 2021 John Wiley & Sons Ltd. Published 2021 by John Wiley & Sons Ltd.

Throat: No swelling or exudates.

Cardiac: Regular rate and rhythm.

Respiratory: Lungs are clear bilaterally.

Abdomen: Soft, nontender, nondistended, and without organomegaly.

Pelvic exam: Inguinal lymph nodes are without swelling or tenderness; vaginal mucosa is moist, pink, and mildly swollen. There is no foul odor; but there is a white, cottage cheese–like discharge at the introitus. The cervix is pink and without friability. There is no cervical motion tenderness (CMT). The pH of the vaginal discharge is within normal range (3.8–4.2).

CRITICAL THINKING

Which diagnostic or imaging studies should be considered to assist with or confirm the diagnosis?
___Pap smear
___Cultures for gonorrhea and chlamydia
___Urine testing for gonorrhea and chlamydia
___Wet mount, including KOH and whiff test
___Urinalysis

If a wet mount were performed, what findings would be expected for the following diagnoses?
• Bacterial vaginosis
• Candidiasis
• Trichomonas

What is the most likely differential diagnosis and why?
___Bacterial vaginosis
___Candidiasis
___Trichomonas
___Gonorrhea
___Chlamydia
___Herpes simplex
___Urinary tract infection

What is the plan of treatment?

What education should be provided to Martha at this visit?

Are any referrals needed?

Is the family history of diabetes relevant to this case?

How can the clinician support the patient regarding her confusion with her sexual preferences?

NOTE: The author would like to thank Leslie Neal-Boylan, PhD, APRN, CRRN, FAAN, FARN for her contribution to this case in the first edition of this book.

Case 6.6 Redness and Swelling in the Breast

By Karen M. Flaherty, MSN, MEd, APRN-BC, CBCN

SUBJECTIVE

Jill is a 26-year-old female who presents today for evaluation of redness, swelling, and pain in her right breast. Three months ago she underwent bilateral nipple piercings while on vacation in the Caribbean. Both sites had healed well until 4 days ago, when she noted "mild" redness on her right lower breast. This has increased in size and depth of color and she began experiencing swelling and pain in the right breast. Last night she noted a small amount of drainage on the right side of bra and felt mildly feverish.

Past medical history: Jill is an otherwise healthy 26-year-old female of Ashkenazi Jewish heritage who had the usual childhood illnesses. Her immunizations are up to date. She's had no chronic illnesses and has no past surgical history.

Family medical history: Jill's mother and father (Ashkenazi Jewish) are alive and well. She has 2 brothers, ages 20 and 18, with no significant medical problems. Her paternal grandmother is age 67 and has Type 2 diabetes mellitus; she was treated for left breast cancer at age 43 and tested positive for the BRCA 1 and 2 gene. Jill's paternal grandfather is age 70 and is alive and well. Her maternal grandmother is age 65 and has high blood pressure; her maternal grandfather is age 67 and alive and well.

Social history: Jill graduated with a degree in art and works as an assistant in an art gallery; she is applying to graduate school. Jill lives in Boston with a female roommate. Her alcohol intake includes 2–3 glasses of wine on the weekend. She has been smoking 3–4 cigarettes per day since age 20. She performs Pilates 2–3 times per week.

Medication: Daily BCP, MVI, Tylenol if needed for headache.

Allergies: Seasonal sllergies (spring), penicillin (rash and hives).

The Family Nurse Practitioner: Clinical Case Studies, Second Edition. Edited by Leslie Neal-Boylan.
© 2021 John Wiley & Sons Ltd. Published 2021 by John Wiley & Sons Ltd.

OBJECTIVE

General: Pleasant young woman, who appears mildly unwell, in moderate discomfort; rates pain 4/10 located in R breast.

Vital signs: Temperature: 100.4°F; P: 90; BP: 100/60.

Cardiac: Rate 96 and regular, no murmurs heard on auscultation.

Respiratory: Rate 16 breaths per minute, lungs clear to auscultation in all lobes.

Skin: Face is flushed. Right breast has marked redness and warmth over the lower half, left breast no redness or increase in temperature.

Breast: Right breast is slightly swollen, with erythema extending over the lower half of the right breast, central area of induration within the area of erythema. Mild skin thickening and edema noted. There is a ring piercing through the right nipple, no drainage seen. Right breast has a tender area of induration within the central portion of the erythema. No other discrete or dominant masses found. No observable drainage seen from right breast. Left breast has a ring piercing through the left nipple, no swelling, erythema, or induration, also with piercing through the left nipple. Left breast is smooth to palpation with no discrete or dominant masses noted, no painful areas on palpation.

Lymph: Left axillary nodes nonpalpable, nontender. Right axilla has 2 mobile, nontender, 0.5 cm, oval palpable nodes.

CRITICAL THINKING

Which diagnostic tests should be considered?

Which differential diagnoses should be considered?

What is the most likely differential diagnosis and why?

What is the plan of treatment?

What is the plan for follow-up?

Would the workup or treatment be different if this patient were a man?

Are any referrals needed?

What health education is important for this patient?

Case 6.7 Sexual Assault

By Meredith Scannell, PhD, MSN, MPH, CNM, CEN, SANE-A

SUBJECTIVE

Aiyata is a 22-year-old female who presents requesting treatment for sexually transmitted infection. She reports she recently graduated from college and was out celebrating the graduation with some friends last night. She reports going to a bar where she met with a male friend who bought her drinks. She has a vague recollection of the night but awoke today naked in the bed with the male friend. She has a vague memory of having sex with the male friend but does not recall many of the details; she is not sure if a condom was used. She is concerned because she has been having vaginal spotting since the event and some pain and discomfort in the vagina.

Past medical history: Depression, childhood sexual abuse, post-traumatic stress disorder.

Past surgical history: None.

Menstrual history: LMP 2 weeks ago; she reports a 28-day cycle and no menstrual irregularities.

Genitourinary: Reports some dysuria that started this morning.

Family history: Aiyata's mother has a history of alcohol abuse and hypertension. Her father's history is unknown.

Social history: Aiyata was raised in a single-parent home with her mother as the primary caregiver. She is currently living in an apartment with college friends. Aiyata recently graduated from college and works part-time as a server. She reports being single since a breakup with her boyfriend. She had been in a mutually monogamous relationship with the boyfriend, but since the breakup, she has had 3 casual sexual partners. She practices safe sex with the use of condoms.

Substance use: She occasionally consumes alcohol 1–2 times a week with 1–2 drinks per setting. She admits to occasional marijuana consumption, but uses no other recreational drugs.

Medications: Oral contraception, Citalopram 20 mg daily.

Allergies: No known drug allergies.

The Family Nurse Practitioner: Clinical Case Studies, Second Edition. Edited by Leslie Neal-Boylan.
© 2021 John Wiley & Sons Ltd. Published 2021 by John Wiley & Sons Ltd.

OBJECTIVE

General: Ayita is sad appearing, talking softly, answering questions appropriately.

Vital signs: Temperature: 98.6°F; BP: 120/74; HR: 99; RR: 18.

Skin: Abrasion on left knee and left elbow.

Neurologic: Alert and oriented × 3

HEENT:

Head: Nontender, without masses, hair normally distributed.

Neck: Lateral neck tender to palpation; dark red ecchymosed areas on right side of neck, trachea midline, no lymphadenopathy. Thyroid nontender, without palpable masses or enlargement.

Eyes: PERRLA and EOMs are intact, left eye small subconjunctival hemorrhage.

Oropharynx: Uvula is midline, no edema, redness, or ecchymosis.

Respiratory: Lung sounds are clear to auscultate.

Cardiac: Regular rate and rhythm.

Breast: Tanner IV, symmetrical.

Abdomen: Soft, nontender, nondistended; active bowel sounds.

Pelvic:

Vulva: No lesions or ecchymosis. The labia minora are red and swollen, tender to palpation; there is a small laceration at the posterior fourchette.

Vagina: No active bleeding, very tender with speculum insertion, white discharge in vaginal vault.

Cervix: Bright red and friable; positive cervical motion tenderness.

Rectal: Rugae normal appearance, no lesions.

CRITICAL THINKING

What is the most likely differential diagnosis in this case and why?
___Sexual assault
___Strangulation
___Pelvic inflammatory disease

Which diagnostic tests are required in this case and why?
___CBC with differential
___Metabolic panel
___LFTs
___Toxicology panel
___HCG
___HIV
___Urinalysis
___NAAT
___CT scan neck

___Transvaginal ultrasound
___Abdominal ultrasound

What are the concerns at this point?

What is the plan of treatment?

What are the plans for referral and follow-up care?

What health education should be provided to this patient?

Are there any standardized guidelines that should be used to assess or treat this case?

Case 6.8 Abdominal Pain

By Leslie Neal-Boylan, PhD, APRN, CRRN, FAAN, FARN

SUBJECTIVE

Rachel is a 17-year-old Caucasian female who presents with complaints of decreased appetite, fatigue, nausea, and intermittent abdominal pain for the past 2–3 weeks. She describes the abdominal pain as sharp and focused in the right epigastric area. She also reports some new-onset pain in her right shoulder but attributes this to carrying around her baby more than usual. She denies vomiting, diarrhea, or constipation. Her typical diet consists of pizza, hot dogs, and salads. Rachel denies any association of her symptoms with food or hunger. Her last normal menstrual period was 3 weeks ago, and she has had 2 negative pregnancy tests at home.

Past medical history: She delivered her son 6 months ago vaginally without complications. Her only other medical history includes a kidney infection 4 months ago.

Social history: She smokes 7 cigarettes a day but admits, "I really don't need them. I am bored." Rachel lives with her boyfriend (the father of her child) and his parents. She moved in, far away from her home, only recently. Her parents made her leave their house when she told them she was pregnant, and they have no contact with her. She states that she feels safe at home and is enjoying her baby. Her boyfriend helps with the baby but often goes out at night with his friends and leaves her at home with the baby. She feels a little isolated because everyone works during the day and she has no access to transportation. She is dependent on her in-laws if she needs to go anywhere by car, and they do not often support her need to go anywhere. Otherwise, she walks. She walked here today for her appointment.

Medication: She is not allergic to any medication and only takes birth control pills.

OBJECTIVE

Vital signs: Rachel is afebrile. BP is 120/80. Pulse is 68 and regular.

Eyes: PERRLA. EOMs are intact. Optic disks are sharp.

Cardiac: Cardiac exam reveals regular rate and rhythm.

Respiratory: Respirations are 12, steady, and unlabored. Lungs are clear.

The Family Nurse Practitioner: Clinical Case Studies, Second Edition. Edited by Leslie Neal-Boylan.
© 2021 John Wiley & Sons Ltd. Published 2021 by John Wiley & Sons Ltd.

Abdomen: Soft with mild tenderness to palpation (TTP) in the RUQ with a positive Murphy's sign. There is no CVA tenderness.

Genitourinary: A urine dipstick reveals positive protein. A urine HCG is negative.

Rachel is diagnosed at this first visit with possible cholecystitis and is given Antivert 12.5 mg for her nausea.

Blood is drawn and sent to the lab. Her urine is sent for analysis, and she is told to return in 1 week.

Rachel returns 1 week later. Her bloodwork reveals a blood glucose of 45 mg/dL. Her other bloodwork is within normal limits. Her urinalysis returns with few bacteria and no protein. Rachel reports that the abdominal pain has worsened and she now has headaches. She denies a history of migraines or frequent headaches. Her nausea is still present but decreased.

Her exam remains unchanged.

CRITICAL THINKING

What is the most likely differential diagnosis in this case and why?
__Cholelithiasis
__Gastroenteritis
__Diverticulitis
__Insulin tumor
__Gastric tumor
__Cholecystitis

Which diagnostic tests are required in this case and why?
__Abdominal ultrasound
__Abdominal CT scan
__Head CT scan
__KUB X-ray
__CBC
__Metabolic panel
__LFTs
__Insulin level
__C-peptide
__OGGT
__Gastrin level

What is the plan of treatment?

Are any referrals needed?

Does the patient's home situation influence the plan?

Are there any standardized guidelines that should be used to treat this case?

Case 6.9 Urinary Frequency

By Leslie Neal-Boylan, PhD, APRN, CRRN, FAAN, FARN

SUBJECTIVE

Susan is a 42-year-old female who presents with a report of burning pain on urination for the past 2 days. She has been urinating frequently and finds that she has to run to make it to the bathroom in time to void in the toilet. She vaguely remembers similar symptoms once in college but doesn't remember what she was diagnosed with or how she was treated for it. She denies flank pain but does have some mild suprapubic pain. She admits to mild dyspareunia in the past few days. Susan is otherwise well but admits to being thirsty more frequently than usual. Her menses are regular, and her LNMP was 10 days ago. She denies vaginal itching, foul odor, or discharge. Her 2 children were born via vaginal deliveries without complications. She does not recall when she last had a pelvic exam or Pap smear and recalls a remote history of an abnormal Pap smear. She thinks she had a colposcopy at that time and after 1 year, she was told to resume a normal Pap smear schedule.

Social history: Susan is a recently divorced mother of 2 young children. Her ex-husband was "fooling around" while they were married, so Susan is worried that she might have a sexually transmitted infection. Since the divorce, Susan has had 1 new male sexual partner. They began their sexual relationship about 1 week ago and did not use condoms because Susan was on birth control pills and "I trust this new man." She works full-time as a preschool teacher and takes care of her children, ages 12 and 15, by herself and without financial support from her ex-husband. Susan does not smoke but has an occasional (1 per month) glass of wine. She admits to having used marijuana in college.

Family medical history: Notable for diabetes Type 2 (mother) and hypertension (father).

Medications: Birth control pills.

OBJECTIVE

General: The patient is in no acute distress and is pleasant and cooperative.

Vital signs: Oral temperature is 98°F. BP is 116/74. HR is 64 and regular.

Respiratory: Respirations are 14 and regular. Lungs are clear bilaterally.

The Family Nurse Practitioner: Clinical Case Studies, Second Edition. Edited by Leslie Neal-Boylan.
© 2021 John Wiley & Sons Ltd. Published 2021 by John Wiley & Sons Ltd.

Back: There is no CVAT.

Cardiac: RRR S1/S2; without murmurs, clicks, gallops, or rubs.

Abdomen: Soft, nontender, nondistended, without organomegaly. Bowel sounds are active in all 4 quadrants.

Reproductive: Pelvic exam reveals no inguinal lymphadenopathy; moist pink vaginal mucosa, negative chandelier sign, and pink anterior cervix without friability. Cervical discharge is thin, white, and odorless. Samples are obtained for culture. This patient could also have provided a urine sample to test for gonorrhea and chlamydia. However, given her history with a new partner and an ex-husband who had other partners, as well as the length of time since her last pelvic exam, it is reasonable to do a pelvic exam at this time. A Pap smear is also performed because Susan cannot recall when she last had one and there is none noted in the electronic record. The test will include HPV testing. The bimanual exam reveals no masses or tenderness.

CRITICAL THINKING

What is the most likely differential diagnosis and why?
__Pregnancy
__Acute cystitis
__Interstitial cystitis
__Diabetes mellitus
__Pyelonephritis
__Pelvic inflammatory disease
__Urinary tract infection (UTI)

Which diagnostic studies should be considered to assist with or confirm the diagnosis?
__Urine dipstick
__Urinalysis
__Urine culture and sensitivity
__CBC
__CMP
__TSH
__Renal ultrasound
__Abdominal and pelvic ultrasound

What is the plan of treatment?

What is the plan for referrals and follow-up?

Would the diagnosis change if the patient had fever and flank pain?

Would the most likely diagnosis change if the patient were male?

What is an important symptom to consider in an older adult?

What if Susan were pregnant?

Case 6.10 Headache

By Leslie Neal-Boylan, PhD, APRN, CRRN, FAAN, FARN

SUBJECTIVE

Sophia is a 35-year-old Latina woman who presents with a complaint of headaches that have been occurring more frequently over the past 2 weeks. She has never had any problems with headaches before. Rarely, she has had a headache after a stressful day but denies premenstrual headaches or frequent headaches until 2 weeks ago. Her headaches are left sided in the temporal area and are severe (7 out of 10 on a 1–10 scale) and throbbing. They occur 3–5 times each week. She occasionally becomes nauseous but rarely vomits. The headaches tend to last several hours and go away if she is able to get sleep. Sophia tries to retreat to a dark and quiet corner when the headaches begin. She sometimes sees "spots in front of her eyes" right before the onset of a headache. Otherwise, she has no trouble with her vision, has had no epistaxis, upper respiratory symptoms, or sinus symptoms. She denies trauma to her head or any neck stiffness. She denies fever, chills, numbness, or weakness.

Past medical history: Sophia has been otherwise well and denies any previous surgeries or hospitalizations other than for 3 vaginal deliveries without complications.

Family history: Migraine headaches in her mother and sister. Her uncle had a benign brain tumor that was successfully treated.

Social history: The patient does not smoke, drinks 1 beer 3 times each week, and denies ever using recreational drugs. She is married and works as an administrative assistant in a busy office. She has 1 preteen and 2 teenagers at home, and their behavior sometimes causes her stress. Her husband is supportive and helpful.

Medications: Sophia's medications include occasional ibuprofen for "aches and pains." She tried the ibuprofen for the headaches without relief. She takes no other medications. She states that her mother told her that she was allergic to penicillin as a child, but she doesn't know why.

The Family Nurse Practitioner: Clinical Case Studies, Second Edition. Edited by Leslie Neal-Boylan.
© 2021 John Wiley & Sons Ltd. Published 2021 by John Wiley & Sons Ltd.

OBJECTIVE

General: Sophia is well groomed. Her manner and speech are appropriate and she is articulate. She is in no apparent distress during the visit.

Vital signs: The patient is afebrile. Her blood pressure is 140/90 (which she says is higher than her normal blood pressure). Pulse is 86, and respirations are regular at a rate of 12.

HEENT: The eye exam reveals clear sclera, conjunctiva without injection, and PERRLA. EOMs are intact. There is no AV nicking or papilledema. Optic disks have clear margins. Nasal mucosa is without erythema or drainage. There is no sinus tenderness to palpation. Cranial nerves II–XII are grossly intact.

Cardiac: Unremarkable.

Respiratory: Unremarkable.

Neurologic: The patient is alert and oriented. Thoughts are coherent and articulation is clear and appropriate. Sensation and proprioception are grossly intact, and the Romberg test is negative. Gait is steady. Brudzinski and Kernig signs are negative.

CRITICAL THINKING

What is the most likely differential diagnosis and why?
___Migraine with aura
___Migraine without aura
___Cluster headache
___Tension headache
___Meningitis
___Temporal arteritis
___Psychogenic headache

Are there tools that can be used to help assess this headache? If so, name two.

Which diagnostic studies should be considered?
___CT scan
___MRI
___CBC
___CMP
___Lipid panel

What is the plan of treatment?

Are any referrals or follow-up needed?

Does the patient's psychosocial history impact how she might be treated?

Is the patient's blood pressure the cause or the result of her headache?

Would the treatment change if the patient were a smoker or on birth control pills?

Case 6.11 Fatigue and Joint Pain

By Leslie Neal-Boylan, PhD, APRN, CRRN, FAAN, FARN

SUBJECTIVE

Aliyah is a 22-year-old African American female who presents with profound fatigue, sore hands and wrists, and frequent episodes of oral and nasal ulcers. She has been told by others that she has a rash across her cheeks when she is exposed to the sun; and she has just begun to notice this herself. Aliyah describes the fatigue as debilitating, and she finds it difficult to work as a legal assistant. When she is home, she frequently naps; but this never fully relieves her fatigue. Her hands and wrists ache, and this further complicates her ability to do her job, as she is expected to type most of the day.

She reports occasional cold sores since she was a teen, but recently these sores have become worse and harder to heal. She has also developed intermittent sores in the nose. Aliyah reports intermittent episodes of fever, and she has been using acetaminophen to control these episodes. She states, "I just don't have any energy, and I really don't feel well."

Aliyah's menses have always been heavy and accompanied by significant dysmenorrhea. The periods started out regular (at age 12) but have gradually become less predictable. Aliyah is a smoker. She has been coughing but denies chest pain, palpitations, dyspnea, swelling of her extremities, seizures, headaches, changes in sensation, weakness, changes in bowel or bladder function, dry eyes or dry mouth, eye pain, or changes in vision.

Past medical surgical history: None.

Family history: No connective tissue or inflammatory diseases, heart disease, diabetes mellitus, or respiratory illness.

Medications: Acetaminophen and a birth control pill.

OBJECTIVE

Vital signs: Temperature: 100.6°F orally; HR: 68 and regular; RR: 12 and regular; BP: 110/64; weight: 110 lbs (down from 120 lbs 4 months ago); height: 5 ft 4 inches.

The Family Nurse Practitioner: Clinical Case Studies, Second Edition. Edited by Leslie Neal-Boylan.
© 2021 John Wiley & Sons Ltd. Published 2021 by John Wiley & Sons Ltd.

HEENT: Mild alopecia is noted. TMs are clear and intact. PERRLA; EOMs are intact; sclera and conjunctiva are clear. Aphthous ulcers are noted in the mouth and nose. Dentition is grossly intact. There is mild bilateral anterior cervical lymphadenopathy.

Cardiac: RRR S1/S2; without murmurs, clicks, gallops, or rubs.

Respiratory: CTA bilaterally.

Skin: An erythematous rash is noted across the cheeks, sparing the nasolabial folds. Livedo is noted on the lower extremities. Nailfold capillaries are positive for loops.

Musculoskeletal: No synovitis or swelling is noted. There is no TTP. There is LROM of wrists fingers bilaterally due to pain.

Neurologic: Mentation is grossly intact. CNs II–XII are grossly intact. Sensation and proprioception are grossly intact. DTRs are +2. Romberg is negative. Heel-toe is negative. RAMs are negative.

CRITICAL THINKING

What is the most likely differential diagnosis and why?
__Rheumatoid arthritis
__Systemic lupus erythematosus
__Vasculitis
__Discoid lupus
__Fibromyalgia
__Osteoarthritis
__Influenza

Which diagnostic studies should be considered to assist with or confirm the diagnosis?
__Urinalysis
__Metabolic panel
__CBC with differential
__Lipids
__TSH
__CK
__ESR or CRP
__U1 ribonucleoprotein (RNP)
__Rheumatoid factor
__CCP
__ANA with reflex
__Anti-DS DNA
__Anti-SM
__Anti-RO/SSA
__Anti-LA/SSB
__Homocysteine
__C3, C4
__HIV
__Hepatitis B
__Hepatitis C
__X-rays (if so, what type?)

__Antiphospholipid antibodies (lupus anticoagulant [LA], IgG and IgM anticardiolipin [aCL] antibodies; and IgG and IgM anti-beta2-glycoprotein [GP] I)
__Urine protein-to-creatinine ratio

What is the plan of treatment?

What is the plan for referrals and follow-up?

Are there other manifestations of this disease?

Would it change the diagnosis or impact the prognosis or treatment if the patient were taking minocycline? What if the patient had a parvovirus?

What are the potential complications of this disease?

Case 6.12 Muscle Tenderness

By Leslie Neal-Boylan, PhD, APRN, CRRN, FAAN, FARN

SUBJECTIVE

Zelda is a 32-year-old female who reports tenderness when anyone or anything touches her. She has experienced these myalgias throughout her body for the past 6 months, and the pain is affecting her quality of life. She describes pain in the back of her head, her neck, her upper chest, upper back, her elbows, backside, and knees. The pain occurs on both sides of her body. "My joints feel swollen, and my skin burns." She feels profoundly fatigued and yet is unable to get a full night's sleep. She has trouble falling and staying asleep. She finds that she is often irritable, and this is affecting her relationships. She denies fever, chills, nausea, vomiting, and diarrhea. She denies changes in her hair, skin, or nails or any change in her menstrual period, which occurs every 28 days and lasts 5 days. Her LNMP was 3 weeks ago. She had unprotected sex 2 weeks ago with an old friend who consoled her after her move here. She denies any joint pain, dry eyes, dry mouth, ulcers, rashes, lesions, or morning stiffness.

Past medical/Surgical history: Hypertension that is controlled; irritable bowel syndrome; and appendectomy age 14 years.

Social history: She moved to this state 2 months ago and had been given opioids by her previous primary care provider. These helped moderately, and she would like some more. "At least they help me get some sleep." Zelda divorced her husband, prompting the move out of state; she moved here with her 2 teenagers, who are getting into trouble and are confused by the recent changes in their lives. Zelda admits to feeling sad often but denies suicidal ideation. She often feels unfocused and unable to concentrate. She denies use of tobacco, alcohol, and recreational drugs.

Zelda grew up in a broken home. Her father was an alcoholic and was occasionally abusive to her. She has worked since age 15 and currently works in the school cafeteria so she can be around her children and be home when they come home. She receives some financial assistance from her ex-husband.

Family medical history: Mother had rheumatoid arthritis. Father died of colon cancer at age 65 years.

Medications: Lisinopril 10 mg; Percocet 10/325 mg every 6 hours as needed for pain; MVI. The patient has been out of Percocet for 4 weeks.

The Family Nurse Practitioner: Clinical Case Studies, Second Edition. Edited by Leslie Neal-Boylan.
© 2021 John Wiley & Sons Ltd. Published 2021 by John Wiley & Sons Ltd.

OBJECTIVE

Height: 5 ft 3 inches; weight: 150 lbs; temperature: 98.7°F oral. HR is 68 and regular. RR is 12 and regular. BP is 124/70.

General: Teary, appears anxious.

HEENT: Head: Normocephalic, mild tenderness to palpation (TTP) of occiput. Eyes: PERRLA, EOMs intact. Nose: No polyps, no erythema. Mouth and throat: No oral ulcers, no erythema, no exudates; tonsils are +2. Neck: TTP, LROM on rotation due to pain; thyroid is nonpalpable.

Cardiac: S1/S2; RRR without murmurs, gallops, clicks, or rubs.

Lungs: Clear to auscultation bilaterally.

Abdomen: Soft, no bruits; positive for bowel sounds; nontender; nondistended. No organomegaly.

Neurologic: Mentation grossly intact; CNs II–XII grossly intact; DTRS +2 UEs and LEs; negative Romberg; negative RAMs; proprioception and sensation grossly intact.

Musculoskeletal: There is FROM, and strength is 5/5 throughout. There is no synovitis, and there are no effusions.

Skin: No rashes or lesions noted.

CRITICAL THINKING

What is the most likely differential diagnosis and why?
__Rheumatoid arthritis
__Systemic lupus erythematosus
__Fibromyalgia
__Sjögren's syndrome
__Osteoarthritis
__Thyroid disease
__Pregnancy
__Mononucleosis
__Celiac serology
__Vitamin D

Which diagnostic studies should be considered to assist with or confirm the diagnosis?
__TSH
__CBC with differential
__Metabolic panel
__ESR and CRP
__Rheumatoid factor
__Anti-CCP
__ANA
__SS-A and SS-B
__X-rays
__MRIs

__HCG
__Urine dipstick
__None

What is the plan of treatment?

What is the plan for referrals and follow-up?

6.13 Insomnia

By Leslie Neal-Boylan, PhD, APRN, CRRN, FAAN, FARN

SUBJECTIVE

Iris, a 48-year-old Asian female, presents with a report of insomnia and impaired concentration. She has not slept through the night for approximately 6 weeks and finds that while she can fall asleep readily, she is too restless to stay asleep. At work (she works as an office manager), she is unable to concentrate and has found herself making simple mistakes. Iris is easily fatigued and states that she frequently feels warm and flushed, but she attributes this to "the time of life." Her menstrual periods have become irregular. Her LNMP was 2 months ago. It lasted 10 days and was slightly heavier than usual. Iris states that she occasionally feels her heart "fluttering" when she feels anxious. She is surprised at this because she has always felt that she coped well with life and was generally happy. "Now, the littlest things seem to bother me and I feel my heart start to flutter. Oh, the change of life. I have dreaded it. Can you give me something for it?" Iris denies fever, chills, pain, weakness, or tremors.

Elimination: Iris has not noticed any changes in her weight or loose stools.

Past medical history: Iris had a hospitalization for a Cesarean section without complications 15 years ago. She also had a hemorrhoidectomy 7 years ago without complications.

Family medical history: Iris has a husband and 1 son who are alive and well. Her mother, age 67, has stage 1 Alzheimer's disease and hypothyroidism. Her father has diabetes mellitus Type 2 and a history of colon cancer. Both are alive.

Social history: Iris lives with her husband and son and states that she is happily married and comfortable financially. She stopped using any form of birth control since her periods became irregular 6 months ago. She is a smoker, takes no medications, and has been generally healthy.

OBJECTIVE

The patient appears anxious but is pleasant and cooperative. Her weight is 136 lbs; she comments that this is 10 lbs less than the last time she checked her weight 3 months ago. Oral temperature is 100° F. BP is 148/94. HR is 96 and regular. Respirations are 12 and regular.

The Family Nurse Practitioner: Clinical Case Studies, Second Edition. Edited by Leslie Neal-Boylan.
© 2021 John Wiley & Sons Ltd. Published 2021 by John Wiley & Sons Ltd.

HEENT: Hair is shiny and soft. No exophthalmos is observed. There is no lid lag or retraction. Sclerae are clear and conjunctivae are without injection. PERRLA and EOMs are intact. CNs II–XII are grossly intact. There is no cervical lymphadenopathy. Trachea is midline. The thyroid is mildly palpable with a bruit. There are no nodules.

Skin: The patient's skin is warm and moist.

Cardiac: HR: 96; RRR: S1/S2; no murmurs, clicks, gallops, or rubs. EKG reveals NSR without abnormalities.

Pulmonary: Lungs are clear bilaterally.

Abdomen: Soft without tenderness or distention. No organomegaly, no bruits. Bowel sounds are active throughout.

Neurologic: There are no tremors. Sensation and proprioception are grossly intact. DTRS are +3 in upper extremities and lower extremities. Romberg is negative. RAMs are negative. Gait is steady.

Musculoskeletal: FROM and strength of 5/5 in all extremities.

CRITICAL THINKING

What is the most likely differential diagnosis in this case and why?
__Hyperthyroidism
__Hypothyroidism
__Menopause
__Pregnancy
__Anxiety/depression
__Infection

Which diagnostic tests are required in this case and why?
__TSH
__CBC
__CMP
__HCG
__CXR
__Radionucleotide uptake scan with iodine (RAI)
__Ultrasound of thyroid
__FSH
__T3
__T4
__Free T4
__Thyrotropin receptor antibody (TRAb)
__Antithydroperoxidase antibody (TPO)
__ANA
__LDL
__HDL

What is the plan of treatment?

What is a likely diagnosis if this patient returns with severe tachycardia, confusion, vomiting, diarrhea, high fever, and dehydration?

What if this patient's lab results return and the TSH is low with normal results for free T4 and T3?

Would the plan be any different if Iris were unemployed?

Are there any standardized guidelines that should be used to assess and treat this case?

Section 7

Men's Health

Case 7.1 Fatigue

By Leslie Neal-Boylan, PhD, APRN, CRRN, FAAN, FARN

SUBJECTIVE

Fred, a 62-year-old male, presents to the primary care clinic with the chief complaint of fatigue. Upon further questioning, he also reports some difficulty concentrating and a decreased sex drive.

Further review of symptoms reveals dry skin, left-knee weakness, occasional heartburn, polyuria, and wheezing on exertion. He denies chest pain or palpitations. He reports being on antidepressants in the past but did not take them as directed. He is easy to get along with, forthcoming in his complaints, and describes his fatigue as a little bit more pronounced in the past couple of months. He also complains of erectile dysfunction, which he has noticed is worse in the past few years, especially since his diabetes is out of control.

Past medical and surgical history: Significant for uncontrolled type 2 diabetes, insulin dependent. The patient reports a last hemoglobin A1c of 10.2. He also has hypertension, gout, obstructive sleep apnea (with refusal to wear CPAP), and hyperlipidemia. His past surgical history includes a deviated septum repair 20 years ago.

Family history: Fred's mother died at the age of 81 of Parkinson's disease; his father died at the age of 56 of Hodgkin's lymphoma; and he has 1 sister who is alive and well at the age of 58.

Screening: He had a negative colonoscopy in 2008. His most recent PSA value was 3.1 in 2007.

Social history: Fred reports drinking 2 drinks of hard liquor daily. He quit smoking 20 years ago and drinks 4 cups of coffee daily. He reports not adhering to his prescribed diabetic diet and has many financial and marital stressors at home. He is self-employed with some college education.

Medications:

Humalog, 75/25, 20 units in the morning and 20 units at night
Nexium, 40 mg daily
Crestor, 10 mg daily
Allopurinol, 300 mg daily
Trazodone, 150 mg at night
Lopid, 600 mg twice daily

The Family Nurse Practitioner: Clinical Case Studies, Second Edition. Edited by Leslie Neal-Boylan.
© 2021 John Wiley & Sons Ltd. Published 2021 by John Wiley & Sons Ltd.

Baby aspirin, 81 mg daily
Micardis, 40/12.5 daily
Actos, 30 mg daily

Allergies: Fred has no known drug, food, or environmental allergies; and his immunizations are up to date.

OBJECTIVE

Vital signs: T: 98°F; P: 72; RR: 20; B/P: 138/90. His weight is 312 lbs, and his height is 58 inches.

General: He has a very pleasant attitude. He is a morbidly obese male, calm, pleasant, and in no acute distress.

Skin: His color is pale. His skin is clear. Small senile keratosis is noted on his left arm.

HEENT: Negative.

Neck: He appears to have short neck syndrome. He has no palpable nodes, no JVD.

Cardiovascular: Regular rate and rhythm. S1 and S2 are normal.

Respiratory: Chest is clear to auscultation.

Abdomen: Obese, nontender; and bowel sounds are present.

Musculoskeletal: Full range of motion.

Genital: He has normal genitalia. There is no evidence of swelling. His testicular exam is normal, and there is appropriate hair growth.

CRITICAL THINKING

Which diagnostic studies should be considered to assist with or confirm the diagnosis?
___CBC
___Comprehensive metabolic panel
___Lipid profile
___Urinalysis with microalbumin and microanalysis
___Total serum testosterone
___Free serum testosterone
___FSH and LH
___Gonadotropin
___Prolactin
___Transferrin saturation
___Hemoglobin A1C

What is the most likely differential diagnosis and why?
___Primary hypogonadism
___Secondary hypogonadism
___Sexual dysfunction
___Depression
___Parkinson's disease

What is the plan of treatment?

What is the plan for referrals and follow-up?

What would be relative and absolute contraindications to the treatment plan of testosterone therapy?

Are there standardized guidelines that would help in this case?

NOTE: The author would like to acknowledge the contributions of Geraldine F. Marrocco, EdD, APRN, CNS, ANP-BC and Amanda La Manna, RN, ANP to this case in the first edition of this book.

Case 7.2 Testicular Pain

By Leslie Neal-Boylan, PhD, APRN, CRRN, FAAN, FARN

SUBJECTIVE

Richard is a 45-year-old male who is an established patient. He arrives at the primary care office with the chief complaint of "extremely painful" right testicular pain for 3 hours. He reports no history of trauma. He reports that the pain came on gradually over the last 3 hours and is associated with some mild dysuria, but no urethral discharge. Pain is described as a 9 on a 0–10 scale. He denies fever, nausea, or vomiting. He reports a loss of appetite due to extreme pain.

Past medical/surgical history: Significant for COPD, GERD, hypertension, and chronic tendonitis in right elbow since fracture in 2007. He also reports a gastrointestinal infection that responded very well to Cipro. His past surgical history includes only a cervical laminectomy in 1996.

Family history: His mother is alive at the age of 87 and has diabetes mellitus type 2. His father died at the age of 79 from leukemia and prostate cancer. He has 4 sisters and 2 brothers who are all alive and well.

Social history: Richard works as a plumber and has been married for 20 years. He reports being in a monogamous sexual relationship with his wife. He lives in a single-family home and has smoked 1 pack of cigarettes per day for the past 30 years. He denies alcohol or substance use and drinks tea daily.

Medications:

Nexium, 40 mg in a.m.
Advair Inhaler, 250/50 1 puffs twice daily
Atacand, 16/12.5 mg
Spiriva inhaler, 1 puff daily

Allergies: No known drug allergies, but has seasonal allergies and an allergy to peanuts.

The Family Nurse Practitioner: Clinical Case Studies, Second Edition. Edited by Leslie Neal-Boylan.
© 2021 John Wiley & Sons Ltd. Published 2021 by John Wiley & Sons Ltd.

OBJECTIVE

General: Visibly grimacing and teary eyed, not smiling. His skin is flushed.

Vital Signs: T: 98.2°F; P: 80; BP: 136/84; RR: 18.

Respiratory: CTA bilaterally.

Cardiac: RRR: S1/S2; no murmurs, clicks, gallops, or rubs.

Genitourinary: Scrotal exam reveals obvious edema and redness of the right scrotal area. The area is very painful to touch or lift. There is no evidence of urethral discharge. The testes are tender to palpation; but the position of the testes is consistent and normal. When in the supine position, with elevation of the testes, Richard notes a slight decrease in pain, which is called Phren's sign. Transillumination of the testes is negative for masses. He has a normal cremasteric reflex. There are no inguinal hernias. The rectal exam reveals some prostate tenderness.

CRITICAL THINKING

What is the most likely differential diagnosis and why?
__Sexually transmitted infection
__Testicular torsion
__Epididymitis
__Testicular tumor
__Trauma

Which diagnostic studies should be considered to assist with or confirm the diagnosis?
__Doppler ultrasound
__Urinalysis
__Urine culture and sensitivity
__Gram stain
__Urine for gonorrhea and chlamydia

What is the plan of treatment?

Are there any referrals or follow-up care needed?

NOTE: The author would like to acknowledge Geraldine F. Marrocco, EdD, APRN, CNS, ANP-BC, who wrote the original version of this case in the first edition of this book.

Case 7.3 Prostate Changes

By Clara Gona, PhD, FNP-BC, RN

Stanley is a 64-year-old Black male who has been at the clinic regularly for health maintenance. He had an unremarkable physical exam 10 months ago. Routine labs, including a CBC, lipid profile, stool for occult blood, and EKG, were normal. He called requesting to be seen by his primary care provider because he has been having some "personal problems." He refused to disclose the nature of the problem and only wants to see his regular provider.

On further questioning Stanley reports problems with urination over the past 6–8 months. The symptoms are getting worse. He reports occasional "leaking" of urine after urination that has been embarrassing. He also reports getting up at least 3 times a night to urinate. Sometimes he has difficulty initiating urination and reports a weaker than usual urinary stream. On further questioning he reports urinary urgency and occasional urinary frequency but denies pain or burning on urination, blood in the urine, abdominal pain, fever, discharge from his penis, or sexual dysfunction.

Past medical history: Osteoarthritis in both knees; insomnia.

Past surgical history: None.

Family history: Stanley's father had diabetes mellitus Type 2 and high blood pressure; his brother has prostate problems. His mother has stage 2 dementia.

Social history: Stanley is a retired teacher and has been married to his wife Ella for 42 years. They have 2 sons and 10 grandchildren. He does not smoke, but does drink 2 shots of Cognac on most nights.

Medications: Ibuprofen as needed; Benadryl PRN for sleep.

Allergies: NKDA.

The Family Nurse Practitioner: Clinical Case Studies, Second Edition. Edited by Leslie Neal-Boylan.
© 2021 John Wiley & Sons Ltd. Published 2021 by John Wiley & Sons Ltd.

OBJECTIVE

General: Stanley is sitting in a chair, in no acute distress.

Vital signs: Weight is 175 lbs; height is 5 ft 10 inches; oral temperature is 98.5°F; BP is 125/80; heart rate is 74; respirations are 14.

Cardiac: Regular rate and rhythm, no murmurs.

Pulmonary: Clear to auscultation in all areas.

Abdomen: Positive bowel sounds in all quadrants, soft and nontender on palpation.

Genitourinary: No suprapubic tenderness; bladder nonpalpable. Symmetric, enlarged, nontender prostate without nodules. No discharge from penis.

Neuro: Anal sphincter is normal tone, normal perineal sensation.

CRITICAL THINKING

What tool might be useful to evaluate Stanley's symptoms?

What are the top three differential diagnoses in this case and why?

Which diagnostic tests are required in this case and why?

What are the concerns at this point?

What is the likely diagnosis?

What is the plan of treatment?

What are the plans for referral and follow-up care?

What health education should be provided to this patient?

Does the patient's psychosocial history impact how you might treat him?

Are there any standardized guidelines that should be used to treat this case? If so, what are they?

Section 8

General Adult Health

Case 8.1 Substance Use Disorder (SUD)

By Jason R. Lucey, DNP, FNP-BC

SUBJECTIVE

Chan Ming, a 26-year-old woman, presents with her partner requesting assistance to "get off pills." She reports a gradual progression from "partying" with alcohol and marijuana, starting at age 15, to using opioids, leading to a variety of legal and social problems. She has tried to quit on her own but experiences withdrawal symptoms (nausea, diarrhea, chills, runny nose, achiness).

Past medical history: Attention-deficit hyperactivity disorder (ADHD) (diagnosed at age 10), anxiety.

Past surgical history: Right knee anterior cruciate ligament repair (at age 24).

Family history: Father, age 48, is "alcoholic"; paternal uncle, age 43, has depression and has attempted suicide.

Social history: Chan Ming works at a local gym but recently lost her job due to repeated tardiness and absences. She was going to community college until about 6 months ago but stopped due to poor grades and financial restrictions. She used to smoke about 1 pack per day of cigarettes but transitioned to vaping nicotine pods about 3 months ago. She reports drinking alcohol (6–8 drinks) multiple days per week (Thursday–Sunday). She also reports near-daily cannabis use (smokes or vapes 1–2 "bowls" daily at night). For the past $2^1/_2$ years, she reports she has been taking "pills" (hydrocodone, oxycodone) daily. Initially, she was given prescriptions for these medicines due to knee pain and post-surgical pain but during a later visit, she reports that she is now purchasing them illicitly. She also reports that within the past month, she began snorting "heroin" (likely fentanyl, based on regional prevalence) because the price of pills was so high, and she was having severe withdrawal symptoms when she tried to cut back and stop on her own. She reports that when she finally admitted how often she was using these drugs and how she was unable to stop on her own, her partner became scared and insisted that they needed help.

Medications: Methylphenidate extended-release, 60 mg daily.

Allergies: NKDA.

The Family Nurse Practitioner: Clinical Case Studies, Second Edition. Edited by Leslie Neal-Boylan.
© 2021 John Wiley & Sons Ltd. Published 2021 by John Wiley & Sons Ltd.

OBJECTIVE

General: Chan Ming appears restless, irritable, and mildly diaphoretic.

Vital signs: Heart rate is 105 beats per minute. Blood pressure is 136/88 mmHG. Respiratory rate is nonlabored and 20 breaths per minute. Temperature is 98.7° F.

Skin: Mild diaphoresis (clammy skin) is present. There are no rashes, bruises, or areas of redness.

HEENT: Skull is normocephalic. Pupils are 3 mm, round, and reactive. Conjunctivae are moist. There is no icterus. There is mild rhinorrhea in both nares. Otherwise, the remaining HEENT exam is unremarkable.

Neck: There is no jugular venous distention, thyromegaly, or any palpable lymph nodes.

Cardiac: Mild tachycardia (rate 105) is present. Rhythm is regular. There is no murmur, rub, or gallop.

Respiratory: Lungs are clear to auscultation.

Abdomen: Abdomen is nontender. There is no hepatosplenomegaly.

Neurologic: Cranial nerves 2–12 are intact. Romberg sign is negative. Gait is smooth and coordinated.

CRITICAL THINKING

What are the top three differential diagnoses in this case and why?

Which diagnostic tests are required in this case and why?

What are the concerns at this point?

What are the options for the medicinal management of acute opioid withdrawal?

What are the three FDA-approved medicines for maintenance therapy for opioid use disorder (OUD) and which may be prescribed in primary care?

What are health promotion/health prevention/harm reduction topics that should be addressed with this patient?

What is the plan of treatment?

What are the plans for referral and follow-up care?

What health education should be provided to this patient?

What demographic characteristics might affect this case?

Does the patient's psychosocial history impact how you might treat him?

What if the patient lived in a rural (or urban) setting?

Are there any standardized guidelines that should be used to treat this case? If so, what are they?

What other professionals might you collaborate with to best provide comprehensive care for substance use disorder?

If you discovered that the patient was using substances intravenously, what other concerns/testing/treatment would you want to consider?

Case 8.2 Foot Ulcer

By Susan M. Jussaume, MSN, APRN, FNP-BC, AHN-BC

SUBJECTIVE

George is a 62-year-old gentleman presenting to primary care with complaints of newly developed right great toe pain with redness, swelling, and discharge. One week ago, while George was performing his routine foot care, he decided to remove a callus on the bottom of his right great toe. The callus had a lifted edge and the patient thought it would be better removed so as to not catch the skin and have it tear away. After gently pulling away the callus using tweezers George noted the skin underneath to be pink and intact. He reports the region where the callus had been removed was visibly indented slightly below the surrounding dermis.

Five days ago George began to develop tenderness and pain (6/10) on the underside of his right great toe with weightbearing and walking activity. George wrapped the toe with a gauze dressing in an effort to pad the great toe, thinking this would help him with pain management while he went about his daily activities. Three days ago, George noted increasing pain and redness in the right great toe and he now had a scant amount of blood-tinged discharge on the dressing when he took the dressing off that evening.

George continued with self-care, washing the affected great toe with antibacterial soap daily, applying a clean, dry gauze dressing during daytime hours and open to air at bedtime. The pain and redness continued and discharge was becoming more abundant. Now, George reports that within the past 24 hours his pain has increased to a 8/10, redness is extending to lateral regions of the great toe with swelling, and he notes the discharge during the evening dressing removal has changed to yellow and blood tinged. George, concerned about worsening symptoms, presents today for evaluation of the right great toe wound.

Family history: Heart disease: PGM, PGF, MGM, MGF, mother, father, and brother; peripheral vascular disease (PVD): mother, brother; hypertension: mother, brother; stroke and TIAs: mother; colon cancer: PGM; colitis: mother; ovarian cancer: mother; diabetes mellitus Type 2: MGM, mother; brain aneurysm: PGF.

Past medical history: Idiopathic thrombocytopenic purpura (ITP) (chronic type), diagnosed at age 33; low back pain (three herniated discs auto accident rear-ended) age 35; duodenal ulcer (resolved), diagnosed at age 40; diaphragmatic hernia, diagnosed at age 40; mixed hyperlipidemia, diagnosed

The Family Nurse Practitioner: Clinical Case Studies, Second Edition. Edited by Leslie Neal-Boylan.
© 2021 John Wiley & Sons Ltd. Published 2021 by John Wiley & Sons Ltd.

at age 48; diabetes mellitus Type 2, diagnosed at age 50; peripheral vascular disease, diagnosed at age 53; sleep apnea, diagnosed at age 53; heart disease (peripheral arterial disease and mild aortic stenosis), diagnosed at age 60.

Social history: George is 62 years old, married for 42 years, father of 4 adult children and grandfather of 4 grandchildren. He is a college graduate and has been employed 49 years in a professional, white-collar position. He has spent most of those years in an executive managerial position, working 40-plus hours weekly. There have been no known occupational hazards or chemical exposures. George is active in his community and a practicing Catholic who attends weekly services. His hobbies include fine woodworking and professional cooking. He says his interpersonal relationships are satisfying and supportive. George reports that his finances are very good; he lives an upper-middle-class lifestyle. George lives in a single-family home in a safe to moderately safe suburban neighborhood. He has never smoked. He rarely drinks alcohol and when he does, he drinks wine.

Medications:

- Atorvastatin, 80 mg one tablet PO at bedtime
- Irbesartan, 150 mg one tablet daily
- Lantus (insulin pen), 12 units SQ daily
- Metformin HCL, 1,000 mg one tablet PO twice a day with meals
- Torsemide, 20 mg one tablet daily every morning
- Potassium chloride ER, 20 MEQ two tablets daily every morning
- Epipen, as directed PRN for bee sting allergy/anaphylaxis
- Senna (stool softener), one tablet daily as directed
- Multivitamin (Centrum Silver), one tablet daily every morning
- Vitamin D3, 2,000 IU one tablet every morning with a meal
- Osteo Bi-Flex (glucosamine chondroitin), 750 mg two tablets daily
- Ultra CoQ10 (Qunol brand), 100 mg one soft gel daily
- Tylenol Extra Strength, 500 mg two tabs daily as needed for pain
- Kaprex (selective kinase response modulator), 350 mg one soft gel daily for low back pain

Allergies:

Prednisone/steroids (high doses cause significant muscle weakness).

Bee sting – Anaphylaxis – carries Epipen and has allergy notification in wallet.

No known food allergies.

Immunizations: Up to date.

OBJECTIVE

George is a well-developed, well-nourished adult male in no acute distress. He is dressed appropriately for the season with excellent hygiene. He is alert and oriented times three. George is engaging and interactive; his speech is clear and articulate. George's gait is steady, but he walks bearing weight on the outer edge of the right foot; his posture is upright.

Vital Signs:

Height: 6 ft 5 inches; weight: 298 lbs (BMI = 35.3); temperature: 98.9°F (temporal); pulse: 84/minute (apical) RRR; respirations: 16 BPM (breaths per minute); blood pressure: 118/72; pulse xx: 99% on room air; pain: 6/10 (foot pain/right great toe).

Integumentary: Intact without rashes or lesions; warm and dry. There are scattered varicosities on the legs bilaterally. There is brownish discoloration to the skin of the lower legs bilaterally, predominantly over the shins and dorsum aspects of the feet. There is no edema.

Right great toe: Plantar aspect of right great toe reveals broken skin integrity with a wound of 2.0 cm × 1.5 cm (length × width), a depth of 2–3 mm. There is a small amount of serosanguinous discharge, some yellow crusting on the edges of the wound; mild redness and swelling are noted on the lateral regions of the right great toe. The toe is warm and tender to palpation. The patient reports pain at 6/10 with passive and active ROM.

HEENT:

Eyes: PERRLA, EOMs intact, visual acuity grossly intact.

Ears: External canals patent, TMs pearly gray, intact. Hearing is intact to whispered voice 3 feet bilaterally.

Nares: Patent, pink mucosa intact; inferior turbinates visible, no discharge.

Throat: Oral mucosa pink, tongue well papulated, no lesions; no swelling or exudate in pharynx; teeth in good repair.

Respiratory/Thorax: Easy breathing, no use of accessory muscles, no retractions. Lungs clear throughout all fields, no crackles, no wheezes.

Cardiac: No lifts or heaves visible; S1, S2 RRR, without murmurs, clicks, gallops, or rubs.

PV: Pulses 2+ bilaterally (brachial, radial, dorsalis pedis, and posterior tibial).

Abdomen: Moderately protuberant, soft nontender throughout, tympany predominant, normoactive bowel sounds all 4 quadrants, no tenderness, Blumberg's negative, no guarding.

Musculoskeletal: Tenderness to palpation and moderate pain with ROM of right great toe joint. Full ROM of all major joints, upper and lower extremities

Neurological: Cranial nerves I–XII grossly intact, alert and oriented ×3, gait steady and balanced, alternating arm swings.

CRITICAL THINKING

Which diagnostic or imaging studies should be considered to assist with or confirm the diagnosis?
___CBC with differential
___HBA1c
___CMP
___Blood cultures
___X-ray (right foot)
___MRI (right foot)

Identify and explain three differential diagnoses.
___Diabetic foot ulcer
___Nonhealing skin wound with secondary bacterial infection
___MRSA infection
___Cellulitis with or without osteomyelitis

What is the plan of treatment?

Are there any standardized guidelines to consider?

What health education should be provided to the patient?

What complicating factors specific to this case should be considered?

What collaborative assessment and care might the patient require? Include your rationale.
___Referral to a wound specialist
___Referral to Podiatry
___Visiting nurse with a wound specialist nurse for follow-up with home care
___Orthopedic or physical therapy consult

Case 8.3 Abdominal Pain and Weight Gain

By Leslie Neal-Boylan, PhD, APRN, CRRN, FAAN, FARN

SUBJECTIVE

Annette, a 28-year-old female, presents to the primary care practice for an initial visit. She presents with two major concerns. First, she is concerned because she was told she had gallstones by ultrasound and was advised by another primary care provider (PCP) that she needed her gallbladder removed. She has had several bouts of abdominal pain and some dyspepsia, but no nausea, vomiting, diarrhea, or any other gastrointestinal symptoms. She points to an area in her abdomen that has been painful, especially when she eats high-fat foods. She has no other gastrointestinal complaints.

Her second complaint is weight gain. Her diet has not changed over the past few years; however, she has noticed a change in the way her clothes fit as well as a 15-pound increase in her weight over the past year. Also over the past year, she has had irregular menses. She often "skips months," and she reports 7 cycles of menstruation over the past year. When she does have her period, "it lasts for over 2 weeks." At one point she did not have a period for 3 months, and she thought that she might be pregnant. Her review of systems is negative except for increased hair growth across the sides of her face, her chin, and the middle of her chest, arms, and upper thighs, which she has had since she was an adolescent. She also complains of acne.

Further review of systems reveals no dizziness, no headache, no problems with her vision, no ringing in her ears; she is not short of breath. She has no complaints of cough, no palpitations, no chest pain. She has no genitourinary complaints. She has no musculoskeletal complaints. She has no weakness, no paresthesia, and no numbness or tingling of the extremities.

Past medical history: Noncontributory.

Past surgical history: None.

Family medical history: Annette's mother has Type 2 diabetes and hypertension. Her father died at age 50 due to lung cancer and had a positive smoking history. Her brother is alive and well at age 26, and her sister is alive and obese at age 22.

Social history: Annette was born in Brazil and reports no tobacco, alcohol, or substance abuse. She drinks 1 cup of coffee daily and lives at home with her mother, brother, and sister in a single-family home in a suburban town. She works full-time as an administrative assistant and is a

---

The Family Nurse Practitioner: Clinical Case Studies, Second Edition. Edited by Leslie Neal-Boylan.
© 2021 John Wiley & Sons Ltd. Published 2021 by John Wiley & Sons Ltd.

part-time student finishing a bachelor's degree in science at a state college. She has a network of friends and family and her hobbies include traveling and theater. She is currently in a sexual relationship with 1 partner and does not practice any form of contraception. Her LMP was 2 months ago, and her last Pap smear was 4 years ago and negative.

Medication and allergies: She has no medication allergies but reports allergies to pork and cats. She is not on any regular medications but takes Tylenol 2 tablets as needed for headache (approximately twice a week). Her immunizations are up to date.

OBJECTIVE

Vital signs are within normal limits with a blood pressure of 110/80 and a temperature of 98.2°F. Pulse is 76 and regular, and respiratory rate is 18. Height is 62 inches, and weight is 200 lbs (BMI 36.6). Annette is a well-developed, obese female who is in no acute distress. She is coherent, alert, and pleasant.

Skin: She has fine, dark hair on her chin and on the sides of her face. There is increased hair growth on her forearms, sternal area, and upper thighs. Acne is present on her forehead and lateral cheeks bilaterally.

Neck: Goiter, thyroid is palpable, nontender; no nodules are palpable or appreciated. Neck is supple and without lymphadenopathy.

Respiratory: Her lungs are clear, and the chest is symmetrical.

Cardiac: Regular heart rate and rhythm. S1 and S2 are present and normal.

Abdomen: Obese and soft; bowel sounds are present; and there is tenderness in the epigastric area. Liver and spleen are nonpalpable.

Musculoskeletal: Extremities are without edema. There is full range of motion and good strength. Carotid, femoral, dorsalis pedis, and post-tibial pulses are all +2.

Neurologic: DTRs are 2+ in the biceps, triceps, brachioradials, patella, and Achilles. Cranial nerves II–XII are grossly intact.

CRITICAL THINKING

Which diagnostic studies should be considered to assist with or confirm the diagnosis?
___Androgen elevation, testosterone level
___Lipids
___LH
___FSH
___Insulin level
___Urea breath test
___Serum *H. pylori*
___TSH, free T4
___LFTs
___HCG
___Vitamin D
___HIV

___Urinalysis
___Transvaginal ultrasound
___Abdominal ultrasound
___CBC with differential
___Metabolic panel
___Prolactin level
___DHEA

What are the most likely differential diagnoses and why?
___Gastroesophageal reflux disease (GERD)
___Cholecystitis
___*Helicobacter pylori* infection/peptic ulcer disease
___Polycystic ovarian syndrome (PCOS)
___Hypothyroidism
___Hyperprolactinemia

What is the plan of treatment?

Are any referrals or follow-up needed?

What if the patient had a positive pregnancy test?

What if the patient were trying to conceive?

Are there any standardized guidelines that should be used to assess or treat this case?

NOTE: The author would like to acknowledge Geraldine Marrocco, EdD, APRN, CNS, ANP-BC who write the case for the first edition of this book.

Case 8.4 Burning Leg Pain

By Antonia Makosky, DNP, MPH, ANP-BC, ANP

SUBJECTIVE

Robert is a 74-year-old gentleman who resides in an assisted living facility. He was referred today by the visiting nurse for evaluation of right leg pain and a new ulcer on the right lower extremity for the past week. The pain is worse when he has his feet up at night for sleep. He describes the pain as "burning," not associated with exercise. The pain improves if he dangles his legs at night. In the daytime, the pain is unchanged if he sits or stands. He is unable to walk very far and uses a walker. He reports having lower extremity swelling for several years.

Robert says he is feeling okay today. He reports chest pain "when I get upset about something" although not with exertion. He denies shortness of breath or palpitations. He reports urinary frequency and alternating constipation (most of the time) and diarrhea (if he takes too much medication for constipation). He is not sexually active.

Past surgical history: Aortic valve replacement

Past medical history: Notable for hypertension; he is a former smoker (40 pack-years). Robert has Type 2 diabetes mellitus, hyperlipidemia, mitral stenosis, atherosclerosis of the coronary arteries, carotid stenosis, atrial fibrillation, constipation, neuropathy of the left hand and both feet, lower extremity edema, and heart failure with preserved ejection fraction (HFpEF). Robert is obese. He ambulates with a walker.

Family history: Robert's father has hypertension and coronary artery disease; his mother and brother are both obese and have Type 2 diabetes mellitus.

Social history: Robert describes himself as having a learning disability. He worked as a garbage collector for many years. His brother visits him at the assisted living apartment building and helps with clothes shopping and other necessities. Robert is well known to visiting nurses for blood pressure checks and medication management. Robert denies alcohol or illicit or recreational drug use. He does not currently have a romantic partner. He enjoys his meals at the assisted living community.

Medications: Acetaminophen, aspirin, atorvastatin, docusate sodium, furosemide, gabapentin, lisinopril, insulin detemir (long acting), insulin lispro (short acting), metoprolol, multivitamin, miralax, ranitidine, warfarin.

Allergies: Oycodone: mental status change.

The Family Nurse Practitioner: Clinical Case Studies, Second Edition. Edited by Leslie Neal-Boylan.
© 2021 John Wiley & Sons Ltd. Published 2021 by John Wiley & Sons Ltd.

OBJECTIVE

General: Unshaven. Well developed, well nourished. Afebrile and in no distress.

Vital Signs: BP: 138/64; heart rate: 68 and regular; RR: 18 and regular; Temp: 97.7°F; SpO$_2$: 100%.

Skin: Tattoos are noted on upper and lower extremities. Lower extremities are almost hairless on the lower legs and feet.

HEENT: Head is normocephalic and nontender. Pupils are equal, round, and reactive to light; EOMs intact. Ear canals clear with TMs intact. Nares patent. Oropharynx is clear with no masses or exudate. Poor dentition.

Neck: Carotids with 2+ bruits bilaterally. No JVD. No lymphadenopathy. Thyroid nonpalpable.

Cardiovascular: AP 68, RRR. Mechanical click appreciated on auscultation. Upper extremity pulses 1+. Femoral pulse is palpable. Popliteal pulse difficult to palpate. Lower extremity pulses are nonpalpable.

Abdomen: Soft. Obese. Nontender. No bruits. Bowel sounds present. No AAA or organomegaly, although exam is limited due to body habitus.

Extremities: Lower legs with dependent rubor. 1 cm well-demarcated open ulcer on right lateral heel. Skin is cool and dry. No clubbing.

CRITICAL THINKING

Which diagnostic or imaging studies should be considered to assist with or confirm the diagnosis?
___Ankle brachial index (ABI)
___Toe brachial index (TBI)
___Exercise ABI
___Six-minute walk test
___Arterial duplex ultrasound
___Abdominal ultrasound

What is the most likely differential diagnosis and why?
___Venous insufficiency
___Venous stasis ulcer
___Peripheral artery disease
___Spinal stenosis
___Nerve root compression
___Diabetic neuropathy

What is the plan of treatment?

Are any referrals needed?

What are the differences between arterial and venous disease?

How should the clinician differentiate between venous ulcers and arterial ulcers?

Case 8.5 Difficulty Breathing

By Rebecca Hill, DNP, RN, FNP-C, CNE

SUBJECTIVE

Janis, a 59-year-old female, presents with tachypnea, dyspnea on exertion, and mild chest discomfort. She was diagnosed with emphysema 4 years ago and was placed on bronchodilator therapy. She has an 80 pack-year history of smoking. Janis states: "I feel short of breath when I walk, and my chest is sore." She describes her chest soreness as mild pressure, rated as 2 on a 1–10 scale. The pain is over the anterior thorax, more pronounced in the ribs, which she believes has developed from coughing hard. She states that she has had a nonproductive cough for 4 days and feels more fatigued than usual. She denies fever, chills, or recent international travel.

Past medical history: She has osteoarthritis in the hands and knees. She has a surgical history of appendectomy and cholecystectomy. In the past year, she has had 2 exacerbations of her COPD and has attempted to stop smoking, using nicotine gum replacement unsuccessfully.

Family history: Noncontributory.

Social history: She lives with her husband, who also smokes 2 packs of cigarettes per day, and cares for her elderly mother, who lives with them and is frail but ambulatory.

Medications: Albuterol MDI, 90 mcg/inhalation, 2 puffs as needed every 4–6 hours; ipratropium bromide MDI, 18 mcg/inhalation, 2 puffs 4 times/day; ibuprofen, 600 mg TID as needed for arthritic pain.

Allergies: Penicillins and cephalosporins (hives).

OBJECTIVE

General: Janis is dyspneic at rest, sitting. Use of accessory muscles evident, pursed lip breathing noted, able to speak in 3-word sentences.

Vital signs: BP: 122/64; P: 92; R: 26; T: 100.2°F; SpO2: 88%. AP to transverse ratio is 1:1.

Skin: Warm and dry.

The Family Nurse Practitioner: Clinical Case Studies, Second Edition. Edited by Leslie Neal-Boylan.
© 2021 John Wiley & Sons Ltd. Published 2021 by John Wiley & Sons Ltd.

HEENT: Negative.

Cardiovascular: RRR: S1/S2; no murmurs, clips, rubs, or gallops. No peripheral edema. Posterior tibial and dorsalis pedis pulses 2+/4.

Respiratory: Lungs have diffuse expiratory wheezing and crackles in the right upper lobe. Tenderness to palpation along intercostal spaces on right and left anterior and lateral thorax from 2nd to 5th intercostal spaces. PFT conducted 2 months prior to visit showed obstructive flow patterns and reduced FEV1/FVC.

Abdomen: Soft, with active bowel sounds in all quadrants.

CRITICAL THINKING

Which diagnostic or imaging studies should be considered to assist with or confirm the diagnosis?
___Spirometry
___Chest X-ray
___CBC
___ABGs
___ECG
___Echocardiogram
___CT of the chest

What is the most likely differential diagnosis and why?
___COPD exacerbation
___Pneumonia
___Asthma
___Pulmonary neoplasm

What is the plan of treatment?

What is the plan for follow-up care?

Are any referrals needed?

What additional risk factors are evident for this patient?

Are there any standardized guidelines that should be used to treat this patient?

NOTE: The author would like to acknowledge Kathy J. Booker, PhD, RN for her contribution to this case in the first edition of this book.

Case 8.6 Burning Epigastric Pain after Meals

By Leslie Neal-Boylan, PhD, APRN, CRRN, FAAN, FARN

SUBJECTIVE

Meredith is a 63-year-old female who presents with worsening epigastric pain. She describes it as burning pain that starts over the sternum and radiates upward to her neck. The pain occurs approximately 30–45 minutes after every meal and continues for about 4.5 hours thereafter. Heavy meals, coffee, and spicy foods make the discomfort worse; she is most uncomfortable when she lies down at night. She has to prop herself on 3 pillows every night to decrease the pain, so she refrains from eating close to bedtime. Meredith also describes a sour taste in her mouth when she lies down and has awakened occasionally with coughing and regurgitation. The pain has been worsening over the past 3 months and occurs daily. The discomfort interferes with her quality of life. She has had some mild relief with Maalox and Tums. Meredith also reports an intermittent nonproductive cough and feeling hoarse when she talks. She denies any fevers, chills, dysphagia, odynophagia, weight loss, fatigue, shortness of breath, abdominal pain, nausea, changes in bowel habits, blood in the stool, or urinary symptoms.

Past medical history: Hyperlipidemia.

Family history: Noncontributory.

Social history: Meredith has smoked ½ ppd for 30 years; drinks a bottle of wine by herself each Friday and Saturday night. She has a history of marijuana use when in college but none currently. She is widowed and works as an elementary school teacher.

Medications: HCTZ, 12.5 mg PO daily; Lipitor: 10 mg.

Allergies: Penicillin.

OBJECTIVE

General: Meredith is well appearing, in no apparent distress, and is moderately obese.

Vital signs: She is afebrile. BP is 160/100. HR is 86 and regular. Respirations are 14 and regular, and oxygen saturation is 96% on room air.

The Family Nurse Practitioner: Clinical Case Studies, Second Edition. Edited by Leslie Neal-Boylan.
© 2021 John Wiley & Sons Ltd. Published 2021 by John Wiley & Sons Ltd.

HEENT: Unremarkable except for some moderate erythema in the posterior pharynx and some dental erosion. Her teeth are stained, as well. There are no abscesses.

Neck: There is no cervical lymphadenopathy, and the thyroid is nonpalpable. Carotids are +2 without bruits.

Cardiac: Regular rate and rhythm without murmurs, clicks, gallops, or rubs.

Respiratory: Lungs are clear bilaterally.

Abdomen: Soft and obese without bruits; positive bowels sounds. There is mild epigastric tenderness on palpation but without rebound guarding. There is no organomegaly.

Rectal: Brown stool with a trace of positive on guaiac testing.

Skin: No rashes, lesions, or ulcers.

CRITICAL THINKING

What is the most likely differential diagnosis and why?
___Angina
___Myocardial infarction
___Gastroesophageal reflux disease (GERD)
___Gastric ulcer
___Duodenal ulcer
___Cholecystitis
___Gastrointestinal bleed

Which diagnostic studies should be considered to assist with or confirm the diagnosis?
___CBC with differential
___Metabolic panel
___Liver function tests
___Urinalysis
___ECG
___Chest X-ray
___*H. pylori* testing
___Endoscopy
___Colonoscopy
___FIT test
___Esophageal manometry and pH monitoring
___Lipids

What is the plan of treatment?

What is the plan for referrals and follow-up?

What are the patient's risk factors for this condition?

What are the possible complications of this condition?

Case 8.7 Chest Pain and Dyspnea without Radiation

By Rebecca Hill, DNP, RN, FNP-C, CNE, and Leslie Neal-Boylan, PhD, APRN, CRRN, FAAN, FARN

SUBJECTIVE

Zachary, a 60-year-old man, presents to the primary care office with sharp chest pain relieved by leaning forward. Zachary reports that he has had increasing chest pain over the past 3 days. His pain is rated as +5/10 and is accompanied by dyspnea, especially when walking. His pain is lessened by sitting upright and leaning forward. He has no radiation of the pain to his jaw, back, or arms. He denies cough or recent international travel. With the development of the dyspnea and a mild fever, he became worried and sought treatment.

Past medical history: Zachary has been well for the past 2 years, aside from a recent upper respiratory infection (2 weeks ago) and a history of gout.

Family history: His father died at age 58 of an MI. His mother had COPD and died at age 75.

Social history: He works as a commodities broker. He commutes to the city daily from out of state and is married and has 3 children, ages 16–25. He is a nonsmoker. He drinks 2–3 beers every evening.

Medications: Zachary is on allopurinol, 300 mg daily, for gout and takes ibuprofen regularly for joint stiffness and pain in his right elbow and both knees. He also takes a daily Ecotrin and supplemental glucosamine.

Allergies: No known allergies.

OBJECTIVE

General: Zachary is dyspneic at rest. He is completely upright and sitting forward on the exam table. His color is ashen.

Vital signs: BP: 142/94; P: 92; R: 28; T: 100.8°F. Height is 6 ft 4 inches. Weight is 247 lbs.

Skin: Cool and dry.

The Family Nurse Practitioner: Clinical Case Studies, Second Edition. Edited by Leslie Neal-Boylan.
© 2021 John Wiley & Sons Ltd. Published 2021 by John Wiley & Sons Ltd.

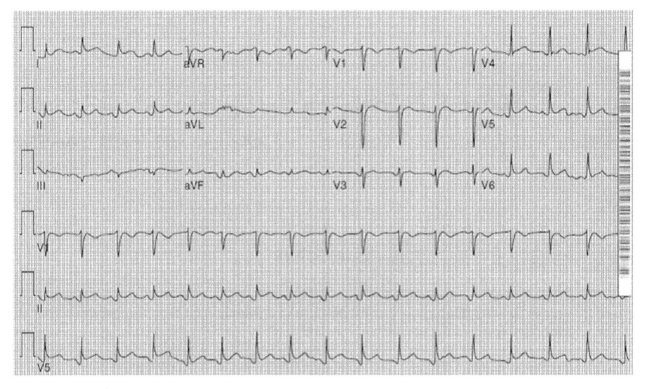

Figure 8.7.1 Zachary's ECG.

HEENT: Negative.

Cardiovascular: He has 6-cm jugular venous distention at 90 degrees. Heart tones: S1/S2 strong, with audible pericardial friction rub; no murmurs. He has trace ankle edema. Pedal and posterior tibial pulses are 1+/4.

Respiratory: CTA bilaterally.
    An ECG is obtained (Figure 8.7.1).

CRITICAL THINKING

Which diagnostic or imaging studies should be considered to assist with or confirm the diagnosis?
___Measure blood pressure for pulsus paradoxus
___Repeat ECG
___Echocardiogram
___CBC with differential
___Electrolytes
___ Lipids
___Blood glucose
___LFTs
___TSH
___BUN and creatinine
___PT and INR

___Urinalysis
___Sedimentation rate
___Serial troponins (stat, 12 and 24 hours)
___Cardiac catherization
___Chest X-ray
___Cardiac MRI

What is the most likely differential diagnosis and why?
___Acute myocardial infarction (MI)
___Pericarditis
___Infectious cardiomyopathy

What is the plan of treatment?

What is the plan for follow-up care?

Are any referrals needed?

What if this patient had recently sustained an acute myocardial infarction?

Are there any standardized guidelines that should be used to assess/treat this case?

NOTE: The author would like to acknowledge Kathy J. Booker, PhD, RN for her contribution to this case in the first edition of this book.

Case 8.8 Chest Pain with Radiation

By Rebecca Hill, DNP, RN, FNP-C, CNE

Oliver, a 48-year-old male, presents to the office with mild-to-moderate chest pressure with radiation to his back. Oliver reports that he was awakened from sleep at 7:00 a.m. with chest pressure, initially described as soreness across his anterior chest and through to his back. He rates his pain as +6/10. He felt as though, if he could just belch, he would feel better. He also reports a nonproductive cough for the past 2 days. His wife drove him to the office to be here when it opened at 9:00 a.m. She tried to convince Oliver to go to the emergency room, but he emphatically refused, insisting on going to the office first. Upon arrival to the office, Oliver is escorted to an examination room and the receptionist is instructed to call 911.

Past medical/surgical history: Diabetes mellitus Type 2. Oliver's last hemoglobin A1c 2 months ago was 7.4%.

Family history: He has a family history of premature coronary artery disease. His father died of acute myocardial infarction (AMI) at age 45. One brother died of AMI at age 49.

Social history: He has smoked for 25 years but has reduced his smoking to 1 pack per day since his brother's death 2 years ago. He has put on 25 pounds in the past 2 years and is generally sedentary.

Medications: Metformin, 500 mg once daily.

Allergies: Latex (anaphylaxis).

General: Oliver is anxious and shows Levine's sign as you enter the examination room. He is slightly diaphoretic. He took one oral aspirin (325 mg) on the way to the office.

Vital signs: BP: 192/96; P: 102; R: 22; T: 97.8°F. His SpO2 is 90%.

ECG: His ECG shows ST-segment depression and T-wave inversion in leads II and III.

The Family Nurse Practitioner: Clinical Case Studies, Second Edition. Edited by Leslie Neal-Boylan.
© 2021 John Wiley & Sons Ltd. Published 2021 by John Wiley & Sons Ltd.

Cardiovascular: His heart tones are muffled with an S3 gallop. His hands and feet are cool on palpation. Radial pulses are 2+. Pedal and posterior tibial pulses are 1+. He has jugular vein distention of 5 cm with head of bed at 90 degrees. He has no carotid bruits, heaves, or thrusts. His PMI is at the 5th ICS, left mid-clavicular line.

Respiratory: He has harsh rhonchi in the upper lobes bilaterally.

CRITICAL THINKING

What is the most likely differential diagnosis and why?
___Acute coronary syndrome
___Pulmonary embolism (PE)
___Gastroesophageal reflux

Which diagnostic or imaging studies should be considered to assist with or confirm the diagnosis?
___Electrocardiogram
___Troponin
___Hemoglobin and hematocrit
___Electrolytes
___BUN and creatinine
___Transfer to emergency services with cardiac catheterization

What is the plan of treatment?

Are any referrals needed?

Does the patient's family history impact how you might treat him?

What are the primary health education issues?

What if this patient were female?

What if the patient lived in a rural, isolated setting?

Are there any standardized guidelines that should be used to assess/treat this case?

NOTE: The author would like to acknowledge the contribution of Kathy J. Booker, PhD, RN to this chapter in the first edition of this book.

Case 8.9 Persistent Cough and Joint Tenderness

By Rebecca Hill, DNP, RN, FNP-C, CNE

SUBJECTIVE

Alice, a 42-year-old female, presents with a persistent dry cough and joint tenderness. She was treated for an upper respiratory infection 1 month ago with only slight improvement in upper respiratory symptoms. At the time of the onset of symptoms, she also had flu-like symptoms, including vomiting and chills, which have resolved. The cough persisted and the joint tenderness has worsened over the past week. She reports a low-grade fever and chills, and notes that both elbows are painful with any arm movement. She reports night sweats for 1 week duration. She has been taking ibuprofen, alternating with acetaminophen, every 4 hours. She has also noted gradual dyspnea with activities.

Past medical history: She has a history of breast cancer, treated with bilateral mastectomy and chemotherapy, and GERD.

Family history: Noncontributory.

Social history: She lives in a rural farming community in the Southeast.

Medications: Omeprazole 20 mg QD, ibuprofen 400–600mg Q8 hours PO PRN, and acetaminophen 650 mg Q6 hours PRN.

Allergies: No known allergies.

OBJECTIVE

General: Coughing.

Vital signs: BP: 122/64; P: 92; R: 26; T: 100.8°F.

Skin: Warm and dry.

HEENT: Negative.

Neck: No JVD or lymphadenopathy.

The Family Nurse Practitioner: Clinical Case Studies, Second Edition. Edited by Leslie Neal-Boylan.
© 2021 John Wiley & Sons Ltd. Published 2021 by John Wiley & Sons Ltd.

Cardiovascular Heart tones bounding; no thrills, rubs, or murmurs. No peripheral edema. All pulses 3+/4.

Respiratory: Bronchovesicular breath sounds audible over anterior chest; posterior breath sounds diminished. Course crackles audible in posterior bases. Harsh, nonproductive cough is evident during lung assessment.

Abdomen: Soft, with active bowel sounds.

Neuromuscular: Limited range of motion of elbow and wrist due to pain. Patellar deep tendon reflexes hyperactive bilaterally.

CRITICAL THINKING

Which diagnostic or imaging studies should be considered to assist with or confirm the diagnosis?
___Chest X-ray
___CBC
___ABGs
___X-ray
___MRI
___CT of chest

What is the most likely differential diagnosis and why?
___Pneumonia
___Bronchitis
___Tuberculosis
___Blastomycoses dermatitidis (BD)
___Osteomyelitis

What is the plan of treatment?

What further diagnostic tests are needed?

What is the plan for follow-up care?

Are any referrals needed?

Are there any standardized guidelines that should be used to assess/treat this case?

NOTE: The author would like to acknowledge Kathy J. Booker, PhD, RN for her contribution to this case in the first edition of this book.

Case 8.10 Morning Headache

By Leslie Neal-Boylan, PhD, APRN, CRRN, FAAN, FARN

Andrew is a 42-year-old African American male who presents with BP 168/92 and morning headaches. Andrew reports headaches upon arising approximately 2 times per week. This morning prompted his coming to the office for evaluation, as he felt some lightheadedness and chest tightness that resolved following his shower. He has never been told that his blood pressure was high, but he has not been seen in the office for 6 years. His last visit was for bronchitis and treatment with antibiotics.

Past medical/surgical history: He has no surgical history.

Family history: His father is deceased at age 65 from an acute MI; one brother died at age 50 with acute MI, following abdominal aortic aneurysm surgery. He has 4 other siblings in good health.

Social history: Andrew has been dealing with several life issues, including the death of a child and a reduction in his work hours at a local manufacturing plant. He smokes 2 packs of cigarettes per day, leads a sedentary life outside of work, and is overweight at 6 ft 2 inches and 255 pounds (BMI = 33). He reports generally good health. His smoking history is 44 years. He is married and has 3 remaining children, ages 12, 15, and 17. His oldest son was killed in a car accident 2 months ago. He drinks moderately, generally 2–3 beers 4–5 times per week. He reports drinking more heavily on the weekends. He and his wife are active in their church. He is a high school graduate and makes approximately $50,000 annually. His wife has a full-time position that supplements the family income to approximately $90,000. For the past 3 months, his business has experienced a downturn and there have been mandatory furlough days, which have required their family spending to be seriously curtailed, although they are able to meet their financial obligations at this time.

Medications: Andrew takes a daily aspirin and a multivitamin, but he is on no prescription medications at this time.

Allergies: No known allergies. He reports being lactose intolerant.

The Family Nurse Practitioner: Clinical Case Studies, Second Edition. Edited by Leslie Neal-Boylan.
© 2021 John Wiley & Sons Ltd. Published 2021 by John Wiley & Sons Ltd.

OBJECTIVE

General: Patient appears older than his stated age; frowning.

Vital signs: BP on arrival is 188/110. After 20 minutes, repeat BP is 180/90. P: 94; R: 20; T: 98.2°F.

HEENT: Cranial nerves intact. EENT exam negative.

Neck: No lymphadenopathy.

Skin: Skin warm and dry.

Respiratory: Lung sounds vesicular over peripheral fields; harsh, bronchial breath sounds in upper lobes bilaterally; moist cough audible; no adventitious breath sounds.

Cardiovascular: No jugular venous distention at 30 degree elevation. Heart sounds strong 3/4; grade 2/6 systolic murmur at left sternal border, 5th ICS. Abdominal and peripheral vascular assessments negative; pedal and post tibial pulses 2+/4+.

Abdomen: Tender over right upper quadrant. Tympany predominates. Liver border WNL, spleen and kidneys nonpalpable.

Neuromuscular: Romberg's sign negative; gait relaxed and symmetrical; no pronator drift. Full ROM all extremities.

CRITICAL THINKING

Which diagnostic studies should be considered to assist with or confirm the diagnosis?
___Electrocardiogram
___Troponin
___CBC
___Comprehensive metabolic panel
___Serum cholesterol panel

What is the most likely differential diagnosis and why?
___Obstructive sleep apnea
___Hypertension
___Dyslipidemia
___Cardiovascular disease
___Diabetes mellitus
___COPD

What is the plan of treatment?

What is the plan for referrals and follow-up care?

What if this patient were female?

What if this patient were also diabetic?

Are there any standardized guidelines that should be used to assess or treat this case?

NOTE: The author would like to acknowledge Kathy J. Booker, PhD, RN for her contribution to this case in the first edition of this book.

Case 8.11 Facial Pain

By Leslie Neal-Boylan, PhD, APRN, CRRN, FAAN, FARN

SUBJECTIVE

Henry, a 32-year-old male, presents with a report of facial pain for 5 days. He reports that he has a headache, especially when he bends down, and that his teeth hurt sometimes. On further questioning, Henry states that he had a cold about 14 days ago. He had rhinorrhea with clear drainage, mild sore throat, ear pressure, and mild headache. The symptoms cleared up after 1 week, and he felt fine, but then some of the symptoms returned about 5 days ago. Now he describes facial pain, headache upon waking, dental discomfort, and blood-streaked thick yellow nasal drainage. His sense of smell seems diminished. He has a history of seasonal allergic rhinitis.

Past medical history: Chicken pox at age 5 years; testicular torsion at age 15 years (no complications).

Family history: His family is well, although his mother and sister have migraine headaches.

Social history: He is happily married with 2 children. Henry works as a supermarket manager, is a nonsmoker, and denies other substance use.

Medications: Advil sinus with no relief.

Allergies: Seasonal hay fever.

OBJECTIVE

General: NAD.

Vital signs: Henry is 6 ft 1 inch tall and weighs 165 pounds. His oral temperature is 99.5°F. BP is 128/84. Pulse is 74 and regular. Respirations are 12 and regular.

HEENT: Sclera are clear; PERRLA; EOMs intact. Tympanic membranes are clear and intact; there is no fluid. There is tenderness to palpation of the frontal and maxillary sinuses. Nares are erythematous and swollen. There is no obvious discharge. Attempts to transilluminate the sinuses

---

The Family Nurse Practitioner: Clinical Case Studies, Second Edition. Edited by Leslie Neal-Boylan.
© 2021 John Wiley & Sons Ltd. Published 2021 by John Wiley & Sons Ltd.

indicate an absence of light. There is cobblestoning in the throat, but no erythema. Tonsils are +2. There are no exudates.

Neck: There is no lymphadenopathy, and the thyroid is nonpalpable.

Cardiac: RRR, S1/S2; no murmurs, clicks, gallops, or rubs.

Respiratory: Clear to auscultation.

CRITICAL THINKING

Which diagnostic studies should be considered to assist with or confirm the diagnosis?
___CT scan of sinuses
___X-ray of sinuses
___CT scan of brain
___CBC
___CMP
___None

What is the most likely differential diagnosis and why?
___Viral upper respiratory infection (URI)
___Acute sinus infection
___Asthma
___Migraine
___Allergic rhinitis
___Nonallergic rhinitis
___Vasomotor rhinitis
___Rhinitis medicamentosa

What is the plan of treatment?

What is the plan for referrals and follow-up treatment?

Is the family history of migraines relevant?

Case 8.12 Fatigue, Confusion, and Weight Loss

By Leslie Neal-Boylan, PhD, APRN, CRRN, FAAN, FARN

SUBJECTIVE

Maryanne, a 78-year-old female widow, presents to the primary care clinic with the chief complaint of feeling very tired lately. She also complains of some nasal congestion. She arrives with her daughter, who provides some gaps in the medical history. The daughter notes that Maryanne's fatigue has been a complaint for about 16 months.

Further review of systems provided by the daughter reveals a concern that her mother seems to have slight confusion, increased fatigue, poor appetite, and a bitter taste sensation when eating. Maryanne eats 3 small meals daily, and she's had some unintentional weight loss over the past few months. She reports a marked decrease in energy level. She denies nausea, vomiting, or emotional lability. She does not eat red meat.

Past medical history: Significant for hypertension for many years; Type 2 diabetes mellitus that is not well controlled on oral meds; high cholesterol for many years; lymphedema in lower extremities bilaterally since adolescence; benign lung densities per chest X-ray; and a report of "Mediterranean anemia." She had cataract removal surgery 5 years ago. She sees a podiatrist every 3 months and sees a retinologist periodically. Her last visit was today, and her exam was negative.

Family history: Her mother died at age 81 with diabetes and hypertension. Her father died of lung cancer. She has two brothers, ages 81 and 83, both with hypertension and one with prostate cancer.

Social history: Maryanne was born in California and has 4 children; does not use tobacco currently; quit smoking over 20 years ago. She denies alcohol use or history of other substance use. She does not drink coffee and does not exercise. Her typical day includes watching television and doing housework. She lives independently in an adult community in Alabama and has a homemaker 3 times weekly. She is a retired cook. She has 1 daughter who lives nearby.

Allergies: No known drug allergies and is up to date on her immunizations.

Skin: Complains of dry skin.

The Family Nurse Practitioner: Clinical Case Studies, Second Edition. Edited by Leslie Neal-Boylan.
© 2021 John Wiley & Sons Ltd. Published 2021 by John Wiley & Sons Ltd.

HEENT: Denies any dizziness or blurry vision. No headaches except for + right ear pain. Sometimes has difficulty swallowing.

Cardiovascular: Denies chest pain or palpitations.

Respiratory: Occasional cough and has noticed more shortness of breath recently. Sleeps on 2 pillows.

Gastrointestinal: Denies abdominal pain or bloating. She does not have any regurgitation. No nausea or vomiting. She has a bowel movement daily that is normal, brown in color, and normal consistency. She does not report any blood in her stool.

Musculoskeletal: Reports joint pain in her knee, especially her left knee.

Psyche: Generally happy, social, but most recently not engaged due to fatigue and weakness.

Medications:

- Glucophage, 1,000 milligrams twice daily
- Avandia, 4 mg daily
- Protonix, 40 mg daily
- Glucotrol, 10 mg daily
- Aricept, 10 mg daily at night
- Cardia, 240 mg daily in morning
- Lisinopril, 10 mg daily
- Diovan, 160/12.5 BID
- Aspirin, 81 mg daily
- Crestor, 5 mg daily
- Zetia, 10 mg daily
- Coreg, 12.5 mg BID
- Lasix, 20 mg daily
- Potassium, 10 mEq daily
- Actonel, 35 mg weekly
- Multivitamin, over the counter
- B12
- Tylenol, as needed for pain

OBJECTIVE

General: Maryanne is a 78-year-old female who is pleasant, slightly confused, and moderately anxious. Her daughter is present during the visit. The patient defers to her daughter for clarification of events and details. Daughter and mother have a positive working relationship with evidence of support and caring.

Vital signs: T: 98.2°F; P: 86; RR: 28; SaO$_2$: 93; B/P: 140/70. Her weight is 191 pounds, and her height is 64 inches.

Skin: Clear, slightly grayish color.

HEENT: Hair thinning, gray at roots, silky texture. Sclera nonicteric, pupils dilated since she just came from the retinologist (examination of her eyes deferred). Oral mucosa, pink moist intact.

Neck: Supple, no JVD, no bruits. Thyroid nonpalpable. No lymphadenopathy.

Cardiovascular: Heart regular rate and rhythm. PMI is at 5th intercostal space left sternal border; + systolic murmur II/VI. Pulses positive all extremities. There is bilateral lower leg edema; chronic lymphedema; no ulcerations; skin intact; no hair growth; no pitting.

Respiratory: Lungs clear to auscultation. Transverse/AP diameter 2/1.

Abdomen: BS+, obese, soft, nontender. No hepatomegaly; no splenomegaly; no hernia.

Neurological: CN I–XII grossly intact. Mental status 30/30 (Folstein Mini Mental Status Exam).

Geriatric depression screen: No evidence of depression.

Musculoskeletal: Walks with a cane; s/p right knee replacement 9 years ago. Full range of motion; no deformities; muscle strength appropriate for age.

CRITICAL THINKING

Which diagnostic studies should be considered to assist with or confirm the diagnosis?
___CBC
___FBS
___CMP
___HbA1c
___TSH
___Ultrasound
___Urea breath test
___Iron studies

What is the most likely differential diagnosis and why?
___Chronic kidney disease
___Anemia (type?)
___COPD
___Obstructive sleep apnea
___Dementia
___Depression
___Gastric ulcer

What is the plan of treatment?

What is the plan for referrals and follow-up care?

Are there standardized guidelines that should be used to assess or treat this case?

NOTE: The author would like to acknowledge Geraldine F. Marrocco , EdD, APRN, CNS, ANP-BC for her contribution to this case in the first edition of this book.

Case 8.13 Hand Numbness

By Leslie Neal-Boylan, PhD, APRN, CRRN, FAAN, FARN

SUBJECTIVE

Timothy is a right-hand dominant, 45-year-old Caucasian male. He presents with a complaint of intermittent "right-hand numbness." He first noticed the numbness about 8 months ago, but it was so slight that he thought nothing of it. Some mornings he wakes up with tingling in his right arm. He then shakes his hand, and the tingling goes away. He now complains of sharp, shooting pains going up his right arm over the past month; and last week, he dropped his hammer a few times while working. He denies any redness, swelling, weakness, or recent trauma to his right hand. He denies symptoms in his left hand.

Past medical history: He dislocated his right shoulder playing basketball in high school. He occasionally has lower back pain and knee pain from all the sports he did in high school. He denies history of arthritis or fractures to the hands, arms, or neck.

Family history: His mother is 67 years old and has a history of hypothyroidism and osteoarthritis. She was diagnosed with hypothyroidism at age 45 and is being treated with levothyroxine on a daily basis. His father is 70 years old and had a stroke at age 50. After extensive rehabilitation, his father exhibits few deficits. His sister is 48 years old and obese with diabetes mellitus Type 2. Timothy denies a family history of rheumatoid arthritis, osteoarthritis, gout, or carpal tunnel syndrome.

Social history: Timothy is a carpenter by trade. He owns a furniture repair business. He is right-hand dominant. He is married to a schoolteacher and lives in a house that he built in the country. He states he makes a decent living and is very concerned with his right hand, as this will impact his livelihood. He has smoked about ½ to 1 pack of cigarettes per day for the past 15 years. He has tried to quit many times but has been unsuccessful. He drinks about a six-pack of beer on the weekends.

Medications: He takes ibuprofen, 200 mg, 2–3 tablets, every few days for knee and back pain. Otherwise, he denies use of any prescription, supplemental, or herbal medications.

Allergies: He reports he gets a nonitchy rash when he takes amoxicillin. He can take penicillin without any problems. He denies any known allergies to food, latex, or the environment.

The Family Nurse Practitioner: Clinical Case Studies, Second Edition. Edited by Leslie Neal-Boylan.
© 2021 John Wiley & Sons Ltd. Published 2021 by John Wiley & Sons Ltd.

OBJECTIVE

General: Timothy is a slightly overweight male, sitting comfortably, in no apparent distress.

Vital signs: Blood pressure: 135/80; pulse: 64 and regular; respirations: 14; temperature: 98.6°F; height: 5 ft 10 inches; weight: 180 lbs; BMI: 25.

Skin: Pale pink without rashes, lesions, or ulcers.

Respiratory: Clear without wheezes or crackles.

Cardiac: S1/S2 intact without murmurs, rubs, or gallops.

Peripheral vascular: Skin pink, warm, and dry without edema, lesions, or ulcers. Brachial, radial, and ulnar pulses 2+ equal and strong bilaterally. Nailbeds pink with capillary refill <2 seconds bilaterally.

Musculoskeletal: Neck with full range of motion (FROM) without pain. Vertebral column in "S" shape without deformity or tenderness to palpation or percussion. No pain, tingling, or numbness with compression of the head onto the cervical neck. Shoulders and elbows aligned with FROM bilaterally, without erythema, swelling, bruising, deformity, crepitus, or pain. Muscle strength 5/5. Forearms, wrist, and hands symmetrical without erythema, swelling, bruising, or deformity bilaterally. Palms without thenar wasting with FROM intact bilaterally. Hand grip strength 5/5 bilaterally. Right thumb abduction strength 4/5; left 5/5.

Neurological: Wrist and hands: Right wrist with pain first and second digit with direct compression of right median nerve; positive Phalen's test with pain and numbness. Negative Tinel's test. Sensation to light touch and 2-point discrimination intact in forearm and fingers equal bilaterally. Deep tendon reflexes: triceps, biceps, brachioradialis, patella, Achilles 2+ bilaterally.

CRITICAL THINKING

What are the three most likely differential diagnoses and why?
___Amyotrophic lateral sclerosis
___Multiple sclerosis
___Carpal tunnel syndrome
___CVA
___Pronator syndrome
___Osteoarthritis

Which diagnostic or imaging studies should be considered to assist with or confirm the diagnosis?
___CBC
___Metabolic panel
___FBG
___TSH
___X-ray of wrists
___Nerve conduction velocity studies (NCV)
___Electromyography (EMG)
___MRI of neck
___X-ray of elbows
___X-ray of neck

What is the plan of treatment?

What is the plan for referrals and follow-up?

What specific activities do you want to ask about?

What other important history questions must you ask so as not to miss an important differential diagnosis?

Why do you inspect for thenar atrophy?

Would your diagnosis change if Timothy complained of acute onset of paresthesias of the upper arm?

Why would you be concerned if Timothy's pain were past his elbows?

What significance does thumb strength have?

When would you consider referring Timothy?

What would you do if this patient were female and pregnant?

Are there any standardized guidelines available to be used to assess or treat this case?

Case 8.14 Chronic Diarrhea

By Clara M. Gona, PhD, FNP-BC, RN, and Leslie Neal-Boylan, PhD, APRN, CRRN, FAAN, FARN

SUBJECTIVE

Amelia, a 25-year-old Caucasian female, presents to the primary care clinic with the chief complaint of abdominal bloating and diarrhea, worsening over the past 2–3 months. Amelia reports that she thinks she has lost weight during that time. Occasionally she comes to the clinic for acute illnesses. Her last visit was almost a year ago with flu-like symptoms. She goes to her gynecologist annually and considers this her routine health maintenance; her last visit was 6 months ago with no significant findings. She has a self-described long history of nonspecific gastrointestinal malaise. She feels nauseous and bloated and has inconsistent voiding patterns with a tendency toward loose stools. Over the past 2 months, however, more than 60% of her stools have been loose, double the usual. She has not noticed any change in her voiding pattern. Generalized abdominal bloating has been increasing in frequency and intensity, now occurring 4–5 times per week, generally 1 hour after eating. There is associated generalized cramping and pain that she rates as a 6/10, though she is in no pain right now. She has vomited 3 times in as many weeks without resolution of symptoms. The patient denies making herself vomit. She reports that she had to leave work numerous times because of the pain and discomfort. Lying down and applying heat make her symptoms more tolerable, but this is an unsustainable management technique; she is worried and frustrated. She has not done any recent traveling.

Past medical and surgical history: Allergic rhinitis.

Family history: Mother and father are alive and well, both with hypertension. Brother, 20, is alive and well with Type 1 diabetes, which he manages well.

Social history: Amelia is a college graduate currently working 50 hours per week for a community development nonprofit organization. She loves her job and sleeps well—though admittedly not enough—usually 6 or 7 hours per night. She goes to the gym for an hour 3–4 times per week, has an active social life, is applying to graduate school, and is generally pleased with her life. If she could change anything, "I'd add a couple hours to the day so I could slow down a little and still get things done. I'm pretty type A, which is why this stomach thing is bothering me so much." She drinks 2–3 cups of coffee a day; skips breakfast; eats a bagel, yogurt, and fruit for lunch; and usually goes out or eats "healthy" takeout for dinner. She drinks socially ~1 time per week, but denies tobacco or other drug use.

The Family Nurse Practitioner: Clinical Case Studies, Second Edition. Edited by Leslie Neal-Boylan.
© 2021 John Wiley & Sons Ltd. Published 2021 by John Wiley & Sons Ltd.

Medications: Lo Ovral, daily (birth control); multivitamin daily; OTC Claritin, 1 tab PRN for allergy symptoms; OTC Mucinex, PRN for cold symptoms.

Allergies: Seasonal. No known drug or food allergies.

Screening and immunizations: Routine blood work last year WNL, but showed borderline iron deficient anemia. Negative Pap smear last year. She is up to date on immunizations including the HPV series.

OBJECTIVE

General: Well-developed and well-nourished but thin, 25-year-old female who looks her stated age. She is in no acute distress.

Skin: Rash on the elbows and extensor surface of the arms.

HEENT: Unremarkable.

Neck: No lymphadenopathy.

Respiratory: Chest, clear to auscultation.

Cardiac: Regular sinus rhythm. No ectopy.

Abdominal: Symmetrical, nondistended, positive BS; nontender; no organomegaly.

CRITICAL THINKING

Which diagnostic studies should be considered to assist with or confirm the diagnosis?
___CBC
___Comprehensive metabolic panel
___TSH
___Tissue transglutaminase antibodies, IgA
___Duodenal biopsy
___Bone mineral density
___Endoscopy
___Skin biopsy
___EMA
___anti-tTG

What is the most likely differential diagnosis and why?
___Irritable bowel syndrome (IBS)
___Celiac disease
___Inflammatory bowel disease (IBD)

What are other possible differential diagnoses?

What is the plan of treatment?

What is the plan for referrals and follow-up?

Are there standardized guidelines or resources that would help in this case?

What demographic characteristics might affect this case?

If this patient had no insurance or lived in a rural area without access to health care (difficult to get to a clinic), how would that change management, or would it change management?

NOTE: The author would like to acknowledge the contribution to this case of Geraldine F. Marrocco, EdD, APRN, CNS, ANP-BC in the first edition of this book.

Case 8.15 Intractable Pain

By Leslie Neal-Boylan, PhD, APRN, CRRN, FAAN, FARN

SUBJECTIVE

Roger, a 43-year-old male, presents to the primary care clinic with the chief complaint of intractable pain. Six months ago, Roger was riding a motorcycle when he was hit by a car and thrown. His right leg was severed below the knee, and he had extreme facial injuries. At the hospital, leg reattachment surgery was unsuccessful; so an above-the-knee amputation was done. He was transferred to a level I trauma center, where he was intubated and trached during his 3-week hospitalization. He is now walking with crutches at home; he does not yet have prosthetics. His nose was fractured and repaired.

He complains of leg pain that is extremely severe and uncontrollable. He reports being "at his wit's end" because nothing is treating his pain. While in the hospital, he was prescribed Percocet for pain; but at the moment he is using over-the-counter analgesics with no effect.

Past medical and surgical history: Significant for esophageal fundoplication for severe GERD five years ago.

Family history: Both parents are alive and well, ages 70 (mother) and 75 (father). His mother has hypertension, and his father has dyslipidemia. He is an only child.

Social history: He reports drinking 2–3 beers weekly and smoking 1 pack of cigarettes daily. He does not use any street drugs. He works as a parcel-delivery truck driver, but he is now on disability from work and collecting unemployment. He lives at home with his wife and 2 small children.

Medications: Ibuprofen, 600 mg every 4 hours for pain; Tylenol, 650 mg every 6 hours for pain.

Allergies: He has no known drug, food, or environmental allergies; and his immunizations are up to date.

The Family Nurse Practitioner: Clinical Case Studies, Second Edition. Edited by Leslie Neal-Boylan.
© 2021 John Wiley & Sons Ltd. Published 2021 by John Wiley & Sons Ltd.

OBJECTIVE

General: Trying to smile, but obviously in pain. Alert, with a child-like stoic look on his face.

Vital signs: T: 97.8°F; P: 76; RR: 18; B/P: 120/84. His weight was not checked as he could not stand and be stable on the scale.

Skin: Good color, no lesions.

HEENT: Obvious facial deformity with missing teeth. Fullness under right eye where plate was placed surgically. Severed palate is healing.

Neck: No lymphadenopathy. Thyroid nonpalpable. Tracheotomy wound healing.

Cardiovascular: Regular rate and rhythm. S1 and S2 are normal.

Respiratory: Chest is clear to auscultation.

Abdomen: Soft, nontender, and bowel sounds are present.

Musculoskeletal: Full range of motion in upper extremities. Stump is wrapped with an Ace bandage. Upon inspection, the incision is clean and well healed. There is no edema.

Genital: He has normal genitalia. There is no evidence of swelling. His testicular exam is normal, and there is appropriate hair growth.

CRITICAL THINKING

Which diagnostic studies should be considered to assist with or confirm the diagnosis? If you choose imaging studies, state what part of the body you will image.
___X-ray
___MRI
___CT scan
___CBC
___CMP

What is the most likely differential diagnosis and why?
___Phantom limb pain
___Neuropathic pain
___Chronic pain related to trauma

What is the plan of treatment?

What is the plan for referrals and follow-up?

Are there standardized guidelines or resources that would help in this case?

NOTE: The author would like to acknowledge the contribution of Geraldine F. Marrocco, EdD, APRN, CNS, ANP-BC to this case in the first edition of this book.

Case 8.16 Wrist Pain and Swelling

By Leslie Neal-Boylan, PhD, APRN, CRRN, FAAN, FARN

SUBJECTIVE

Rosa, a 29-year-old Latina woman, presents for evaluation of wrist pain and swelling. She developed symptoms about 3 months ago and has noted progressive worsening since that time. In addition, she has tenderness across the balls of her feet with any weight bearing. The pain is worse when she is inactive and improves with activity. The symptoms have significantly impacted her ability to perform her job as a receptionist in a busy office. She denies any recent trauma to her hands or feet or other joint pain.

She notes stiffness in the feet and ankles as well as 4 hours of overall morning stiffness that improves only marginally for the rest of the day. She has noted increased fatigue and weakness in the last few months. She often naps when she gets home from work and has curtailed her social activities significantly. Rosa denies fever, chills or other systemic symptoms. Rosa denies dry eyes or dry mouth, changes in her vision, neck or shoulder stiffness, chest pain or difficulty breathing. She denies ever having previous episodes of these symptoms. Rosa denies any rashes, lesions or ulcers, any changes in her hair, skin or nails, any polyuria, polydipsia, or polyphagia. She does not recall being bitten by any insects recently and spends most of her time indoors. Rosa denies any weight loss, history of pregnancy or any memory changes. She is not aware of having any recent infection, nor has she experienced any problems with her bowel or bladder function. She denies numbness or tingling in any part of her body.

Past medical history: None.

Family history: No family history of any inflammatory or autoimmune disease, except for a cousin with systemic lupus erythematosus.

Social history: Rosa is single, but several family members live nearby. She barely supports herself without assistance, but her parents occasionally give her money for extras. She denies a history of smoking or drug use. She drinks with friends on the weekends, consuming 1–2 mixed drinks or beers on Friday and Saturday evenings. She states that she is generally happy but would like to settle down with someone in a monogamous relationship. She verbalizes her fear of having a serious disease during the visit today.

Medications: Rosa takes only birth control pills and a multivitamin daily.

The Family Nurse Practitioner: Clinical Case Studies, Second Edition. Edited by Leslie Neal-Boylan.

OBJECTIVE

General: Rosa appears to be in no apparent distress.

Vital signs: Rosa weighs 110 lbs, and her height is 63 inches. She has an oral temperature of 100 degrees Fahrenheit. BP is 120/70. HR is 64 and regular. Respiratory rate is 12 and regular.

HEENT: Her head is normocephalic and nontender. There are no scalp lesions or apparent alopecia. PERRLA, with EOMs intact. Sclerae are clear without visible scleritis. There is no malar rash or any lesions or ulcers on her face or buccal mucosa.

Neck: There is no cervical or other lymphadenopathy. Her thyroid is nonpalpable. CNs II–XII are grossly intact.

Cardiac: The cardiac exam reveals RRR S1/S2 with no murmurs, clicks, gallops, or rubs.

Respiratory: Lungs are clear bilaterally.

Skin: The skin is clear.

Abdomen: Soft without organomegaly, tenderness, or bruits.

Neuromuscular: There is moderate synovitis (swelling) of the MCP and PIP joints bilaterally and of the MTP joints bilaterally. The patient has limited ROM of the UE and LE digits due to pain. There are no nodules noted on any extremity. The Phalen's, Finkelstein's, and Tinel's tests are negative. There is no warmth or redness of any joint. DTRs are +2 throughout.

CRITICAL THINKING

What is the most likely differential diagnosis and why?
___Osteoarthritis
___Rheumatoid arthritis
___Systemic lupus erythematosus
___Carpal tunnel syndrome
___Sjögren's syndrome

Which diagnostic studies should be considered to assist with or confirm the diagnosis?
___Rheumatoid factor
___ESR
___CRP
___CCP
___ANA, C3, and C4
___Anti-DS DNA
___CMP
___CBC
___HLA-B27
___SS-B
___SS-A
___Imaging studies

What is the plan of treatment?

What is the plan for referrals and follow-up?

Would the primary diagnosis be different if the patient were 55 years old?

Would there be treatment considerations if the patient had a history of tuberculosis?

Section 9

Mental Health

Case 9.1 Sad Mood

By Sheila Swales, MS, RN, PMHNP-BC

SUBJECTIVE

Julia is an 18-year old college student of Hispanic descent who presents with "sad mood": episodes of unexplained tearfulness, low energy, difficulty concentrating, increased appetite, and hypersomnia (sleeping 10–12 hours per night). She reports experiencing these symptoms throughout the day and that they have persisted for the past 5–6 weeks. Julia reports that she has fallen behind in her coursework and is at risk of failing two classes. She has been less engaged socially and reports missing a recent gathering to celebrate her best friend's birthday because she couldn't motivate herself to shower and get dressed for the occasion. She admits that she no longer feels comfortable in most of her clothes due to a recent weight gain of 8 pounds. She denies any precipitating stressors but discloses that adjusting to college life and living away from her family have been more difficult than she anticipated. She misses the support and structure of family life. Julia denies experiencing suicidal ideation. Her PHQ-9 score is 19 and she indicates that symptoms have made it "very difficult" for her to engage academically and socially. Julia states that she may have been a little depressed during her junior year of high school when a close friend abruptly distanced himself and stopped returning her calls. She has never sought treatment for depressive symptoms or any other mental health issues.

Past medical history: Julia has no history of seizures or traumatic brain injuries.

Family history: Julia's mother is being treated for hypertension and depression.

Social history: Julia was raised in an intact family. She has close relationships with her parents and two younger siblings. She has friends, including her best friend, Amelia. She reports no current or past history of romantic relationships. Julia enjoys watching old movies and spending time outdoors in nature. She exercises several times per week. Julia describes herself as "not religious." She denies using alcohol, nicotine, or other substances.

Medications: None.

Allergies: No known allergies.

The Family Nurse Practitioner: Clinical Case Studies, Second Edition. Edited by Leslie Neal-Boylan.
© 2021 John Wiley & Sons Ltd. Published 2021 by John Wiley & Sons Ltd.

OBJECTIVE

General: Cooperative, appears tense with mildly pressured speech and psychomotor agitation.

Vital signs: BP: 118/76; P: 80; R: 20; T: 98.6°F; height: 5 feet 4 inches; weight: 142 lbs; BMI: 24.4.

HEENT/Neck: There is no JVD.

Cardiovascular: There is a 2+ carotid, no bruit. Regular rate and rhythm, S1 and S2.

Respiratory: Lungs are clear to auscultation and percussion.

Musculoskeletal: Full range of motion of the neck and trunk. Abdomen is soft, nontender, and nondistended. Extremities show no edema, clubbing, or cyanosis.

CRITICAL THINKING

What are the top three differential diagnoses in this case and why?

Which diagnostic tests are required in this case and why?

What are the concerns at this point?

What are 3–5 case-specific questions to ask?

What is the plan of treatment?

What are the plans for referral and follow-up care?

What health education should be provided to this patient?

What demographic characteristics might affect this case?

Does the patient's psychosocial history impact how you might treat her?

What if the patient lived in a rural (or urban) setting?

Are there any standardized guidelines that should use to treat this case?

Case 9.2 More Than Depression

By Sara Ann Jakub, MA, SYC, LPC, and Anna Goddard, PhD, APRN, CPNP-PC

SUBJECTIVE

Marc is a 19-year-old Hispanic male, and a senior in high school. Marc presents to the school-based health center for a routine physical exam. The Patient Health Questionnaire (PHQ-2) administered to Marc at the start of the physical reveals a reported feeling of hopeless nearly all the time. Marc denies loss of interest in activities but reports calling out sick from his part-time after-school job several times a month. The school reports a high number of school absences and grades shifting from Bs to Ds during this marking period.

Past medical history: Early childhood onset asthma, history of obesity in childhood, history of self-injurious behavior (SIB) in the form of superficial scratching skin with use of fingernails.

Family history: Maternal history is positive for heart disease, high blood pressure, episodic depression, and alcohol and tobacco dependence. First-degree relative (maternal side) positive for migraine headaches. Paternal history is unknown.

Social history: Marc denies current use of drugs or alcohol. He is the oldest of 4 children, father unknown, with early childhood exposure to domestic violence (DV) between mother and boyfriend, episodes of housing insecurity (multiple moves between friends' homes and stays at motels), mother works 3 jobs to provide for family, resulting in the patient providing supervision to his younger siblings.

Sleep history: Difficulty initiating sleep with frequent waking throughout night, denies nightmares; average 5–6 hours per night per personal fitness tracker (Fit-Bit) recording.

Medications: Albuterol MDI .083% inhaler PRN; Xopenex (nebulizer) PRN wheeze, Cetirizine 10 mg QD.

Allergies: Environmental allergies, allergy-induced eczema, penicillin.

Review of Systems:

HEENT: Ongoing congestion, no changes in hearing, no vision changes, wears glasses.

Skin: No rashes.

The Family Nurse Practitioner: Clinical Case Studies, Second Edition. Edited by Leslie Neal-Boylan.
© 2021 John Wiley & Sons Ltd. Published 2021 by John Wiley & Sons Ltd.

Cardiovascular: No shortness of breath, no chest pain, no history of cardiac anomalies, no murmurs.

Respiratory: No shortness of breath, last used inhaler over 6 months ago, last nebulizer use unknown.

Gastrointestinal: No nausea, vomiting, or diarrhea, no constipation, loss of appetite.

Genitourinary: No increased frequency of pain or increased urination.

Muscoskeletal: No swelling or joint tenderness.

Heme: Denies easy bruising.

OBJECTIVE

General: The patient appears tired, is slow in responsiveness (verbally and behaviorally) to most requests, and fidgets with his clothing. He presents disheveled with dirty jeans and stains on his hooded sweatshirt; his hair is unbrushed. While placing a blood pressure cuff on Marc's arm, several thin linear scars approximately 2 inches long and 2 centimeters thick are visible. Some scars appear white; silvery in tone; one mark is pink in tone with minimal scabbing.

Vital signs: Temperature: 98.3°F; heart rate: 102; blood pressure: 128/84; RR 22.

Eyes: PERRLA, EOM intact.

ENT: Normal appearance of posterior oropharynx, clear rhinorrhea bilateral.

Lymph: No lymphadenopathy.

Cardiovascular: Tachycardia, no JVD, no carotid bruits, no murmurs, regular rhythm.

Lungs: Clear to auscultation bilaterally, no accessory muscle use, no crackles or wheezes.

Skin: Several thin linear scars approximately 2 inches long and 2 centimeters thick were visible. Some scars appeared white, silvery in tone; one mark was pink in tone with minimal scabbing.

Abdomen: Normal bowel sounds, abdomen soft and nondistended.

Genitourinary: Not examined.

Musculoskeletal: No edema, cyanosis, 5/5 strength with normal range of motion, no swollen joints.

Neurological: Alert and oriented X 3, CN II–XII grossly intact.

CRITICAL THINKING

What are the top three differential diagnoses in this case and why?
__Major depressive disorder
__Other specified depressive disorder
__Other specified trauma disorder
__Personal history of self-harm
__Hypothyroidism
__Adjustment sleep disorder (acute insomnia)

What diagnostic tests are required in this case and why?
__Patient Health Questionnaire-9 (PHQ-9)
__Beck Depression Inventory
__Non-Suicidal Self-Injury Assessment Tool (NSSI-AT)
__Columbia Suicide Severity Rating Scale (C-SSRS)
__CBC with differential
__Thyroid panel

What are the concerns at this point?

What is the plan of treatment?

What health education should be provided to this patient?

What demographic characteristics might affect this case?

Does the patient's psychosocial history affect how you might treat him?

What if the patient were elderly or under age 13?

Case 9.3 Postpartum Depression

By Nancy M. Terres, PhD, RN

Jake, 4 weeks old, presents to a pediatric practice in January for a weight check. He is accompanied by his mother, Laura. Laura says she experienced no perinatal complications, and was discharged 2 days postpartum, while Jake remained in the hospital for another 5 days for feeding and weight gain. Laura has been bringing Jake into the primary care office twice a week for weight checks, but this is the first time he is being seen by the nurse practitioner in the practice.

Birth history: Jake was the full-term product of a spontaneous vaginal delivery after a 10-hour labor to a Gr 3, P1, SAB 2, 40 y.o. mother. Laura underwent several years of fertility interventions, which included two first-trimester spontaneous pregnancy losses. During this recent pregnancy Laura received regular prenatal care, was healthy, and took no medications except for prenatal vitamins. She neither smoked any substances nor drank any alcoholic beverages during her pregnancy. Jake's Apgar scores were 9 at 1 minute, 9 at 5 minutes, and 10 at 10 minutes. His birth weight was 4 lbs., 10 oz. (2.098 kg). He had an uneventful extended hospital course focused on feeding and gaining weight with breastfeeding, plus bottle feedings/day of fortified pumped breast milk or formula fortified for 24 calories/oz. every other feeding for catch-up growth. After an initial postnatal weight loss, Jake started gaining about 30–40 gms/day while still hospitalized. His discharge weight was 4 lbs. 5 oz. (1.9561 kg). Jake's hospital discharge plan was:

- Keep Jake warm, check his temperature several times a day.
- Breastfeed every 2 hours around the clock.
- Reinforce pumped milk bottle feeding with a teaspoon of human milk fortifier for each 3 oz. of breast milk for 24 calories/oz. three times a day.
- Twice-weekly weight checks.

Social history: Before Jake was born Laura was an executive for a biomedical company, and her husband Craig is an executive for a global investment company. They live in a single-family home in an upscale suburb of a large northeastern city. When Laura became pregnant she and

Craig decided that the time commitment involved with both of their careers would not be conducive to attentive parenting, so they made the mutual decision that Laura would stay home with Jake. Craig works long hours. He also travels regularly for work. He currently carries the health care benefits in his job, so Laura feels she cannot complain about his being away so often. Craig is a member of the local country club, and is part of a group that trains for marathons, while Laura tends to be more reserved, preferring her small circle of friends mostly from her work. None of Laura's friends are at home with babies, and Laura does not see them regularly since leaving work. Laura's parents, besides living a distance away, are elderly and in poor health, and not a direct source of support. She has a brother who lives close to her parents, but no other siblings. The paternal grandparents live in the southwest United States and are retired. When asked who she considered her main support to be, Laura said it was Craig. However, Craig is not available much of the time to help Laura with Jake. Jake's frequent feeds have created tension between the parents because Craig cannot get a full night's sleep to go into work the next day with Jake in a bassinet in the room. Laura eventually moved into Jake's room to remain close to him and to make her available for his frequent feeds without disturbing Craig. Laura has a previous history of depression since her teens that worsened during her struggles with infertility and pregnancy losses. She had an eating disorder in high school and in the early years of college, but denies any issues with eating since then. She has periodically taken Citalopram, but not in several years, and was resistant to medication while going through infertility treatments and while breastfeeding. She believes that all medications prescribed or over the counter while breastfeeding are unsafe for the baby. Laura is continuing with prenatal vitamins but is taking no medications.

Diet: Laura is continuing with every-2-hour breastfeeding. She tried to pump milk to provide time for bottle feeding when Jake was first discharged from the hospital, but experienced trouble obtaining more than 1 oz. of pumped milk in total at a time, which she didn't believe was enough for his supplemental increased calorie bottles. She decided to nurse Jake every 2 hours through the night, since he is an avid feeder. She is not supplementing feedings with fortified formula at this time, since she felt it affected her milk supply to not be nursing every 2 hours. Laura is unsure if she misses any of her own meals because Jake's care is so absorbing, and Laura feels she has no time to herself to care for her own needs.

Elimination: Jake has small amounts of yellow loose stools with most feedings, and has about 8–10 wet diapers/day.

Sleep and feeding behavior: Jake is difficult to awaken for the frequent feedings, falls asleep during feedings, and mostly sleeps when not feeding. When awake he can be difficult to comfort even to latch on for feeding, but once latched on will settle well into the feeding. If Jake is fussy Laura tends to offer the breast more often than the recommended 2 hours. Jake nurses 10 minutes on one breast and 30–50 minutes on the other breast. He requires frequent stimulation to remain awake during feedings.

Family medical history: Both parents are in good physical health. Craig has seasonal allergies, but no history of chronic respiratory problems. Both parents are of average height and weight by report. Neither Craig nor Laura are smokers, nor do they allow Jake near smokers. The maternal grandparents are in their 80s, with a history of heart disease, Type 2 diabetes, and arthritis. The paternal grandparents are in their late 70s, with a history of arthritis, hypertension, and hyperlipidemia. There is a history of breast cancer in paternal extended family members, and seasonal allergies in both maternal and paternal extended family.

Medications: Jake was given his first dose of Hepatitis B (Hep B) vaccine upon hospital discharge. He has had no other immunizations, nor is he currently taking any medications.

Allergies: No known allergies. No untoward reaction to the Hep B vaccine.

OBJECTIVE

General: Jake appears very small for his age. He sleeps quietly during the visit until being undressed for the weight check. Once becoming fussy he is difficult to comfort, and seems to resist cuddling, arching away and escalating rapidly in his distress, which Laura says is typical for him. Throughout the appointment Laura has a noticeably flat affect. She vacillates between a passive posture often looking off out the window and not observing the baby during the exam, to reacting with anxiety, especially as he becomes inconsolably fussy.

Vital signs: Jake's temperature is 36.3°C, AP is 110, R is 40, BP is 50/40.

Measurements: Weight 5 lbs. (<5th percentile), head circumference 33 cm (< 10th percentile), and length 18.5 inches (10th percentile).

Skin: Pink, some sagging skin still on his thighs, with some flaking skin, lips moist, good skin turgor, occasional milia on his facial cheeks and nose.

Nose: Clear, no discharge.

Mouth: Palate intact, some white patches on left side of his mouth, easily removed with a cotton swab.

Abdomen: Soft, small, easily reducible umbilical hernia.

Cardiorespiratory: Chest clear, no murmurs.

Genitourinary: Circumcised, testicles descended, normal urine stream observed.

Neurologic: Movements smooth, symmetrical. Poor state control moving from active sleep to full-out crying. Jake does not respond readily to the usual comfort measures such as holding, position changes, or walking while softly bouncing or rocking. Somewhat hyperactive Moro reflex, strong sucking and rooting, and asymmetrical tonic neck reflexes present. Two-beat ankle clonus is noted bilaterally. He can be brought into the quiet alert state slowly. Once he calmed, he fixed on a bright red ball and visually tracked the ball 180 degrees. He was attentive to his mother's voice briefly. No vocalizations were heard this appointment aside from fussing, but Laura stated she has heard the beginnings of some cooing recently.

CRITICAL THINKING

What is the diagnosis and its contributing factors?

- **For Jake**
- **For Laura**

Why must concerns about Laura be addressed at this appointment?

What additional information is needed?

What are the treatment options?

- **For Jake**
- **For Laura**

What are the plans for referral and follow-up care? Include resources that may be needed to determine treatment options.

What demographic characteristics might affect this case?

Are there any standardized guidelines that should be used to treat this case? If so, what are they?

Case 9.4 Anxiety

By Sheila Swales, MS, RN, PMHNP-BC

SUBJECTIVE

Jonathan is a 28-year-old single Caucasian male who works as a systems analyst for a financial services company. He presents complaining of a tense and irritable mood that has worsened in the past few weeks. He also reports feeling anxious and having trouble sleeping. He notes having more frequent headaches, stomach upset, and diarrhea. He often feels tired and complains of difficulty concentrating at work. He worries that his new boss will notice that he's more forgetful and taking longer to complete projects. He enjoys his work, but also finds it stressful. He has difficulty unwinding in the evening unless he has a couple of beers, which has become a regular occurrence.

Past medical history: Jonathan reports a history of anxiety that first emerged in high school and recalls worrying needlessly about being late with assignments, disappointing his parents, and losing important friendships. He has no history of treatment for anxiety or other psychiatric disorders.

Family history: Jonathan's father has untreated anxiety. His mother has hypertension and diabetes mellitus Type 2.

Social history: Jonathan lives with a roommate; they have a good relationship. He has a group of friends and usually sees them on weekends to watch sports. Jonathan is close to his parents and younger sister, who live out of state. He completed a graduate degree 1 year ago and has been employed in financial services for 1 year. He admits to no regular exercise and drinks 2–3 beers daily in the evening. His caffeine intake is 2–3 twelve-ounce Red Bull energy drinks per day. He denies using other substances.

Medications: None.

Allergies: No known allergies.

The Family Nurse Practitioner: Clinical Case Studies, Second Edition. Edited by Leslie Neal-Boylan.
© 2021 John Wiley & Sons Ltd. Published 2021 by John Wiley & Sons Ltd.

OBJECTIVE

General: Cooperative, in no apparent distress.

Vital signs: BP: 126/82; P: 84; R: 22; T: 98.6°F; height: 5 ft 11 inches; weight: 188 lbs; BMI: 26.2.

HEENT/Neck: There is no JVD.

Cardiovascular: There is a 2+ carotid, no bruit. Regular rate and rhythm, S1 and S2.

Respiratory: Lungs are clear to auscultation and percussion.

Musculoskeletal: Full range of motion of the neck and trunk. Abdomen is soft, nontender, and nondistended. Extremities show no edema, clubbing, or cyanosis.

CRITICAL THINKING

What are the top three differential diagnoses in this case and why?

Which diagnostic tests are required in this case and why?

What are the concerns at this point?

What is the plan of treatment?

What are the plans for referral and follow-up care?

What health education should be provided to this patient?

What demographic characteristics might affect this case?

Does the patient's psychosocial history impact how you might treat him?

What if the patient lived in a rural (or urban) setting?

Are there any standardized guidelines that should be used to treat this case? If so, what are they?

Case 9.5 Trauma

By Erin Patterson Janicek, LCSW, and Anna Goddard, PhD, APRN, CPNP-PC

SUBJECTIVE

Brittany is a 12-year-old biracial female in the 7th grade. She presents twice in 1 week to the school-based health center (SBHC) for stomachaches. At the second visit, in a discussion about nutrition and sleep hygiene, Brittany reports difficulty with falling asleep due to being worried something bad will happen, especially to her mom, as well as disrupted sleep due to nightmares. Brittany reports her family moved homes 3 months ago because "stepdad is gone and isn't allowed around us anymore." After the move, Brittany states "I thought I would feel better, but I felt worse instead." She quit gymnastics because it did not feel fun anymore. She also reports difficulty focusing, which has had a negative impact on her grades. The school counselor also reports recent concerns relating to Brittany's concentration and her leaving the classroom frequently for breaks. Brittany acknowledges difficulty focusing and that "my mind won't stop when a room is quiet, so I try to distract myself." When asked about her thoughts during those times or the content of her distressing dreams, Brittany quietly says "I'm not ready to talk about it." Her school counselor also notes some recent social isolation and an increasingly more serious nature, and comments that this is a shift for a once "smiley and engaging" student.

Past medical history: Brittany has a past history of gastroesophageal reflux disease (GERD), which has resolved; she no longer takes medications. She denies any history of prior hospitalizations or surgery. She has seen a gastroenterologist in the past but otherwise does not see any specialists nor does she see her primary care provider regularly. She denies any recent weight gain or loss. She denies sexual activity and had a negative PHQ-9 and CRAFFT as part of her annual screening at the SBHC.

Family history: Her family history is positive for maternal alcohol use and a first-degree relative with a history of substance use. Paternal history is unknown.

Social history: Brittany is the oldest of 2 siblings, both sisters. Her biological parents divorced when she was 3 years old and her biological father lives several states away. He visits on holidays and occasionally in the summer. Her mother remarried and is currently in a domestically violent relationship with Brittany's stepfather. All 3 children witnessed ongoing physical and verbal abuse toward the biological mother. As of 3 months ago, Brittany's stepfather is currently in prison with a no contact order in place for all of the children.

The Family Nurse Practitioner: Clinical Case Studies, Second Edition. Edited by Leslie Neal-Boylan.
© 2021 John Wiley & Sons Ltd. Published 2021 by John Wiley & Sons Ltd.

Sleep history: She reports difficulty initiating sleep and waking throughout the night. She gets an average of 6–7 hours nighttime sleep, per self-report. She will sometimes take a Tylenol PM from the medicine cabinet to help fall asleep but reports it "doesn't help her stay asleep."

Medications: None.

Allergies: No known drug allergies.

Review of Systems:

Constitutional: Lack of energy, no weight gain or loss.

HEENT: Reports no changes in hearing or vision, no runny nose, postnasal drip, or any URI symptoms.

Skin: No itching, dry skin, or rashes.

Cardiovascular: No chest pain, no history of cardiac anomalies, no murmurs.

Respiratory: No shortness of breath or difficulty breathing, no night sweats, no wheezing or history of RAD.

Gastrointestinal: No nausea, vomiting, or diarrhea/constipation. Occasional heartburn with certain foods.

Genitourinary: Unremarkable.

Musculoskeletal: No join pain or muscle pain.

Neurological: Frequent headaches, no double vision, no balance issues, or dizziness.

Hematologic: Denies bruising or easy bleeding.

OBJECTIVE

General: Well-appearing with age-appropriate clothing and good hygiene; initially shy but now more talkative.

Vital signs: T: 98.3°F; heart rate: 68; blood pressure: 110/68; RR: 18; height: 5 ft 4 inches; weight: 169 lbs; BMI: 29.

Eyes: PERRLA, EOM intact, dark circles under eyes.

ENT: Normal appearance of posterior oropharynx, nares patent, no postnasal drip, TMs gray pearly and visible ossicles.

Lymph: No lymphadenopathy.

Cardiovascular: No JVD, no carotid bruits, no murmurs, regular rate and rhythm, femoral pulses equal +2.

Lungs: Clear to auscultation bilaterally, no accessory muscle use, no crackles or wheezes.

Skin: Unremarkable.

Abdomen: Normal bowel sounds, abdomen soft and nondistended, no HSM.

Genitourinary: Not examined.

Musculoskeletal: Full range of motion in all 4 extremities.

Neurological: Alert and oriented × 3, CN 2–12 grossly intact.

CRITICAL THINKING

What are the most likely differential diagnoses in this case and why?
__Post-traumatic stress disorder
__Unspecified trauma- and stressor-related disorder
__Child-affected by parental relationship distress
__Major depressive disorder
__Generalized anxiety disorder
__Hypothyroidism

Which diagnostic tests are required in this case and why?
__PHQ-9
__Beck Depression Inventory
__The Non-Suicidal Self-Injury Assessment Tool (NSSI-AT)
__Columbia–Suicide Severity Rating Scale (C-SSRS Screener)
__CBC with differential
__Thyroid panel
__CMP

What are the concerns at this point?
__Suicide risk assessment
__Self-harm risk assessment
__Safety of going home
__Headaches
__Sleep hygiene
__Hypothyroidism

What is the plan of treatment?

What is trauma-informed care?

What are the plans for referral and follow-up care?

What demographic characteristics might affect this case?

Does the patient's psychosocial history impact how you might treat her?

If this patient were male (instead of female), how might that change management and treatment?

The Older Adult

Case 10.1 Forgetfulness

By Amy Bruno, PhD, RN, ANP-BC

SUBJECTIVE

Sophie is a 62-year-old female who presents today with her son, Taylor, for a chief complaint of "forgetfulness." Sophie is somewhat withdrawn during the appointment and offers very little information. She gives her son permission to share her history. Her son Taylor tells you that for the past 2 months he has noticed that his mother is becoming increasingly forgetful and more withdrawn. She has forgotten appointments and to pick up her grandson at school 4 times over the past 2 months. She previously was able to take her medications independently but now her son notes he has to remind her daily and has started to organize her medications for her. Taylor also notes that his mother is not sleeping well and is up at 4 a.m. most mornings and then will nap for about 4 hours during the day. She has also stopped going to her weekly knitting group and is not participating in weekly meetings at her church anymore.

Sophie does admit today to feeling "down" and simply states, "I don't feel like doing anything." She attributes her forgetfulness to being "stressed out" about her daughter and her father's medical condition. She reports she has frequent nighttime wakening because "I worry about my family and my legs hurt." When asked how often she is taking her prescribed Alprazolam, she states, "I have to take it 2–3 times a day for my nerves."

Sophie has not had any trouble getting dressed, making meals, or showering independently. She has not gotten lost with driving.

Sophie does not have a mental health counselor or a psychiatrist at the present time. Her former psychiatrist retired 2 years ago and her PCP has been prescribing her psychiatric medications.

Past medical history: Type 2 diabetes mellitus, diabetic peripheral neuropathy (DPN), hypertension, hyperlipidemia, depression, anxiety, post-traumatic stress disorder, chronic insomnia

Family history:

- Mother age 82: Coronary artery disease (CAD), Type 2 diabetes mellitus, hypertension, hyperlipidemia
- Father, age 88: Hypertension, hyperlipidemia, prostate cancer, diagnosed with Alzheimer's disease at age 80
- Brother, age 66: Hypertension, myocardial infarction (MI) at age 65, Type 2 diabetes mellitus

The Family Nurse Practitioner: Clinical Case Studies, Second Edition. Edited by Leslie Neal-Boylan.
© 2021 John Wiley & Sons Ltd. Published 2021 by John Wiley & Sons Ltd.

- Son, age 40: Hypercholesterolemia
- Grandson, age 10: Asthma

Social history:

- Lives with her son, Taylor, and her 10-year-old grandson, Joseph, in a suburban house.
- Taylor assists Sophie with her medications and appointments. Taylor is 40 years old and works full-time as a math teacher at the local high school. He is divorced and has full custody of his son, as his ex-wife has a substance use disorder and is currently incarcerated.
- Retired (worked as a receptionist for a dental office for over 40 years).
- Highest education completed: high school.
- Divorced for over 10 years and ex-husband physically and emotionally abused her for over 20 years; ex-husband now deceased due to lung cancer.
- Her daughter, Cynthia, has a substance-use disorder and a history of homelessness and incarceration.
- No history of smoking or illicit drug use, and she does not drink alcohol.

Medications:

- Metformin 1000 mg po twice daily
- Gabapentin 1200 mg po three times daily
- Lisinopril 20 mg po daily
- Rosuvastatin 20 mg po daily
- Citalopram 20 mg po daily
- Buproprion XR 150 mg po bid
- Alprazolam 0.5 mg three times daily PRN
- Trazodone 400 mg po at night

Allergies: Sulfa: rash

OBJECTIVE

General: 62-year-old female, well-dressed, well-nourished, in no apparent distress.

Vital signs: Blood pressure: 136/82; HR: 72; RR 20.

Cardiac: AP RRR, no murmurs, rubs, gallops, no JVD, no carotid bruits bilaterally.

Pulmonary: Lung sounds clear to auscultation bilaterally, no use of accessory muscles

Neurological: Patient is alert/oriented to person, time, and place; flat affect and depressed mood; has difficulty maintaining eye contact during exam; poor effort during physical exam and screening questionnaires; normal insight and judgment, speech clear. CN II–XII grossly intact. Normal tone to all 4 extremities; no cogwheel rigidity noted. Reflexes: 2+ bilaterally to biceps, triceps, and brachioradialis, hypoactive bilateral knee and Achilles reflexes; no clonus, toes downgoing bilat. Coordination: F-N-F testing WNL, RAM WNL, Romberg negative. Sensory exam: Decreased pinprick, light touch, and vibratory sense to lower extremities in a stocking-like distribution; proprioception intact. Gait: Slightly wide-based, normal speed, stride, and arm swing intact, no ataxia observed.

Montreal Cognitive Assessment (MoCA) Screening = 22

Patient Health Questionnaire-9 (PHQ-9) = 15

CRITICAL THINKING

What are the top three differential diagnoses in this case and why?

Which diagnostic tests are required in this case and why?
__CBC
__TSH
__Vitamin B12
__CMP
__RPR or FTA testing
__HgA1C
__Lipids
__ESR

What are the concerns at this point?

What are 3–5 case-specific questions to ask the patient?

What is the plan of treatment?

What are the plans for referral and follow-up care?

What health education should be provided to this patient?

What demographic characteristics might affect this case?

Does the patient's psychosocial history impact how you might treat her?

Case 10.2 Behavior Change

By Sheila L. Molony, PhD, APRN, GNP-BC, FGSA, FAAN

SUBJECTIVE

Antonio is an 84-year-old male resident of a continuing care retirement community (CCRC). The residential director admitted him to the respite care wing of the nursing home last evening due to behavior changes including agitation, disorientation, and wandering outside without appropriate clothing. The director brings him to the on-site clinic the next morning. She reports that the on-call provider last evening ordered 1 mg of IM haloperidol, which was given soon after the resident came to the unit. The residential director reports that Antonio had a poor appetite for a few days before this and was found napping in the lounge, which is not unusual. He fell on his way to the dining room the previous morning, but sustained no apparent injury. During his last annual health maintenance visit 3 months prior, he scored 22/30 on the Montreal Cognitive Assessment (MoCA) and was diagnosed with mild cognitive impairment (MCI). He is usually alert and oriented to season, year, place, and person and has no difficulty navigating inside or outside his residence.

His only complaint today is a new complaint of frequent heartburn that he has been treating with over-the-counter (OTC) pills (he can't remember the name). He denies pain, cough, shortness of breath, or changes in bladder/ bowel habits.

Past medical history: Coronary artery disease (CAD) with angioplasty/stent placement ×2, hypertension (HTN), benign prostatic hypertrophy (BPH), asthma, hyperlipidemia (HLD), heart failure with normal ejection fraction (HFNEF), mild cognitive impairment (MCI), osteopenia, and osteoarthritis (OA). He had a motorcycle accident in his youth with a left leg injury.

Psychosocial history: Antonio moved to the CCRC 1 year ago with his wife, who died 4 months prior. He cared for her until she died, then stayed in his apartment, complaining of anxiety and difficulty sleeping. He recently became more involved in community activities and has been making friendships in the building. He has been attending two meals per day in the communal dining room, until this week, and has been independent in bathing, dressing, grooming, walking, transferring, eating, and toileting. He does not climb stairs due to poor endurance but is able to walk on level ground over modest distances without fatigue. Before his wife died, he would take the community van to local shops twice a month. He has a daughter-in-law and two nieces who live within 50 miles, call weekly, and visit once or twice a month.

The Family Nurse Practitioner: Clinical Case Studies, Second Edition. Edited by Leslie Neal-Boylan.
© 2021 John Wiley & Sons Ltd. Published 2021 by John Wiley & Sons Ltd.

Medications: Fluticasone propionate 100 mcg/salmeterol 50 mcg (Advair Diskus), one inhalation twice per day; simvastatin, 40 mg by mouth, once daily; atenolol, 100 mg by mouth, once daily; losartan, 50 mg by mouth, once daily; furosemide, 20 mg by mouth, once daily; K-dur, 10 mEq by mouth, once daily; isosorbide mononitrate ER (Imdur), 30 mg by mouth, once daily; alendronate, 70 mg once per week; multivitamin (MVI) with iron, 1 by mouth, once daily; vitamin C, 500 mg by mouth, twice daily; docusate sodium succinate, 1 by mouth, once daily; OTC medication - unknown for heartburn.

Allergies: NKDA.

Health maintenance: Td vaccine 2007. Never had the flu vaccine, pneumococcal vaccine, or shingles vaccine (received education/information on last visit).

OBJECTIVE

Vital signs: Temperature: 100.0°F; pulse: 58 (irregular); respirations: 28; blood pressure: 168/58; weight: 161 (164 last month); height: 72 inches.

Note: His usual vital signs are: Temp: 97.4°F; pulse: 70–80 (regular); BP: 130–140/60–70).

General: Today Antonio appears sleepy, disheveled, restless, and vague. He can walk to the examination room but is unsteady and needs assistance getting undressed for the physical examination. He is unable to fully cooperate with the exam. His skin is dry, especially over the lower extremities.

Mental status: Speech is slow but clear; thought processes are slow and disorganized; irritable mood; distractible; decreased ability to focus. MOCA15/30.

Head: Normocephalic without obvious lesions, masses, depressions, or tenderness. No temporal bruits.

Eyes: Visual acuity 20/40 bilaterally with glasses. Eyelids are symmetrical with no ptosis, but slight ectropion bilaterally. PERRLA. Conjunctiva and sclera clear with slight arcus senilis. EOMs and visual fields WNL with slight decrease in upward gaze bilaterally. He has a few beats of horizontal nystagmus on extreme lateral gaze. Red reflexes intact but incomplete visualization of retinas due to difficulty cooperating with exam and frequent eye closing/sleepiness.

Ears: Unable to cooperate with hearing acuity screen. External ears are without lesions or tenderness. Canals are obstructed with dark cerumen bilaterally. Unable to visualize TMs.

Nose/sinuses: Nares patent with pink mucosa; no lesions, deviations, or discharge. No frontal or maxillary sinus tenderness.

Mouth/throat: Oral mucosa dry and intact. Tongue and uvula midline, and tongue movement is symmetrical. Pharynx clear. No lesions, masses, cavities, or bleeding.

Neck: Supple; no carotid bruits or thyromegaly. No cervical lymphadenopathy.

Chest: No skin lesions, deformities, tenderness, crepitus, axillary lymphadenopathy, or breast masses. No rubs or thrills. PMI nonpalpable.

Heart: Regular rhythm with frequent pauses. No murmurs or obvious gallops.

Lungs: Symmetrical chest wall expansion. Resonance on percussion throughout all fields. Fremitus palpable and symmetrical. Fine crackles at left base, and coarse inspiratory crackles and expiratory rhonchi over right lower lung field. No egophony, bronchophony, or whispered pectoriloquy.

Abdomen: Soft, nontender, with quiet bowel sounds in all quadrants; no palpable masses, organomegaly, or bruits. Soft stool in rectum; hemoccult negative. Slightly enlarged prostate, symmetrical. No palpable masses.

Neurologic: Gait shuffling with small steps. Slightly unsteady, leaning to one side. Unable to stand with feet together without swaying. No pronator drift. No postural or intention tremor. CNs II–XII grossly intact. Reflexes 3+ and symmetrical in both upper extremities. Lower extremities: 2+ patellar reflex, 1+ Achilles reflex. Plantar reflex ↓. Able to detect pain in all extremities, but unable to cooperate with full sensory or coordination testing.

Musculoskeletal: Muscle strength 4/5 in upper and lower extremities bilaterally.

Peripheral vascular: Bounding radial and brachial pulses: 2+. Femoral and popliteal: 2+. Pedal: 1+. Unable to detect posterior tibial pulse. Ankle edema bilaterally with left > right: 2-3+.

CRITICAL THINKING

Which diagnostic or imaging studies should be considered to assist with or confirm the diagnosis?
___Head CT or MRI
___Chest X-ray
___Abdominal X-ray
___Urinalysis
___EKG
___CBC with diff
___Complete metabolic panel (includes: albumin, blood urea nitrogen, calcium, carbon, chloride, creatinine, glucose, potassium, sodium, total bilirubin and protein, and liver enzymes
___Ammonia level
___Arterial blood gas or pulse oximetry
___TSH, free T4, T3
___Toxic screen of blood or urine
___Orthostatic blood pressure
___Depression screening
___Rapid plasma reagin (RPR)
___HIV
___B12/folate
___Lumbar puncture
___Electroencephalogram (EEG)
___Cultures (urine, sputum or blood)

Which differential diagnoses should be considered at this point?
__Dementia
__Depression
__Delirium
__CVA/TIA
__Psychiatric/mental health condition

What is the treatment plan?

Are any referrals needed?

What aspects of the health history require special emphasis in older adults?

What if this patient were under age 65? Would that change the management plan?

What patient, family, and/or caregiver education is important in this case?

Are there any standardized guidelines that should be used to assess or treat this case?

What are some of the possible contributors to this patient's hypotension? Are any referrals needed? What management strategies should be considered?

Case 10.3 Tremors

By Amy Bruno, PhD, RN, ANP-BC

SUBJECTIVE

Mr. Alfredo Suarez is a right-handed 68-year-old male who presents to the office with tremors to bilateral hands. His daughter, Maria, accompanies him to this visit and is worried he has "Parkinson's." Mr. Suarez reports that he first noticed "shaking" to his hands about 2 years ago but was not bothered by it and attributed it to "getting old." Over the past 2 months, the hand shaking has started to interfere with his ability to play cards and prepare meals. Maria interjects and states "his hands shake all the time now and he can't even hold a fork." Maria goes on to report that her father is an avid woodworker and is no longer working in his shop because he kept "dropping tools."

Mr. Suarez states the tremors are consistently present all of the time and he most notices them when he tries to hold objects or read his book. He is most annoyed by these symptoms because they are interfering with hobbies. He reports, "people notice it and bring it up and then it gets worse." He says that his brother has "shaky hands" and that he thinks his paternal grandmother had "Parkinson's" because "she always shook." He reports that tremors increase during stress and anxiety. He reports he also feels "more anxious lately" and doesn't know if his medication is working. He notes increased anxiety about attending social events and worrying about his granddaughter, who was diagnosed with epilepsy last year. He feels his hands are becoming "very clumsy." He denies any alleviating factors. He denies any numbness or weakness to extremities. Denies any changes in gait or falls.

Past medical history: Hypertension (HTN), hyperlipidemia (HLD), generalized anxiety disorder, GERD, asthma/COPD overlap syndrome

Family history:

- Mother: HTN, HLD, CAD
- Father: Stroke, HTN, Type 2 DM
- Brother: HTN, Type 2 DM, "shaky" hands

Social history:

- Patient is widowed and lives alone. He lost his wife 2 years ago due to breast cancer. He has 1 daughter, Maria, and 2 grandchildren who he sees regularly and who live nearby.
- He retired at age 65 and worked as a carpenter.

The Family Nurse Practitioner: Clinical Case Studies, Second Edition. Edited by Leslie Neal-Boylan.
© 2021 John Wiley & Sons Ltd. Published 2021 by John Wiley & Sons Ltd.

- Hobbies: Woodworking, cooking, spending time with family, and reading.
- Nonsmoker; no illicit drug use.
- Drinks a "shot" of bourbon 3–4 nights per week.

Medications:

- Lisinopril 20 mg po daily
- Rosuvastatin 20 mg po daily
- Fluoxetine 60 mg po daily
- Omeprazole 20 mg po daily
- Albuterol MDI 2 puffs every 4 hours as needed
- Tiotropium inhaler 2 puffs once a day

Allergies: NKDA

OBJECTIVE

General: Pleasant, cooperative, NAD.

Vital signs: BP: 142/88; HR: 72; RR: 20; T: 98.9°F; height: 72 inches; weight: 210 lbs; BMI: 27.

Systems approach listed by system:

Cardiovascular: Apical pulse RRR, no murmurs, rubs, gallops, no S3, S4.

Pulmonary: Lung sounds clear to auscultation bilaterally; respirations unlabored and regular.

Musculoskeletal: FROM to all 4 extremities, normal muscle bulk noted, no edema, redness to joints, strength 5/5 to all 4 extremities.

<u>**Neurological:**</u> Patient is alert/oriented to person, time, and place; normal affect and mood; normal insight and judgment, speech clear. CN II–XII intact. Normal tone to all 4 extremities; no cogwheel rigidity noted. Reflexes: 2+ bilaterally to biceps, triceps, and brachioradialis, 1+ to bilateral knees and Achilles; no clonus, toes downgoing bilaterally. Coordination: F-N-F testing WNL, RAM WNL, Romberg negative. Sensory exam: Normal pinprick, light touch, and vibratory sense to all 4 extremities; proprioception intact. Tremor exam: Bilateral course action and postural tremor noted to both hands that relieves at rest, right is slightly more prominent than left; there is no intention or resting tremors on exam; no other adventitious movements noted. Spiral drawing, done with right hand.

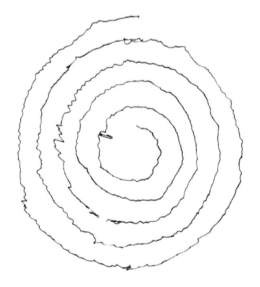

Gait exam: Patient able to arise from a sitting to standing position without using arms; demonstrates normal speed, stride, and turn, arm swing intact bilaterally, slightly stooped posture, no reemergence of hand tremors with ambulation.

CRITICAL THINKING

What are the top three differential diagnoses in this case and why?

Which diagnostic tests are required in this case and why?

What are the concerns at this point?

What is the plan of treatment?

What are the plans for referral and follow-up care?

What health education should be provided to this patient?

What demographic characteristics might affect this case?

Does the patient's psychosocial history impact how you might treat him?

What if the patient lived in a rural (or urban) setting?

Are there any standardized guidelines that should be used to treat this case? If so, what are they?

Are there other history questions that are pertinent when assessing a patient with tremors?

If this patient did not have insurance, would that change the management strategy?

Case 10.4 Weight Gain and Fatigue

By Leslie Neal-Boylan, PhD, APRN, CRRN, FAAN, FARN

SUBJECTIVE

Maxwell is a 70-year-old homosexual African American male and retired corporate lawyer who first came to the health maintenance organization 3 years ago. At that time, he had not been to a primary care provider since he retired from full-time work at age 60. Maxwell continues to consult and does occasional part-time work for his previous law firm. He admits to a sedentary lifestyle, a weight gain of 25 pounds within the past 2 years, and occasional fatigue and headache.

Past medical history: None significant.

Past surgical history: Significant for a tonsillectomy at the age of 7.

Family history: Significant for thyroid disease, hypertension, coronary artery disease, Type 2 diabetes mellitus, hyperlipidemia, and obesity. Father died from a myocardial infarction at age 69.

OBJECTIVE

VISIT THREE YEARS AGO

Vital signs: 220 lbs with a height of 6 ft 1 inch and a body mass index of 29. Blood pressure: 140/88; radial pulse: 78; temperature: 98.7°F; respiratory rate: 16.

Physical examination: Significant for acanthosis nigricans and central adiposity.

Diagnostic test results: Fasting lipids revealed a total cholesterol of 182, a low-density lipoprotein level of 106, a high-density lipoprotein level of 57, and a triglyceride level of 95. His fasting blood glucose was 95, and the Hemoglobin A1c was 5.6. His thyroid-stimulating hormone level was 8.0 mU/L. A routine electrocardiogram documented normal sinus rhythm and rate.

Diagnoses: Hypertension and hyperthyroid disease.

The Family Nurse Practitioner: Clinical Case Studies, Second Edition. Edited by Leslie Neal-Boylan.
© 2021 John Wiley & Sons Ltd. Published 2021 by John Wiley & Sons Ltd.

Plan: The patient is started on hydrochlorothiazide 25 mg, aspirin 81 mg, and Norvasc 2.5 mg by mouth daily and levothyroxine 0.50 mcg by mouth daily. He is counseled regarding lifestyle modifications, inclusive of preparing and eating a low-sodium and low-fat diet. Maxwell was encouraged to start a routine exercise program of at least 30 minutes of modest aerobic activity such as walking as if to catch a bus. He was also encouraged to lose 5–7% of his body weight. These lifestyle modifications have proven effective in diabetes prevention and maintenance, as well as in control of blood pressure and lipid levels. The patient is informed regarding the mechanism of action of the medications, duration of action, contraindications, and adverse effects. The patient is also instructed to take the levothyroxine on an empty stomach first thing in the morning.

THREE-MONTH FOLLOW-UP VISIT

Vital signs: Blood pressure of 128/76.

Diagnostic test results: Thyroid-stimulating hormone level is 4.50. Basic metabolic panel: blood urea nitrogen level of 14; creatinine level of 0.98; sodium level of 137; potassium level of 3.8; and a chloride level of 104.

Plan: The patient was given a list of potassium-containing foods and reminded to eat 1 or 2 items daily due to his low potassium level. He is instructed to continue to take his medications.

TODAY'S VISIT

SUBJECTIVE

Maxwell has been very busy in his semi-retirement and has not been in for a physical examination or labwork for more than 2 years. Now he presents with complaints of extreme fatigue for the past 2 months and low libido. He states that he feels fatigued all the time, and sleep does not seem to relieve it. He is able to work around the house, but has cut back on his legal work and has limited socialization and participation in outside activities due to fatigue. He reports sleeping for 8–10 hours a night, with his sleep interrupted by a need to go to the bathroom at least twice. He awakens fatigued.

Sexually, he has a morning erection but not as strongly as in previous months. He has limited sexual desire. He is able to have an erection with intercourse, but it is less of an erection than previously. He states that he has been in a monogamous relationship for the past 2 years. He admits to a 15-pound weight gain over the past 2 years. He reports that he experiences occasional constipation and some cold intolerance. He reports feeling "shaky" on occasion, especially when he has not eaten in a while. He denies fever, night sweats, and tobacco or drug use and reports socially drinking several glasses of red wine per week.

Past medical history: Remains significant for hypertension and hypothyroidism.

Past surgical history: Remains the same.

Family history: Unchanged.

Medications: Hydrochlorothiazide 25 mg by mouth daily, Norvasc 2.5 mg by mouth daily, levothyroxine 0.50 mcg by mouth daily, aspirin 81 mg by mouth daily, multivitamin, 1 capsule and fish oil capsules, 2000 mg by mouth daily. There are no known drug allergies and no known food allergies.

OBJECTIVE

Vital signs: Temperature: 98.6°F; radial pulse: 76; blood pressure: 134/80; oxygen saturation: 99%; height: 6 ft 1 inch; weight: 235 lbs (15-lb weight gain); body mass index: 31. Physical exam is unremarkable except for the following findings:

Skin: Poor skin turgor; acanthosis nigricans.

Mouth: Dry oral mucosa.

Cardiac: NSR, No ectopy.

Respiratory: CTA bilaterally.

Abdomen: Central adiposity.

Lymph: No significant lymphadenopathy.

Rectal: Hemoccult negative for occult blood.

CRITICAL THINKING

Which diagnostic studies should be considered to assist with or confirm the diagnosis?
___FIT test
___Complete blood count
___Thiamine
___Iron studies
___Complete metabolic panel
___Rapid HIV test
___HIV viral load test
___HbA1c
___Thyroid-stimulating hormone
___Testosterone
___Urine analysis
___Tuberculosis testing
___Urine microalbumin/creatinine ratio
___FSH and LH
___Prolactin
___Chest X-ray

What is the most likely differential diagnosis and why?
___HIV and/or AIDS
___Pernicious anemia
___Hypothyroidism uncontrolled
___Secondary hypogonadism
___Diabetes mellitus

What is the plan of treatment?

What is the plan for referrals and follow-up?

Does the patient's psychosocial history impact how you might treat him?

What if this patient were a premenopausal female?

What if the patient were over the age of 80?

Are there standardized guidelines that should be used to assess and treat this patient?

NOTE: The author would like to acknowledge the contribution of Vanessa Jefferson, MSN, BCANP, CDE to this case in the first edition of this book.

Case 10.5 Visual Changes

By Millie Hepburn, PhD, RN, ACNS-BC, SCRN

SUBJECTIVE

Marion is an 85-year-old woman of European descent who lives alone and comes to the office every 3–6 months for monitoring of hypertension and hyperlipidemia. Today she presents with a concern about vision changes. Marion reports some vision changes including increased sensitivity to glare; increased difficulty with dark adaptation, with colors seeming not as vivid as they used to; and increased difficulty with reading, but that she does not have any "floaters" as her friend reported to her last week. She states that she needs bright light to read comfortably. She mentions that this has worsened over the past few years and has become increasingly bothersome. She denies any eye pain or discharge, diplopia, or halos. She has no history of eye trauma. She mentions that her last eye exam was 5 years ago. She denies any history of glaucoma but thinks she may have had some early cataracts on her last exam. Marion states that she maintains an independent lifestyle and requires no assistance in her day to day activities.

Past medical/surgical history: Hypertension; hyperlipidemia; peripheral arterial insufficiency; osteoporosis; generalized anxiety disorder; osteoarthritis; status post hip fracture with repair/pinning at age 82.

Family history: Mother: died at age 78, lung cancer; had age-related macular degeneration and migraines. Father: died at age 65, MI; had coronary artery disease, diabetes, and stroke.

Social history: Marion was widowed 10 years ago and lives alone in a 1-bedroom, first-floor apartment with 5 steep stairs to enter the building. She is dating socially and attends the senior dances at the local community center about once a week. She maintains the flower gardens in her front yard and states that she walks a half mile most days with her friend. Marion states that she falls asleep without difficulty most nights, but often awakens during the night and has difficulty falling back asleep. She states that she actually sleeps about 5.5 hours per night, but experiences some daytime sleepiness. She states that she has 1–2 drinks after her dance class and occasionally when on a date. She quit smoking 25 years prior (smoked 1 pack of menthol cigarettes per day for 40 years).

Diet: Marion's typical diet includes toast with butter and jam for breakfast with black coffee; soup and sandwich with a glass of milk for lunch; roast beef, potatoes with gravy, and green beans with butter and salt for dinner; and no snacks. She eats dinner out with friends about 2 or 3 nights per

---

The Family Nurse Practitioner: Clinical Case Studies, Second Edition. Edited by Leslie Neal-Boylan.
© 2021 John Wiley & Sons Ltd. Published 2021 by John Wiley & Sons Ltd.

week at the diner or a restaurant and usually has some type of meat, potato or white rice, and a cooked vegetable. She does not drive, as she uses public transportation.

Medications: She has brought all of her medication bottles with her. Her medications include lisinopril, atorvastatin, citalopram, and alendronate. She has an expired prescription/bottle of hydroxyzine that she states that she uses occasionally for "nerves." She also takes acetaminophen as needed for arthritis pain.

Allergies: Penicillin (causes rash to chest and arms).

Marion admits to some gradual visual changes; difficulty hearing (mostly in crowded restaurants); postnasal drip; and occasional arthritis pain in her shoulders, fingers, hips, and knees. She admits to occasional leakage of urine when she has a cold/cough. She denies headache, falls, head trauma, cough, dyspnea, chest discomfort, abdominal pain, and change in appetite or weight, polyuria, polydipsia, polyphagia, weakness, numbness, and dizziness.

OBJECTIVE

Eyes: Visual acuity: 20/40 in both eyes (with corrective eyeglasses). The outer one-third of her eyebrows is absent. Slight ectropion bilaterally. Conjunctiva/sclera clear. No crescentic shadow. Positive for arcus senilis. PERRLA. EOMs intact with mild decrease in upward gaze; visual fields full. Positive for red reflex bilaterally; suboptimal retinal visualization.

The remainder of the physical examination is unchanged since her last visit.

CRITICAL THINKING

Which diagnostic studies should be considered to assist with or confirm the diagnosis?
___Amsler grid
___MacuFlow
___National Eye Institute Visual Functioning Questionnaire 25
___Ophthalmological referral for testing

Which of the symptoms or signs related to Marion's eyes or vision represent pathological changes versus normal aging?

Which differential diagnoses should be considered at this point? What are the three most common diagnoses/conditions affecting vision in older adults? Are Marion's signs and symptoms similar to the clinical presentations of these conditions?
___Macular degeneration
___Glaucoma
___CVA
___Cataracts

Based on this exam, what is the plan of care? Would you seek any referrals from the interprofessional team?

If Marion were under 65 years of age, would the management plan change?

What patient, family, and caregiver education is most important in this case?

A few weeks after the visit described above, you receive a phone call from Marion's friend, who calls the clinic with news that Marion experienced a brief episode of slurred speech and

right-sided weakness that lasted a few minutes. These symptoms occurred about 30 minutes ago. What is your priority recommendation? Her friend reports that Marion is feeling fine now but she is frightened. What is your advice?

What diagnostic evaluation should be completed?

What education is needed?

What is the management plan?

What are some of the most important domains of nursing assessment and management (physical, psychological) during these first few hours after symptoms? In the early post-stroke period?

Case 10.6 Back Pain

By Ivy M. Alexander, PhD, APRN, ANP-BC, FAANP, FAAN

SUBJECTIVE

Mary is a 63-year-old female who presents with upper midback pain that began after lifting her 3-year-old granddaughter 3 days ago. She says the pain began right after she lifted her granddaughter up over her head and then placed her into the high chair. Her granddaughter weighs about 25 pounds. Mary says she has done this many times without any pain or problems in the past. Mary cares for her granddaughter during the day while her daughter is working. She describes the pain as sharp and notes that it radiates into her lower chest and around to her abdomen. Mary's pain is constant and heavy but does wane a little bit with rest (5–7 on a 1–10 scale). It is unaffected by nonsteroidal anti-inflammatory drugs (NSAIDs), acetaminophen, or topical rub, each of which she tried once. She feels slightly short of breath, described as "it is hard to take a full breath in, because it hurts." She found it difficult to put on a turtleneck shirt this morning.

Mary describes her overall health as "good." She says that she is enjoying retirement and caring for her granddaughter. She reports stable weight for the past 5–6 years; she had gained 5–10 pounds in the first 2–3 years after menopause. She identifies her usual weight as 120–125 pounds. She reports good energy and that she usually sleeps well but has not slept well since this pain began. She denies any substantive premenstrual syndrome (PMS) symptoms when she was having regular menses. She denies having had symptoms of premenstrual dysphoric disorder (PMDD).

Mary reports her usual mood as "excellent!" Mary denies moodiness, nervousness, anxiety, irritability, or feeling quick to anger. She denies feeling depressed and says, "I laugh a lot. I have loads of fun caring for my granddaughter, and my husband is always quick with a joke." Mary denies anhedonia and says that she enjoys gardening, reading, and social activities with her husband, friends, and daughter and her family. Mary denies eating disorders. She says she has had to reduce her intake lately to keep her weight stable.

Mary denies problems with concentration, memory, or cognition. She says she uses a calendar to keep track of activities, especially appointments or play dates and preschool for her granddaughter. Mary reports no specific systemic complains. She denies general fatigue and says she did not have terrible hot flashes like her sister did with the change of life. She feels well.

The Family Nurse Practitioner: Clinical Case Studies, Second Edition. Edited by Leslie Neal-Boylan.
© 2021 John Wiley & Sons Ltd. Published 2021 by John Wiley & Sons Ltd.

HEENT: Mary denies problems with headaches. However, she has sinus headaches when her seasonal allergies are bothersome. Mary uses bifocals, which she has had for many years. She has annual ophthalmologic exams with her optometrist. She denies changes in hearing, smell, taste, or swallowing. She reports some dry-eye symptoms and needs to use eye-lubricating drops only rarely. She has seasonal allergies that cause light rhinorrhea, sneezing, and itchy eyes in the fall.

Respiratory: Mary denies cough or wheeze. She describes a sensation of being short of breath since the pain began, saying, "It is not that I can't breathe; it is that I cannot take in a full, deep breath because it hurts."

Cardiovascular: Mary denies prior chest pain, palpitations, dyspnea on exertion (DOE), peripheral edema, or a history of blood clots. She says that the pain she has now radiates into her lower chest but is definitely coming from her upper midback area. She denies problems with cold hands and feet. She reports being diagnosed with high blood pressure about 8 years ago. She has been treated with HCTZ, which she tolerates well.

Breast: Mary reports that she does regular self–breast exams. She usually does them at the beginning of the month when she changes the calendar to the new month. She denies any concerns or recent breast changes. She denies any discharge, pain, or tingling. She breastfed her daughter.

Gastrointestinal: Mary denies heartburn or persistent abdominal pain. She reports daily regular bowel movements, without constipation or recent changes in color, consistency, or pattern of stools. Specifically, she denies seeing any blood or experiencing fecal incontinence. She describes some pain radiating into her abdomen but again states that it is definitely coming from her upper midback.

Genitourinary: Mary reports some urgency and occasional leakage of small amounts of urine, especially with coughing or laughing. She denies urinary frequency, history of recurrent urinary tract infections, pyelonephritis, renal stones, and urine dribbling or outright incontinence. She says she does not have dysuria. She reports occasional nocturia of once or twice at night. She says this is usual for her over many years and that she goes right back to sleep after using the toilet.

Gynecological: Mary reports no abnormal Pap smears or GYN surgeries. She denies vaginal or vulvar discharge, itching, irritation, soreness, burning, abnormal bleeding, or lesions. She denies pelvic pain or rash. She reports some vaginal dryness, especially noticed with sexual activity.

Pregnancy history: Mary has been pregnant twice. She is P2, G1, TAB 1 (for fetal demise at 11 weeks). Her daughter is healthy at age 32. Mary reports that she breastfed her daughter for 13 months.

Menstrual history: Mary reports that her LMP was 11 years ago. She reports that her menses were regular, lasting for 6–7 days with 2 days of light flow, followed by 3 days of heavier flow, and then 1–2 days of light flow again. She experienced menarche at 12 years of age; and after the first few years, she had very regular periods occurring about every 28 days. Her menses remained regular right up until her last period.

Menopause: Mary reports that her experience with the transition to postmenopause was fairly smooth. She had some hot flashes during the day and rarely at night. She did not experience drenching sweats. She never took hormone therapy or other medications for her symptoms. She has some vaginal dryness, and she and her husband do use lubricant when having sexual intercourse.

Contraception: Mary reports that she used oral contraceptive pills for contraception in the past. She stopped using oral contraceptive pills after her last pregnancy; she and her husband used either male condoms or withdrawal after that. She says that she would not have minded getting pregnant again, but it never happened.

Sexual: Mary reports that she is sexually active with her husband of 35 years. She is mostly satisfied, but she notes that it has become harder to get adequately lubricated and that it takes longer to achieve orgasm. She reports she has had 6 lifetime partners and has been monogamous with her husband for over 38 years. They have intercourse about once a week. She reports that her desire/libido is satisfactory but is less strong than it was when she was younger. She denies dyspareunia. She reports their usual sexual practices include initiation by her husband, cuddling and kissing, then foreplay that includes genital manipulation, and then vaginal intercourse with penile penetration. They regularly use over-the-counter (OTC) lubricants, due to her dryness. She says she feels good during sex and enjoys sex with her husband. She reports their relationship quality as "Wonderful. He is my partner and my best friend." She says that, due to the pain in her upper back, she did not engage in sex last night when her husband tried to initiate.

Musculoskeletal: Mary reports that she felt good up until 3 days ago. She has had rheumatoid arthritis (RA) for many years, and it is well controlled on her current DMARD (disease-modifying antirheumatic drug). She has used steroids for about the past 6 years (oral prednisone 5–10 mg daily depending on her symptoms) and then started DMARDs. She now takes a new DMARD, leflunomide; and she has not had a significant flare for a few years with this new medication. She does have some morning stiffness that is mostly relieved with a warm shower and movement. She gets regular exercise and is quite active in caring for her granddaughter with daily walks, often pushing the stroller, getting her in and out of the high chair, and playing with her on the swings at the park.

Endocrine: Mary denies polydipsia, polyuria, polyphagia, and symptoms of diabetes mellitus Type 2 (DMT2).

Skin/hair: Mary denies any recent skin changes or lesions of concern. She has noticed some increased dryness and wrinkles and dry/thinning hair, especially on her head. She denies hirsutism or facial hair.

Hematologic: Mary denies any bleeding or bruising that doesn't correlate to a specific injury. She says she is a bit surprised that there is no bruising on her back as it feels like there should be something visible.

Neurologic: Mary denies numbness, tingling, fainting, dizziness (vertigo), feeling off balance, or difficulty walking. She had some numbness in her right shoulder-blade region the day after her pain began; that numbness has subsided.

Sleep: Mary's usual bedtime routine includes nighttime washing and tooth brushing followed by reading for about 20 minutes. She denies using stimulants except for coffee each morning. She wakes every night to urinate and reports that she falls right back to sleep. Since her back pain began, she has had trouble sleeping. She is able to fall asleep but then awakens in pain and finds it very hard to get back to sleep because she cannot get comfortable. She usually goes to bed around 10 p.m. and falls asleep around 10:30 p.m. She gets up around 6:30 a.m. most days. She reports that she usually feels refreshed when she wakes up but has not since her back pain began.

Past medical/surgical history: Rheumatoid arthritis (RA), well controlled at present; history of oral steroid use in the past 6 years; + hypertension, controlled; + seasonal allergies (fall). Wisdom teeth excisions at age 18; TAB at age 33.

Family history: Mother: deceased from breast cancer; father: DMT2, HTN, some dementia; sister: A+W.

Social history: Mary lives with her husband of 35 years and the family cat in a private home that they own. She is a retired elementary schoolteacher and currently provides day care for her granddaughter while her daughter works. She reports that she enjoys caring for her granddaughter very much and is thrilled that she can help her daughter and son-in-law by caring for her grand-daughter. She reports no important recent life events; the most recent was her granddaughter's birth 3 years ago. She describes her usual day as follows: She awakes around 6:30 a.m., makes breakfast for herself and her husband, showers and dresses, greets her granddaughter and pre-pares her breakfast, reads a book with her granddaughter, and then they watch *Sesame Street* on TV. Some mornings they have a play date or go to the library for reading circle or music. She feeds her granddaughter lunch around noon and then settles her to nap from about 1–3 p.m. In the afternoons they might have a play date, go to the park, read, or play some games at home. Her daughter usually picks up the granddaughter around 5:30 p.m. Mary makes dinner most evenings and spends time in the evening with sewing, TV, playing cards with her husband, or doing household chores. She starts getting ready for bed around 10 p.m. She reports walking for about 1 mile most days with her granddaughter in the stroller. On the weekends she also goes to a water aerobics class. Her 24-hour diet recall reveals: cereal with 1% milk and coffee (black) for breakfast; tuna salad on toast for lunch; grilled chicken with garden salad for dinner; and carrot sticks for an afternoon snack. She reports that she eats out about once per week and enjoys dessert on occasion. She denies use of tobacco. She reports alcohol use as 1 glass of red wine most evenings. She denies use of recreational/illicit drugs. She reports feeling safe at home and with her husband and family. She denies ever having been hit, slapped, kicked, or otherwise physically hurt by someone (except her granddaughter who occasionally will "fight" when it is time to change clothes). She denies ever being forced to have sexual activities when she did not want to. She uses seatbelts and sunblock regularly and has working smoke and carbon monoxide detectors at home. There are no guns in the home, and she denies any concerns for her granddaughter's or her personal safety. She denies having any current concerns about HIV.

Medications: OTC antihistamines for allergies PRN; nasal spray for allergies PRN; MVI daily; calcium (when she remembers); HCTZ, 25 mg daily; glucosamine sulfate with chondroitin, 1500 mg in divided dose daily; omega-3 supplements (fish oil), 2 g daily; leflunomide, 10 mg daily.

Allergies: NKDA, NKFA (but finds that too much yeast bothers her RA with increased morning stiffness and more joint swelling). Some "hay fever" in the fall.

OBJECTIVE

General: Appears well, but uncomfortable with slow careful movements and limited use of upper extremities; neatly dressed; appropriate affect.

Vital signs: BP: 130/78 (L) sitting; P: 74; RR: 10; weight: 130 lb; height 5 feet 5 inches; BMI 21.6.

Neck: Supple, w/o LAN. Thyroid NT, w/o palpable masses or enlargement. Carotids w/o bruits. Limited neck AROM, especially chin-to-chest, due to pain.

Respiratory: Clear to anterior and posterior; w/o wheezes, rales, rubs, or rhonchi. Patient unwilling to take full inhalation due to pain.

Cardiovascular: RRR, normal S1 and S2 w/o murmurs, rubs, or gallops; +pain with manual com-pression to anterior and posterior chest wall. No cyanosis, edema, or clubbing; +2 pulses bilaterally.

Breasts: Without masses, skin changes, or discharge bilaterally. No lymphadenopathy.

Abdomen: Positive for bowel sounds ×4 quadrants; soft, nondistended. NT with superficial or deep palpation; without HSM, masses, or bruits.

Spine: Good AROM at waist and for twisting with lower spine. Thoracic spine with limited AROM due to pain; +tenderness over T7 and T8.

Musculoskeletal: Positive for FAROM throughout; but limited upper spine mobility and upper extremities for full overhead movements, slight tenderness and swelling over MCP and PIP joints of BIL hands, joints w/o crepitus, no digital ulnar deviation, no swan neck or boutonniere deformities, no nodules. 5/5 motor strength, but with limited effort of bilateral upper extremities (BIL UEs).

Neurologic: CN II–XII grossly intact; gait even; DTRs 2+; Romberg negative.

CRITICAL THINKING

What are the most likely differential diagnoses in this case and why?

Which diagnostic tests are required in this case and why?

What is the plan of treatment?

What are the plans for referral and follow-up care?

What health education should be provided to this patient?

What demographic characteristics might affect this case?

Does the patient's psychosocial history impact how you might treat her?

Are there any standardized guidelines that should be used to treat this case? If so, what are they?

Case 10.7 Acute Joint Pain

By Sara Smoller, RN, MSN, ANP-BC

SUBJECTIVE

Rami is a 72-year-old male presenting with 2 days of acute onset left great toe pain. He complains of pain with any movement or ambulation. He denies trauma or injuries. He woke up with the pain 2 days ago; it began very suddenly. He denies a prior history of foot or leg problems. He has never had symptoms like this before. Rami reports otherwise feeling well; he denies any systemic symptoms including fever or chills; however, he notes that his toe feels warm. He has been taking Tylenol 650 mg every 6 hours with minimal relief. He tried 2 ibuprofen yesterday that helped slightly. He avoids taking this, as it upsets his stomach.

Past medical history: Osteoarthritis, COPD, hypertension.

Family history: Rami's mother and father have diabetes mellitus Type 2. His father has severe osteoarthritis.

Social history: Rami is a retired nurse. He lives alone; his wife died 3 years ago of pancreatic cancer. He has 4 children; they all live in New York where he is from, originally. Rami is a non-smoker and drinks 2 glasses of red wine nightly. He is fairly active, playing pickleball with the town league 1–2 × per week.

Medications: Tylenol 325 mg prn; Spiriva 1 inhalation daily; albuterol 50 mg qd; chlorthalidone 25 mg qd; amlodipine 10 mg qd

Allergies: Sulfa (hives)

OBJECTIVE

General: No apparent distress.

Vital signs: Temperature: 97.9°F (PO); BP: 158/72; pulse: 64 and regular. He is 5 ft 11 inches tall and 195 pounds.

General: Rami is pleasant and cooperative and in no distress.

The Family Nurse Practitioner: Clinical Case Studies, Second Edition. Edited by Leslie Neal-Boylan.
© 2021 John Wiley & Sons Ltd. Published 2021 by John Wiley & Sons Ltd.

Eyes: PERRL. No injection or icterus.

Cardiac: Regular rate and rhythm, no murmurs.

Lungs: Clear bilaterally.

Abdomen: Soft, nontender, nondistended. No palpable masses or hepatosplenomegaly.

MSK: Left great toe swollen with diffuse erythema, warmth, and tenderness to light touch over the metatarsal phalangeal (MTP) joint. Minimal flexion and extension of the great toe due to significant pain. Gait is antalgic due to pain.

Pulses: Bilateral dorsalis pedis and posterior tibial pulses 2+.

Skin: No rashes to the lower extremities, left great toe is diffusely erythematous.

CRITIAL THINKING

What is the most likely diagnosis and why?
___Sprain/strain
___Acute gouty arthritis
___Septic arthritis
___Osteoarthritis
___Rheumatoid arthritis

What are possible differential diagnoses?

Which diagnostic or imaging studies should be considered to assist with or confirm the diagnosis?
___X-ray
___Complete blood count
___BUN/Creatinine (renal function)
___Uric acid
___Joint aspiration

What is the plan of treatment?

Are there any modifiable risk factors or medications Rami is taking that could contribute to this diagnosis?

What are the plans for referral and follow-up care?

What health education should be provided to Rami at this visit?

What if Rami had uncontrolled diabetes mellitus? How would this affect the treatment plan?

Rami recovers from his current symptoms but comes in again in 4 months with a similar problem. What should be done for him at this visit?

Case 10.8 Itching and Soreness

By Sheila L. Molony, PhD, APRN, GNP-BC, FGSA, FAAN

SUBJECTIVE

Rosa is a 74-year-old woman who presents with a complaint of itching and soreness in her left side and upper back. She tells you that she has been gardening and that she thinks she may have a spider or bug bite, but she cannot see this area. She felt an "irritation" 2–3 days ago with intermittent itching. She took some oral OTC Benadryl© without benefit. She now complains of intermittent "shooting pain" and "tingling" sensations around the area of the left shoulder blade. She has been wearing a camisole instead of a bra for comfort. She denies itching in any other location on the body and has no other dermatological complaints. She denies recent trauma to the chest or back. She denies use of new shampoos, lotions, laundry products, clothing, perfumes, or topical agents.

Past medical history: Positive for hypertension (HTN); osteoarthritis (OA, primarily of the knees and fingers); gout; osteoporosis, and polymyalgia rheumatica (PMR).

Medications: Zestoretic, 1 tablet by mouth once per day; alendronate, 70 mg, by mouth, once per week; allopurinol, by mouth, 200 mg po once per day; Prilosec, 20 mg by mouth once per day; and prednisone, 7.5 mg by mouth, once per day. She has been taking these medicines for over 1 year (with varying prednisone dose adjustments).

Allergies: She denies any environmental, contact, or medication allergies.

OBJECTIVE

Head: Abundant, slightly dry hair in normal distribution with no alopecia or breaking. Head is normocephalic and atraumatic.

Lymph nodes: No palpable lymphadenopathy in head, neck, thorax, or axilla.

Skin: Pale with multiple scattered, small, bright-red, pinpoint papules over the chest and back, as well as several irregularly shaped, flat, light-brown macules. She has no visible rash, discoloration,

The Family Nurse Practitioner: Clinical Case Studies, Second Edition. Edited by Leslie Neal-Boylan.
© 2021 John Wiley & Sons Ltd. Published 2021 by John Wiley & Sons Ltd.

or lesion in the affected area, and no obvious insect bite or entry wound. Her skin is very dry in all areas.

Thorax: Exquisite tenderness on palpation in the left subscapular area, extending to the anterior axillary line, lateral to the left breast.

Her remaining physical examination is within normal limits.

CRITICAL THINKING

What is the most likely differential diagnosis and why?
__Bug bite
__Contact dermatitis
__Eczema
__Herpes zoster
__Infestation (lice or scabies)
__Medication-related adverse effects
__Polymyalgia rheumatica (exacerbation)
__Rib fracture
__Seborrheic dermatitis
__Systemic disease
__Xerosis (dry skin)

Which diagnostic or imaging studies should be considered to assist with or confirm the diagnosis?
__Erythrocyte sedimentation rate (ESR or "sed rate")
__Immunoglobin E titer
__Immunoglobin G titer for varicella zoster
__Metabolic (chemical) profile including LFTs, BUN/creatinine, electrolytes, and TSH
__Polymerase chain reaction (PCR) testing
__Skin biopsy
__Skin scraping for microscopy

What is the management plan?

Are any referrals appropriate at this time?

Which of the clinical findings are consistent with normal aging changes?

What are the most common causes of pruritus (itching) in older adults? What are the risks and benefits of antihistamine therapy for pruritus, such as diphenhydramine (Benadryl©)?

If new lesions continue to appear after 1 week, what additional considerations should be addressed?

Which specific vaccines' dates of administration should be included in immunization documentation for older adults?

How can excess disability be prevented?

How can comfort (physical, psychosocial, and spiritual) be enhanced, beginning immediately? How can suffering be reduced?

Case 10.9 Knee Pain

By Leslie Neal-Boylan, PhD, APRN, CRRN, FAAN, FARN

SUBJECTIVE

Sharon, a 68-year-old obese woman, presents with bilateral knee pain described as "aching pain around the knee." The pain is worse going down stairs, with activity, and at night. She denies any recent trauma other than kneeling activities. She denies hearing any popping sounds or experiencing any locking or giving way of the knee. She denies being bitten by a tick, although she does occasionally work in her garden. She denies fever or chills or general malaise or confusion. She is the mother of 4 adult children and 3 young grandchildren and stays very busy babysitting and helping in the children's households. However, the knee pain has recently limited her activities. When she was a young woman, she was athletic and participated in sports; but since her children grew up, she has been in a sedentary office job and rarely exercises. She has felt well and has not seen a health care provider for 5 years. She still gets occasional hot flushes but has not had a period for 16 years. She experiences vaginal dryness and states that she does not participate in sexual activity, as she is a widow.

Past medical/surgical history: Sharon had surgery for carpal tunnel syndrome bilaterally 20 years ago. She also has had several suspicious skin lesions removed that have been benign. She had one episode of nephrolithiasis at age 35. Two of her children were born by cesarean section, and two were born via vaginal childbirth. There were no complications with any of the births.

Family medical history: Her mother had rheumatoid arthritis and died of complications at age 55.

Social history: Sharon is a nonsmoker, drinks "socially" (1 glass of red wine when she goes to a restaurant once each week), and has never used recreational drugs. Sharon lives alone but has her family and many friends to keep her busy. She feels safe at home and is generally happy with her life but a little tired from all of the babysitting and housework she has been doing.

Medications: Her medications include a multivitamin and occasional aspirin or acetaminophen for "aches and pains." These medicines have relieved her knee pain somewhat but not to her satisfaction. Sharon is not allergic to any medications.

The Family Nurse Practitioner: Clinical Case Studies, Second Edition. Edited by Leslie Neal-Boylan.
© 2021 John Wiley & Sons Ltd. Published 2021 by John Wiley & Sons Ltd.

OBJECTIVE

Vital signs: Sharon is afebrile. Her blood pressure is 160/90; HR is regular and 84; respiratory rate is regular at 14. Her weight is 210 lbs.

Cardiac: Regular rate and rhythm with no murmurs, clicks, gallops, or rubs.

Respiratory: Lungs are clear bilaterally.

Abdomen: Obese and soft without organomegaly or bruits.

Musculoskeletal: Sharon's knees are mildly swollen without erythema or warmth. There is no tenderness to palpation. Drawer, McMurray, and Lachman tests are negative. The bulge and ballottement signs are also negative. There is mild nonpitting ankle edema.

Skin: Without any current suspicious lesions or any rashes or ulcers.

CRITICAL THINKING

What is the most likely differential diagnosis and why?
__Ligament strain or tear
__Bursitis
__Osteoporosis
__Osteoarthritis
__Patellofemoral syndrome
__Gout
__Pseudogout
__Lyme disease
__Rheumatoid arthritis

Which diagnostic or imaging studies should be considered to assist with or confirm the diagnosis?
__Lyme titer
__CBC
__CMP
__Lipids
__TSH
__Colonoscopy
__Mammogram
__Pelvic exam
__ESR
__Rheumatoid factor
__CCP
__DEXA scan
__Vitamin D level

What should be the plan of treatment?

What should be the plan for health maintenance testing for this patient?

Does this patient need gynecological care and treatment at this time?

What is the plan for referrals and follow-up?

Case 10.10 Hyperthermia and Mental Status Changes in the Elderly

By Suellen Breakey, PhD, RN, and
Patrice K. Nicholas, DNSc, DHL (Hon), MPH, MS, RN, NP-C, FAAN

This case takes place in early August in the northeast United States. The heat index has exceeded 90°F for 4 days. Judith is an 84-year-old white woman who lives in low-income senior housing in a heavily populated urban area. Her neighbor, who checks on Judith daily, finds Judith in apparent distress. The urgent care clinic is across the street so the neighbor gets one of the other neighbors to help get Judith to the clinic. The nurse practitioner examines Judith and finds her to be febrile with acute neurological changes (lethargic, confused, incoherent, and unable to follow commands), hypotensive, and tachycardic. The neighbor says that the apartment was very hot.

Vital signs: Temperature: 103.3°F PO; HR: 110 ST; BP: 84/50; RR: 30; oxygen saturation 90% on room air. An intravenous line is placed, and a 500 mL bolus of normal saline is given to Judith at the clinic.

Past medical history: HTN, hypercholesterolemia, and mild congestive heart failure (diagnosed 8 years ago); ejection fraction (40%).

Social history: Judith lives alone in low-income urban senior housing. She is a retired U.S. postal worker. Her apartment lacks air conditioning, but she does have a fan. She receives Meals on Wheels 3 times a week. Her husband of 45 years died 6 years ago. She has 3 children who visit approximately every 2 to 3 weeks. Other than family, she has limited social interaction outside the housing complex apart from an occasional visit with neighbors.

Family history: Mother had hypertension and history of a myocardial infarction. Father had diabetes and died from complications of stroke. Adult children with unknown health backgrounds.

Medications: Furosemide 20 mg PO daily; lisinopril 10 mg PO daily; metoprolol SR 50 mg PO daily; simvastatin 20 mg PO daily.

Allergies: No known allergies.

OBJECTIVE

Vital signs: Temp: 102.5°F core; HR: 106 ST; BP: 90/58; RR: 28; oxygen saturation: 96% on 2L nasal cannula.

The Family Nurse Practitioner: Clinical Case Studies, Second Edition. Edited by Leslie Neal-Boylan.
© 2021 John Wiley & Sons Ltd. Published 2021 by John Wiley & Sons Ltd.

General: Judith is an 84-year-old white woman; height 5 ft 1 inch; weight 115 lb; no obvious signs of injury or distress noted; lying on stretcher. She is awake, unable to follow commands consistently, and appears restless (e.g., picking at sheets and oxygen tubing).

HEENT: Lips are pale and dry; buccal mucosa and tongue are dry; no nodes or masses palpated.

Neurological: Oriented to person only; speech slurred; pupils are 3 mm equal and reactive to light and accommodation; no obvious focal deficits noted; difficult to assess systematically due to patient's mental status.

Cardiac: Normal S1, S2; no murmurs or bruits noted. Radial and distal pulses are 1+, equal bilaterally; +CSM; no peripheral edema noted.

Respiratory: Lungs are clear bilaterally; patient tachypneic but does not appear in distress; no nasal flaring or use of accessory muscles noted.

Abdominal/GI: Abdomen soft, nontender; bowel sounds present in all 4 quadrants; no pain; no masses; no bruits noted.

Musculoskeletal: Gait not assessed due to neurological changes. Evidence of crepitus bilaterally in knees on palpation. Hip flexion < 90 degrees.

Skin/Dermatologic: Skin is hot, dry, and intact.

CRITICAL THINKING

What are the top three differential diagnoses in this case and why?

Which diagnostic tests are required in this case and why?

What are the concerns at this point?

The elderly are particularly vulnerable to heat-related illnesses (HRIs), such as heat exhaustion and heatstroke. List the symptoms and treatment associated with each condition.

Identify six risk factors that Judith has for developing heatstroke and explain how each contributes to its development.

Identify and explain three physical assessment findings from the case that support a diagnosis of heatstroke.

Identify and explain three elements from the patient's history that support a diagnosis of heatstroke.

What is the differential diagnosis for heatstroke?

What is the plan of treatment?

What are the plans for referral and follow-up care?

What health education should be provided to this patient?

What demographic characteristics might affect this case?

Does the patient's psychosocial history impact how you might treat her?

How does this patient's living in an urban area impact her risk for heatstroke?

Are there any standardized guidelines that should be used to treat this case? If so, what are they?

Section 11

Resolutions

Case 1.1 Cardiovascular Screening Exam

Which diagnostic or imaging studies should be considered to assist with or confirm the diagnosis?

An electrocardiogram, chest X-ray, and echocardiogram should all be performed.

Results of diagnostic tests: ECG results are normal. CXR is normal. Echocardiogram reveals a patent ductus arteriosus.

What is the most likely differential diagnosis and why?

Patent ductus arteriosus (PDA):

PDA is the most common congenital heart defect seen in premature infants. Intravenous indomethacin (the drug of choice) often stimulates closure of the ductus arteriosus in premature infants. Nonsteroidal anti-inflammatory drugs (NSAIDs) such as ibuprofen may also be used to stimulate closure of the PDA. Prophylaxis for infective endocarditis is required until the PDA is closed. No long-term sequelae usually occur if the PDA is treated before pulmonary vascular disease develops.

What is the plan of treatment, and what should be the plan for follow-up care?

- Monitor weight and other growth parameters at subsequent visits.
- Provide emotional support. Allow the parents to verbalize their concerns about their baby's health maintenance. Facilitate mother-infant attachment.
- Return to clinic in 4 days for 2-week, well-child check and weight check.
- Discuss signs and symptoms of increased work of breathing (increased respiratory rate; intercostal retractions; nasal flaring) with parents and when to call the office (decreased by-mouth intake; decreased urine output; increased work of breathing; increased temperature ≥100.4°F).

Are there any referrals needed?

- Refer to cardiology for consideration of medication or surgery to aid in the closure of the duct.
- Consider referral for genetic counseling regarding future conception.

Does the patient's psychosocial history influence how you might treat her?

Since this mother is a single mother with two other children in the home, it is important for the health care provider to ensure that the family is referred to the appropriate social service agencies.

The Family Nurse Practitioner: Clinical Case Studies, Second Edition. Edited by Leslie Neal-Boylan.
© 2021 John Wiley & Sons Ltd. Published 2021 by John Wiley & Sons Ltd.

The family should be referred to the Women, Infants, and Children (WIC) program for supplemental food and infant formula services. Mothers with a lower socioeconomic status have been found to be more at risk for postpartum depression, so it will be important for the health care provider to screen this mother for postpartum depression at subsequent visits throughout the baby's first year of life.

What if this baby were a girl?

Girls have been noted to be affected by patent ductus arteriosus twice as often as boys.

What if this baby had been born full term?

Functional closure of the ductus occurs within 15 hours of birth in a normal full-term infant, but true closure with the inability to reopen takes about 3 weeks.

What if this baby had been born at a higher altitude?

Babies born at higher altitudes are at increased risk for a patent ductus arteriosus.

Are there any standardized guidelines that should be used to assess or treat this case?

There are no standardized guidelines located in the literature for the assessment and/or treatment of patent ductus arteriosus.

REFERENCES AND RESOURCES

Conrad, C., Newberry, D., Harris-Haman, P., & Zukowsky, K. (2019). Understanding the pathophysiology, implications, and treatment options of patent ductus arteriosus in the neonatal population. *Advances in Neonatal Care, 19*, 179–187.

Havranek, T., Rahimi, M., Hall, H., & Armbrecht, E. (2015). Feeding preterm neonates with patent ductus arteriosus (PDA): Intestinal blood flow characteristics and clinical outcomes. *Journal of Maternal-Fetal & Neonatal Medicine, 28*, 526–530.

Hundscheid, T., van den Broek, M., van der Lee, R., & de Boode, W. (2019). Understanding the pathobiology in patent ductus arteriosus in prematurity—beyond prostaglandins and oxygen. *Pediatric Research, 86*, 28–38.

Lewis, T., Shelton, E., Van Driest, S., Kannankeril, P., & Reese, J. (2018). Genetics of the patent ductus arteriosus (PDA) and pharmacogenetics of PDA treatment. *Seminars in Fetal & Neonatal Medicine, 23*, 232–238.

Case 1.2 Pulmonary Screening Exam

Which diagnostic or imaging studies should be considered to assist with or confirm the diagnosis?

It is important to obtain an arterial blood gas (ABG) to determine the level of gas exchange and acid-base balance. The ABG results reveal mild respiratory and metabolic acidosis.

Chest radiography is the diagnostic standard for transient tachypnea of the newborn. The chest radiograph shows generalized overexpansion of the lung (hypoaeration of alveoli) and flattened contours of the diaphragm, which are consistent with transient tachypnea of the newborn.

What is the most likely differential diagnosis and why?

Transient tachypnea of the newborn (TTN):

Transient tachypnea of the newborn (TTN) is a self-limited disease. Approximately 1% of neonates have some form of respiratory distress that is not associated with infection, such as transient tachypnea of the newborn. TTN results from a delay in clearance of fetal liquid from the lungs. Infants with TTN usually present with tachypnea within the first few hours of life. It has been associated with precipitous deliveries and births by cesarean section. It is also more common in babies born to mothers with diabetes. Medical care of TTN is supportive. As the retained lung fluid is absorbed by the infant's lymphatic system, the pulmonary status of the infant typically improves. TTN resolves over a 24-hour to 72-hour period.

What is the plan of treatment, referral, and follow-up care?

- Begin oxygen therapy in the office.
- Refer the patient and family to the local emergency department for support of the respiratory system, a workup for possible sepsis (complete blood count, blood cultures, lumbar puncture for culture of cerebrospinal fluid, and urine culture), and consultation with a neonatologist. An ambulance should be called to transport the baby from the office to the emergency department so that the baby's airway and respiratory status may be maintained.
- Provide emotional support to the parents. Allow the parents to verbalize their concerns about their baby's health status. Facilitate mother-infant attachment.

The Family Nurse Practitioner: Clinical Case Studies, Second Edition. Edited by Leslie Neal-Boylan.
© 2021 John Wiley & Sons Ltd. Published 2021 by John Wiley & Sons Ltd.

Are there any demographic characteristics that would affect this case?

The risk for TTN is equal in males and females. There has been no association with race or ethnicity reported. TTN presents as respiratory distress in full-term or near-term infants.

What if the patient lived in a rural, isolated setting?

Health care providers practicing in rural, isolated settings should have emergency office plans in place for patients experiencing respiratory distress.

Are there any standardized guidelines that should be used to assess or treat this case?

There were no standardized guidelines located in the literature for the assessment and/or treatment of transient tachypnea of the newborn.

REFERENCES AND RESOURCES

Kayıran, S., Erçin, S., Kayıran, P., Gursoy, T., & Gurakan, B. (2019). Relationship between thyroid hormone levels and transient tachypnea of the newborn in late-preterm, early-term, and term infants. *Journal of Maternal-Fetal & Neonatal Medicine, 32*, 1342–1346.

Li, J., Wu, J., Du, L., Hu, Y., Yang, X., Mu, D., & Xia, B. (2015). Different antibiotic strategies in transient tachypnea of the newborn: An ambispective cohort study. *European Journal of Pediatrics, 174*, 1217–1223.

Omran, A., Mousa, H., Abdalla, M., & Zekry, O. (2018). Maternal and neonatal vitamin D deficiency and transient tachypnea of the newborn in full term neonates. *Journal of Perinatal Medicine, 46*, 1057–1060.

Case 1.3 Skin Screening Exam

Which diagnostic or imaging studies should be considered to assist with or confirm the diagnosis?

Eosinophils will be noted on microscopic examination using a Wright stain. Eosinophilia may also be noted on peripheral blood studies. However, the diagnosis of erythema toxicum is usually made on the basis of clinical findings from the history and physical examination. No diagnostic testing is usually needed.

What is the most likely differential diagnosis and why?

Erythema toxicum:

Erythema toxicum, also called erythema toxicum neonatorum or toxic erythema of the newborn, is a common skin condition seen in newborns. It is self-limited and only occurs in the neonatal period. Herpes usually has more of a clustered and vesicular appearance, whereas the lesions of erythema toxicum are scattered. Milia are whitish, pearly bumps in the skin of newborns. The lesions are not on erythematous bases. Milia lesions typically occur on the cheeks, nose, and chin—and not on the trunk.

The etiology of erythema toxicum is unknown. It may appear in up to 70% of newborns between 3 days and 2 weeks of life. Although the condition is harmless, it can be of great concern to the new parent.

What is the plan of treatment?

Erythema toxicum is not contagious and does not require any medical treatment. It usually resolves within 2 weeks after birth. Follow-up care is not needed unless the condition persists or does not resolve by 2 weeks of life.

Are any referrals needed?

Erythema toxicum neonatorum is often diagnosed easily by pediatricians and family physicians. If the features are atypical, if the newborn appears ill, or if the newborn has risk factors for sepsis, consultation with a pediatric dermatologist may be advisable.

The Family Nurse Practitioner: Clinical Case Studies, Second Edition. Edited by Leslie Neal-Boylan.
© 2021 John Wiley & Sons Ltd. Published 2021 by John Wiley & Sons Ltd.

Does the patient's psychosocial history impact how you might treat her?
The family has a pet dog. The lesions from erythema toxicum may sometimes resemble flea bites. Flea bites also should be considered among the differential diagnoses.

Are there any demographic characteristics that would affect this case?
There have been significant differences noted in the incidence of erythema toxicum based on race or gender. This condition is limited to the neonatal period. If an infant older than 28 days of age has a similar rash, then other diagnoses should be strongly considered.

Are there any standardized guidelines that should be used to assess or treat this case?
There are currently no standardized guidelines for the assessment and/or treatment of erythema toxicum.

REFERENCES AND RESOURCES

Chadha, A., & Jahnke, M. (2019). Common neonatal rashes. *Pediatric Annals, 48*, e16–e22.

Shepard-Hayes, A. (2019). *Pediatric erythema toxicum.* Retrieved from: https://emedicine.medscape.com/article/909671-overview

Weatherspoon, D. (2018). Baby's skin. *International Journal of Childbirth Education, 33*, 13–17.

Case 1.4 Oxygenation

Which diagnostic or imaging studies should be considered to assist with or confirm the diagnosis?

A nasopharyngeal swab should be performed. A complete blood count (CBC) is seldom useful since the white blood cell (WBC) count is usually within normal limits. Chest radiographs are not routinely necessary. The nonspecific findings of hyperinflation and patchy infiltrates may be seen on the chest radiograph.

Results of diagnostic tests: The nasopharyngeal swab was positive for RSV.

What is the most likely differential diagnosis and why?

Bronchiolitis:

The most likely differential diagnosis is bronchiolitis related to an infection with RSV. Matthew's history and physical examination form the primary basis for the diagnosis of bronchiolitis. Bronchiolitis is usually due to a viral infection of the small lower airways (bronchioles). Infection is spread by direct contact with respiratory secretions. Previous infection does not confer immunity. Reinfection can be common. Early symptoms are those of a viral URI, including mild rhinorrhea, cough, and sometimes low-grade fever. It is unlikely to be chlamydial pneumonia since the mother was successfully treated during the pregnancy. Scattered crackles with good breath sounds are characteristic of chlamydial pneumonia, and wheezing is usually absent. Conjunctivitis and middle-ear abnormality may be present in half the infants with chlamydial pneumonia. Chest radiographs will show bilateral interstitial infiltrates with hyperinflation.

What is the plan of treatment, referral, and follow-up care?

- Consider oxygen therapy in the office, and monitor Matthew's cardiac and respiratory status. The American Academy of Pediatrics states that clinicians may choose not to administer supplemental oxygen if the child's oxygen saturation is above 90% on room air.
- Place Matthew in an upright position to facilitate respirations.
- The American Academy of Pediatrics recommends against the use of albuterol in infants and children with bronchiolitis.

The Family Nurse Practitioner: Clinical Case Studies, Second Edition. Edited by Leslie Neal-Boylan.
© 2021 John Wiley & Sons Ltd. Published 2021 by John Wiley & Sons Ltd.

- Refer patient and family to the local emergency department for support of the respiratory system, a workup for possible sepsis (complete blood count, blood cultures, lumbar puncture for culture of cerebrospinal fluid, and urine culture), and consultation with a neonatologist. An ambulance should be called to transport the baby from the office to the emergency department so that the baby's airway and respiratory status may be maintained.
- Provide emotional support to the parents. Allow the parents to verbalize their concerns about their baby's health status. Facilitate mother-infant attachment.

What demographic characteristics might affect this case?

Race and socioeconomic status may affect the frequency of contracting bronchiolitis. Lower socioeconomic status may increase the likelihood of hospitalization. Bronchiolitis occurs as much as 1.25 times more frequently in males than in females. In cases of bronchiolitis, 75% of the cases occur in children younger than 1 year, and 95% occur in children younger than 2 years. Incidence peaks in those aged 2–8 months.

Does the patient's psychosocial history impact how you might treat him?

Matthew's father is a smoker; and the family has 2 cats. Both of these things may be lung irritants.

What if the patient lived in a rural, isolated setting?

Health care providers practicing in rural, isolated settings should have emergency office plans in place for patients experiencing respiratory distress.

REFERENCES AND RESOURCES

Condella, A., Mansbach, J., Kohei, H., Dayan, P., Sullivan, A. Espinola, J., & Camargo, C. (2018). Multicenter study of albuterol use among infants hospitalized with bronchiolitis. *Western Journal of Emergency Medicine: Integrating Emergency Care with Population Health, 19,* 475–483.

Karampatsas, K., Kong, J., & Cohen, J. (2019). Bronchiolitis: An update on management and prophylaxis. *British Journal of Hospital Medicine, 80,* 278–284.

Ralston, S. L., Lieberthal, A. S., Meissner, H. C., Alverson, B. K., Baley, J. E., Gadomski, A. M., Hernandez-Cancio, S. (2014). Clinical practice guideline: The diagnosis, management, and prevention of bronchiolitis. *Pediatrics, 134,* e1474–e1502.

Rivera-Sepulveda, A., Rebmann, T., Gerard, J., & Charney, R. (2019). Physician compliance with bronchiolitis guidelines in pediatric emergency departments. *Clinical Pediatrics, 58,* 1008–1018.

Case 1.5 Nutrition and Weight

Which diagnostic or imaging studies should be considered to assist with or confirm the diagnosis?
No tests are needed based on the history and physical examination.

What is the most likely differential diagnosis and why?
Overfeeding:
Based on the history of the baby taking 5 oz of formula every 2 hours, the significant weight gain in the first 2 weeks of life, and the unremarkable physical examination, the most likely differential diagnosis is overfeeding. Gastroesophageal reflux disease (GERD) is often associated with failure to thrive. Neonates with GERD may also present with respiratory symptoms. Neonates with gastroenteritis may present with diarrhea and fever—which this baby does not have.

What is the plan of treatment and follow-up care?
- Via a Spanish-speaking medical interpreter, provide education about feeding, proper mixing of formula, and signs of satiety in neonates.
- Discuss ways to comfort the baby that do not involve feeding.
- Refer the family to the Women, Infants, and Children (WIC) Program for a consultation with a nutritionist and assistance with obtaining formula.

Does the patient's psychosocial history impact how you might treat this case?
Having a teenage mother who has limited English proficiency is an aspect of the patient's psychosocial history that may affect her treatment. Working with the mother and her family will require extra time during visits to ensure that the patient education and anticipatory guidance are properly understood.

What demographic characteristics might affect this case?
There are no particular race or socioeconomic characteristics that would affect overfeeding.

The Family Nurse Practitioner: Clinical Case Studies, Second Edition. Edited by Leslie Neal-Boylan.
© 2021 John Wiley & Sons Ltd. Published 2021 by John Wiley & Sons Ltd.

Are there any standardized guidelines that should be used to assess or treat this case?

There are no known guidelines that focus on overfeeding in the neonate. The American Academy of Pediatrics has guidelines about the introduction of solids.

REFERENCES AND RESOURCES

Barfield, E., & Parker, M. (2019). Management of pediatric gastroesophageal reflux disease. *JAMA Pediatrics, 173,* 485–486.

Barnhart, D. (2016). Gastroesophageal reflux in children. *Seminars in Pediatric Surgery, 25,* 212–218.

Rostas, S., & McPherson, C. (2018). Acid suppression for gastroesophageal reflux disease in infants. *Neonatal Network, 37,* 33–41.

Singendonk, M., Brink, A., Steutel, N., van Etten-Jamaludin, F., van Wijk, M., Benninga, M., & Tabbers, M. (2017). Variations in definitions and outcome measures in gastroesophageal reflux disease: A systematic review. *Pediatrics, 140,* 1–15.

RESOLUTION

Which laboratory tests should be ordered as part of a 12-month, well-child visit?
According to the American Academy of Pediatrics (AAP) *Recommendations for Preventive Pediatric Health Care* guidelines, there are several tests that are recommended for the 12-month well-child visit. A hemoglobin or hematocrit is recommended at the well-child visit to screen for iron deficiency anemia. A blood lead test is also recommended to screen for an elevated blood lead level. A tuberculin test is recommended if the child has risk factors for contracting tuberculosis, such as travel to an endemic area, residing in a homeless shelter, or visiting someone in jail. Neil's father is incarcerated. If he visits in father in jail, he should receive a screening for tuberculosis.

Other than "well child," what additional diagnoses should be considered for Neil?
Based on the information gathered during his history and on his physical examination, there are several additional diagnoses that may be considered. Related to Neil's nutrition, there are 2 potential diagnoses: at risk for constipation and at risk for iron deficiency anemia. Neil is drinking nearly 40 oz of cow's milk daily. This amount of milk is excessive for his age (recommended amount is 20–24 oz daily). Excessive milk intake is associated with iron-deficiency anemia, as well as constipation. Regarding his weight, Neil is currently in the age range to develop physiologic anorexia of the toddler. Because the rate of growth decreases during the second year of life (between 1 and 2 years of age), this diagnosis signifies that the child needs fewer calories and therefore may be more likely to eat less. Another consideration is that Neil is becoming full from his excessive milk intake and may be less likely to be hungry for solid foods.

What is the plan of treatment, referral, and follow-up care?
The plan of treatment for this visit would be to discuss the excessive milk intake, discuss iron-rich foods, and discuss the decreased caloric needs of the young toddler compared to the young infant. Kayla should be advised to feed Neil solid foods before offering him milk. She should also be advised to wean Neil off the bottle and to feed him liquids from a cup only, limiting juice to 4 oz and cow's milk to 24 oz per day. A daily pediatric multivitamin may also be prescribed for Neil.

Since Kayla already receives TANF and WIC services, she can be referred to the SNAP food stamp assistance program for additional help in acquiring nutritious foods for Neil. If further nutritional concerns arise, the family can be referred to a nutritionist. Neil should return to the

The Family Nurse Practitioner: Clinical Case Studies, Second Edition. Edited by Leslie Neal-Boylan.
© 2021 John Wiley & Sons Ltd. Published 2021 by John Wiley & Sons Ltd.

office for a well-child visit in 3 months for his 15-month checkup. He should return sooner if there are signs and symptoms of illness.

Does this patient's psychosocial history affect how you might treat this case?

Neil's family is likely to be of a lower socioeconomic status (SES) based on their eligibility for governmental subsidies such as WIC, TANF, and Section 8. Because of their SES, the family may be less likely to be able to afford nutritious foods. This could affect Neil's weight and growth patterns.

What if the patient lived in a rural setting?

Living in a rural setting might further limit access to nutritious foods since there may be fewer local facilities where nutritious foods can be readily purchased.

Are there any demographic characteristics that might affect this case?

The family's low income status is the demographic factor in this case. Other demographic characteristics such as gender and ethnicity are not likely to affect this case.

Are there any standardized guidelines that should be used to assess or treat this case?

Refer to the Office of Disease Prevention & Health Promotion and American Heart Association resources in the References and Resources below for guidelines on nutrition and weight that might be used to assess or treat this case.

REFERENCES AND RESOURCES

American Academy of Pediatrics Committee on Practice and Ambulatory Medicine, Bright Futures Periodicity Schedule Workgroup. (2019). 2019 recommendations for preventive pediatric health care. *Pediatrics, 143.*

American Heart Association. (2019). *Dietary recommendations for healthy children.* https://www.heart.org/en/healthy-living/healthy-eating/eat-smart/nutrition-basics/dietary-recommendations-for-healthy-children

Lagemaat, M., Amesz, E., Schaafsma, A., & Lafeber, H. (2014). Iron deficiency and anemia in iron-fortified formula and human milk-fed preterm infants until 6 months post-term. *European Journal of Nutrition, 53,* 1263–1271.

Office of Disease Prevention and Health Promotion. (2015). *Dietary guidelines for Americans 2015–2020* (8th ed.). https://health.gov/dietaryguidelines/2015/guidelines/

Sopo, S., Arena, R., & Scala, G. (2014). Functional constipation and cow's milk allergy. *Journal of Pediatric Gastroenterology & Nutrition, 59,* e34–e34.

U.S. Department of Agriculture Food and Nutrition Services. (2019). *Special supplemental nutrition program for women, infants, and children (WIC).* https://www.fns.usda.gov/wic

U.S. Department of Agriculture Food and Nutrition Services. (2019). *Supplemental nutrition assistance program (SNAP).* https://www.fns.usda.gov/snap/supplemental-nutrition-assistance-program

Case 2.2 Breastfeeding

RESOLUTION

Which laboratory or diagnostic imaging tests should be ordered as part of a 9-month, well-child visit?

According to the American Academy of Pediatrics (AAP) *Recommendations for Preventive Pediatric Health Care* guidelines, there are no recommended laboratory tests or diagnostic imaging tests for the 9-month, well-child visit. However, based on Julio's history of receiving a low-iron formula, the health care provider may consider obtaining a hemoglobin test to screen for iron-deficiency anemia. If the hemoglobin is abnormally low, then the health care provider can obtain a full complete blood count to confirm the diagnosis of iron deficiency anemia. The AAP guidelines recommend that children at risk for lead poisoning (those children living at or below the poverty line who live in older housing) receive a risk-assessment screening for lead poisoning at 9 months of age.

What is the most likely differential diagnosis and why?

Iron deficiency anemia and constipation:

Based on the history provided by Julio's mother, diagnoses to consider would be iron deficiency anemia and constipation.

What is the plan of treatment, referral, and follow-up care?

The plan of treatment would be to discuss nutrition, anticipatory guidance, and safety. For the 9-month visit, the health care provider should discuss safety issues such as car safety (having the child in a rear-facing car seat) and water safety (water temperature < 120 degrees; never leaving the baby in the bathtub alone; keeping the toilet lid and the bathroom door closed; emptying mop buckets after each use). In addition, the health care provider should discuss firearm safety, the prevention of burns, and the need for working smoke and carbon monoxide detectors.

The health care provider should discuss anticipatory guidance topics such as introducing the cup and beginning to wean Julio off the bottle; reading to him each night; and discouraging television watching and encouraging more interactive activities that promote proper brain development, such as talking, playing, singing, and reading together.

Nutrition topics such as the need for iron-fortified formula, not low-iron formula, to prevent iron deficiency anemia should be discussed. Nutritional suggestions should be given to prevent constipation associated with iron intake, such as pureed prunes or prune juice.

The Family Nurse Practitioner: Clinical Case Studies, Second Edition. Edited by Leslie Neal-Boylan.
© 2021 John Wiley & Sons Ltd. Published 2021 by John Wiley & Sons Ltd.

The family may be referred to the WIC (Women, Infants, and Children) program for assistance with obtaining formula and iron-fortified infant cereals. The WIC program has nutritionists on staff who will be able to provide Julio's family with nutritional education.

Julio should follow up for a well-child visit at 1 year of age or sooner as needed for signs and symptoms of illness.

Does this patient's psychosocial history affect how you might treat this case?

The language difference between the health care provider and the patient's family may be a potential barrier to receiving effective health care—even with the use of a certified medical interpreter. Because of this barrier, the health care provider may need to spend extra time when working with this family.

What if the patient lived in a rural setting?

It may be difficult to obtain appropriate medical interpreter services for families living in rural settings. This may prompt health care providers to use family members for interpretation, which could compromise patient confidentiality. Telephone interpreter services are available for use for practices without in-person interpreters. Also, obtaining supplemental nutrition services such as WIC may be difficult because of lack of access to nearby WIC distribution centers.

Are there any demographic characteristics that might affect this case?

Besides being of Hispanic ethnicity and not speaking English, age is a demographic factor that might affect this case. At 9 months of age, Julio likely has no maternal iron stores; and since he is consuming low-iron formula and not taking multivitamins, he is at risk for iron deficiency anemia.

Are there any standardized guidelines that should be used to assess or treat this case?

The American Academy of Pediatrics has issued several clinical practice guidelines that may assist health care providers during well-child visits. For more information, refer to the resources below and their web links.

REFERENCES AND RESOURCES

American Academy of Pediatrics Committee on Practice and Ambulatory Medicine, Bright Futures Periodicity Schedule Workgroup. (2019). 2019 recommendations for preventive pediatric health care. *Pediatrics, 143*.

American Heart Association. (2019). *Dietary recommendations for healthy children*. https://www.heart.org/en/healthy-living/healthy-eating/eat-smart/nutrition-basics/dietary-recommendations-for-healthy-children

Centers for Disease Control and Prevention. (2009). *Lead prevention tips*. http://www.cdc.gov/nceh/lead/tips.htm

Martin-Marcotte, N. (2018). Functional constipation in children: Which treatment is effective and safe? An evidence-based case report. *Journal of Clinical Chiropractic Pediatrics, 17*, 1485–1489.

Powers, J., & Buchanan, G. (2014). Iron deficiency in toddlers to teens: How to manage when prevention fails. *Contemporary Pediatrics, 31*, 12–17.

U.S. Department of Agriculture Food and Nutrition Services. (2019). *Special supplemental nutrition program for women, infants, and children (WIC)*. https://www.fns.usda.gov/wic

Case 2.3 Growth and Development

Which diagnostic or imaging studies should be considered to assist with or confirm the diagnosis?

Many cases of children not gaining weight are nonorganic, so a history and physical examination are normally all that are needed. Certain laboratory tests may help to screen for an underlying pathologic condition. A complete blood count (CBC) can be ordered as well as a urinalysis and urine culture. If an electrolyte imbalance is suspected, electrolytes including blood urea nitrogen (BUN) and creatinine can be ordered. Liver function tests may also be ordered to rule out an underlying liver condition.

If it is suspected that the infant is having a physical problem such as difficulty swallowing, a modified barium swallow may be ordered. This test would be done under the directions of a feeding therapist and a radiologist. During the test, the infant would be given liquids and solids differing in consistency. The infant's swallows would be filmed to determine if there are swallowing difficulties that are contributing to the lack of weight gain. A chest radiograph would be helpful in assessing whether a cardiopulmonary disease is a contributing factor.

What is the most likely differential diagnosis and why?
<u>*Nonorganic failure to thrive:*</u>

With an infant who is not gaining weight, there are several differential diagnoses to consider, including organic failure to thrive, nonorganic failure to thrive (FTT), constitutional growth delay, and fetal alcohol spectrum disorder. We do not know much about Kilah's birth and past history—only that she was removed from her mother's care and placed in foster care. Because it is unknown whether or not she was exposed to substances, including alcohol, in utero, it would be wise to initially consider a diagnosis of fetal alcohol spectrum disorder as a contributing factor to the failure to gain weight. Children with true fetal alcohol syndrome display a failure to gain weight, as well as distinct facial anomalies; and they typically have cognitive/developmental impairment. Those with fetal alcohol spectrum disorder may display growth and cognitive delays but may or may not have the distinct facial features that are associated with fetal alcohol syndrome. Given Kilah's history, there was nothing on the physical examination or in the history to indicate that she has distinct facial anomalies or any delays in development. Based on these findings, it is likely that both fetal alcohol spectrum disorder and fetal alcohol can be ruled out as causes for Kilah's growth impairment.

The Family Nurse Practitioner: Clinical Case Studies, Second Edition. Edited by Leslie Neal-Boylan.
© 2021 John Wiley & Sons Ltd. Published 2021 by John Wiley & Sons Ltd.

Constitutional growth delay may also be considered in the differential diagnoses for a failure to gain weight. Children with constitutional growth delay may have linear growth velocity and weight gain that slows beginning as early as age 3–6 months. We do not have information on this child's linear growth velocity. We have only one length measurement, which would not tell us whether or not the linear growth velocity is stable, increasing, or decreasing. However, most children who have constitutional growth delay do not seek medical attention until puberty, when a lack of sexual development becomes apparent and a discrepancy in height from peers is noted because of the delay in pubertal growth spurt. This makes it likely that Kilah does not have constitutional growth delay and that her care provider should consider other diagnoses.

Organic FTT usually results from problems such as neuromuscular abnormalities, craniofacial abnormalities, or lack of appetite. Other conditions that may result in organic FTT include breathing difficulties, significant developmental delay, and primary gastrointestinal disease or dysfunction. The information obtained in Kilah's history and on her physical examination does not indicate that she suffers from any of the aforementioned problems, making organic FTT an unlikely diagnosis.

Nonorganic FTT usually results from adverse environmental and psychosocial factors. It may be associated with abnormal interactions between the caregiver and the infant. This may result in an inadequate provision of food and/or inadequate intake of food. Nonorganic FTT is most common in the setting of poverty. Its causes may include a combination of poverty and lack of preparation for parenting. An important part of the evaluation of all children is observation of the infant while feeding. Observing infants while they are feeding sheds light on maternal-infant interactions. Given Kilah's history and physical examination and the elimination of the previous diagnoses, nonorganic FTT is the most likely diagnosis at this time. Kilah's caregiver has not cared for an infant in the past, so it may be possible that she is unaware of the caloric needs of a 9-month-old. A 9-month-old infant needs an approximate caloric intake of 140 kilocalories (kcal)/kilogram (kg) per day. Calculating Kilah's daily caloric needs (6.4 kg × 140 kcal) means that she would need 896 kcal per day. Calculating her caloric intake based on her reported history, Kilah's daily caloric intake is less than her calculated caloric needs. Calories in regular infant formula are 20 kcal/oz. Kilah's stated intake is 24 oz of formula daily, which provides her with 480 kcal/day. She also eats 2 jars of stage 1 baby food daily. Stage 1 baby foods typically have 25–50 kcal/jar, providing Kilah with an additional 50–100 kcal per day. Kilah's approximate caloric intake per day is 530–580 kcal, far below her daily caloric need of 896 kcal. Also, Kilah's foster mother does not work outside the home and receives several government housing and food subsidies. Her eligibility for these subsidies makes it likely that she lives at or near the poverty line, a risk factor for nonorganic FTT.

What is your plan of treatment, referral, and follow-up care?

The goal for Kilah would be to provide her with adequate caloric intake for growth. In this case, it would appear that Kilah can be treated for her nonorganic FTT on an outpatient basis. However, frequent follow-up visits are necessary (initially at 2–4 weeks, then at least monthly thereafter). Kilah's weight gain, linear growth velocity, head circumference, and daily caloric intake should be recorded at each follow-up visit. Her weight, length, and head circumference should be plotted on the same age-appropriate growth chart over time. Angela should be instructed on proper caloric intake for Kilah and on ways to increase calories in Kilah's diet. Home visits from the health care provider or an outreach worker may assist in determining the underlying reason for the nonorganic FTT.

If outpatient treatment does not lead to documented weight gain, hospitalization may be necessary for diagnostic and therapeutic reasons. When treating an infant with FTT, a multidisciplinary team approach should be used. A pediatric health care provider, nutritionist, and social worker should be a part of the team. A mental health care professional may also be included. This team should complete a thorough evaluation of the family's psychosocial situation and determine if future support is required. A home visit can help to support the caregiver. The family may also be referred to a local food bank if food affordability is a problem.

Does this patient's psychosocial history affect how you might treat this case?

Kilah's psychosocial history does affect how this case would be treated. Kilah is in foster care. It is essential that her foster care worker be informed of a diagnosis. Through the state's child protective services, Kilah's foster care worker may be able to provide additional support (social and financial) for Angela. They may also need to determine if Kilah would be better cared for in a foster home where the foster mother is knowledgeable about infant nutrition and care.

What if the patient lived in a rural setting?

If this patient and her foster family lived in a rural setting, having frequent follow-up appointments in the office might not feasible. In that case, the health care provider could consider employing the services of a visiting nurse service to visit the home monthly to monitor Kilah's weight and nutritional status. The family's ability to obtain additional food through a source such a food bank may be limited as there may not be one in the area.

Are there any demographic characteristics that might affect this case?

While failure to thrive can occur in any socioeconomic strata, nonorganic FTT is more likely to occur in families living in poverty. There is an increased incidence of nonorganic FTT in children receiving Medicaid, children living in rural areas, and those who are homeless. While the exact reason is unknown, nonorganic FTT is more likely to occur in females than in males. In regard to age in the pediatric population, the most likely age groups to have nonorganic FTT are infants and toddlers.

Are there any standardized guidelines that you should use to assess or treat this case?

Homan (2016) provides guidelines for the detection and treatment of failure to thrive.

REFERENCES AND RESOURCES

Homan, G. (2016). Failure to thrive: A practical guide. *American Family Physician, 94*, 295–300.

Larson-Nath, C., Mavis, A., Duesing, L., Van Hoorn, M., Walia, C., Karls, C., & Goday, P. (2018). Defining pediatric failure to thrive in the developed world: Validation of a semi-objective diagnosis tool. *Clinical Pediatrics, 58*, 446–452.

Sirotnak, A. (2018). *Failure to thrive*. Retrieved from: https://emedicine.medscape.com/article/915575-overview

Vachani, J. (2018). Failure to thrive: Early intervention mitigates long-term deficits. *Contemporary Pediatrics, 35*, 14–27.

Case 2.4 Heart Murmur

Which diagnostic or imaging studies should be considered to assist with or confirm the diagnosis?
Based on the history and physical examination, no imaging studies are needed. However, if any of the listed studies were ordered, no abnormalities would be noted on the test.

What is the most likely differential diagnosis and why?
Still's murmur:
Still's murmur is a murmur that is classified as "functional," "innocent," or "physiologic." It is not a structural defect of the heart and may be a result of noise flowing through a normal heart. There is no known cause. Neither a PDA nor a VSD are position-dependent (heard louder in the supine position). Also, the vibratory quality of the murmur is consistent with a Still's murmur. PDA is more common in infants born prematurely.

What is your plan of treatment, referral, and follow-up care?
- Discuss physiologic murmurs with the parents and explain that no limitation on activity is required.
- Monitor weight and other growth parameters at subsequent visits.
- Allow the parents to verbalize their concerns about their baby's health maintenance.
- Discuss signs and symptoms of increased work of breathing (increased respiratory rate; intercostal retractions; nasal flaring) with parents and when to call the office (decreased by mouth intake; decreased urine output; increased work of breathing; increased temperature).
- Return to clinic in 3 months for well-child check or sooner as needed.

Are there any referrals needed?
Consider a referral to cardiology. However, a referral for a Still's murmur in a child 1 year old or greater is not required.

Does the patient's psychosocial history impact how you might treat him?
There are no known psychosocial factors that would affect the treatment of this patient.

The Family Nurse Practitioner: Clinical Case Studies, Second Edition. Edited by Leslie Neal-Boylan.
© 2021 John Wiley & Sons Ltd. Published 2021 by John Wiley & Sons Ltd.

What if this baby were a girl?

There are no known gender differences in the occurrences of Still's murmur.

What if this baby were 6 months old?

Infants less than 1 year of age should be referred to a cardiologist for evaluation of all murmurs.

Are there any standardized guidelines that should be used to assess or treat this case?

There were no standardized guidelines located in the literature for the assessment and/or treatment of Still's murmur.

REFERENCES AND RESOURCES

Foppa, M., Rao, S., & Manning, W. (2015). Doppler echocardiography in the evaluation of a heart murmur. *JAMA: Journal of the American Medical Association, 313,* 1050–1051.

Lefort, B., Cheyssac, E., Soulé, N., Poinsot, J., Vaillant, M., Nassimi, A., & Chantepie, A. (2017). Auscultation while standing: A basic and reliable method to rule out a pathologic heart murmur in children. *Annals of Family Medicine, 15,* 523–528.

Mitchell, S., Dalal, N., Frank, L., Clauss, S., Aljohani, O., Bradley-Hewitt, T., Harahsheh, A., & Dzelebdzic, S. (2018). Recurrent cardiology evaluation for innocent heart murmur: Echocardiogram utilization. *Clinical Pediatrics, 57,* 1436–1441.

Case 2.5 Cough

Which diagnostic or imaging studies should be considered to assist with or confirm the diagnosis?

Based on the history and physical findings, there are no laboratory or imaging studies needed other than a CXR. However, if a CBC were obtained, the results would show nonspecific findings such as an elevated white blood count. An ABG examination is not necessary since the child does not appear to be in respiratory distress. The CXR reveals a steeple sign; it signifies subglottic narrowing during inspiration.

What is the most likely differential diagnosis and why?

Croup:

Croup is the most likely differential diagnosis based on the history, physical examination findings, and the chest X-ray findings of steeple sign. The presence of inspiratory stridor, low-grade fever, and barking cough support the diagnosis of croup. With epiglottitis, the child usually appears toxic, and the fever is usually 40°C or higher. With epiglottitis, marked restlessness and extreme anxiety may be present. Infants with bronchiolitis are more likely to have expiratory wheezing and rales, as opposed to inspiratory stridor.

What is the plan of treatment, referral, and follow-up care?

Begin oxygen therapy in the office. The child should be kept as comfortable as possible. She should be allowed to remain in her parent's arms. Unnecessary painful interventions that may cause agitation and increased oxygen requirements by the child should be avoided. Monitor heart rate, respiratory rate/effort, and pulse oximetry.

A single dose of dexamethasone should be administered in the office, and the child should be monitored for improvement. If no improvement is seen, refer the patient and family to the local emergency department for support of the respiratory system. An ambulance should be called to transport the baby from the office to the emergency department so that the baby's airway and respiratory status may be maintained. Antibiotics are not indicated. Provide emotional support to the parents. Allow the parents to verbalize their concerns about their baby's health status.

The Family Nurse Practitioner: Clinical Case Studies, Second Edition. Edited by Leslie Neal-Boylan.
© 2021 John Wiley & Sons Ltd. Published 2021 by John Wiley & Sons Ltd.

Are there any demographic characteristics that would affect this case?

Male-to-female ratio for croup is approximately 1.4:1. Croup occurs most frequently between the ages of 7 months and 36 months. While croup is rare after 6 years of age, it may present as late as 15 years.

What if the patient lived in a rural, isolated setting?

Health care providers practicing in rural, isolated setting should have emergency office plans in place for patients experiencing respiratory distress.

REFERENCES AND RESOURCES

April, M., & Long, B. (2019). Do glucocorticoids improve symptoms and reduce return visits or admission rates among children with croup? *Annals of Emergency Medicine, 73*, 459–461.

Gates, A., Johnson, D., & Klassen, T. (2019). Glucocorticoids for croup children. *JAMA Pediatrics, 173*, 595–596.

Newsom, C. (2019). Using glucocorticoids to treat croup in children. *AJN: American Journal of Nursing, 119*, 21–21.

Parker, C., & Cooper, M. (2019). Prednisolone versus dexamethasone for croup: A randomized controlled trial. *Pediatrics, 144*, 1–9.

Smith, D., McDermott, A., & Sullivan, J. (2018). Croup: Diagnosis and management. *American Family Physician, 97*, 575–580.

Case 2.6 Diarrhea

Which laboratory or imaging studies should be considered to assist with or confirm the diagnosis?

A CBC would not provide any clinically useful information in this case. The white blood count (WBC) may be elevated but that is a nonspecific finding as the WBC is likely to be elevated with most infectious processes. A stool culture may provide identification of an infectious organism that is causing the diarrhea. They are not done routinely for acute cases of pediatric diarrhea that are being treated in the outpatient setting. Electrolyte levels can be obtained if there is a concern of dehydration. A hydrogen breath test may be helpful in diagnosing older children with lactose intolerance, but this test is not usually done on babies and very young children because it can cause severe diarrhea. Similarly, a lactose tolerance test can aid in the diagnosis of lactose intolerance, but it is usually not performed on babies and very young children.

What is the most likely differential diagnosis and why?

Viral gastroenteritis:

The complaint of diarrhea can lead to several differential diagnoses. The most common differentials for someone with David's history are viral gastroenteritis, antibiotic-associated diarrhea, and lactose intolerance. Differentiating between these conditions requires a thorough history and review of systems. Viral gastroenteritis should be considered as David has had diarrhea, vomiting, and fever. He also recently started a new day care, which is a risk factor for viral gastroenteritis. David recently finished a course of antibiotics, which could be a possible source of diarrhea. Whole milk was introduced into the diet, which may lead the health care provider to consider lactose intolerance.

Based on the history and physical exam, viral gastroenteritis due to rotavirus is the most likely of the differential diagnoses. The presence of fever likely rules out noninfectious causes of diarrhea. Rotavirus is one of several viruses known to cause gastroenteritis. It commonly affects children in the winter months in the United States but may occur year-round in developing countries. Many children under the age of 5 years have come into contact with this virus at some point in their lives.

The Family Nurse Practitioner: Clinical Case Studies, Second Edition. Edited by Leslie Neal-Boylan.
© 2021 John Wiley & Sons Ltd. Published 2021 by John Wiley & Sons Ltd.

What is the plan of treatment, referral, and follow-up care?

In the majority of cases of viral gastroenteritis infection related to rotavirus, no medications are necessary. Antidiarrheal agents should typically be avoided in young children. Antibiotics are not indicated and may include diarrhea as a side effect—worsening the diarrhea. Hyperosmolar beverages such as sports drinks should be avoided because they may cause infants to develop hypernatremia. Excessive plain water intake may cause infants to develop hyponatremia. Beverages such as Pedialyte® have the correct balance of glucose, sodium, and potassium and should be encouraged in small, frequent feedings for the child with viral gastroenteritis secondary to rotavirus. Because rotavirus is contagious, family members should be encouraged to practice good hand washing after changing diapers and before preparing meals. David's mother should be instructed that the diarrhea may last 1 full week. She should also be instructed about the signs and symptoms of dehydration and told to seek care immediately if any of these signs and symptoms develops. Based on the history and physical findings, no referrals are needed at this time.

David's mother should be allowed to express her concerns regarding his illness status, especially since he is just recovering from acute otitis media and also since she believed that she may have contributed to the diarrhea with the introduction of food with curry or the introduction of whole milk.

Are there any demographic factors that should be considered?

There have been no racial/ethnic factors that contribute to the development of rotavirus, but it has been shown that it is more prevalent among those of lower socioeconomic status.

Are there any standardized guidelines that should be used to assess or treat this case?

The Advisory Committee on Immunization Practices (ACIP) has developed guidelines for the prevention of rotavirus in infants and small children.

REFERENCES AND RESOURCES

Black, R. (2019). Progress in the use of ORS and zinc for the treatment of childhood diarrhea. *Journal of Global Health, 9,* 1–3.

Duncan, D. (2018). Gastroenteritis: An overview of the symptoms, transmission, and management. *British Journal of School Nursing, 13,* 484–488.

Freedman, M. (2019). Probiotics vs placebo against gastroenteritis. *Contemporary Pediatrics, 36,* 2.

Hartman, S., Brown, E., Loomis, E., & Russell, H. (2019). Gastroenteritis in children. *American Family Physician, 99,* 159–165.

Onyon, C., & Dawson, T. (2018). Gastroenteritis. *Paediatrics & Child Health, 28,* 527–532.

Case 2.7 Fall from Height

Which laboratory tests should be ordered as part of a workup after a fall from height?

Since Victor hit his head, any laboratory tests or imaging studies would be geared toward diagnosing an intracranial bleed. There is no clear consensus regarding whether all patients with mild head injuries should have neuroimaging. If imaging is determined to be necessary, a CT scan is the diagnostic study of choice in the evaluation of a head injury because it has a rapid acquisition time, is nearly universally available, is easily interpretable, and is reliable. For those with obvious signs of a traumatic brain injury (TBI), such as evidence of skull fracture on physical exam, or neurologic changes, obtaining a head CT scan has a clear benefit. However, for patients without obvious signs of TBI, the decision to perform a head CT scan requires more consideration, since patients with minor head injuries may receive unnecessary CT scans that provide no clinical benefit.

What is the most likely differential diagnosis and why?

There are several diagnoses that should be considered for a child with a head injury, including minor closed head injury, subdural hematoma, subarachnoid hemorrhage, and epidural hematoma. There are several factors from this case that lead to the diagnosis of minor head injury. Victor's Glasgow Coma Scale (GCS) was 15/15, there were no focal neurological deficits, and there was no seizure activity. These factors support a diagnosis of mild closed head injury. Additional factors that support this diagnosis are that there was no vomiting, no loss of consciousness, the fall was less than 1 meter, and there was no fluid or drainage from Victor's nose or ears. Patients with a subarachnoid hemorrhage typically have vomiting and loss of consciousness. There were no focal neurologic findings, and there was a GCS of 15/15. Patients with a subdural hematoma generally lose consciousness (although this is not an absolute) and typically experience moderate to severe blunt head trauma. Epidural hematoma may present with loss of consciousness, vomiting, and seizures.

What is the plan of treatment, referral, and follow-up care?

Based on Victor's history, physical examination, and likely diagnosis of a mild closed head injury, he should be observed in the office and would likely not need radiographic evaluation or neuroimaging. There will be no limitations on his activity or diet. His mother can be told to apply ice for

The Family Nurse Practitioner: Clinical Case Studies, Second Edition. Edited by Leslie Neal-Boylan.
© 2021 John Wiley & Sons Ltd. Published 2021 by John Wiley & Sons Ltd.

20 minutes at a time (every 2–4 hours as needed) to his head wound for 24 hours. This will help to reduce or prevent swelling of the injured area. Victor can be discharged to home if it is determined that he has a reliable caregiver at home who can monitor him for signs of complications related to his head injury. Victor's caregivers should be given an instruction sheet for head injury care that explains that he should be awakened every 2 hours and assessed neurologically. Victor's caregivers should be instructed to seek medical attention if he develops persistent nausea and vomiting, seizures, unusual behavior, or watery discharge from either the nose or the ears. There are no referrals necessary based on Victor's history and physical examination findings.

Does this patient's psychosocial history affect how you might treat this case?

An aspect of Victor's psychosocial history that might affect the handling of his case is that both of his parents are teenagers. Previous research has shown that children of adolescent mothers (when compared to children of adult mothers) have an increased rate of unintentional injuries during the first 5 years of life.

What if the patient lived in a rural setting?

A patient living in a rural setting may not be able to access a health care center in a timely fashion for assessment and diagnostic testing of a head injury after a fall.

Are there any demographic characteristics that might affect this case?

There are no specific demographics that affect this case. There are no known associations of unintentional head injury with ethnicity or gender in the pediatric population.

REFERENCES AND RESOURCES

Gelernter, R., Weiser, G., & Kozer, E. (2018). Computed tomography findings in young children with minor head injury presenting to the emergency department greater than 24h post injury. *Injury*, *49*, 82–85.

Harris, L., Axinte, L., Campbell, P., & Amin, N. (2019). Computer Tomography (CT) for head injury: Adherence to the National Institute for Health and Care Excellence (NICE) criteria. *Brain Injury*, *33*, 1539–1544.

Miescier, M., Dudley, N., Kadish, H., Mundorff, M., & Corneli, H. (2017). Variation in computed tomography use for evaluation of head injury in a pediatric emergency department. *Pediatric Emergency Care*, *33*, 156–160.

Osmond, M. H., Klassen, T. P., Wells, G. A., Davidson, J., Correll, R., Boutis, K., & Pediatric Emergency Research Canada (PERC) **Head Injury** Study Group. (2018). Validation and refinement of a clinical decision rule for the use of computed tomography in children with minor head injury in the emergency department. *CMAJ: Canadian Medical Association Journal*, *190*, E816–E822.

Case 3.1 Earache

Are there laboratory tests or diagnostic imaging studies that should be ordered as part of a workup for ear pain?

Middle ear effusion may be confirmed with the observation of decreased or absent tympanic membrane mobility with pneumatic otoscopy. Unfortunately, when performing pneumatic otoscopy in infants and young children, it can be very difficult to maintain a tight-fitting seal for the exam. Tympanometry may be performed to determine the presence of fluid (infected or uninfected) in the middle ear. Tympanometry is useful if cerumen makes visualization of the tympanic membrane difficult on otoscopic exam. Tympanocentesis, though not often done, may be performed to acquire a sample of the fluid behind the tympanic membrane for culture and sensitivity if the child is immunocompromised or has failed previous courses of antibiotic therapy.

What is the most likely differential diagnosis and why?

Otitis media:

The complaint of ear pain can lead to several differential diagnoses. Acute otitis media, otitis externa, cholesteatoma, foreign body, and hemotympanum (blood behind the tympanic membrane) are some of the more common causes of ear pain in a child. A thorough history and careful physical exam will help to differentiate among these diagnoses.

Otitis media is the most likely diagnosis for Janice based on the history and physical examination findings. Janice had a fever, sleep and eating disturbances, and a previous history of otitis media. On examination, the left TM was erythematous and bulging. It is unlikely to be otitis externa as there is no ear pain elicited by palpation of the external ear, a characteristic sign of otitis externa. Cholesteatoma should be considered in the differential because of Janice's past diagnosis of otitis media. However, there was no pocket of retraction, keratinous debris, or mass on the tympanic membrane, ruling out a diagnosis of cholesteatoma.

What is the plan of treatment, referral, and follow-up care?

The first-line treatment for uncomplicated otitis media in a child with a temperature less than 39°C (102.2°F) is amoxicillin, 80–90 mg/kg per day for 7–10 days. For children 6 years and older, a 5–7 day course of amoxicillin is appropriate. For children with a temperature over 39°C (102.2°F) or if

The Family Nurse Practitioner: Clinical Case Studies, Second Edition. Edited by Leslie Neal-Boylan.
© 2021 John Wiley & Sons Ltd. Published 2021 by John Wiley & Sons Ltd.

H. influenza or *M. catarrhalis* are suspected, therapy should start with amoxicillin-clavulanate (90 mg/kg per day of amoxicillin and 6.4 mg/kg per day of clavulanate) in 2 divided doses per day.

In patients with non–Type 1 allergic reactions to amoxicillin, a cephalosporin may be used (cefdinir 14 mg/kg per day in 1 or 2 doses, cefpodoxime 10 mg/kg per day once daily, or cefuroxime 30 mg/ kg per day in 2 divided doses). If the child has experienced a Type 1 reaction in the past (anaphylaxis or urticaria), azithromycin (10 mg/kg per day on the first day, then 5 mg/kg for 4 days) or clarithromycin (15 mg/kg per day in 2 divided doses) may be used. Because Janice has had hives in the past when using penicillin, azithromycin is the best choice for her. At 14 kg, her dose on day 1 would be 140 mg and on days 2 through 5, her dose would be 70 mg. Using the 100 mg/5 mL oral suspension, her dose would be 7 mL on day 1, then 3.5 mL for days 2 through 5.

Based on the history and physical exam findings, no referrals are needed at this time.

Janice's mother, Marsha, should be instructed to follow up with a call to the office or to seek medical attention if no improvement is seen in 48–72 hours after the first dose of medication. Janice's fever should be lowered, and her sleeping and eating should also improve in 48–72 hours.

Does this patient's psychosocial history affect how you might treat this case?

Janice's psychosocial history contains elements that may increase her risk for developing otitis media. Her enrollment in a child care center places her at an increased risk for developing otitis media. Janice's father is a smoker. Exposure to passive cigarette smoke has been found to be a risk factor for the development of otitis media in preschool children. This information can be discussed with Janice's parents. Janice's father can be given information on smoking cessation resources.

What if the patient lived in a rural setting?

If Janice lived in a rural setting, her parents would be given clear instructions about when and how to follow up if there is no improvement in the 48- to 72-hour window or if symptoms worsen. If an emergency department is not easily accessible, Janice should be followed closely by her primary care provider to ensure that worsening symptoms are not left unnoticed.

Are there any demographic characteristics that might affect this case?

Otitis media has been found to be more frequent in certain racial groups, such as the Inuit and American Indians. The difference in the frequency of occurrence compared to other racial groups is likely due to anatomic differences in the Eustachian tube. Regarding gender, boys have been found to be affected more commonly than girls. No specific causative factors for this have been found in the literature. Age is a demographic characteristic that affects otitis media. Otitis media occurs more commonly in infants, toddlers, and preschool children between the ages of 6 months and 3 years of age. This age distribution may be due to a combination of several factors. These factors can be immunologic, such as lack of pneumococcal antibodies, and/or anatomic. Younger children have a low angle of the Eustachian tube with relation to the nasopharynx.

REFERENCES AND RESOURCES

Chang, J., Shapiro, N., & Bhattacharyya, N. (2018). Do demographic disparities exist in the diagnosis and surgical management of otitis media? *Laryngoscope, 128,* 2898–2901.

Gaddey, H., Wright, M., & Nelson, T. (2019). Otitis media: Rapid evidence review. *American Family Physician, 100,* 350–356.

Homme, J. (2019). Acute otitis media and group A streptococcal pharyngitis: A review for the general pediatric practitioner. *Pediatric Annals, 48,* e343–e348.

Marom, T., Kraus, O., Habashi, N., & Tamir, S. (2019). Emerging technologies for the diagnosis of otitis media. *Otolaryngology–Head & Neck Surgery, 160,* 447–456.

Medhurst, R. (2018). Homeopathy for the management of otitis media. *Journal of the Australian Traditional-Medicine Society, 24,* 28–30.

Van Wyck, F. (2018). *Tympanocentesis.* Retrieved from: https://emedicine.medscape.com/article/1413525-overview

Case 3.2 Bedwetting

RESOLUTION

What laboratory tests or diagnostic imaging studies should be ordered as part of a workup for bedwetting?

A urine dipstick will provide information on hydration, infection, diabetes insipidus, or diabetes mellitus by measuring the urine specific gravity, nitrites, glucose, and ketones. A urine culture can be done if infection is suspected to identify the organism. In preschool-aged children with enuresis and a urinary tract infection (UTI), consider a renal and bladder ultrasound. If abnormalities are found on the ultrasound, a voiding cystourethrography (VCUG) to identify structural abnormalities and measure bladder filling can be obtained. An X-ray of the kidney, ureters, and bladder can be done if constipation or abnormalities of the spine are suspected. Urodynamic studies measure the flow of urine qualitatively and quantitatively and may be used if a neurological disorder is suspected or in children with daytime wetting who do not respond to traditional therapies.

What is the most likely differential diagnosis and why?

Enuresis:

Bedwetting, or enuresis, has many etiologies. Enuresis refers to involuntary urinary incontinence beyond the expected age of 4 years for daytime dryness and 5 years for night dryness. It may involve genetic factors, changes in vasopressin secretion, sleep factors, structural abnormalities, infection, or psychological factors. Primary nocturnal enuresis (PNE) is defined as a child > 5 years who is incontinent at night with no previous history of dryness at night for an extended period of time. Secondary enuresis refers to episodes of bedwetting after a period of dryness > 6 months and can be precipitated by a stressful event in the child's life.

The most common differentials for enuresis are urinary tract infection, diabetes mellitus, diabetes insipidus, structural abnormalities of the genitourinary tract, constipation, excessive caffeine, spinal cord injury, or psychological stress. A UTI may be the source when there is dysuria, urinary frequency, and a positive urine culture. High glucose or ketones in the urine dip would indicate diabetes mellitus, and a low specific gravity would indicate diabetes insipidus. Abdominal palpation of stool or stool visible on a KUB (kidneys, ureters, and bladders) X-ray would indicate constipation. Abnormal physical exams of the spine or reflexes can indicate an underlying neurologic disorder or spinal cord injury. Structural abnormalities are identified with a renal and bladder ultrasound, VCUG, or urodynamic studies. In the absence of clinical evidence for enuresis, a

The Family Nurse Practitioner: Clinical Case Studies, Second Edition. Edited by Leslie Neal-Boylan.
© 2021 John Wiley & Sons Ltd. Published 2021 by John Wiley & Sons Ltd.

thorough history should review psychological stressors, abuse, or dietary patterns that include caffeine or liquids before bed.

Javier's mother states he has "never been dry at night but has been toilet-trained during the daytime for 2 years." Because enuresis refers to involuntary urinary incontinence beyond the expected age of 4 years for daytime dryness and 5 years for night dryness, Javier is within the normal age range for his bedwetting to be considered nonpathologic.

What is the plan of treatment, referral, and follow-up care?

The plan of treatment would be to provide counseling and reassurance for the family after ruling out any other physiological, psychological, or organic causes of bedwetting. The health care provider can reassure the family that Javier is developmentally appropriate for his age. Bedwetting is more frequent in boys than girls, and 5%–10% of children have primary nocturnal enuresis (PNE) at age 5. It is important to emphasize that Javier might be experiencing stress and embarrassment related to his bedwetting and that this is exacerbated by teasing from his sister, being spanked for wetting the bed by his father, and seeing his mother's frustration. Parents should avoid punishment and criticism of a child's bedwetting and provide positive reinforcement when the child has a night without wetting the bed.

The health care provider may recommend children's books on bedwetting or making a sticker chart to keep track of dry nights. Javier's mother should be reminded to limit nighttime fluids to 2 hours before bed. She can also ensure that Javier has easy access to the toilet. The family can be helped to set a goal for Javier to use the toilet when he has to go to the bathroom at night, rather than staying dry all night. Based on history and physical exam, Javier does not need a referral at this time. Telephone follow-up can be conducted with Javier's family to monitor progress over the course of the next year until his 5-year-old well-child visit. His family should be encouraged to come to the office sooner as needed for signs and symptoms of illness.

For children with true enuresis, there are several options that can be used in the treatment of this condition, such as bedwetting alarms or medications. Bedwetting alarms work best with children 7 years or older and can be very effective. The alarm conditions the child to get up to use the toilet in order to avoid the alarm going off. They must be used every night for 3–4 months, the family must be counseled on proper use, and the family must wake the child if the child does not awaken to the noise of the alarm.

Medications can also help to manage enuresis. First-line treatment is desmopressin acetate vasopressin (DDVAP) in children ages 7 years and older to reduce the volume of urine produced at night. In patients with nocturnal enuresis and daytime incontinence or those who fail with DDVAP alone, adding anticholinergic agents such as oxybutynin chloride or imipramine, a tricyclic antidepressant, in children age 6 years and older can be helpful in reducing uninhibited bladder contractions. Children older than 6 years may also benefit from complementary medicine including chiropractic care, melatonin, acupuncture/acupressure, hypnosis, and biofeedback, although there is limited evidence of the success of these interventions.

Daytime wetting can also be a stressful issue for children. Its origin can be neurologic, anatomic, muscular, or functional, which results in problems with storage or emptying of the bladder. Similar to nocturnal enuresis, a full workup should be done to determine the cause. Daytime enuresis is treated with the same medications and behavioral strategies as nighttime enuresis.

Does this patient's psychosocial history affect how you might treat this case?

In Javier's situation, the health care provider should reinforce with the parents and sibling that Javier should not be teased or punished for bedwetting.

What if the patient lived in a rural setting?

If this patient lived in a rural setting, it might not be convenient for them to return to clinic for a follow-up visit. Telephone follow-up with the family to discuss Javier's bedwetting and to evaluate any strategies the family has tried may be more feasible for families living in a rural setting.

Are there any demographic characteristics that might affect this case?

There is no racial or ethnic predisposition regarding the development of enuresis. In relation to gender, males are affected more than females. The incidence of enuresis decreases as children age. Javier's mother reports frustration with having to wash sheets frequently and buy new mattresses because of bedwetting. Considering the socioeconomic status of the parents, it is possible that this is causing additional financial strain for the family. As the provider, you can suggest plastic coverings for the mattress or plastic reusable underpads to protect the mattress from getting wet, as well as absorbent briefs for Javier to wear at night.

REFERENCES AND RESOURCES

Cheer, B. (2019). In review: Children with nocturnal enuresis. *Nursing in Practice: The Journal for Today's Primary Care Nurse, 108*, 30–32.

Jabbour, M., Abou Zahr, R., & Boustany, M. (2019). Primary nocturnal enuresis: A novel therapeutic strategy with higher efficacy. *Urology, 124*, 241–247.

Kamperis, K., Hagstroem, S., Faerch, M., Mahler, B., Rittig, S., & Djurhuus, J. (2017). Combination treatment of nocturnal enuresis with desmopressin and indomethacin. *Pediatric Nephrology, 32*, 627633.

Kuwertz-Bröking, E., & von Gontard, A. (2018). Clinical management of nocturnal enuresis. *Pediatric Nephrology, 33*, 1145–1154.

Siddiqui, J., Qureshi, S., Allaithy, A., & Mahfouz, T. (2019). Nocturnal enuresis: A synopsis of behavioral and pharmacological management. *Sleep & Hypnosis, 21*, 16–22.

St-Jean, A. (2018). Chiropractic care of a 10-year-old female with primary nocturnal enuresis: A case report. *Journal of Clinical Chiropractic Pediatrics, 17*, 1490–1495.

Waters, K., Prentice, B., & Caldwell, P. (2017). An exploratory study of melatonin in children with nocturnal enuresis. *Australian & New Zealand Continence Journal, 23*, 15–18.

Case 3.3 Burn

RESOLUTION

Are there any laboratory tests or diagnostic imaging studies that should be ordered as part of a workup for a burn?

There are no recommended laboratory or imaging studies for a burn such as the one described in the physical examination.

What is the most likely differential diagnosis?

Partial thickness burn:

When examining a pediatric patient with a burn, it is important to determine the thickness of the burn. Older descriptions of burns were first, second, or third degree. Now burns are classified as superficial, superficial partial thickness, deep partial thickness, and full thickness injuries. Superficial burns (first degree) affect only the surface of the skin (epidermis). The skin will be erythematous and painful but will not develop blisters. Superficial burns usually tend to heal within 1 week without scarring. A partial-thickness (second-degree) burn damages not only the epidermis but extends down into the dermis. These burns will typically be painful. Partial-thickness burns are subdivided into two categories: superficial partial-thickness burns and deep partial-thickness burns. Superficial partial-thickness burns develop blisters within approximately 2 to 3 weeks. Superficial partial-thickness burns usually heal without significant scarring. Deep partial-thickness burns are at risk for significant scarring due to the depth of the injury. Healing time for deep partial-thickness burns is weeks to months. Full-thickness burns (third degree) require an extensive healing time if not excised and grafted. Full-thickness burns may not be painful because the nerves are damaged. These burns have a poor cosmetic outcome.

Based on the history and physical examination, it appears that Faye has a partial-thickness burn to her right hand.

What is your plan of treatment, referral, and follow-up care?

Immediate treatment of the injury in the home environment should be documented. It is preferable to cool a partial-thickness burn for approximately 20 minutes to diminish the burning of the skin. Evaluation of a burn includes an investigation as to the type of heat source, estimation of temperature, and duration of contact. Ascertaining this information may give insight into the depth of burn.

The Family Nurse Practitioner: Clinical Case Studies, Second Edition. Edited by Leslie Neal-Boylan.
© 2021 John Wiley & Sons Ltd. Published 2021 by John Wiley & Sons Ltd.

The initial management of a burn involves determining the burn depth and total body surface area (TBSA) affected. Only partial- and full-thickness burns are included in the calculation. The TBSA may be calculated using either the rule of nines burn chart (Table 3.3.1) or the Lund and Browder burn chart (Tables 3.3.2 and 3.3.3). For the pediatric patient, the Lund and Browder burn chart is preferred. Calculating the percentage of TBSA affected is important when deciding the need for hospitalization versus outpatient management. Criteria for determining whether a burn can be treated at home vary based on the experience and resources of the treating health care center. Burns that *may* be treated on an outpatient basis include those that affect less than 15% TBSA and those that have no airway involvement. The ability of the child to drink and tolerate oral fluids and having a dependable family able to transport the patient for clinic appointments are also key factors. If the burn is the result of suspected abuse, the patient may not be treated on an outpatient basis.

For small burns, a rough estimate of the affected BSA can be made by comparing the burn with the size of child's palm (which represents approximately 1% of the BSA). Since Faye's burn is only on her right palm, it is estimated that her burn represents only 1% of her TBSA. Although the burn represents only a minute portion of Faye's TBSA, all burns of the hands, mouth, or genitals require immediate medical attention. Hand burns are susceptible to functional limitations, as a consequence of scar formation and contractures. The treatment of hand burns in the pediatric patient should involve careful follow-up to gauge not only the healing and restoration of function to the hand but

Table 3.3.1. Rule of Nines Burn Chart.

Body Part	Percent of Body Surface Area		
	Infant	Child	Adolescent/Adult
Head	18%	13%	9%
Anterior trunk	18%	18%	18%
Posterior trunk	18%	18%	18%
Upper extremity (each one)	9%	9%	9%
Lower extremity (each one)	14%	16%	18%
Genitalia	1%	1%	1%

Table 3.3.2. Lund and Browder Burn Chart (Part 1).

Body Part	Percent of Body Surface Area
Head	See chart below (Part 2) as this measurement changes with age
Neck	1%
Anterior trunk	13%
Posterior trunk	13%
Upper extremity (each one)	5%
Buttocks	5%
Lower extremity (each one)	See chart below (Part 2) as this measurement changes with age
Genitalia	1%

Table 3.3.3. Lund and Browder Burn Chart (Part 2).

Age (years)	0	1	5	10	15	Adult
1/2 of head	9½%	8½%	6½%	5½%	4½%	3½%
1/2 of one thigh	2¾%	3¼%	4%	4¼%	4½%	4¾%
1/2 of one leg	2½%	2½%	2¾%	3%	3¼%	3%

also to assess for psychological and emotional trauma. Current American Burn Association (2006) guidelines recommend burn unit referral for burns involving the hands. However, many hand burns are treated in primary care settings, such as the emergency room, primary care office, or an urgent care center.

Goals of treatment for Faye's partial-thickness (second-degree) burn are to reduce pain and prevent infection. Pain relievers such as acetaminophen or ibuprofen can help with inflammation and pain and should be used according to directions. Children under the age of 18 years should not be given aspirin for the relief of pain or inflammation because of the risk of developing Reye syndrome. Topical antimicrobials of choice include bacitracin and neomycin for partial-thickness burns. Since this is a hand burn at risk for contractures, the primary care health care provider in this case should refer Faye to the local emergency department or to a burn specialist if one is accessible.

Faye's mother should be educated regarding the signs and symptoms of infection and when to call or return to the primary care office. She should also be educated about the prevention of burns.

Does this patient's psychosocial history affect how you might treat this case?

An aspect of Faye's psychosocial history that might affect the handling of her case is that her mother is a teenager. Research has shown that when compared to children of adult mothers, children of adolescent mothers have an increased rate of unintentional injuries during the first 5 years of life. It would be important to provide extensive education regarding safety to prevent future unintentional injuries. It would also be important to have close follow-up to ensure that the family follows up as necessary.

What if the patient lived in a rural setting?

If Faye and her family lived in a rural setting, gaining rapid access to a health care provider skilled in treating hand burns in pediatric patients might be delayed. Also, the family may experience barriers in attending follow-up appointments to monitor the healing. For this reason, if Faye's family lived in a rural setting, she might have to be hospitalized for the initial treatment of her burn.

Are there any demographic characteristics that might affect this case?

Both age and ethnicity are demographic factors that may affect the incidence of burns in the pediatric patient. Children less than 6 years of age are more likely to suffer from burns than children over 6 years of age. This may be due to a natural curiosity on the part of the younger child, coupled with their slower reaction time when contacting a hot object. African American children are most commonly affected by burns, followed by Caucasians, Hispanics, and Asians.

Are there any standardized guidelines that should be used to assess or treat this case?

The American Burn Association has listed guidelines for the management of burns and burn centers. See the reference listed below.

REFERENCES AND RESOURCES

Aghaei, A., Soori, H., Ramezankhani, A., & Mehrabi, Y. (2019). Factors related to pediatric unintentional burns: The comparison of logistic regression and data mining algorithms. *Journal of Burn Care & Research, 41,* 606–612.

American Burn Association. (2006). *Burn referral criteria.* Retrieved from: http://ameriburn.org/wp-content/uploads/2017/05/burncenterreferralcriteria.pdf

Hawkins, L., Centifanti, L., Holman, N., & Taylor, P. (2019). Parental adjustment following pediatric burn injury: The role of guilt, shame, and self-compassion. *Journal of Pediatric Psychology, 44,* 229–237.

Nelson, S., Conroy, C., & Logan, D. (2019). The biopsychosocial model of pain in the context of pediatric burn injuries. *European Journal of Pain, 23*, 421–434.

Padalko, A., Cristall, N., Gawaziuk, J., & Logsetty, S. (2019). Social complexity and risk for pediatric burn injury: A systematic review. *Journal of Burn Care & Research, 40*, 478499.

Parrish, C., Shields, A., Morris, A., George, A., Reynolds, E. Borden, L., . . . Ostrander, R. (2019). Parent distress following pediatric burn injuries. *Journal of Burn Care & Research, 40*, 79–84.

Rosado, N., Charleston, E., Gregg, M., & Lorenz, D. (2019). Characteristics of accidental versus abusive pediatric burn injuries in an urban burn center over a 14-year period. *Journal of Burn Care & Research, 40*, 437–443.

Sheckter, C., Kiwanuka, H., Maan, Z., Pirrotta, E., Curtin, C., & Wang, N. (2019). Increasing ambulatory treatment of pediatric minor burns—The emerging paradigm for burn care in children. *Burns, 45*, 165–172.

Case 3.4 Toothache

RESOLUTION

Which diagnostic or imaging studies should be considered to assist with or confirm the diagnosis?

Unless a systemic infection is suspected, there are no laboratory tests needed for a diagnosis associated with tooth pain. Imaging studies such as a dental X-ray will be able to detect caries not visible to the naked eye.

What are the most likely differential diagnoses and why?
Gingivitis and dental caries:

When considering the symptom of tooth pain, there are several differential diagnoses to consider, including gingivitis, dental caries, and periodontitis. Gingivitis is an inflammatory process of the gum tissues surrounding the teeth. With gingivitis, the gingiva (gums) may appear to be erythematous and swollen. This is prevalent in people with inadequate oral hygiene, inadequate plaque removal, poor nutrition, and lack of periodic dental examinations. Caries (cavities) are decayed areas of the teeth that develop into openings or holes. Caries are caused by a combination of factors, including not cleaning the teeth well, eating frequent sugary snacks, and drinking sugary drinks. Periodontitis is a serious gum infection that damages the soft tissues and bones that support the teeth. Like gingivitis and caries, periodontitis is usually the result of poor oral hygiene. People who have periodontitis will likely have receding gums. They may also display pus between their teeth and gums. Based on the history of erythematous and edematous gums and holes in his teeth, it would appear that Lamont has both gingivitis and dental caries. He was not reported to have any receding of his gums, so it is unlikely that he has developed periodontitis.

What is the plan of treatment, referral, and follow-up care?

Treatment for Lamont's tooth pain related to his gingivitis and caries will encompass several aspects. Proper oral hygiene (including brushing and flossing) should be stressed. Because of a probable lack of hand dexterity in a 5-year-old, Lamont's parents should assist him in brushing his teeth at least once daily and flossing the teeth that are in contact with other teeth. Using a power toothbrush with an oscillating motion has been shown to be better at removing plaque than a manual toothbrush. These actions will help to reduce plaque associated with gingivitis and caries. Lamont should use a warm saline rinse several times per day to help resolve his gingival

The Family Nurse Practitioner: Clinical Case Studies, Second Edition. Edited by Leslie Neal-Boylan.
© 2021 John Wiley & Sons Ltd. Published 2021 by John Wiley & Sons Ltd.

inflammation. An oral rinse with a hydrogen peroxide 3% solution may also help. Nonsteroidal anti-inflammatory drugs (NSAIDs) have been shown to assist with the resolution of pain and inflammation associated with gingivitis and caries. Prevention of dental disease through good oral hygiene and regular dental checkups should be discussed with Lamont's parents. Proper nutrition, including foods that do not contain simple sugars, should be stressed. Research has shown that foods containing milk or milk components (e.g., yogurt) may have cariostatic properties. These foods should be encouraged as part of a balanced diet for Lamont. Drinking from the bottle should be discontinued. Lamont should be referred to a dentist for a professional cleaning of his teeth and for the management of his caries. He should follow up in the primary care office if his tooth pain worsens or if he develops a fever before his dental appointment.

Does this patient's psychosocial history affect how you might treat this case?

Children who immigrate to the United States tend to have a higher rate of dental disease and lower rates of dental health care utilization than do children born in the United States. Lamont's family may not have had access to preventive dental care and teaching about good dental hygiene in their home country. In addition, Lamont has a cariogenic diet. His history revealed that he eats quite a bit of junk food. Lamont also still drinks sugary drinks from a bottle.

What if the patient lived in a rural setting?

Children in rural locations may have decreased access to dental care based on the lack of availability to a nearby dentist. However, research reveals that children in rural settings have fewer cavities than children in urban areas.

Are there any demographic characteristics that might affect this case?

Preschool age is a common time for the development of dental problems because the responsibility of oral hygiene (such as tooth brushing) shifts to the child. The preschool-age child does not always have the manual dexterity to brush and floss correctly. Therefore, they are at risk for developing dental problems such as gingivitis and dental decay. It is estimated that 9%–17% of children aged 3–11 years have gingivitis and 70%–90% adolescents have gingivitis. In adults, gingivitis is slightly more common in males than in females, because females are more likely to have better oral hygiene.

Are there any standardized guidelines that should be used to assess or treat this case?

The American Academy of Pediatric Dentistry has developed guidelines for pediatric dental health. See their reference below.

REFERENCES AND RESOURCES

American Academy of Pediatric Dentistry (AAPD). (2018). *Guideline on periodicity of examination, preventive dental services, anticipatory guidance/counseling, and oral treatment for infants, children, and adolescents.* Retrieved from: https://www.aapd.org/globalassets/media/policies_guidelines/bp_periodicity.pdf

Bidwell, J. (2018). Fluoride mouth rinses for preventing dental caries in children and adolescents. *Public Health Nursing, 35,* 85–87.

Cheng, L. L. (2017). Limited evidence suggests fluoride mouth rinse may reduce dental caries in children and adolescents. *Journal of the American Dental Association (JADA), 148,* 263–266.

Chieh, T., Badger, G., Acharya, B., Gaw, A., Barratt, M., & Chiquet, B. (2018). Influence of ethnicity on parental preference for pediatric dental behavioral management techniques. *Pediatric Dentistry, 40,* 265–271.

Karami, S., Ghobadi, N., & Karami, H. (2017). Diagnostic and preventive approaches for dental caries in children: A review. *Journal of Pediatrics Review, 5,* 1–7.

Ogawa, J., Kiang, J., Watts, D., Hirway, P., & Lewis, C. (2019). Oral health and dental clinic attendance in pediatric refugees. *Pediatric Dentistry, 41,* 31–34.

Peres, M., Ju, X., Mittinty, M., Spencer, A., & Do, L. (2019). Modifiable factors explain socioeconomic inequalities in children's dental caries. *Journal of Dental Research, 98,* 1211–1218.

VanMalsen, J., & Compton, S. (2017). Effectiveness of early pediatric dental homes: A scoping review. *Canadian Journal of Dental Hygiene, 51,* 23–29.

Case 3.5 Abdominal Pain

RESOLUTION

Are there laboratory tests or diagnostic imaging studies that should be ordered as part of a workup for abdominal pain?

An abdominal radiograph may be helpful if constipation is suspected. It may reveal a full rectal vault and fecal loading. There would be no signs of obstruction. A stool test for occult blood would reveal the presence of blood in the stool and may suggest rectal or anal tearing during stooling. Anorectal manometry evaluates internal sphincter relaxation with rectal distention. This test would be used if Hirschsprung disease is suspected. A digital rectal exam should reveal a full rectal vault in functional constipation, while Hirschsprung disease is more likely to present with an empty rectum on physical exam. Patients with constipation and failure to thrive should be evaluated with a celiac panel for celiac disease and a thyroid function test for hypothyroidism. While Jennifer's history and physical are not consistent with Crohn's disease, it would be important to consider this diagnosis if her abdominal pain were persistent and unrelieved by treatment, given the family history for this disease. In a patient with Crohn's disease, ESR may be elevated. An endoscopy and colonoscopy would be warranted if this diagnosis was suspected.

What is the most likely differential diagnosis and why?
Constipation:
While the differential diagnosis for abdominal pain is extensive, it is important to bear in mind that the majority of abdominal pain in children is functional and not the result of an underlying pathological process. Included in the differential diagnosis for functional abdominal pain are functional dyspepsia, functional constipation, irritable bowel syndrome, cyclic vomiting syndrome, abdominal migraine, and functional abdominal pain syndrome.

Organic etiologies of abdominal pain include gastrointestinal infection, anatomic abnormalities such as Hirschsprung disease or intussusception, inflammatory diseases such as celiac disease, Crohn's disease, and dietary intolerances. Red flags for organic etiologies of abdominal pain include pain that occurs at night and awakens the child; pain that is distant from the umbilicus; pain accompanied by fever, dysuria, or hematuria; joint pain or swelling; significant vomiting; a change in bowel movement habits; weight loss; or slowed growth. Constipation, with or without abdominal pain, may also be the result of cystic fibrosis, neurological dysfunction, and

---

The Family Nurse Practitioner: Clinical Case Studies, Second Edition. Edited by Leslie Neal-Boylan.
© 2021 John Wiley & Sons Ltd. Published 2021 by John Wiley & Sons Ltd.

321

hypothyroidism, which should be ruled out in cases of constipation that do not respond to standard interventions. Given Jennifer's history of increased cow's milk intake, her habit of having a bowel movement only 2–3 times per week, and mild tenderness in left lower quadrant, the mostly likely diagnosis is constipation.

What is the plan of treatment, referral, and follow-up care?

Initial management of constipation requires a "cleanout," which can be achieved using oral or rectal medications, including enemas, osmotic laxatives, stimulant laxatives, and polyethylene glycol. Polyethylene glycol (PEG) and stool softeners are safe and effective for long-term treatment and should be considered in patients with recurrent functional constipation. PEG is especially useful in the pediatric population, as it is tasteless and can be dissolved easily in any beverage.

Because much of the management for constipation involves behavior modification and lifestyle changes, it is important to take the time to educate families. Jennifer's parents should be educated about constipation, including management guidelines and when to seek medical care. While there is limited support for dietary and exercise interventions for constipation, these lifestyle changes are healthy choices for all patients and may offer some relief for select patients. Jennifer's parents should be encouraged to provide her with a low-fat, high-fiber diet and ensure that she gets plenty of regular exercise. Jennifer's mother should be told to decrease Jennifer's cow's milk intake to no more than 24 oz per day since excessive intake of cow's milk has been associated with constipation. Adequate water intake may help prevent constipation as well.

In preschool-aged children with a history of constipation, toileting is often met with fear and frustration. Scheduled toileting can help to normalize toilet time as a relaxing and painless activity. Jennifer's parents should be instructed to have her sit on the toilet for 15 to 20 minutes at a time, 2 to 3 times a day, even if she does not have a bowel movement. Due to the gastrocolic reflex, timing this toileting for 15 to 20 minutes after the completion of meals may prove helpful. During toilet time, Jennifer should sit with both feet firmly on the floor and should be encouraged to relax. A parent should be present with Jennifer during toilet time to provide reassurance and to observe bowel movements. Information obtained about the size and shape of Jennifer's stools can provide both her parents and her health care provider information about the success or failure of her treatment. A reward system (such as a sticker chart) for successful toileting efforts and bowel movements may help to encourage future success, while failures should simply be ignored.

Based upon the history and physical exam, there is no indication for referral at this time. It is important that Jennifer and her parents follow up with her health care provider by telephone in 1 to 2 weeks to assess the effectiveness of the recommended interventions. This time will also allow Jennifer's parents to express any questions, concerns, or frustrations that may have arisen regarding her symptoms and treatment. The family should follow up in the office in 1 month or sooner if necessary. Prolonged constipation that does not respond to treatment or recurrent abdominal pain that appears to be unrelated to functional constipation may require a referral to a pediatric gastroenterologist.

Does this patient's psychosocial history affect how you might treat this case?

Treatment for constipation does not vary significantly based on psychosocial history, but it is important to bear in mind a family's access to fresh produce, as well as their dietary preferences, when offering nutritional recommendations. Furthermore, constipation may be more prevalent during periods of transition, such as starting school, the arrival of a new sibling, or moving to a new home. When these transitions exist, interventions may require more time before they are successful. Parents should be encouraged in their efforts, allowed to air frustrations, and offered regular support from health care providers.

What if the patient lived in a rural setting?

Residence in a rural setting should not affect the treatment of Jennifer's constipation. However, if a more serious etiology were suspected and access to health care were limited by location, more aggressive diagnostics at the time of presentation may be warranted.

Are there any demographic characteristics that might affect this case?

Constipation is a very common complaint in childhood. In fact, it is estimated that 3%–5% of pediatric health care visits are the result of constipation. The prevalence of constipation is equal among girls and boys during childhood, but it occurs more frequently in females than in males following puberty. While constipation occurs throughout infancy, childhood, and adulthood, it appears to be more prevalent during weaning and toilet training, and also in school-aged children. Many children with constipation have a family member who also has constipation.

REFERENCES AND RESOURCES

Bruce, J., Bruce, C., Short, H., & Paul, S. (2016). Childhood constipation: Recognition, management and the role of the nurse. *British Journal of Nursing, 25,* 1231–1242.

Ferrara, L., & Saccomano, S. (2017). Constipation in children: Diagnosis, treatment, and prevention. *Nurse Practitioner, 42,* 30–34.

Howarth, L., & Sullivan, P. (2016). Management of chronic constipation in children. *Paediatrics & Child Health, 26,* 415–422.

Khan, L. (2018). Constipation management in pediatric primary care. *Pediatric Annals, 47,* e180–e184.

Seidenfaden, S., Ormarsson, O., Lund, S., & Bjornsson, E. (2018). Physical activity may decrease the likelihood of children developing constipation. *Acta Paediatrica, 107,*151–155.

RESOLUTION

Which diagnostic or imaging studies should be considered to assist with or confirm the diagnosis?

To rule out a microbial cause, a swab of the skin under the foreskin and of any discharge should be analyzed for culture and sensitivity. Gram staining may be used to identify the causative microorganism and guide treatment. Dark field microscopy may be ordered to observe the presence of spirochetes, specifically *Treponema pallidum*. A potassium hydroxide test may be performed to look for hyphae if candida is suspected. In addition, a urinalysis should be performed for the detection of microorganisms from the bladder, urethra, meatus, or glans penis and to rule out a urinary tract infection and diabetes.

What is the most likely differential diagnosis and why?

Balanoposthitis:

Conditions to consider in the differential diagnosis of erythema and swelling of the foreskin include balanitis, phimosis, paraphimosis, and balanoposthitis. Balanitis refers to the inflammation of the glans penis. The foreskin is not swollen in balanitis, thus it may occur in both circumcised and uncircumcised males. Balanitis often presents in conjunction with diaper dermatitis. In phimosis, the foreskin cannot be retracted due to adhesion between the prepuce and glans penis, which becomes chronically swollen. This condition is physiologic at birth and should resolve between 3 and 6 years of age. Paraphimosis is a less likely diagnosis for Lydell, but it is one that should be considered for patients with swollen foreskin. In this condition, the foreskin is retracted past the coronal sulcus. Venous stasis results in swelling and pain of the foreskin.

Balanoposthitis refers to any infection of the foreskin. *Staphylococcus* and *Streptococcus* are the most common bacterial causes of posthitis. *Candidiasis* is a common fungal origin of posthitis and often occurs in conjunction with fungal diaper dermatitis. In addition, patients may develop irritant non-specific balanoposthitis from poor hygiene, especially related to smegma or prolonged contact with wet diapers. Based on the history and physical examination, Lydell has most likely developed a form of balanoposthitis.

The Family Nurse Practitioner: Clinical Case Studies, Second Edition. Edited by Leslie Neal-Boylan.
© 2021 John Wiley & Sons Ltd. Published 2021 by John Wiley & Sons Ltd.

What is your plan of treatment, referral, and follow-up care?

In addition to Lydell's diagnosis of balanoposthitis, he will likely have a concurrent diagnosis of physiologic phimosis. Because there is no discharge present, it is likely that the cause of Lydell's balanoposthitis is irritation from his diaper. The best treatment for Lydell at this time is a daily bath with a weak salt solution to alleviate inflammation and the application of bacitracin antibiotic ointment to the affected area 2–3 times daily. Lydell's parents should also be instructed to permit him to be without a diaper for 5–10 minutes after each diaper change to allow air to the area and to allow his diaper area to fully dry. His parents should also be told not to try to retract the foreskin fully as this may result in paraphimosis. Lydell's parents should be further educated to reinforce proper hygiene of the genital area. Lydell's family should follow up by phone in 2 days to report progress and healing. They should return to the office if his condition worsens or if there is no improvement in 48 hours after beginning the salt baths and bacitracin treatment. Health care providers should be aware that circumcision is not a preventative treatment of balanoposthitis in children younger than 3 years old. For chronic or recurrent balanoposthitis, a referral to a pediatric urologist should be considered.

Does this patient's psychosocial history affect how you might treat this case?

Though Lydell's father is involved in his care, his father does not reside with Lydell. Because there is no male figure directly caring for Lydell, it is important to educate the mother and grandmother in male genitourinary health. Proper hygiene of the glans penis and foreskin should be discussed, emphasizing that Lydell's foreskin will not likely be fully retractable at 2 years of age and that they should not forcibly retract the foreskin under any circumstances.

What if the patient lived in a rural setting?

Care of balanoposthitis would not change in a rural setting. Education regarding hygiene should be emphasized as before. For patients living in agricultural settings, hand hygiene after contact with animals should be discussed.

Are there any demographic characteristics that might affect this case?

When considering ethnicity, balanoposthitis has been noted to occur twice as often in African Americans and Hispanics. The difference in occurrence rates compared to Caucasians is likely related to different circumcision rates between the ethnic groups. Age is not necessarily a factor in the development of balanoposthitis. This condition can occur in males at any age, and the etiologies will vary depending on the age of the patient.

REFERENCES AND RESOURCES

Paquin, R., & Burstein, B. (2017). Comparison of outcomes for pediatric paraphimosis reduction using topical anesthetic versus intravenous procedural sedation. *American Journal of Emergency Medicine, 35*, 1391–1395.

Randjelovic, G., Otasevic, S., Mladenovic-Antic, S., Mladenovic, V., Radovanovic-Velickovic, R., Randjelovic, M., & Bogdanovic, D. (2017). *Streptococcus pyogenes* as the cause of vulvovaginitis and balanitis in children. *Pediatrics International, 59*, 432–437.

Toole, K. (2018). Balanoposthitis in a toddler. *Urologic Nursing, 38*, 237–239.

Case 4.1 Rash without Fever

Which diagnostic or imaging studies should be considered to assist with or confirm the diagnosis?

- Bacterial culture
- Bacterial culture of the nares
- Examination of Tzanck smear
- Fluorescent antibody testing of smears
- Fungal culture
- Gram stain
- KOH examination
- Viral culture

Results of testing:

- Bacterial culture: Positive for *Staphylococcus aureus* +/− *Streptococcus pyogenes*
- Bacterial culture of the nares: Positive for *Staphylococcus aureus*
- Examination of Tzanck smear: Negative
- Fluorescent antibody testing of smears: Negative
- Fungal culture: Negative
- Gram stain: Gram-positive
- KOH examination: Negative
- Viral culture: Negative

What is the most likely differential diagnosis and why?
Impetigo:
Impetigo is the most common bacterial skin infection in children. It occurs most commonly between 2 and 5 years of age, although it can appear at any age. Impetigo is caused by a superficial bacterial invasion of the epidermis via breaks in the normal skin barrier. Although *Streptococcus pyogenes* was once the leading cause of impetigo, the incidence of *Staphylococcus aureus* has risen steadily since the 1980s, and the majority of cases of childhood impetigo are now caused by *Staphylococcus aureus*. Methicillin-resistant *Staphylococcus aureus* (MRSA) accounts for up to 80% of

---

The Family Nurse Practitioner: Clinical Case Studies, Second Edition. Edited by Leslie Neal-Boylan.
© 2021 John Wiley & Sons Ltd. Published 2021 by John Wiley & Sons Ltd.

all cases of impetigo in some areas of the country. Most of these strains are community acquired and often affect healthy children with normal immune function, whereas historically MRSA is typically seen in hospitalized patients. Children are most often infected by direct contact with infected individuals, but fomites also pose a risk of infection spread.

Classic impetigo begins as erythematous macules or papules that quickly evolve to become vesicles with fragile roofs. The vesicles easily rupture, and the fluid inside dries to form honey-colored crusts on the eroded skin. Impetigo most often occurs on exposed areas of skin more susceptible to trauma, such as the face and extremities. The incidence is greatest in the summer months. Superficial breaks in the epidermis predispose an individual to develop impetigo. For that reason, impetigo frequently occurs overlying insect bites, atopic dermatitis, and other conditions that lead to skin abrasions. The differential diagnosis includes atopic or other forms of dermatitis, herpes simplex infections, a kerion caused by dermatophyte infection, varicella, Sweet's syndrome, scabies, pemphigus foliaceus, insect bites, ecthyma, discoid lupus erythematosus, and candidiasis.

Another form, bullous impetigo, accounts for approximately 30% of all cases of impetigo. Superficial vesicles also occur in bullous impetigo, but they rapidly enlarge to create bullae with sharp margins and no surrounding erythema. The bullae also rupture and develop honey-colored crusts as in classic impetigo. Bullous impetigo is more common in neonates and represents a localized variation of staphylococcal scalded skin syndrome caused by a toxin-producing form of *Staphylococcus aureus*. Bullous impetigo typically occurs in areas prone to friction and moisture such as the diaper area, axillae, and neck folds. The differential diagnosis includes second-degree burns, fixed drug eruptions, immunobullous diseases such as immunoglobulin A dermatosis, bullous pemphigoid, epidermolysis bullosa, and erythema multiforme. Bullous impetigo can be mistaken for cigarette burns, so child abuse is sometimes included in the differential diagnosis.

Although a bacterial culture and Gram stain are useful tools in diagnosing impetigo, the diagnosis can often be made clinically. Bacterial cultures will typically show *Staphylococcus aureus* with or without *Streptococcus pyogenes*. In rare instances, *Streptococcus pyogenes* impetigo can lead to poststreptococcal glomerulonephritis. Bacterial cultures are more useful when nephritogenic strains of *Streptococcus pyogenes* or drug resistance are suspected in a patient. In one study, carriage of *Staphylococcus aureus* was reported in the nasal passage of up to 42% of children between 7 and 19 years of age. A higher incidence has been reported in patients who actually have impetigo. Decisions to treat an individual should not be made based on the presence or absence of *Staphylococcus aureus* in the nasal passage, because a large percentage of unaffected individuals will test positive; and, conversely, an individual with impetigo may not be a nasal carrier. Other sites of the body may less commonly be colonized with *Staphylococcus aureus*.

Rare complications of impetigo include sepsis, osteomyelitis, arthritis, endocarditis, pneumonia, cellulitis, lymphadenitis, toxic shock syndrome, poststreptococcal glomerulonephritis, and generalized staphylococcal scalded skin syndrome. If an individual has recurrent MRSA infections, it may be useful to treat the patient and household members with intranasal mupirocin twice daily for 5 days a few times per year in an attempt to reduce the risk of nasal carriage.

What the treatment plan for this diagnosis?

Impetigo is usually self-limiting, localized, and heals without scarring, even without treatment. Small patches of impetigo will typically respond to topical antibiotics such as mupirocin applied twice daily for 5–7 days or retapamulin applied twice daily for 5 days. There is now documentation of mupirocin-resistant strains of staphylococci. Although most topical antibiotics cause at least partial clinical improvement, they may prolong the carriage state of the bacteria on the skin surface. Healthy children with impetigo that is widespread or recalcitrant to topical therapy may require oral antibiotics. Preferred oral antibiotics include amoxicillin-clavulanate, clindamycin, dicloxacillin, cephalosporins, and macrolides. If MRSA is recovered from a culture, bacterial sensitivities should guide drug selection.

What would the appropriate treatment plan for this diagnosis be if the patient were febrile and/or showing other signs of systemic illness?

Infants and children with extensive disease, signs of progressive cellulitis, and systemic symptoms may need hospitalization for parenteral antibiotic therapy and close observation.

What is the plan for follow-up care?

A follow-up appointment in 7–10 days to assess response to treatment may be helpful. However, the high rate of cure and low rate of complications related to impetigo may render follow-up unnecessary except in recalcitrant cases.

Are any referrals needed?

Not typically, but some serious or special cases (as mentioned above) may need hospitalization.

Should the patient stay out of school and/or day care during treatment? If so, for how long?

Children should be treated for a minimum of 24 hours before returning to school or other group settings such as day care in order to avoid spread.

What, if anything, should be recommended to unaffected household members?

It is important to emphasize good hygiene to the patient and family members in order to prevent further autoinoculation and spread to previously unaffected contacts. Good hand washing with antibacterial soap and disinfection of fomites is useful.

REFERENCES AND RESOURCES

Kosar, L., & Laubscher, T. (2017). Management of impetigo and cellulitis: Simple considerations for promoting appropriate antibiotic use in skin infections. *Canadian Family Physician*, *63*, 615–618.

Romani, L., Steer, A., Whitfeld, M., & Kaldor, J. (2015). Prevalence of scabies and impetigo worldwide: A systematic review. *Lancet Infectious Diseases*, *15*, 960–967.

Schachner, L. (2018). Ozenoxacin cream 1% for the topical treatment of impetigo in adults and children is effective & safe & offers advantages vs other antibiotics. *Dermatology Times*, *39*, 41–41.

VanRavenstein, K., Smith, W., O'Connor-Durham, C., & Williams, T. (2017). Diagnosis and management of impetigo. *Nurse Practitioner*, *42*, 40–44.

Case 4.2 Rash with Fever

RESOLUTION

Which diagnostic or imaging studies should be considered to assist with or confirm the diagnosis?

Diagnostic studies to identify a truncal rash can include tests for viruses, bacteria, or fungi. A Tzanck smear of a vesicle scraping would show multinucleated cells if the rash is due to varicella or herpes simplex virus. Additionally, viral culture and direct fluorescent antigen testing (DFA) can be done to differentiate between the two. DFA is more sensitive and much faster than viral culture. If the rash is found to be varicella, polymerase chain reaction (PCR) will assist in determining whether the rash is a wild-type varicella virus or vaccine-induced varicella. If there is any suspicion of a fungal infection, a potassium hydroxide (KOH) smear test can be performed to assess for the presence of hyphae. However, the description of Aubrey's vesicular rash does not appear to be fungal in origin. In the presence of a sore throat and rash, a bacterial culture for group A beta-hemolytic streptococcus (GABHS) may be performed. No imaging studies are required.

What is the most likely differential diagnosis and why?

Breakthrough varicella zoster virus (VZV), also known as chickenpox:

Key diagnostic clues are the description of the rash as maculopapular with vesicles; the history of a low-grade fever, cough, and rhinitis; and the absence of cervical lymphadenopathy. Aubrey did not get her second VZV vaccine, and a single dose is only 70%–90% effective for preventing VZV.

As always, other possible diagnoses must be considered. A truncal rash could be shingles, but it is also caused by VZV and only develops after prior infection with chickenpox. Furthermore, the distribution would most likely be limited to one dermatome. Since Aubrey reported a sore throat, scarlet fever associated with strep pharyngitis would be part of the differential diagnosis. However, the scarlet fever rash is often described as a "sandpaper rash," and lacks vesicles. With Aubrey's symptoms, the rash could also be a viral exanthema. But in the case of a viral exanthema, Aubrey would likely have a more generalized truncal rash. Lyme disease, with its classic "bull's-eye" rash, must be considered—but this rash is not vesicular. Finally, tinea corporis would be a possible diagnosis; however, Aubrey's rash does not have erythematous raised edges or central clearing as is common with tinea infections.

The Family Nurse Practitioner: Clinical Case Studies, Second Edition. Edited by Leslie Neal-Boylan.
© 2021 John Wiley & Sons Ltd. Published 2021 by John Wiley & Sons Ltd.

Wild-type chickenpox, caused by the varicella zoster virus, is an easily identifiable disease. It is typically a maculopapular rash with vesicles, characteristically with lesions beginning on the trunk and spreading distally. The lesions may be in different stages of healing. It is currently recommended that children get 2 doses of the VZV vaccine. It has been estimated that approximately 7% of children who received only one dose of the VZV vaccine developed VZV over a 10-year period, while only 2.2% of children who received 2 doses developed VZV. In cases of breakthrough VZV, there are often less than 50 lesions, and many times there are less than 10 lesions. Furthermore, in breakthrough varicella, the rash may be primarily maculopapular with few, if any, vesicles. Typically, the unvaccinated child who contracts chickenpox will have an average of 300–400 vesicles and, perhaps, up to 1000 vesicles. It is important for the health care provider to understand that breakthrough varicella infections present differently, and much less acutely, than classic wild-type VZV. If the history and physical presentation of the rash are consistent with VZV, no diagnostic tests are usually done.

What is the plan for treatment, referral, and follow-up care?

Breakthrough VZV is a self-limiting disease. The management is primarily supportive: diphenhydramine for itching and acetaminophen for fever and pain management. Oatmeal baths can be used to ameliorate itching. Aubrey should stay home from school until all of her lesions have dried and crusted. Aspirin should be avoided due to the risk of Reye syndrome in children. Acyclovir will not be helpful in Aubrey's case because her rash appeared more than 24 hours before she presented to the office. The health care provider should inquire about the vaccination status of Aubrey's brother and whether her parents have positive VZV titers, indicating immunity to the virus.

Does this patient's psychosocial history affect how you might treat this case?

Aubrey has no psychosocial characteristics that would alter management of her breakthrough VZV.

What if the patient lived in a rural setting?

If Aubrey lived in a rural setting, the consideration of tick-borne disease might be higher on the differential. However, living in an urban or suburban environment, excursions into rural places need to be considered.

Are there any demographic characteristics that might affect this case?

If Aubrey were immunocompromised or had contact with an immunocompromised patient, her VZV would be treated more aggressively.

REFERENCES AND RESOURCES

Dubey, V., & MacFadden, D. (2019). Disseminated varicella zoster virus infection after vaccination with a live attenuated vaccine. *CMAJ: Canadian Medical Association Journal, 191*, E1025–E1027.

Harpaz, R., & Leung, J. (2019). The epidemiology of herpes zoster in the United States during the era of varicella and herpes zoster vaccines: Changing patterns among older adults. *Clinical Infectious Diseases, 69*, 345–347.

Lopez, A. S., LaClair, B., Buttery, V., Zhang, Y., Rosen, J., Taggert, E., . . . Marin, M. (2019). Varicella outbreak surveillance in schools in sentinel jurisdictions, 2012–2015. *Journal of the Pediatric Infectious Diseases Society, 8*, 122–127.

Ludman, S., Powell, A., MacMahon, E., Martinez-Alier, N., & du Toit, G. (2018). Increased complications with atopic dermatitis and varicella-zoster virus. *Professional Nursing Today, 22*, 27–31.

Marin, M., Leung, J., & Gershon, A. (2019). Transmission of vaccine-strain varicella-zoster virus: A systematic review. *Pediatrics, 144*, 1–9.

Weinberg, A., Popmihajlov, Z., Schmader, K. E., Johnson, M. J., Caldas, Y., Salazar, A. T., . . . Levin, M. J. (2019). Persistence of varicella-zoster virus cell-mediated immunity after the administration of a second dose of live herpes zoster vaccine. *Journal of Infectious Diseases, 219*, 335–338.

RESOLUTION

What are the top three differential diagnoses in this case and why?

Bacterial conjunctivitis:

Acute bacterial conjunctivitis typically presents with complaint of unilateral eye redness, although it can be bilateral, along with purulent discharge. Mild discomfort may be reported, but pain and itch are generally absent. Discharge is copious and often yellow, green, or white in coloration. Patients may report history of "crusty, eyelids being stuck closed or glued together" in the mornings. This history detail was previously highly predictive of bacterial conjunctivitis. However, caution is advised relying on this specific detail, as several types of conjunctivitis present with variations of discharge leading to formation of dried crusts overnight. An important detail that can assist in differentiating bacterial conjunctivitis from other etiologies is the presence of purulent discharge continuing throughout the day, often reappearing minutes after cleansing/wiping eye. Upon examination, the conjunctiva will appear injected and the inner canthus (inner corner of eyes), along with lid margins, may reveal purulent discharge. Vision remains normal.

Common pathogens of bacterial conjunctivitis are _Staphylococcus aureus_, _Streptococcus pneumonia_, _Haemophilus influenza_, and _Moraxella catarrhalis_. Transmission is facilitated by contact with patient's discharge and or contaminated surfaces. Bacterial conjunctivitis is considered extremely contagious.

Viral conjunctivitis:

Viral conjunctivitis typically presents with complaint of unilateral redness, watery to mucoserous discharge, and burning or sandy sensation. Itch is not commonly reported. Although symptoms can remain unilateral, the second eye often becomes involved within 48 hours of initial onset. Often but not always, the occurrence of a viral prodrome precedes or shortly follows emergence of conjunctivitis, with spontaneous resolution between 1 to 2 weeks. Associated symptoms may include pharyngitis, upper respiratory infection, congestion, and fever.

Upon examination, the conjunctiva will appear injected without presence of purulent discharge. Discharge often appears watery or mucoserous. Excessive tearing may be present along with an enlarged and tender pre-auricular node. Further inspection directed to the tarsal conjunctiva may reveal follicular prominence or a "bumpy" appearance. Vision remains normal.

The Family Nurse Practitioner: Clinical Case Studies, Second Edition. Edited by Leslie Neal-Boylan.
© 2021 John Wiley & Sons Ltd. Published 2021 by John Wiley & Sons Ltd.

Common viral pathogens are adenovirus, enterovirus, and their subtypes. Transmission is facilitated by direct contact with the patient and their secretions, as well as contaminated fomites. Viral conjunctivitis is considered highly contagious. Treatment is supportive with application of cool compress and artificial tears. Antibiotics are not indicated for treatment of viral conjunctivitis.

Allergic conjunctivitis:
Allergic conjunctivitis typically presents with bilateral injection, watery drainage, and the distinct symptom of itch, which is not commonly present with bacterial and viral etiologies. Patients often report history of atopy whether seasonal rhinitis, eczema, asthma, or to specific allergens such as pet dander. Reports of prior exposure to allergens in combination with symptom of itch can aid in distinguishing etiologies. Associated symptoms would be consistent with common allergy symptoms of congestion, rhinorrhea, sneezing.

Upon examination, the conjunctiva will appear injected with copious epiphora (tearing). Discharge will be watery, thin, and often stringy. Similar to viral etiologies, follicular prominence to the tarsal conjunctiva may be present. In select presentations conjunctival edema, chemosis, can be noted. Vison remains normal.

Allergic conjunctivitis is caused by an allergen-induced, Immunoglobulin E (IgE)-mediated hypersensitivity response. Treatment hinges on reducing exposure to known allergens and over-the-counter antihistamine medications. Topical ophthalmic drops can be added for more moderate to severe responses.

What are the diagnostic tests required in this case and why?

A diagnosis of conjunctivitis is typically clinical through process of exclusion. Important aspects of history and examination include ensuring normal vision acuity and ruling out any recent history of trauma. Any vision-threatening findings should warrant further evaluation before a diagnosis of conjunctivitis is made.

Diagnostic testing is not routinely ordered. Cultures to identify bacteria and antibiotic sensitivity are reserved for more complex presentations, such as patients with compromised immune systems, contact lens wearers, neonates, and treatment failures.

What is the plan of treatment?

Bacterial conjunctivitis is frequently a self-limited process, but topical antibiotics, either drops or ointment, are recommended in order to provide quicker recovery, limit the spread of infection, and reduce the risk of further complication. Topical antibiotics are preferred due to their direct application to the ocular surface, which ensures a higher concentration of delivered medication. Empirical treatment with broad-spectrum antibiotics, such as polymyxin B sulfate and trimethoprim sulfate, 0.3% gentamycin, 0.5% erythromycin, and 0.3% tobramycin, can be utilized, as comparative studies have not shown one ophthalmic antibiotic to be superior to another. Ointment is preferred over drops as a treatment consideration for younger children, as it may be difficult to administer drops. Ointments can have a blurring effect and, as a result, are not recommended for adults who require clear vision for activities of daily living. Medication choice should focus on cost effectiveness and local bacterial resistance pattern, if known.

Are there any standardized guidelines that should be used to treat this case? If so, what are they?

The American Academy of Ophthalmology created a guideline on preferred practice patterns of conjunctivitis. The guideline showcases aspects of initial history collection through comprehensive medical examination. Referral guidelines are also presented. This guideline can be found at http://www.aao.org.

What are the plans for follow-up care and referral?

As mentioned previously, bacterial conjunctivitis is often self limiting with use of antibiotic medication serving to shorten the clinical course, limit the spread of infection, and reduce the risk of complications. If symptoms do not resolve or improve within 1 week of treatment, further evaluation is warranted. Educational guidance focusing on decreasing transmission through meticulous hand hygiene and avoidance of sharing personal objects should be provided to the patient/family. Referral to ophthalmology is warranted for any history and or findings related to sight-threatening conditions. Examples include decreased visual acuity, significant photophobia, severe eye pain, suspected foreign body, recurrent episodes, or corneal opacity.

Are there any special examination and or treatment considerations that may affect this case?

Regarding this case, the patient reported wearing glasses. In presentations of conjunctivitis it is important to inquire about contact lens use. There are recommendations as to the treatment of bacterial conjunctivitis in those who wear contact lenses. Soft, extended-wear lenses carry a greater risk of pseudomonal keratitis. Findings include acute red eye, discharge, and ulcerative keratitis marked by an inability to open or keep open the eye due to severe foreign body sensation. If keratitis is ruled out and bacterial conjunctivitis is diagnosed, patients may be treated with topical antibiotics. Due to the risk of pseudomonas, fluoroquinolones are the medications of choice. It is recommended that contact lens use be discontinued until 24 hours post resolution of discharge.

REFERENCES AND RESOURCES

American Academy of Opthalmology Cornea/External Disease Panel, Preferred Practice Patterns Committee. (2018). *Conjunctivitis*. San Francisco, CA: American Academy of Opthalmology (AAO).

Cronau, H., Kankanala, R. R., & Mauger, T. (2010). Diagnosis and management of red eye in primary care. *American Academy of Family Physicians, 81*(2), 137–144.

Eltis, M. (2011). Contact-lens-related microbial keratitis: Case report and review. *Journal of Optometry, 4*(4), 122–127.

Hovding, G. (2008). Acute bacterial conjunctivitis. *Acute Opthalmologica, 86*(1), 5–17.

Spering, K. A. (2011). CME/CE: Therapeutic strategies for bacterial conjunctivitis. *Clinical Advisor, 14*(8), 31–40.

Case 4.4 Sore Throat

Which diagnostic or imaging studies should be considered to assist with or confirm the diagnosis?

When evaluating a sore throat, several tests may be helpful to determine the cause of the illness and to decide the treatment plan. If group A beta-hemolytic streptococci (GABHS) is suspected, a rapid antigen detection test (rapid strep test) and a throat culture should be performed. Both tests are needed because the rapid test provides a preliminary result, while the culture provides the final result after 48 hours. The benefits of using the rapid strep test along with the culture are avoiding unnecessary antibiotic usage and treating the patient in an appropriate and timely manner. If the Epstein-Barr virus (EBV) is suspected, a CBC, monospot, and LFTs should be ordered.

If other viral etiology is suspected, diagnostic testing is not needed. Imaging studies are usually not needed unless a retropharyngeal, parapharyngeal, or peritonsillar abscess is suspected. In that case, a plain lateral neck film may be ordered as an initial screening tool.

What is the most likely differential diagnosis and why?

GABHS:

Several differential diagnoses should be considered when evaluating a sore throat. Viral etiologies cause 40% of cases of sore throats, with enteroviruses, adenoviruses, and EBV being the most common. Bacterial pathogens cause 30% of sore throats, which are usually caused by GABHS, although other pathogens such as *Staphylococcus aureus* or *Haemophilus influenzae* should also be considered. Pharyngitis caused by the fungus *Candida albicans* is another differential diagnosis that should be considered, especially for immunosuppressed individuals. Other more urgent diagnoses such as peritonsillar abscess or retropharyngeal abscess need to be ruled out. Given the patient's history of fever of 101°F, sore throat, and headache, along with the physical exam findings of erythematous tonsils with exudates, palatal petechiae, and cervical adenopathy, the most likely diagnosis is GABHS. In addition to this patient's classic symptoms, many children may also experience nausea or vomiting and/or a scarlatiniform rash.

The Family Nurse Practitioner: Clinical Case Studies, Second Edition. Edited by Leslie Neal-Boylan.
© 2021 John Wiley & Sons Ltd. Published 2021 by John Wiley & Sons Ltd.

What is the plan for treatment, referral, and follow-up care?

Penicillin or amoxicillin is the drug of choice for treating GABHS. They are effective and do not contribute to antibiotic resistance and the complication of rheumatic fever will be avoided. In penicillin-allergic patients, recommended courses of treatment include narrow-spectrum cephalosporins (cephalexin, cefadroxil), clindamycin, azithromycin, or clarithromycin. Whether the pharyngitis is viral or bacterial in origin, the use of antipyretics for pain and fever is beneficial, as are other symptomatic treatments such as increasing liquid intake.

Referral to an ear, nose, and throat (ENT) specialist is only necessary should complications arise. Follow-up care is needed if the patient's symptoms worsen or persist for more than 48 hours while on antibiotics.

Does this patient's psychosocial history affect how you might treat this case?

There is nothing in this patient's psychosocial history that would affect how this case is treated.

What if the patient lived in a rural setting?

No changes in diagnosis or treatment are required if the patient lives in a rural setting. However, if the patient has emigrated from or traveled to a high-risk area for diphtheria, other testing and treatment should be considered.

Are there any demographic characteristics that might affect this case?

There is no racial or ethnic predisposition for the development of GABHS. Regarding age, the majority of children who develop GABHS are between 5 and 10 years of age. Socioeconomic status is not known to be associated with GABHS.

REFERENCES AND RESOURCES

Berkley, J. (2018). Management of pharyngitis. *Circulation, 138*, 1920–1922.

Farrer, F. (2018). OTC treatments for tonsillitis and pharyngitis. *Professional Nursing Today, 22*, 8–11.

Homme, J. (2019). Acute otitis media and group a streptococcal pharyngitis: A review for the general pediatric practitioner. *Pediatric Annals, 48*, e343–e348.

Norton, L., Lee, B., Harte, L., Mann, K., Newland, J., Grimes, R., & Myers, A. (2018). Improving guideline-based streptococcal pharyngitis testing: A quality improvement initiative. *Pediatrics, 142*, 1–9.

Case 4.5 Disruptive Behavior

Which diagnostic or imaging studies should be considered to assist with or confirm the diagnosis?

Selected lab evaluations help to convince parents that the child is physically healthy and that other conditions may be important to consider. A CBC and lead screening assures that there is no anemia, infection, or elevated lead level. Hyperactive thyroid would be very unlikely to present this constellation of symptoms and need not be obtained unless the mother is very concerned because of her own thyroid disorder. Vision and hearing screening are essential to assure that Jason has intact sensory systems so he is able to respond appropriately to directions and facial cues.

Jason's hearing screen was normal. Vanderbilt ADHD screening indicated no concerns with inattentiveness or combined-type ADHD. Information gathered from the school suggested that Jason started the year as a capable student who has begun to lag behind his peers, especially in reading and social skills. Jason's mother completed the Pediatric Symptom Checklist. Scoring revealed that Jason has trouble obeying his teacher, is often irritable and angry, fights with other children, does not listen to rules, does not understand other people's feelings, blames others for his troubles, teases others, and refuses to share.

What is the most likely differential diagnosis and why?

Oppositional defiant disorder:

To arrive at a working diagnosis, much more information needs to be gathered from Jason's teacher and from standardized screening tools and possibly school assessments of learning issues. Based on the test results and further history from his mother and teacher, it appears that Jason meets the *DSM-5* diagnostic criteria for oppositional defiant disorder (ODD). This diagnosis is more likely than depression. Jason's behavior is more extreme than his peers', and it interferes with his social and academic development. Jason also has numerous risk factors for this disorder, including financial problems in the family, family instability, a parent with a substance abuse disorder, parents with a history of ADHD, lack of positive parental involvement, and inconsistent discipline.

The Family Nurse Practitioner: Clinical Case Studies, Second Edition. Edited by Leslie Neal-Boylan.
© 2021 John Wiley & Sons Ltd. Published 2021 by John Wiley & Sons Ltd.

What is the plan of treatment?

Discuss the diagnosis with his mother and father. Reinforce that this is a manageable condition and that primary care will provide support to the family in their efforts to make change. Discuss that early intervention is critical and has the greatest possibility of preventing ODD from progressing to conduct disorder. Address parental concerns and assure them that effective, consistent discipline can make significant improvements.

- Recommend parent-focused discipline literature such as *1-2-3 Magic* by Thomas Phelan.
- Refer for parent-management training such as Russell Barkley's Parent Management Training or Ross Greene's Collaborative Problem-Solving.
- Refer to conduct clinic, if available in community or university setting.
- Refer for family therapy or individual play therapy for Jason.
- Consider social skills training if peer relationships deteriorate.
- Encourage close communication with his teacher to assure consistent approaches to behavior changes.
- If comorbid ADHD develops at a later time, stimulant medications may be helpful.

What is the plan for follow-up care?

Follow up in the primary care setting to reinforce strategies learned in therapy and to offer continued support for family efforts. Encourage the grandparents' participation in visits so they will utilize the same approaches that the parents are learning.

Are there any demographic factors that might affect this case?

This condition can occur in any socioeconomic or racial group. Risk factors are noted above.

REFERENCES AND RESOURCES

de la Osa, N., Penelo, E., Navarro, J., Trepat, E., & Ezpeleta, L. (2019). Prevalence, comorbidity, functioning and long-term effects of subthreshold oppositional defiant disorder in a community sample of preschoolers. *European Child & Adolescent Psychiatry, 28*, 1385–1393.

El Ouardani, C. (2017). Innocent or intentional?: Interpreting oppositional defiant disorder in a preschool mental health clinic. *Culture, Medicine & Psychiatry, 41*, 94–110.

Katzmann, J., Görtz-Dorten, A., & Döpfner, M. (2018). Child-based treatment of oppositional defiant disorder: Mediating effects on parental depression, anxiety and stress. *European Child & Adolescent Psychiatry, 2*, 1181–1192.

Miller, R., Gondoli, D., Gibson, B., Steeger, C., & Morrissey, R. (2017). Contributions of maternal attention-deficit hyperactivity and oppositional defiant disorder symptoms to parenting. *Parenting: Science & Practice, 17*, 281–300.

Ter-Stepanian, M., Martin-Storey, A., Bizier-Lacroix, R., Déry, M., Lemelin, J., & Temcheff, C. (2019). Trajectories of verbal and physical peer victimization among children with comorbid oppositional defiant problems, conduct problems and hyperactive-attention problems. *Child Psychiatry & Human Development, 50*, 1037–1048.

NOTE: The author would like to acknowledge Patricia Ryan-Krause, MSN, APRN, who co-authored this case in the first edition of this book.

Case 4.6 Cough and Difficulty Breathing

What diagnostic or imaging studies should be considered to assist with or confirm the diagnosis?

The nasal pharyngeal swab for direct fluorescent antibody (DFA) was positive for influenza type A. Oxygen saturation is 94%, which is an indication of poor exchange of oxygenation. Chest X-ray was negative for pneumonia; and there is no peribronchial cuffing, which is more often seen in bronchiolitis. There was no mediastinal shift or collapsed lung seen with foreign body aspiration.

What are the top differential diagnoses and why?

Foreign body aspiration: Always consider when seeing a patient with acute wheezing, even if they have a diagnosis of asthma.

Bronchiolitis: Consider if the child is less than 2 years of age and develops wheezing with a viral illness.

Asthma: Consider if there is a family history of asthma, allergies and/or eczema, and recurrent episodes of wheezing.

GERD: Children can aspirate and symptoms can mimic asthma.

What is the most likely differential diagnosis and why?
Asthma:

Asthma is one of the most prevalent chronic diseases facing American children today. The diagnosis of asthma is based on the exclusion of alternative diagnoses, as well as the history of recurrent and transient airflow obstructive symptoms, the patient's subjective experience of symptoms, and objective clinical manifestations. These criteria will vary among patients and in the same patient over time. The important signs and symptoms needed to diagnose asthma include (1) recurrent wheeze, (2) improvement of symptoms after treatment with a bronchodilator, (3) recurrent cough or shortness of breath, (4) impaired peak flow performance when compared to the expected value based on height and age, and (5) exclusion of alternative differential diagnoses.

A differential diagnosis still requires consideration in any patient who is wheezing, including one with a known diagnosis of asthma and a history of exacerbations. Several conditions may lead to a presentation similar to acute asthma. Some of these include congestive heart failure, vocal cord

The Family Nurse Practitioner: Clinical Case Studies, Second Edition. Edited by Leslie Neal-Boylan.
© 2021 John Wiley & Sons Ltd. Published 2021 by John Wiley & Sons Ltd.

dysfunction, gastroesophageal reflux, acute bronchitis or bronchiolitis, pulmonary emboli, or the presence of a foreign body.

After the diagnosis of asthma has been made, the severity of the patient's asthma can be classified, based in part on the frequency of symptoms, findings on physical exam, and severity of exacerbations. Severity ranges from intermittent to severe persistent, depending on the frequency of daytime symptoms, nighttime symptoms, interference with normal activity, lung function, and number of exacerbations requiring oral corticosteroids in the past year. Accurate classification of asthma severity is critical because treatment goals and pharmacological management are based on the individual's asthma classification. Because individuals may manifest different symptoms over time, periodic reevaluation and adjustment of the patient's medications are necessary.

Information gathered during the initial asthma assessment will serve as baseline data, by determining the patient's respiratory status and the severity of the current exacerbation. After an intervention is implemented, repeat assessments are recommended. These serial assessments can be compared against the baseline data so that trends in the patient's response to treatment can be revealed. Next, the health care provider can assess the severity of the current exacerbation through auscultation of the lung fields, noting the movement of air and presence of abnormal breath sounds. Treatment should be initiated as soon as the diagnosis of an asthma exacerbation is confirmed.

What is the plan of treatment?

An asthma exacerbation should be treated with an early intensification of an inhaled beta$_2$-agonist and the administration of oxygen and an oral or systemic steroid when medically necessary. The inhaled beta$_2$-agonists, known as quick-relief or rescue medications, should be given to all patients regardless of the severity of their exacerbation. Exacerbation therapy should begin with up to 3 treatments of a short-acting beta$_2$-agonist, given at 20-minute intervals over an hour. The minimum dose should be 2.5 mg, or 0.15 mg/kg of body weight. The alternative is to give 2–6 puffs of albuterol, 90 mcg/puff by metered dose inhaler (MDI) with a spacer attachment. However, if no improvement is demonstrated after the initial treatment, the exacerbation severity can be classified as moderate or severe, and a steroid should be given in conjunction with the bronchodilator. The recommended child dose for an oral steroid such as prednisolone is a loading dose of 2 mg/kg of body weight, followed by 2 mg/kg/day 1 to 2 times a day (maximum dose of 60 mg/day). Additionally, an inhaled beta$_2$-agonist should be given every 4 hours as needed for wheezing.

What is the plan for follow-up care?

After the treatment goals have been met, the patient can continue therapy and monitoring independently at home with a short-term intensification of their treatment. For most patients, this means an increase in the frequency of beta$_2$-agonist use and the addition of a systemic steroid. Patients should not leave the health care setting without receiving educational information, an asthma action plan, a follow-up appointment to take place within 3 days of the exacerbation, and a clear understanding of how to contact the provider should their condition deteriorate. It is recommended that children who have experienced an exacerbation should follow up with their health care provider 2–3 days after the acute episode to (1) monitor the response to treatment, (2) encourage continued patient compliance with their medication regimen, (3) prevent a relapse of symptoms, and (4) provide an educational review of information discussed during previous visits.

Are any referrals needed at this time?

No. The provider should consider a referral to a pulmonologist or allergist if symptoms cannot be managed using standard approaches or if the provider thinks that there may be additional factors that complicate the case.

Are there any standardized guidelines that should be used to assess or treat this case?

The following approach to acute asthma treatment is based on the findings of the National Heart, Lung, and Blood Institute Expert Report Panel (2007) and the Global Initiative for Asthma (GINA)

(2019). This information is meant to serve as a guide to exacerbation treatment. Strict adherence to general guidelines should never supersede individual response to therapy, which is monitored through patient report of symptoms, continuous skilled assessment, and accurate data collection. Adjustments may need to be made initially and ongoing during treatment depending on the patient's prior exacerbation history, present respiratory abilities, and response to treatment. The lowest and simplest dosing regimen that effectively controls the individual's acute asthma should be selected to encourage patient compliance.

REFERENCES AND RESOURCES

Albassan, S., Hattah, Y., Bajwa, O., Bihler, E., & Singh, A. C. (2016). Asthma. *Critical Care Nursing Quarterly, 39*(2), 110–123.

Global Initiative for Asthma (GINA). (2019). 2019 GINA Report: Global strategy for asthma management and prevention. Retrieved from: https://ginasthma.org/

Meadows-Oliver, M., & Banasiak, N. C. (2005). Asthma medication delivery devices. *Journal of Pediatric Health Care, 19*(2), 121–123.

National Asthma Education & Prevention Program. (2007). Expert panel report 3: Guidelines for the diagnosis and management of asthma. Bethesda, MD: National Institute of Health.

Voorend-van Bergen, S., Vaessen-Verberne, A. A., de Jongste, J. C., & Pijnenburg, M. W. (2015). Asthma control questionnaires in the management of asthma in children: a review. *Pediatric pulmonology, 50*(2), 202–208.

Zahran, H. S., Bailey, C. M., Damon, S. A., Garbe, P. L., & Breysse, P. N. (2018). Vital signs: Asthma in children—United States, 2001–2016. *Morbidity and Mortality Weekly Report, 67*(5), 149.

Case 4.7 Left Arm Pain

RESOLUTION

Which diagnostic or imaging studies should be considered to assist with or confirm the diagnosis?
Based on the history and physical examination, a radiograph of the left arm and clavicle is needed to rule out a fracture.

What is the most likely differential diagnosis and why?
Suspected child physical abuse:
Physical abuse of Jair should be considered. He has a physical injury and his parents are providing inconsistent stories about the origin of his injuries. Additionally, Jair has injuries (bruising and an abrasion) on the right side of his body—the side opposite of his fall. Abused children often present with multiple types of injuries (bruising, abrasions, and fractures). Multiple types of injuries decrease the likelihood of a single medical condition being the cause of the injuries.

What is the plan for treatment, referral, and follow-up care?
- Refer this child to the local emergency department for further evaluation, consultation with a social worker, and possible in-patient admission.
- Call child protective services to report a suspected case of child physical abuse.
- Allow the parents to verbalize their concerns about their baby's health.

Are there any referrals needed?
A referral to the local child protective services agency is warranted. Health care providers can receive help and resources from the Childhelp National Child Abuse Hotline. The Childhelp National Child Abuse Hotline is dedicated to the prevention of child abuse. The hotline is staffed 24 hours a day, 7 days a week with professional crisis counselors who can provide assistance in over 170 languages through the use of interpreters. They can be reached at https://www.childhelp.org/hotline/ or by telephone at 1-800-4-A-CHILD.

The Family Nurse Practitioner: Clinical Case Studies, Second Edition. Edited by Leslie Neal-Boylan.
© 2021 John Wiley & Sons Ltd. Published 2021 by John Wiley & Sons Ltd.

Does the patient's psychosocial history impact how you might treat him?
Adolescent mothers have been shown to exhibit higher rates of child abuse than do older mothers. Other psychosocial factors such as lower economic status, lack of social support, and high stress levels may also contribute to the link between adolescent parents and child abuse (Children's Bureau, n.d.).

REFERENCES AND RESOURCES

Children's Bureau. (n.d.). *Teen parenting*. https://www.childwelfare.gov/topics/can/factors/parentcaregiver/teen/

Fréchette, S., Zoratti, M., & Romano, E. (2015). What is the link between corporal punishment and child physical abuse? *Journal of Family Violence, 30*, 135–148.

Ho, G., Gross, D., & Bettencourt, A. (2017). Universal mandatory reporting policies and the odds of identifying child physical abuse. *American Journal of Public Health, 107*, 709–716.

Johnson, M. (2017). Imaging and diagnosis of physical child abuse. *Radiologic Technology, 89*, 45–67.

Teeuw, A., Kraan, R., Rijn, R., Bossuyt, P., Heymans, H., & van Rijn, R. (2019). Screening for child abuse using a checklist and physical examinations in the emergency department led to the detection of more cases. *Acta Paediatrica, 108*, 300–313.

Case 4.8 Nightmares

RESOLUTION

Which diagnostic or imaging studies should be considered to assist with or confirm the diagnosis?

An EEG may reveal altered consciousness during night terror episodes. An EEG will also help to diagnose nocturnal seizures. Polysomnography can help to diagnose parasomnias such as sleep-walking, nightmares, and night terrors. An MRI may show if a brain lesion is causing the problem of night awakening and screaming. A CT scan and skull radiographs are usually not helpful in the testing for sleep disturbances.

What is the most likely differential diagnosis and why?

Night terrors:

Nightmares happen during REM (rapid eye movement) sleep. Children with nightmares awaken and will recall having vivid dreams. A child who is having a nightmare is fully awake and often will seek comfort from a caregiver. Nocturnal seizures, which occur only during sleep, can cause the victim to cry, scream, walk, run about, or curse. Like other seizures, these are usually treated with medication. With nightmares, the child may also scream and cry. Night terrors (sometimes known as sleep terrors) in stage IV of the sleep cycle. Stage IV is also known as slow-wave sleep (SWS) and usually occurs during the first third of the night. Although appearing to be awake, children experiencing a night terror are still in a light sleep. A child suffering from a night terror will be unable to be calmed by a caregiver. Each episode will generally last for less than 5 minutes, although some children experience multiple terrors each night. A child who experiences night terrors will usually have no memory of the event in the morning, while a child with a nightmare may or may not have a memory of the dream but will almost certainly remember being awake. Night terrors are the most likely diagnosis when taking the history and physical examination into account.

What is the plan for treatment, referral, and follow-up care?

Several factors have been theorized to contribute to night terrors, such as lack of a regular bedtime, a full bladder, and extra noise or lights in the sleeping environment. A treatment plan would encompass education on each of these aspects. Daniel's lack of a set bedtime may contribute to his being overtired but neither clinical exam nor history suggest that he struggles with daytime fatigue or lack of energy. However, the health care provider should question the mother about this

The Family Nurse Practitioner: Clinical Case Studies, Second Edition. Edited by Leslie Neal-Boylan.
© 2021 John Wiley & Sons Ltd. Published 2021 by John Wiley & Sons Ltd.

possibility further. A full bladder at the time of a night terror cannot be ruled out and should also be further explored. It should be noted that Daniel shares a bedroom with his younger brother. It is unknown whether the brother uses a nightlight, snores, or otherwise contributes to environmental pollution through music or television.

When providing education, parents should be reminded that the night terror episodes, while disturbing to them, are not remembered by the child. When a child is experiencing a night terror, a parent should check on him to confirm his safety. Although difficult, parents are discouraged from picking up the child or providing other comfort measures. For the child experiencing a night terror, consoling from a parent can cause greater distress and result in full awakening.

The health care provider may suggest that Daniel's mother maintain a sleep diary and observe him throughout several night terror episodes, noting the amount of time after he falls asleep that the night terror begins. After Daniel's sleep-wake pattern is determined, his mother should wake him up approximately 15 minutes before the usual time of the night terror and keep him awake and out of bed for a full 5 minutes. This process should continue for approximately for 5–10 days. By waking up the child before the night terror actually begins, the sleep cycle is consistently disturbed and is then able to be reestablished—typically without the resumption of the night terrors. This may help to break the disruptive sleep pattern that has resulted in the night terrors. Upon awakening the child, the parents can also coax the child to use the bathroom if a full bladder is a suspected contributor to the night terrors.

Prior to sleep, there are other steps that parents can take to reduce the occurrence of night terrors. A consistent bedtime and sleep hygiene routine may reduce the occurrence of night terrors. Daniel's mother can begin by establishing a consistent time for bed along with a regular bedtime routine. Maintaining quiet time without sudden unsettling noises near bedtime may minimize some of the external stimuli that are thought to contribute to night terrors. Since night terrors might be triggered by a full bladder, having Daniel use the toilet prior to bedtime and even during the course of the night might be beneficial in reducing reoccurrence of night terrors. In extreme cases of night terrors, benzodiazepines (known to suppress the stage IV level of deep sleep) have been prescribed, although this is not a standard recommendation. Pharmacological options are controversial and are generally not considered in children under the age of 7 years. Alternative options such as hypnosis, biofeedback, and various relaxation techniques have been used with some success to reduce or eliminate occurrence of childhood night terrors. Calming music or bedtime stories may also assist with the reduction of night terrors.

Follow-up can be done by telephone in 1–2 weeks to ascertain if the recommendations to reduce the night terrors have been effective. Daniel's family should also follow up in the office if Daniel exhibits drooling, jerking, or stiffening of the body during the night terror. If the episodes have continued without improvement, consider referring Daniel to a sleep specialist and for a polysomnography test to assist with the diagnosis of a parasomnia.

Does this patient's psychosocial history affect how you might treat this case?

Daniel lives in a home with several family members. With 3 generations of family members in the home, bedtime may not be a quiet time. Including Daniel's grandmother in the treatment plan may also help to reduce or lessen the occurrence of night terrors.

What if the patient lived in a rural setting?

The treatment of night terrors would not vary based on residence in a rural area. However, if Daniel's night terrors continued and he needed to be referred to a specialist, the family might have difficulty accessing specialty services if they do not reside near a major medical center that employs a sleep specialist.

Are there any demographic characteristics that might affect this case?

Children between the ages of 3 and 5 years of age are most likely to experience night terrors with the prevalence decreasing with increasing age. There is no clear indication regarding gender and the occurrence of night terrors. Some studies say that the occurrence is nearly equal. Studies show that 49% of affected children were boys, and 51% were girls. Others studies report that childhood night terrors occur more frequently in boys.

REFERENCES AND RESOURCES

Ellington, E. (2018). It's not a nightmare: Understanding sleep terrors. *Journal of Psychosocial Nursing & Mental Health Services, 56*, 11–14.

Moreno, M. (2015). Sleep terrors and sleepwalking: Common parasomnias of childhood. *JAMA Pediatrics, 169*, 704–704.

Petit, D., Pennestri, M.-H., Paquet, J., Desautels, A., Zadra, A., Vitaro, F., . . . Montplaisir, J. (2015). Childhood sleepwalking and sleep terrors: A longitudinal study of prevalence and familial aggregation. *JAMA Pediatrics, 169*, 653–658.

Richarde, S. (2018). Night terrors and sleepwalking in children and adults: Pathophysiology and potential therapies. *Journal of the American Herbalists Guild, 16*, 59–67.

NOTE: The author would like to acknowledge the contribution of Allison Grady, MSN, RN to this case in the first edition of this book.

Case 4.9 Gastrointestinal Complaint

RESOLUTION

What are the top three differential diagnoses for this patient? What tests would help to confirm your suspicions?

Given the vagueness of the symptoms—essentially several months of diarrhea and abdominal pain—there should be many potential diagnoses on your list of differentials. Initially, irritable bowel syndrome (IBS), celiac disease, functional abdominal pain, food allergy, failure to thrive, autoimmune disease, and eating disorder all come to mind. These are some of the first thoughts because Katie is having ongoing, but still relatively new, abdominal symptoms that are affecting her quality of life. This list of possibilities includes gastrointestinal focus but also includes other systems such as immune, genetic, and psychological. Important pieces of the patient's history that might help to narrow the possibilities include that Katie expanded her palate around the same time that her growth began to slow, which might point more to celiac disease, food allergy, or autoimmune disease and may suggest against an eating disorder. Taking a careful history can guide the provider by revealing potential clues and new information about the condition. If the patient has identified any stressful triggers (e.g., situations at home or school) or changes to bowel patterns (for example, periods of diarrhea and then periods of constipation), this might point more toward irritable bowel syndrome (IBS). Skin changes such as hives, eczema, or dermatitis herpetiformis or gastrointestinal complaints around mealtimes might suggest food allergy or celiac disease. A detailed and specific family history in combination with information about any recent illnesses that Katie has experienced might help to better understand the risk of an autoimmune or genetic disease.

Katie's diagnosis, however, is celiac disease. Although celiac is only present in less than 2% of the population (Lebwohl, Sanders, & Green, 2018), the main symptoms are gastrointestinal in nature, family history of a second-degree relative with the condition (Fedewa et al., 2019, in press), and a mother with a history of multiple miscarriages all raise the suspicion of celiac disease (Nahar & Avani, 2019) (see Table 4.9.1).

Celiac disease:

Celiac disease (CD) has been described as "a chronic, small-intestinal immune-mediated enteropathy initiated by exposure to dietary gluten in genetically predisposed individuals and characterized by specific autoantibodies against tissue transglutaminase 2, endomysium, and/or deamidated gliadin

The Family Nurse Practitioner: Clinical Case Studies, Second Edition. Edited by Leslie Neal-Boylan.
© 2021 John Wiley & Sons Ltd. Published 2021 by John Wiley & Sons Ltd.

Table 4.9.1. Classification of Symptoms.

Category of Symptom	Symptoms/Conditions				
Gastrointestinal	Abdominal pain	Diarrhea or Constipation	Vomiting		
Nongastrointestinal	Failure to thrive	Loss of dental enamel	Dermatitis herpetiformis	Iron-deficiency anemia	Osteoporosis/ Osteopenia
Common co-occurring conditions	Type 1 diabetes	Thyroid conditions	Down syndrome	First-degree relatives with celiac disease	Family member with Multiple miscarriages

Source: From Nahar et al. (2019) Sealing the Diagnosis of Celiac Disease in Pregnancy. *The Medicine Forum*: Vol. 20, Article 9.

peptide" (Leonard, Sapone, Catassi, & Fasan, 2017, p. 647). In more conventional terms, celiac disease is an autoimmune condition that is triggered by the environmental exposure to gluten, which is found in wheat, rye, and barley. The affected individual develops autoantibodies to the gluten, which in turn cause inflammation and small villous atrophy of the small bowel. Over time, this recurrent injury to the small bowel can result in chronic inflammation, increased risk for infection, and numerous other anatomical and clinical changes that interfere with quality of life and threaten overall health.

Celiac disease typically presents with gastrointestinal symptoms but the effects of the disease is not limited to this corporal system. Nongastrointestinal features such as skin rash (dermatitis herpetiformis), fatigue, anemia, dental abnormalities, failure to thrive, and nutritional abnormalities also are common presenting symptoms for patients with celiac disease (Leonard et al., 2017; Khatib, Baker, Ly, Kozielski, & Baker, 2016). In fact, most patients with celiac disease have zinc, folate, and vitamin D deficiencies (Mager et al., 2019). Celiac is most often diagnosed in the fourth to sixth decades of life, but can be present from any time that gluten ingestion occurs—often, shortly after the introduction of solids in infancy (U.S. Preventive Services Task Force, 2017).

The European Society for Pediatric Gastroenterology, Hepatology, and Nutrition (ESPGHN) released a set of guidelines for the diagnosis of celiac disease in 2012. If celiac disease was suspected based on history and physical, the provider was encouraged to draw a serum tTG and a total Immunoglobulin A (IgA). If the tTG comes back negative, this patient is thought *not* to have celiac disease and other conditions should be explored. If the tTG comes back positive, the recommendation is to transfer to a pediatric GI specialist, as celiac is a likely diagnosis (Husby et al., 2012). Other blood tests that help to guide the diagnosis include serum endomysial antibody (EMA) and HLA-DQ2 and HLA-DQ8, which are generally ordered by DNA testing and interpreted by gastroenterologists (Husby et al., 2012). ESPGHAN notes that "HLA-DQ2/HLA-DQ8 typing has a role in the case finding strategy in individuals who belong to groups at risk for CD. A negative result for HLA-DQ2/HLA-DQ8 renders CD highly unlikely in these children, and hence there is no need for subsequent CD antibodies testing in such individuals" (Husby et al., 2012, p. 145). Those who have HLA-DQ2/HLA-DQ8 positivity should note that while its absence is sensitive to *not* having celiac disease, it is not specific for *having* celiac disease. In such a circumstance, results of blood tests previously noted, specifically the results of the EMA test (a positive test in addition to positive HLA testing would indicate celiac disease), a duodenal endoscopy, and a work-up for other ailments should be taken into consideration before confirming a diagnosis of celiac disease (see Figure 4.9.1, Husby, 2012, p. 153).

A duodenal endoscopy remains a gold standard in the diagnosis of celiac disease, albeit a controversial one. Because celiac disease typically is associated with "an increased number of intraepithelial lymphocytes (>25 per 100 enterocytes), elongation of the crypts, and partial to total villous atrophy" in the small intestine, biopsies have been recommended to both grade the severity of the disease (using the Marsh scale) and monitor for improvement over time (Leonard et al., 2017, p. 651). Recently, ESPGHAN has stated that a biopsy can be omitted if a patient has "signs and symptoms suggesting celiac disease, a positive anti-tTG antibodies finding with a level greater

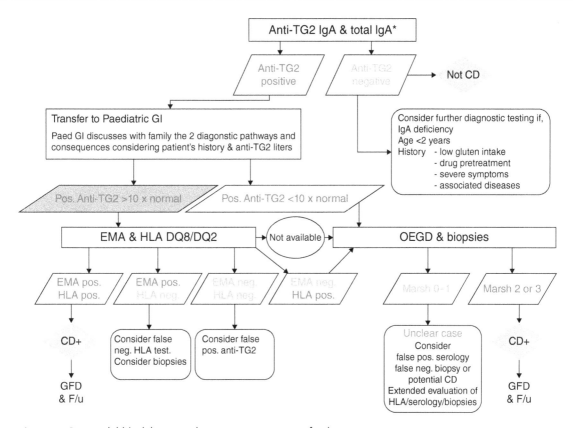

Anti-TG2 IgA & total IgA*

Anti-TG2 positive

Anti-TG2 negative → Not CD

Transfer to Paediatric GI

Paed GI discusses with family the 2 diagnostic pathways and consequences considering patient's history & anti-TG2 liters

Consider further diagnostic testing if,
IgA deficiency
Age <2 years
History - low gluten intake
        - drug pretreatment
        - severe symptoms
        - associated diseases

Pos. Anti-TG2 >10 x normal

Pos. Anti-TG2 <10 x normal

EMA & HLA DQ8/DQ2 → Not available → OEGD & biopsies

EMA pos. HLA pos.

EMA pos. HLA neg.

EMA neg. HLA neg.

EMA neg. HLA pos.

Marsh 0–1

Marsh 2 or 3

CD+

↓

GFD & F/u

Consider false neg. HLA test. Consider biopsies

Consider false pos. anti-TG2

Unclear case Consider
false pos. serology
false neg. biopsy or
potential CD
Extended evaluation of
HLA/serology/biopsies

CD+

↓

GFD & F/u

Figure 4.9.1. Child/Adolescent with Symptoms Suggestive of Celiac Disease.

than 10 times the upper limit of normal, a positive antiendomysial antibody finding obtained at a different time than the anti-tTG antibodies finding, and a HLA genotype compatible with celiac disease" (Leonard et al., 2017, p. 651). It is no longer recommended to monitor improvement in diagnosis status or adherence to gluten-free diet through serial endoscopies as villous changes may take long to heal, risk to the patient may outweigh the benefit, and simple blood tests provide adequate markers, usually at a lower costs and risks to patients.

What other information gathered through noninvasive methods would help to confirm the diagnosis?

A detailed history might be the most important aspect of diagnosing celiac disease. Specific questions that a primary care provider might ask include:

- When did Katie begin expanding her food preferences? What types of foods did she enjoy before? What type of food does she prefer now?
- When did Katie first begin to have GI symptoms? Do the symptoms seem related to meals/mealtime? Is it always diarrhea or are there other complaints?
- What is Katie's general stooling pattern (e.g., Does she stool daily? Does she have a history of constipation? Any history of blood in the stool?)
- Does Katie have a history of food allergy? Does anyone else in the house have a history of a food allergy? What happens when that person ingests that food?
- Have you kept a food diary or tried to track symptoms to time of day, meals, schoolwork, and so on? If so, have you noticed any patterns?
- What is school like? Does Katie have friends? Participate in activities? Is she making good grades? Have teachers expressed any concerns?
- Does Katie take naps during the day? If so, for how long? How does she sleep at night?

- What other symptoms is Katie experiencing?
- What have you tried to make her symptoms better? Does anything help? Does anything make it worse?
- Review of her growth chart: Is there a true slowing of growth? When did it start? How severe is it? Is it only height that has slowed? Only weight? Both? Is there a family history of plateaued or diminished growth?

Beyond a solid history, a careful clinical exam is also warranted. Special attention should be paid to the following:

- Evidence of dental enamel changes
- Pallor (suggestive of anemia)
- Evidence of malnutrition: examine hair, skin, nails
- Abdominal exam, as this is the greatest single source of discomfort. Take note of distention, localized pain, and hyper or decreased bowel sounds.
- Abnormal thyroid (celiac and thyroid conditions are often co-occurring conditions)
- If examining genitalia, look for delayed development via Tanner staging.
- Phenotypic evidence of genetic diseases such as Down syndrome, Turner syndrome, Williams syndrome, which have an association with CD.

What information from the family history helps to guide your differentials?

Family history is an important consideration in celiac disease. Those at greatest risk for celiac are those with first-degree relatives with the disease. Outside of that group, ESPGHAN suggests that "Testing should be offered to . . . children and adolescents with the otherwise unexplained symptoms and signs of chronic or intermittent diarrhea, failure to thrive, weight loss, stunted growth, delayed puberty, amenorrhea, iron-deficiency anemia. . ." as well as to patients with "type 1 diabetes mellitus, Down syndrome, autoimmune thyroid disease, Turner syndrome, Williams syndrome, selective immunoglobulin A deficiency, autoimmune liver disease, and first-degree relatives with CD" (Husby et al., 2012, p. 137). In our case, Katie does not have a first-degree relative with celiac, although her mother could have asymptomatic disease given that her sister has it .

It is also useful to consider any symptoms of Katie's siblings when assessing potential risk for celiac disease. Katie's mother's history of miscarriage is also common in celiac disease and may help to support the decision to test for the disease. There is disagreement within the medical community whether those without any symptoms, regardless of risk factors, should be screened. The U.S. Preventive Services Task Force recommends against this practice because of the risks associated with false positive results and the emotional strain that can come from testing. (U.S. Preventive Services Task Force, 2017). Alternatively, ESPGHAN has an algorithm dedicated to "the Child Without Symptoms Suggestive of CD Who Belongs to a High-Risk Group" (Husby et al., 2012, p. 154). It is the opinion of this group that the potential damage to the body and the high risk of celiac is adequate rationale for pursuing confirmation testing.

Once the diagnosis is established, what other multidisciplinary support would you offer the patient and family? What other medical specialties/subspecialties would you engage?

Pediatric celiac disease is one that is best diagnosed and ultimately managed by a pediatric gastroenterologist. The only available treatment for this disease is a lifelong, strict adherence to a gluten-free diet. While many have dabbled in this diet, helping to elevate it to fad status, when it is being undertaken for medical reasons, it is a difficult and costly one to maintain. As a primary care provider, it should be stressed to patients and their families that a gluten-free diet should *not* be initiated until a positive diagnosis has been made, as low levels of ingestion atypical to the patient's presenting diet during a work-up may give false-negative test results. When patients are diagnosed with celiac disease the following may be useful to provide both concurrent and supportive care within the primary care space:

- **Nutrition:** Registered dieticians can provide guidance on a gluten-free diet, teach patients and families how to read and interpret labels, and can help correct nutritional deficiencies (e.g., vitamin supplementation and/or electrolyte correction) that may have existed prior to the diagnosis. Recent studies have demonstrated that gluten-free diets are often high in carbohydrates and fat and lack micronutrients. A review of several diets demonstrate a near-universal lack of folate (Mager et al., 2019). For patients with special considerations, including vegetarianism or food allergies, a registered dietician is an invaluable resource.
- **Psychology/Mental health:** Children with celiac disease can experience an impaired quality of life due to their diet restrictions, uncomfortable symptoms, anxiety related to "tainted" food, and bullying related to their condition. Having a mental health provider who can normalize feelings and teach strategies to overcome stressors at different developmental milestones is an important aspect to holistic care. See, for example, Cadenhead et al. (2019) for more information on coping with a chronic illness. A provider who can expertly identify and address concerns related to eating disorders is also a welcome resource. There are associations between anorexia and celiac disease, which should be screened for and further researched. Having a knowledgeable resource to help with the complexity of a restricted diet due a chronic health condition and the psychological and deleterious effects of anorexia will benefit patients and family alike (Cadenhead et al., 2019; Marild et al., 2017).
- **School nurses/Resources:** Children with celiac disease that is suboptimially managed may experience greater school absences due to disease flairs and accidental gluten ingestion has a greater chance of happening outside of a more-controlled home setting. As such, students—especially young ones—need to have a resource person at school whom they can disclose their symptoms to, create a plan for management of said symptoms (e.g., using the bathroom in the nurse's office), and coordinate missed work with teachers. Educating teachers about the effect of gluten ingestion and collaborating with the student to discreetly leave the room, if necessary, can help decrease the stigma and embarrassment of celiac disease. If patients have numerous hospitalizations or medical appointments, an IEP may be necessary to prevent the child from falling behind in school.

As Katie ages, further discussion and emphasis on the importance of adherence to the gluten-free diet and ownership of food choices will need to be had. Teenagers are at a high risk for poor diet compliance, which can result in a decreased quality of life due to worsening symptoms and social isolation. As Mager and colleagues write,

> . . . the major factors influencing adherence to the GFD [gluten free diet] included the presence of GI symptoms, age of the child, and ethnicity. This was particularly important to adolescents with CD where consideration of the school environment, thoughts of feeling different and social settings were drivers of reduced adherence to the GFD. (Mager et al., 2018, p. 947)

Subspecialties: Beyond pediatric gastroenterologists, other subspecialists might be necessary based on other symptoms and co-morbidities. For example, if a patient has a microcytic anemia, a referral to a hematologist might be warranted. If there is evidence suggestive of osteoporosis or osteopenia, a referral to an orthopedist might be appropriate. If there are concerns related to diabetes or thyroid conditions, endocrinology would also be a necessary service to engage. And finally, if there are reasons to suspect other genetic conditions, a referral to a genetic counselor should be considered to help understand underlying pathologies and their possible consequences. All of these recommendations, however, are made with the assumption that a large, pediatric hospital is accessible to the patient. If a pediatric facility is not available, the family may be required to travel long distances to access one or the primary care provider may be tasked with reviewing recommendations, seeking out consultations, and managing co-morbidities for which they do not have specialized knowledge and training. This type of complex care requires a lot of time and energy of the primary care specialist but also deprives the patient of experts in pediatric subspecialties. As such, initial consultation by the patient and their families complete with an individualized plan for treatment and follow-up with a pediatric specialist is always preferable, even if long-term management is not possible.

Special considerations: People who are diagnosed with celiac disease face a life of gluten-free eating. Failure to adhere to this diet can lead to clinical manifestations such as abdominal pain, bloating, diarrhea, and constipation. If severe, short-term complications from these side effects can include dehydration, hypovolemic shock, and infection. Long-term consequences include damage to the intestinal tract and villous, chronic inflammation; loss of bone mineral density, which increases the risk of fracture; damage to teeth; and chronic anemia, to name a few. As such, strict adherence to this diet is an imperative. However, socioeconomic and sociocultural realities must be faced and addressed (see, e.g., Mager, 2018; Mager, 2019). Discussing access to appropriate food, willingness to potentially change the patient's diet to include foods that are foreign or otherwise not eaten by the rest of family, affordability of food, and ability to attend multiple medical appointments and undergo numerous medical tests should all be considered when providing comprehensive care. Creating plans that are realistic and of maximum benefit to the patient must be made and establishing a partnership with families and subspecialists may also improve adherence.

REFERENCES AND RESOURCES

Cadenhead, J. W., Wold, R. L., Lebwohl, B., Lee, A. R., Zybert, P., Reilly, N. R., . . . Green, P. H. R. (2019). Diminished quality of life among adolescents with coeliac disease using maladaptive eating behaviours to manage a gluten-free diet: A cross-sectional, mixed-methods study. *Journal of Human Nutrition and Dietetics* 32, 311–320.

Fedewa, M. V., Bentley, J. L., Higgins, S., Kindler, J. M., Esco, M. R., & MacDonald, H. V. (2019). Celiac disease and bone health in children and adolescents: A systematic review and meta-analysis. *Journal of Clinical Densitometry: Assessment and Management of Musculoskeletal Health* (in press): 1–11.

Husby, S., Koletzko, S., Korponay-Szabo, I. R., Mearin, M. L., Phillips, A., Shamir, R., . . . Zimmer, K. P. for the European Society for Pediatric Gastroenterology, Hepatology, and Nutrition. (2012). European Society for Pediatric Gastroenterology, Hepatology, and Nutrition guidelines for the diagnosis of coeliac disease. *Journal of Pediatric Gastroenterology and Nutrition, 54*(1), 136–160.

Khatib, M., Baker, R. D., Ly, E. K., Kozielski, R., & Baker, S. (2016). Presenting pattern of pediatric celiac disease. *Journal of Pediatric Gastroenterology and Nutrition, 62*, 60–63.

Lebwohl, B., Sanders, D. S., & Green, P. H. R. (2018). Coeliac disease. *Lancet, 391*, 70–81.

Leonard, M. M., Sapone, A., Catassi, C., & Fasano, A. (2017). Celiac disease and nonceliac gluten sensitivity: A review. *Journal of the American Medical Association, 318*(7), 647–656.

Mager, D. R., Macron, M., Brill, H., Liu, A., Radmanovich, K., Mileski, H., . . .Turner, J. M. (2018). Adherence to the gluten-free diet and health-related quality of life in an ethnically diverse pediatric population with celiac disease. *Journal of Pediatric Gastroenterology and Nutrition, 66* (6), 941–948.

Mager, D. R., Liu, A., Macron, M., Harms, K., Brill, H., Mileski, H., . . . Turner, J. M. (2019). Diet patterns in an ethnically diverse pediatric population with celiac disease and chronic gastrointestinal complaints. *Clinical Nutrition ESPEN, 20*, 73–80.

Marild, K., Stordal, K., Bulik, C. M., Rewers, M., Ekbom, A., Liu, E., & Ludvigsson, J. F. (2017). Celiac disease and anorexia nervosa: A nationwide study. *Pediatrics, 139*(5), e20164367.

Nahar, R., & Avani, A. (2019). Sealing the diagnosis of celiac disease in pregnancy. *The Medicine Forum, 20*(9). https://doi.org/10.29046/TMF.020.1.008; available at: https://jdc.jefferson.edu/tmf/vol20/iss1/9

North American Society for Pediatric Gastroenterology, Hepatology, and Nutrition. (2005). Guideline for the diagnosis and treatment of celiac disease in children: Recommendations of the North American Society for Pediatric Gastroenterology, Hepatology, and Nutrition. https://www.naspghan.org/files/documents/pdfs/position-papers/celiac_guideline_2004_jpgn.pdf

U.S. Preventive Services Task Force. (2017). Screen for celiac disease: U.S. Preventive Services Task Force recommendation statement. *Journal of the American Medical Association, 317*(12),1252–1257.

Case 4.10 Food Allergies

RESOLUTION

What are the top three differential diagnoses? What testing will confirm the diagnosis?

The differential diagnosis for this patient would include: celiac disease, food protein–induced enteropathy, food allergy, or food intolerance. Celiac disease typically presents with abdominal pain, diarrhea, and reflux (Khatib, Baker, Ly, Kozielski, & Baker, 2016). Some patients may experience nongastrointestinal symptoms, but these do not include respiratory compromise or hives as a result of gluten ingestion. Thus, James's symptoms of hives and respiratory distress would suggest against celiac. Food protein–induced enteropathy is a non-IgE moderated food allergy most commonly associated with milk protein intolerance (Nowak-Wegrzyn, 2015). This condition usually presents in infancy and is relatively rare. Based on the type of foods that James was eating and his age, this also seems like a less likely diagnosis. That leaves food allergy and food intolerance on our list of differentials.

Anaphylaxis is defined as

> An acute, severe, life-threatening allergic reaction in presensitized individuals, leading to a systemic response caused by the release of immune and inflammatory mediators from basophils and mast cells. At least two organ systems are involved, such as the skin, the upper and lower airways, and the cardiovascular, neurologic, and gastrointestinal systems, in this order of priority or in combination. (Andreae & Andrea, 2019)

Based on this definition, what James experienced was an anaphylactic reaction, which occurs only with allergy—not intolerance. Therefore, we can feel confident that James experienced an allergic reaction, most likely to something that he was eating. The next question is, what is James allergic to? James was eating a peanut butter and jelly sandwich, but there are a lot of details that are left out. For example, what type of jelly? What type of bread (e.g., nut bread? Whole wheat?)? What type of peanut butter—does it include any other type of nut? Time to reaction (while eating? Minutes-to-hours later)? What else was he eating or drinking at the time (another potential source of allergen)? These details of the history will help to guide the testing for the source of the allergen. The most common sources of food allergy are egg, milk, peanuts, soy, tree nuts, wheat, and shellfish (Guandalini & Newland, 2011, p. 428). Willitis and colleagues note that the most common

The Family Nurse Practitioner: Clinical Case Studies, Second Edition. Edited by Leslie Neal-Boylan.
© 2021 John Wiley & Sons Ltd. Published 2021 by John Wiley & Sons Ltd.

childhood allergy in their study was the tree nut. This may help James's provider feel more confident in labeling peanut butter as the culprit for James's allergy (Willits et al., 2018, p. 1425).

Peanut butter allergy:

According to the National Institute for Allergy and Infectious Diseases, the gold standard for diagnosis of food allergy includes history; physical; skin prick test with associated skin and organ findings; allergen-specific serum IgE; and oral food challenge, which can be open label or blinded (Boyce, Assa'ad, & Burks, 2012, pp. 10–12). These methods of testing should be used in combination as opposed to singular approaches, as this gives the highest levels of specificity and sensitivity. It is the job of the pediatric primary care provider to give a referral to a qualified pediatric allergist who can supervise the testing and interpret the findings.

Another piece of the history that the primary care provider should recognize as a possible connection to a food allergy is James's history of eczema. "It is well known that family history of atopy and atopic dermatitis are risk factors in the development of IgE mediated food allergies with the coexistence of asthma being the most commonly identified factor for severe reactions" (Guandalini & Newland, 2011, p. 428). Performing a careful clinical exam to learn the extent of the skin changes and monitoring for worsening eczema will be important for the provider moving forward. In addition, reviewing past medical records and history with James's mother to look for indications of asthma, reactive airway disease, or other concerns with regard to the respiratory system may help to narrow the differential diagnoses.

How should the provider educate the mother about the seriousness of anaphylaxis and the risk of it occurring again?

James's mother is hopeful that her son does not have a true, anaphylactic allergy to peanuts. This is an understandable position; it can be overwhelming to care for children with severe allergies. Children and families must learn to read labels, carry emergency medications, and avoid triggers, and the patients are often the target of bullies in school (Feng & Kim, 2018). It is the role of the primary care provider to explain the life-threatening nature of anaphylactic food allergies, provide resources and education related to the reading and interpretation of food labels, coordinate with school administration to create a safe environment, and help the family to create an appropriate home setting for the food-allergic child. The primary care provider or their staff should take the time to review with the parents and patient the proper use and timing of single-use, injectable epinephrine (usually an EpiPen) and subsequent emergency management of anaphylaxis.

On the flip side, parents will sometimes believe that their child has a food allergy when, in fact, they do not. ". . . self-reported allergy typically overestimates true allergy.. . . In one meta-analysis, the rate of self-reported food allergy among children was 12%, compared with 3% when confirmatory testing was performed (Sichereret al., 2017, p. 3). Parents and children will believe that signs of an intolerance, such as flatulence or gastrointestinal discomfort when consuming milk products, indicates an allergy requiring that specific foods be avoided and changes to the school and home setting must be made. Educating parents and caregivers about the specific symptom and treatment differences between intolerances and allergies is an important job for the primary care provider. This can provide ease of mind for those without allergies and bring greater awareness to the seriousness of IgE mediated allergies.

How can the provider help the school manage a child with food allergies?

One role of the primary care provider is to be a public health advocate in their community. This can be accomplished through several means with regard to food allergies. For example, the American Academy of Pediatrics (AAP) recommends that physicians teach caregivers and teachers to: recognize the symptoms of anaphylaxis versus simple allergy and how to manage each; the proper use and timing of an EpiPen or its equivalent; provide epinephrine prescriptions for schools to be used for unexpected reactions as local and state laws allow (i.e., not associated with any particular student); and provide families with known allergies a prescription that allows for a supply of EpiPens that cover both school and home settings" (Sicherer, Mahr, & Section on Allergy and Immunology, 2010). The AAP also provides templates for providers to use when completing allergy action plans to be used in school or similar settings that has simple instructions for what to do during an allergic and/or anaphylactic reaction (Wang, Sicherer, & Section on Allergy and Immunology, 2017).

If this family does not have insurance, what is the expected out-of-pocket expense for an EpiPen? Likely more than one will be needed, so how can a family navigate this barrier?

The cost of injectable, single-use epinephrine can be very high, even with prescription drug insurance coverage. In fact, there has been national press spotlighting both its cost and lack of availability (see, e.g., Kaplan, 2018). Although there are now several options for single-use injectable epinephrine, some require private insurance while others are hampered by lack of availability for the smaller doses.

If access to medication proves to be a barrier for James and his family, the primary care provider has several options. First, they can attempt to procure samples directly from the drug company. While this seems like an obvious fix to a problem, in-office drug samples are often not allowed due to ethical concerns with regard to the relationship between pharmaceutical companies and physicians. If this route is not an option for James's provider, they can next attempt to negotiate with pharmacies and/or insurance companies. While providers may not perform this task directly, case managers and nursing staff within the practice will need to take time and resources out of a clinic to perform this exercise. Ultimately, it may be the responsibility of the provider to conduct a peer-to-peer consultation with insurance to confirm the medical necessity of a product. A third option would be to provide vials of epinephrine along with a syringe that the family would be responsible for drawing up as needed. While this is very cost effective, it is also not ideal for most families, as the ability to think clearly and quickly draw up medication into a syringe in the setting of an emergency can be overwhelming for nonmedically trained parents. In addition, schools may not accept vials and syringes if there is no school nurse present, as the liability may be too great.

What is the essential information that all caregivers (not just parents) need to know when caring for James?

The most essential information is twofold: First, the only way to prevent an allergic reaction is to completely avoid the allergen. Reading labels, knowing what other nontraditional products may contain the allergen, and teaching the child to avoid the trigger is vital.

The second piece of information is the swift recognition and treatment of an allergic reaction. Teaching caregivers the signs and symptoms of anaphylaxis and empowering them to use the epinephrine is the best way to help halt a reaction. "Researchers suggest that epinephrine is safe but often underutilized and that there is poor recognition about both how and when to use epinephrine autoinjectors" (Sicherer et al., 2017, p. 4). While no one wants to cause pain or suffering by giving a deep, intramuscular injection, the overall health, safety, and life of a child outweighs these risks. Adults must be willing to use the epinephrine and call emergency personnel for further management in the setting of anaphylactic reactions. The side effects of epinephrine, including tachycardia, nausea, and tremors, are all temporary and generally are not dangerous. Again, these side effects outweigh the anoxia and damage caused by lack of perfusion during an anaphylactic allergic reaction. As such, providers should consider using some of their time to teach caregivers the signs of anaphylaxis (see Table 4.10.1) as compared to simple allergy (see Table 4.10.2). Allowing caregivers the opportunity to use the epinephrine "trainer" (an EpiPen without the needle or medication that can be used to practice the injection) to familiarize themselves with the setup and force needed to activate the pen can go a long way in fostering an environment that is supportive, educated, and empowered. Caregivers can also be taught to give antihistamines such as Benadryl or Zyrtec for simple hives or uncomplicated itching. It should be impressed upon caregivers that for patients who are prescribed emergency epinephrine, it must be carried on the person who has the allergy (or by

Table 4.10.1. Symptoms of Anaphylaxis.

Anaphylaxis Symptom	Clinical Manifestations
Respiratory ristress	Wheezing, throat closing, bronchospasm
Skin manifestations	Diffuse hives, wheals
Edema	Periorbital or perioral edema
Gastrointestinal distress	Diarrhea, vomiting, severe abdominal cramping

Table 4.10.2. Allergy Symptoms.

Allergy Symptom	Clinical Manifestation
Itching	Itching, with or without discrete hives
Gastrointestinal changes	Loose stools, cramping, flatulence

an accompanying responsible adult) at all times. Lack of epinephrine leads to delays in treatment that can result in fatal outcomes (Warren, Zaslavsky, Kan, Spergel, & Gupta, 2018). Normalizing the carrying of epinephrine and knowing when to use it will help the child feel empowered to participate in activities with peers. The child with an allergy will also feel secure knowing that there is a plan and readily available medication should it be necessary, which might allow them to venture outside the confines of their allergen-controlled environment.

What advice should the mother be given regarding introduction of peanut-based products to the youngest child now that food allergies are known to be in the family?

Primary care providers should be able to anticipate that parents of a child with an allergy will also want to know about the risks of allergies to their other children. In a seminal study published in 2015, DuToit and colleagues demonstrated that rather than delaying the introduction of peanuts in high-risk populations, as had previously been recommended by the AAP, there is actually a protective factor in the *early* introduction of the potential allergen (DuToit et al., 2015). The findings from the Learning Early About Peanut (LEAP) study warned, however, that these results were not generalizable to all types of food allergens. "The authors concluded that, in children at high risk for allergy, the early introduction of peanuts significantly decreased peanut allergy. Furthermore, authors pointed out that early consumption of peanut in high-risk infants is allergen specific and does not prevent the development of other allergic disease" (Ferraro, Zanconato, & Carraro, 2019, p. 1131). Specifically, it should be noted that "there is no need to delay the introduction of allergenic foods beyond 6 months of age and that they should not be introduced before 4 months of age" (Greer, Sicherer, Burks, & Committee on Nutrition, Section on Allergy and Immunology, 2019, p. 4). Indeed, with limited exception to the child at highest risk for allergy, no testing is necessary prior to administration. Primary care providers should take the time to review sibling risk factors, including the presence of eczema, allergies, and family history before making a recommendation to seek testing for siblings. Parents should be counseled about the risk of keeping known allergens in the house and the danger associated with giving "just a little peanut butter" to siblings or friends with severe allergies. Siblings can be taught how to recognize signs of anaphylaxis in their siblings with allergies.

For mothers of newborns, "no conclusions can be made about the role of breastfeeding in either preventing or delaying the onset of specific food allergies" (Greer et al., 2019, p. 4). As such, it is generally advised that mothers continue to breastfeed as they had planned without modifications to diet or duration. Similarly, there has been speculation that the use of hydrolyzed formula would help prevent atopy and, possibly, later food allergy. "The overall results of these new studies have weakened previous conclusions that there was modest evidence that the use of either partially or extensively hydrolyzed formula prevents atopic dermatitis in high-risk infants who are formula fed or initially breastfed after birth" (Greer et al., 2019, p. 4).

Finally, there are advances being made in the treatment of food allergies. For families with access to pediatric allergists, desensitization through food oral immunotherapy can be an option. This is a process that must be closely supervised by an allergist, requires a significant amount of time, and comes with the risk of severe reactions during the process. "The objectives of this therapy is to have the patient become less sensitive to the allergen and to potentially eliminate adverse reactions to the food allergen" (Sitton & Temples, 2017, p. 101). Other potential treatments include sublingual immunotherapy, epicutaneous immunotherapy, food allergen modifications, and anti-IgE medications. To date, oral desensitization has been the most successful technique, but depending on the goals and resources of families the other options may be beneficial.

REFERENCES AND RESOURCES

Andreae, D. A., & Andrea, M. H. (2019). Anaphylaxis. *BMJ Best Practice*. Last reviewed: June 2019. Available at: https://bestpractice.bmj.com/topics/en-us/501

Boyce, J. A., Assa'ad, A., & Burks, A. W. (2012). *Guidelines for the diagnosis and management of food allergy in the United States*. Washington, DC: U.S. Department of Health and Human Services.

DuToit, G., Roberts, G., Sayre, P. H., Bahnson, H. T., Radulovic, S., Santos, A. F., . . . Lack, G. for the LEAP Study Team. (2015). Randomized trial of peanut consumption in infants at risk for peanut allergy. *New England Journal of Medicine, 372*(9), 803–813.

Feng, C., & Kim, J. H. (2018). Beyond avoidance: The psychosocial impact of food allergies. *Clinical Reviews of Allergy and Immunology*. Published online September 1, 2018. Retrieved from: https://doi.org/10.1007/s12016-018-8708-x.

Ferraro, V., Zanconato, S., & Carraro, S. (2019). Timing of food introduction and the risk of food allergies. *Nutrients, 11*, 1131.

Greer, F. R., Sicherer, S. H., Burks, A. W., & Committee on Nutrition, Section on Allergy and Immunology. (2019). The effects of early nutritional interventions on the development of atopic disease in infants and children: The role of maternal dietary restriction, breastfeeding, hydrolyzed formulas, and timing of introduction of allergenic complementary foods. *Pediatrics, 143*(4), e20190281.

Guandalini, S., & Newland, C. (2011). Differentiating food allergies from food intolerances. *Current Gastroenterology Reports, 13*(5), 426–434.

Kaplan, S. (2018, August 16). FDA approves generic EpiPen that may be cheaper. *New York Times*. https://www.nytimes.com/2018/08/16/health/epipen-generic-drug-prices.html

Khatib, M., Baker, R. D., Ly, E. K., Kozielski, R., & Baker, S. S. (2016). Presenting pattern of pediatric celiac disease. *Journal of Pediatric Gastroenterology and Nutrition, 62*(1), 60–63.

Nowak-Wegrzyn, A. (2015). Food protein-induced enterocolitis syndrome. *Allergy and Asthma Proceedings, 36*(3), 172–184.

Sicherer, S. H., Allen, K., Lack, G., Taylor, S. L., Donovan, S. M., & Oria, M. (2017). Critical issues in food allergy: A national consensus report. *Pediatrics, 140*(2), 3.

Sicherer, S. H., Mahr, T., & Section on Allergy and Immunology. (2010). Clinical report—Management of food allergy in the school setting. *Pediatrics, 126*, 1232–1239.

Sitton, C., Temples, H. S. (2017). Practice guidelines for peanut allergies. *Journal of Pediatric Health Care, 32*(1), 101.

Wang, J., Sicherer, S. H., & Section on Allergy and Immunology. (2017). Guidance on completing a written allergy and anaphylaxis emergency plan. *Pediatrics, 139*(3), e20164005. https://pediatrics.aappublications.org/content/pediatrics/139/3/e20164005.full.pdf

Warren, C. M., Zaslavsky, J. M., Kan, K., Spergel, J. M., & Gupta, R. S. (2018). Epinephrine auto-injector carriage and use practices among US children, adolescents, and adults. *Annals of Allergy, Asthma & Immunology, 121*, 479–489.

Willits, E. K., Park, M. A., Hartz, M. F., Schleck, C. D., Weaver, A. L., & Joshi, A. Y. (2018). Food allergy: A comprehensive population-based study. *Mayo Clinic Proceedings, 93*(10), 1425.

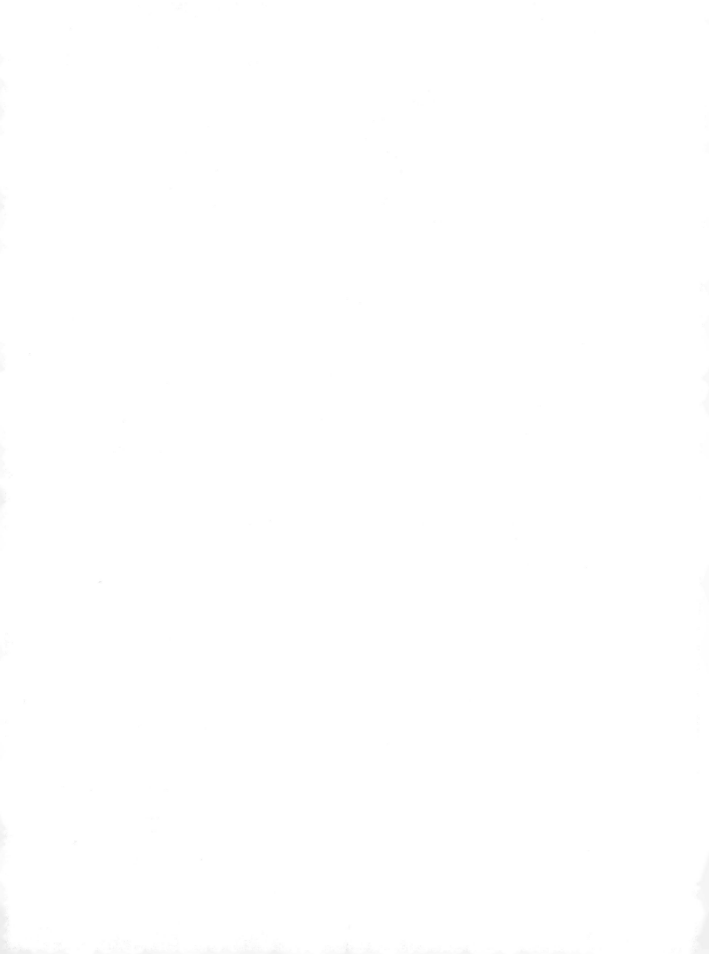

Case 4.11 Obesity

RESOLUTION

Which diagnostic or imaging studies should be considered to assist with or confirm the diagnosis?

A lipid profile, oral glucose tolerance test, and insulin levels would provide a basis to determine if Tamika currently has risk factors for hypercholesterolemia, insulin resistance, or Type 2 diabetes. Sleep apnea should also be considered due to the history of snoring and its association with obesity. A sleep study should therefore be considered.

BMI: Body mass index is a surrogate for adiposity. It is a number calculated from a person's weight in kilograms to their square height in meters. It provides an indicator of adiposity and is used to screen for weight categories that may lead to health problems.

Oral glucose tolerance test (OGGT): This is a standard laboratory method to determine how the body metabolizes sugar. It is used to diagnose impaired glucose tolerance, a frequent precursor to type 2 diabetes.

Insulin Resistance: Insulin, made in the pancreas, helps the body use glucose for energy. In insulin resistance, muscle, fat, and liver cells do not respond properly to insulin; and, as a result, the body requires more insulin to help glucose enter the cells. The pancreas eventually fails to keep up leading to elevated blood glucose levels and Type 2 diabetes.

Cholesterol Screen: Cardiovascular disease risk factors are fairly common among obese children. These include elevated cholesterol levels, high blood pressure, and Type 2 diabetes.

Sleep Study: Sleep apnea is a complication of obesity. It is associated with loud snoring and labored breathing.

Psychosocial Evaluation: Psychosocial issues are a fairly common consequence of childhood obesity. Obese children are frequent targets of social discrimination and stigmatization. This can contribute to low self-esteem that may hinder academic and social functioning over time.

What is the most likely differential diagnosis and why?

Exercise intolerance associated with obesity:

The patient is a 12-year-old, Hispanic female with a primary complaint of shortness of breath with exertion. She denies any other symptoms and is taking no medications. Her physical exam is remarkable only for an elevated BMI of 34, which places her in the obese range at greater than the

The Family Nurse Practitioner: Clinical Case Studies, Second Edition. Edited by Leslie Neal-Boylan.
© 2021 John Wiley & Sons Ltd. Published 2021 by John Wiley & Sons Ltd.

95th percentile for her age group, and darkly pigmented areas around her neck called acanthosis nigricans, a known risk factor for insulin resistance. Cardiovascular disease risk would be another major consideration in Tamika's health assessment. In addition to physical concerns, it is important for the provider to also monitor social and emotional development.

Are any referrals needed at this time?

Referral to a dietitian may be helpful. Referral to an ear, nose, and throat specialist would rule out any mechanical breathing difficulties due to enlarged tonsils or adenoids.

Can the school be of assistance?

A referral to the school nurse to counsel and support Tamika between office visits may be beneficial.

What community resources are available to this family?

Tamika would likely benefit from participation in an after-school activity. Helping her to research programs at her school, her local Boys and Girls Clubs, or her YMCA may assist her on the way to a more active lifestyle. Use of Internet resources like Let's Move may provide ideas to find ways to be more active at home as well.

What type of nutrition support may aid this family?

Involving the entire family in discussing ways to improve eating habits and activity will likely provide much needed guidance. Calorie and fat content lists from local fast-food restaurants will offer guidance in making better food choices.

REFERENCES AND RESOURCES

Durbin, J. (2018). Pediatric obesity in primary practice: A review of the literature. *Pediatric Nursing, 44,* 202–206.

Gaffney, K., Kitsantas, P., Brito, A., & Kastello, J. (2014). Baby steps in the prevention of childhood obesity: IOM guidelines for pediatric practice. *Journal of Pediatric Nursing, 29,* 108–113.

Nelson, C., Colchamiro, R., Perkins, M., Taveras, E., Leung-Strle, P., Kwass, J., & Woo Baidal, A. (2018). Racial/ethnic differences in the effectiveness of a multisector childhood obesity prevention intervention. *American Journal of Public Health, 108,* 1200–1206.

Reed, M., Cygan, H., Lui, K., & Mullen, M. (2016). Identification, prevention, and management of childhood overweight and obesity in a pediatric primary care center. *Clinical Pediatrics, 55,* 860–866.

Santos, M., Cadieux, A., Gray, J., & Ward, W. (2016). Pediatric obesity in early childhood. *Clinical Pediatrics, 55,* 356–362.

NOTE: The author would like to acknowledge Elaine Gustafson, MSN, PNP, who co-authored this case in the first edition of this book.

RESOLUTION

What are the most likely differential diagnoses in this case and why?
Substance use/abuse:
While Natalie is not admitting to drug or frequent alcohol use, she does admit to social drinking and has been caught with marijuana and juuling. Her symptoms and behaviors as well as teacher reports indicate possible substance use and abuse.

Major depressive disorder (MDD):
Natalie is demonstrating several symptoms of MDD, including a loss of interest in activities and diminished ability to think or concentrate in class. She also presents with symptoms congruent with depression-related problems including fatigue, difficulties feeling motivated and reduced functioning in grades over a period of months, and decreased school attendance and grades. Further assessment is needed to refine a diagnosis of MDD, and with Natalie refusing to complete standardized screening tools including the Patient History Questionnaire (PHQ) 9 and CRAFFT, the health care provider does not have full criteria for MDD at his time. However, depression should be of strong concern and is often comorbid with drug and alcohol use.

School phobia:
Refusal to go to school or school avoidance is a form of severe anxiety often referred to as "school phobia." School phobia is a chronic fear of attending school that interferes with normal life and can last weeks or more. Adolescents with school phobia often have trouble engaging in school, forming relationships or friendships, and are often correlated with being bullied in the school environment. While school phobia is more commonly reported in elementary school, high school students can also have severe school phobia. The health care provider should assess for possible bullying or life changes such as moving, parental divorce or conflict, or difficulty with peers. Academic difficulties or struggles should also be a concern at this point, especially in a 17-year-old who is near graduation.

Students with school phobia often demonstrate physiological symptoms (vomiting, headaches, or gastrointestinal issues such as diarrhea). Students with school phobia can feel dizzy or cry uncontrollably at the possibility of having to attend school. While Natalie has been missing a considerable amount of school, she currently denies any of these symptoms. Natalie's presentation

The Family Nurse Practitioner: Clinical Case Studies, Second Edition. Edited by Leslie Neal-Boylan.
© 2021 John Wiley & Sons Ltd. Published 2021 by John Wiley & Sons Ltd.

is that she is showing little interest in doing well in school and would prefer to be doing other things: possibly marijuana and juuling, as indicated in her disciplinary reports from the school.

Sleep problems:
Natalie's fatigue is most likely related to drug and alcohol use with comorbid depression. Poor sleep hygiene is often common in adolescents and sleep problems are symptomatic for a variety of mental health disorders. It is important to obtain more information about sleep patterns and hygiene; however, this can be prioritized to a future visit.

Thyroid disorder:
When diagnosing depression, organic causes should also be considered in the differential. Hypothyroidism can cause depression, fatigue, weight gain, lack of energy, memory loss, and difficulty processing information.

What are the top diagnostic tests required in this case and why?
Toxicology screen:
Drug testing has been recommended in different clinical settings as a way to identify or avert drug use, or as part of treatment. However, there is very little consensus to date on indications for when to offer and require drug testing, as well as disagreement on how useful the results are. The common drug assays are urine, blood, breath, saliva, sweat, and hair. The cost, ease of collection, test type, time frame (results back and time since last use), as well as indications for testing, all vary wildly. Clinical practices and labs must be certified by the Clinical Laboratory Improvement Amendment (CLIA).

Toxicology blood tests are the most useful for detecting drugs and alcohol but limitations include testing requirements within 2–12 hours of impairment and high cost, trained personnel, and equipment. Blood testing is rarely used in primary care settings; however, in high-school SBHCs it is common for teachers, administration, and parents to request the provider to "run a toxicology screen" on a student.

Beyond these limitations, the patient needs to consent for a toxicology screen of any kind, and the parent/guardian to additionally be involved in that conversation if the patient is under 18 years of age. Therefore, with Natalie's presentation and background at this visit, a toxicology screen is not one of the top diagnostic tests needed at this time.

Thyroid panel:
A blood panel that includes thyroid-stimulating hormone (TSH), T3 and T4 hormone levels for specific indicators of a thyroid condition, can rule this out as a contributor to the Natalie's decreased mood. Natalie's presentation has changed from past years, and she does not regularly access care by a primary care provider who can track changes over time in development and presentation; therefore, a thyroid blood panel should be considered.

Suicide assessment:
Treatment should include an immediate assessment for suicide risk. Natalie presents with enough indicators of depression that the provider should consider suicide ideation as a possibility.

What are the concerns at this point?
Natalie is presenting abnormally and with changes in behavior, demeanor, and attitude than in the past, including frequent visits to the SBHC, which include not wanting to be in school and signs for depression. She is describing sleep problems, which can compound mental health issues, and is at risk for early school dropout before graduation from her decline in academics.

The physical examination revealed no obvious concerns for organic causes of depression or tiredness; however, Natalie is not followed by a primary care provider and utilizes emergency rooms and urgent care clinics for her care. Therefore, the provider should still consider a laboratory studies, including a thyroid panel, for a baseline and include a thorough physical assessment as part of her plan today.

While Natalie is not admitting to drug use at this visit, she has a history of juuling in class and marijuana possession, both of which require further assessment and education on the risks of juuling and marijuana use.

She has a past history of noncompliance with a low dose of an SSRI, Lexapro. While this isn't necessarily a concern at this point, it is important to note that Natalie was treated with pharmaceuticals for either depression, anxiety, or both in the past.

What is the plan of treatment?

The health care provider can utilize motivational interviewing techniques in order to elicit further response from Natalie or to engage in discussion about possible drug/alcohol use. Use open-ended questions and if Natalie engages in conversation, ask for elaboration or more detail if she is willing to engage. Use affirming statements, when possible, commenting positively on her statements. Reflect on any change talk, for example, if she makes any statements indicating that she wishes her circumstances were different. The health care provider can ask about peer drug use and then try to engage in conversation on whether Natalie has tried the same substances. Be direct and nonjudgmental in conversation. Do not force answers if Natalie does not engage in the conversation. If Natalie admits to further substance use, try to determine the frequency and amount and whether any adverse effects have previously occurred.

What are the plans for referral and follow-up care?

Ask Natalie if she has ever been to a therapist for counseling and assess where, with whom, and for long, as well as her feelings about engaging in therapy. Asking about her previous experience in therapy will help the referral process. Because Natalie is under the age of 18, reaching out to Natalie's parent or guardian on concerns for signs of depression and referral for counseling would be appropriate at this time. However, it is important to maintain Natalie's confidentiality at this point regarding anything specific she confides to the health care professional. Therapists are trained in further identifying substance use as a secondary diagnosis in mental health concerns and can further refer to a substance use counselor if indicated. At this point, we are not sure if Natalie is using frequently or engaging in social experimentation and exploration of substances.

Follow-up regarding Natalie's lack of sleep and fatigue are also beneficial to this case. Disrupted sleep is a symptom of many mental disorders but also can exacerbate mental disorders, including depression. Assess for inadequate levels of sleep including the quantity, quality, and satisfaction with sleep. Review sleep hygiene (caffeine consumption later in the day, bedtime routine, etc.), as well as a sleep schedule. If sleep continues to be a concern, ask the patient to complete a sleep log (see an example at www.brightfutures.org/mentalhealth/pdf/families/ec/diary.pdf).

What health education should be provided to this patient?

Anticipatory guidance in a supportive manner should be given, including written handouts on either a specific substance or an overview of substance use. There are many recommended 1- page handouts for teens that can be found through the Drug Enforcement Agency (DEA), National Institute on Drug Abuse (NIDA), and National Institute of Alcohol Abuse and Alcoholism (NIAAA) websites.

The majority of substance use begins in adolescence, when developing brains are most vulnerable. Early identification and treatment prevent long-term consequences, such as academic difficulties and future mental health and substance use disorders.

Many teens, and even adults, think marijuana is safe because it is now used medicinally and becoming decriminalized. Marijuana, whether smoked or vaped, can increase heart rate, make the veins in the eyes expand and look bloodshot, as well as affect coordination, driving, learning, and memory. The active ingredient, THC, affects the brain and causes dopamine release, which gives the feeling of a "high." However, this can also create feelings of worry, fear, and paranoia, and cause delusions, hallucinations, and loss of senses. Studies have found that marijuana can make depression worse and some studies have found that heavy use of marijuana in youth can lead to schizophrenia for people who are already at risk and raise the risk of depression later in life. Because THC affects the brain's ability to make choices, teens who are using marijuana are also at risk for unsafe sex (and therefore HIV and STIs) or getting in the car with someone under the influence. Marijuana use and then withdrawal includes symptoms of irritability, not sleeping, not wanting to eat, anxiety, and craving more marijuana.

Natalie asks, "Are you going to tell my mom about this?" How do you respond?

Consult the local consent laws, as most states in the United States allow minor sto consent for care for alcohol and drug use. The health care provider should take this opportunity to discuss confidentiality with the patient, which includes needing to break confidentiality if the patient is: (1) at risk of harming themselves; (2) at risk of harming someone else; or (3) someone else harming them. Depending on how Natalie responded to the assessment for suicidality, the health care provider may decide to break confidentiality and reach out to the parent/guardian.

Conversation with Natalie should include that you would like to refer her for counseling at this time, and parental consent will be needed. Reassure Natalie that nothing you've discussed so far will be shared with her mom, but that you need to let her mom know that you are concerned about signs of depression including chronic fatigue, struggling academics and engagement with peers, as well as loss of interest in things that she used to enjoy. Calling her mom with Natalie present and letting Natalie hear the conversation is another way to build trust with Natalie that specific details of their discussion are not shared but that concern for her mental health and well-being is communicated to her caregiver.

Should Natalie's age be different, practitioners would additionally need to account for mandated reporting laws for populations at risk (elderly or under age 13). Clinicians are to review the restrictions to confidentiality with the patient while engaged in risk assessments as described above and should also be familiar with the reporting laws in the state where they practice.

Does the patient's psychosocial history impact how you might treat her?

We know that Natalie has several risk factors, including living in a single-parent household and having one sibling in prison and another who has unknown whereabouts. She admits to high-risk behaviors, including sexual promiscuity and therefore engaging in discussion of STI testing and safe-sex practices should also be considered.

While we do know that Natalie lives at home with her mother, we do not know details about their relationship, her working status, or if any protective factors at home are present. Natalie's mom might work long hours or be absent in other ways since Natalie is now a teenager, which can also lead to patient feelings of abandonment. Gentle and nonjudgmental further assessment of her home life and social history can provide more details on how to best proceed.

Finally, Natalie's medical history includes no history of depression, anxiety, or substance use disorder. However, we know that she was previously treated with an SSRI, which is used to treat depression and anxiety. Because Natalie does not utilize a primary care medical home for her care, this history may be difficult to untangle.

Can minors seek substance abuse counseling without parental consent?

The SBHC setting allows adolescents confidentiality for seeking certain health care services that are protected by law, such as reproductive care or substance abuse counseling and treatment. However, most adolescents still receive insurance benefits under their parent/guardian's insurance, and if said insurance is commercial insurance, an explanation of benefits (EOB) is sent home to the parent/guardian. Therefore, follow the agency or place of practice guidelines in billing for medical confidential visits. Some practices may have a grant or alternative billing options for patients who are under 18 years of age seeking this care, while some practices may write off these visits in order to assure confidentiality and that an EOB is not sent home.

Are there any standardized guidelines that should be used to treat this case? If so, what are they?

The Patient Health Questionnaire-9 (PHQ-9) and the Columbia–Suicide Severity Rating Scale (C-SSRS) are recommended for use in primary care to further screen for concerns related to depression and anxiety. These screening tools have been recommended by the American Academy of Pediatrics (AAP), the School-Based Health Alliance, and the National Association of Pediatric Nurse Practitioners (NAPNAP) for routine use for screening students for mental health concerns.

SBIRT (Screening, Brief Intervention, and Referral for Treatment) can clinically benefit youth, adolescents, and adults with mild to moderate substance use (not yet showing signs of dependence). SBIRT utilization has already been endorsed and recommended at the federal level by the Substance Abuse and Mental Health Services Administration (SAMHSA), the Veterans Administration (VA), the Department of Defense (DoD), the White House Office of National Drug Control Policies, different managed care providers, and the School-Based Health Alliance.

SBIRT involves four different components for implementation, including:

1. Screening: Administer a validated screen tool recommended for adolescents (such as the S2BI or the CRAFFT) in order to identify youth who engage in substance use and may have possible substance use disorders. It is recommended to also screen for depression and anxiety as they are comorbid with substance use (i.e., PHQ-9, GAD-7).
2. Brief intervention: The provider then engages a patient who scores positive (above the screening tool threshold) in what is referred to as a "brief intervention" using motivational interviewing (MI) techniques and can range from a brief conversation to future counseling sessions. Discuss the advantages and disadvantages of substance use. Determine if substance use reduction or even abstinence is a goal of the patient and begin problem-solving to reach that goal.
3. Referral to treatment: After screening and a brief intervention, the patient may still need a referral for treatment for either moderate or severe substance use or for depression and/or anxiety. MI can be used to accept the need for treatment and engage in counseling. Substance dependence may require referral for outpatient individual or group counseling for specialized substance abuse or even medically managed intensive treatment, which is often in-patient.

REFERENCES AND RESOURCES

Adolescent SBIRT: Screening Brief Intervention & Referral to Treatment. (2019). *At-Risk in primary care: Adolescents:* SBI with adolescents. Training available. https://kognito.com/products/sbi-with-adolescents.

BNI-Art Institute: Boston University School of Public Health. (2019). Adolescent Brief Negotiated Interview (BNI) algorithm. Retrieved from https://www.bu.edu/bniart/files/2011/10/Bilingual-ADOLESCENT-ALGORITHM_3.15.11.pdf;http://www.ct.gov/dmhas/lib/dmhas/adpc/(7)_adolescent_sbirt.pdf

Center for Adolescent Substance Use Research. (2018). The CRAFFT 2.1 manual. http://crafft.org/wp-content/uploads/2018/08/FINAL-CRAFFT-2.1_provider_manual_with-CRAFFTN_2018-04-23.pdf

Curtis B. L., McLellan, A. T., & Gabellini, B. N. (2014). Translating SBIRT to public school settings: An initial test of feasibility. *Journal of Substance Abuse Treatment, 46,* 15–21.

Kroenke, K., Spitzer R. L., & Williams, J. B. (2001). The PHQ-9: Validity of a brief depression severity measure. *Journal of General Internal Medicine, 16*(9), 606–613.

Levy, S., Weiss, R., Sherritt, L., Ziemnik, R., Spalding, A., Van Hook, S., & Shrier, L. A. (2014). An electronic screen for triaging adolescent substance use by risk levels. *JAMA Pediatrics, 168*(9), 822–828. doi:10.1001/jamapediatrics.2014.774

Maslowsky, J., Capell, J. W., Moberg, D. P., & Brown, R. L. (2017). Universal school-based implementation of screening, brief intervention and referral to treatment to reduce and prevent alcohol, marijuana, tobacco, and other drug use: Process and feasibility. *Substance Abuse: Research and Treatment,11,* 1–10.

Mitchell, S. G., Gryczynski, J., O'Grady, K. E., & Schwartz, R. P. (2013). SBIRT for adolescent drug and alcohol use: Current status and future directions. *Journal of Substance Abuse Treatment*, *44*(5), 463–472.

National Center for Mental Health Checkups at Columbia University. (n.d.). PHQ-9 modified for teens. *Incorporating Mental Health Screening into Adolescent Office Visits*. https://mmcp.health.maryland.gov/epsdt/healthykids/AppendixSection4/PHQ-9%20Modified.pdf

Oregon Health and Science University. (2019) SBIRT Oregon: Clinic tools. http://www.sbirtoregon.org/clinic-tools/

Paschall, M. J., & Bersamin, M. (2018). School-based mental health services, suicide risk and substance use among at-risk adolescents in Oregon. *Preventive Medicine*,*106*, 209–215.

Quanbeck, A., Lang, K., Enami, K., & Brown, R. (2010). A cost-benefit analysis of Wisconsin's screening, brief intervention, and referral to treatment program: Adding the employer's perspective. *WMJ*, *109*(1), 9–14.

Tanner-Smith, E. E., & Lipsey, M. W. (2015). Brief alcohol interventions for adolescents and young adults: A systematic review and meta-analysis. *Journal of Substance Abuse Treatment*, *51*, 1–18. doi:10.1016/j.jsat.2014.09.001

Case 5.2 Weight Loss

What are the top differential diagnoses in this case and why?

Eating disorder:

An eating disorder is defined by an unhealthy attitude toward food that involves eating too much or too little, or becoming obsessed with weight and body shape. Symptoms of eating disorders including avoiding socialization when food is involved, eating very little food, making oneself sick after eating, constant worrying about weight and body shape, exercising too much, and/or very strict habits or routines around food.

The most common eating disorders are:

1. *Anorexia nervosa*, which is defined by keeping weight as low as possible by not eating enough food, exercising too much, or both.
2. *Bulimia nervosa*, which is defined by loss of control and eating a large amount of food in a short amount of time (binging) and then deliberately making oneself sick such as using a laxative, making oneself throw up, or overexercising to keep from gaining weight.
3. *Binge-eating disorder*, in which the individual loses control of eating and eats large portions of food to the point of feeling uncomfortable, upset, guilty, or sick.
4. *Other specified feeding or eating disorder* is when an individual does not meet the exact symptoms of anorexia, bulimia, or binge-eating disorder.

At this point, we know that Roseanne's mother is concerned about her weight but we do not know if Roseanne is concerned or is just strongly influenced by her mother or even her coach. She is a Division I athlete and is on a strict and constant exercise regimen. At this point she has a low BMI and does not get her periods (which can also be attributed to her birth control), which are symptoms of an eating disorder. Other physical symptoms are constantly feeling cold, tired, or dizzy and problems with digestion, all of which she denies.

Excessive exercise:

Compulsive exercise is common in athletes; compulsive exercisers are also sometimes referred to as "exercise addicts" or "obligatory athletes." High-performance runners, professional athletes, and body builders are all reported to have exercise addiction. Excessive exercise can lead to injuries,

The Family Nurse Practitioner: Clinical Case Studies, Second Edition. Edited by Leslie Neal-Boylan.
© 2021 John Wiley & Sons Ltd. Published 2021 by John Wiley & Sons Ltd.

exhaustion, depression, and even suicide. Excessive exercisers will organize their lives around the exercise routine. At this time, excessive exercise is a concern, including the history of injuries from cheerleading.

Malnutrition:
Malnutrition occurs from an inadequate diet or problems absorbing nutrients from food. The most common causes of malnutrition are long-term health conditions, low income, or a restricted diet. Unintentional weight loss (losing 5–10% of one's body weight over 3–6 months) is the most common symptom of malnutrition. Signs of malnutrition include weak muscles, chronic fatigue, low mood, frequent infections, or illnesses. An indicator of possible or high risk of malnutrition is a BMI under 18.5, which means Roseanne is a candidate.

Malabsorption:
Causes of malabsorption are cystic fibrosis (or diseases that affect the pancreas), lactose intolerance, or intestinal disorders (such as celiac disease). Symptoms include abdominal discomfort (gas and bloating), frequent diarrhea, loose stool or stools that are light in color or bulky, weight loss, and frequent skin rashes. Roseanne's review of symptoms and physical examination makes malabsorption less of a concern.

Thyroid disorder:
Hyperthyroidism from an overactive thyroid can cause unintentional weight loss (when appetite and food intake is the same or increased but the individual continues to lose weight), tachycardia, arrhythmias, heart palpitations, increased appetite, nervousness, anxiety, irritability, hand or finger tremors, sweating, changes in menstrual patterns, heat sensitivity, changes in bowel patterns, enlarged thyroid goiter), fatigue, muscle weakness, difficulty sleeping, skin thinning, and fine, brittle hair. While we know Roseanne is excessively exercising and has abnormal menstrual patterns that are most likely from her frequent exercise, it is important to consider thyroid health at this point as well.

Anxiety:
Some adolescents have high standards and personal goals with disciplined behavior that can lead to anxiety surrounding control and perfectionism. However, when these behaviors interfere with social, emotional, and occupational functioning (including school performance or pressure) they can lead to an anxiety disorder. The most common somatic symptoms of pediatric anxiety disorders include restlessness, feeling sick to stomach, blushing, palpitations, muscle tension, sweating, trembling and shaking, easily fatigued, feeling paralyzed, chills, and hot flashes. At this time, neither Roseanne nor her mother is stating that any of these symptoms are a concern or problem.

Female athlete triad:
Female athlete triad is a medical condition in physically active females involving: (1) low energy, with or without disordered eating; (2) menstrual dysfunction (usually amenorrhea); and (3) osteoporosis. Long-term consequences may not be reversible, making prevention, early diagnosis, and intervention important. Tracking menstruation is often useful for identifying athletes at risk and should be part of the preparticipatory sports physical. At this point, female athlete triad is a concern and one of the most likely primary diagnoses.

What are the diagnostic tests required in this case and why?
Laboratory evaluation of the amenorrheic athlete includes a pregnancy test, follicle-stimulating hormone, thyroid-stimulating hormone, and prolactin levels. Estradiol levels may also be helpful. Roseanne is currently on a birth control pill where she does not get her period, which is often preferred for female teenage athletes. However, even though she is on birth control, other causes of secondary amenorrhea should still be considered, including weight changes, pregnancy, stress, hypothyroidism, and prolactinoma. If Roseanne is sexually active, screening for sexually transmitted infections should also be included.

What are the concerns at this point?

Concern about her weight is the main priority at this time, as Roseanne has a low body mass index and is a competitive athlete. She also has a history of broken bones requiring surgery, and while she is a competitive athlete in which these injuries are likely, early osteoporosis and her bone mineral density are a concern.

Further exploration around when weight first became a concern and what her weight was a year ago at her last physical would be helpful. A full diet history of what Roseanne eats including how many calories she consumes should also be explored.

As seen in female athlete triad, hypothalamic amenorrhea may result from the decrease in estrogen levels, which has a negative effect on bone density. Estrogen is involved in osteoclast and osteoblast activity, bone formation and resorption, and inhibits bone turnover. Adolescence is a time of peak bone mass accrual and therefore, this effect of estrogen during this developmental period is critical. Helping Roseanne, her mother, and possibly her coaches understand the long-term effects on low bone density is important.

A systemic review of randomized control trails and cohort studies show that bone loss reduction can be addressed through oral contraceptive pills (OCPs), which Roseanne is already taking. OCPs with 20–35 micrograms of ethinyl estradiol may help maintain bone mineral density. However, only the restoration of spontaneous menses through restoring energy balance offers best reversal of low bone mineral density concerns.

Roseanne's mental well being is also a concern, including a lack of regular sleep (less than 8 hours on average) as well as the stress and pressure of maintaining a 4.0 grade average and competing in a rigorous exercise schedule of being a Division I athlete. The provider can administer a standardized screening instrument for depression and anxiety (such as the PHQ-9 or the SCARED) to help elicit further conversation around Roseanne's mental health.

Should Roseanne's mother be asked to leave the room at this time? Why or why not?

Roseanne's mother should be asked to leave the room so that you can ask and gather further information from Roseanne that she may not feel comfortable discussing in front of her mother. Confidentiality should be reviewed/explained to Roseanne. Areas that should be further explored include:

Sexual activity: The provider should ask Roseanne about her current or past sexual activity including contraceptives beyond the birth control pill. Depending on her answers, health education surrounding STIs and HIV including possible testing and treatment should be explored.

Social pressure: It would also be helpful to ask Roseanne about her competitive cheerleading. Use open-ended, nonconfrontational questions such as "Can you tell me more about your cheerleading?" Ask if she enjoys cheerleading without her mother present and further explore if she has a choice in her full schedule and constant practice. Try to elicit discussion on Roseanne's need for perfection and competitive nature. Ask what other activities she enjoys or participates in.

Weight: While Roseanne's mother is concerned about her weight, ask Roseanne if she is concerned as well without her mother present. Inquire about her family and family dynamics between herself and her mom and dad. Ask if she snacks throughout the day and if she ever vomits after eating or takes laxatives or other diet pills or supplements. Ask if she ever eats in private when no one else is around or feels ashamed in eating or gaining weight.

What is the plan of treatment?

Long-term risks for the female athlete triad include osteoporosis (and fracture), psychological effects of disordered eating, and eventually diminished athletic performance. Balancing energy availability, bone health, and menstrual function are indicators of a healthy athlete. The goal of treatment for the female athlete triad is adjusting energy expenditure and energy availability. Family-based therapy and cognitive behavioral therapy are both effective for disordered eating.

Recommending a nutritionist (or a sports nutritionist) can help Roseanne (and her mother) determine the quantity and quality of foods consumed as well as dietary supplementation. Daily intake of 1000–1300 mg of calcium and 600 units of Vitamin D is recommended.

What are the plans for referral and follow-up care?

Depending on Roseanne's answers, further assessment may be necessary. The provider should assess the parotid gland, tooth enamel erosion, the palms for carotenemia, skin fold thickness and mid-upper arm circumference, or the presence of Russell sign (calluses on the knuckles or back of hand due to repeated self-induced vomiting over long periods of time). Roseanne's weight and eating patterns should be closely monitored in future visits and continued conversation should occur after her laboratory results come back. The female athlete triad takes a team approach and involving the sports nutritionist, coaches, parents, and a mental health care provider, if indicated, is critical.

What health education should be provided to this patient?

Discuss Roseanne's weight with both Roseanne and her mother. Emphasize that her body mass index is in the 6th percentile for weight and that this is low for her height and age. While her physical examination was normal, recommend that laboratory tests be ordered today and that no other medical problems exist.

Provide education on nutrition, including maximizing bone density during adolescence and the importance of calcium and vitamin D supplementation. A food diary or journal can be suggested for recording weight, diet, and exercise. Long-term consequences of osteoporosis and bone health are often not reversible. Dancers, gymnasts, and runners are usually at the highest risk of the triad and for long-term effects and consequences.

Often the low energy availability from restrictive eating of athletes is related to lack of proper nutrition knowledge as well as not making time to eat adequately.

What demographic characteristics might affect this case?

Certain regions of the country have what is sometimes referred to as extreme athletics at the secondary school level where youth and adolescents compete in rigorous sportsmanship in middle and high school (such as cheerleading, football, and bull riding in the Southern states).

Are there any standardized guidelines that should be used to treat this case? If so, what are they?

The American College of Obstetricians and Gynecologists (2017) have published recommendations for screening the female athletes triad, which include the following:

1. Do you worry about your weight or body composition?
2. Do you limit or carefully control the foods that you eat?
3. Do you try to lose weight to meet weight or image/appearance requirement in your sport?
4. Does your weight affect the way you feel about yourself?
5. Do you worry that you have lost control over how much you eat?
6. Do you make yourself vomit or use diuretics or laxatives after you eat?
7. Do you currently or have you ever suffered from an eating disorder?
8. Do you ever eat in secret?
9. What age was your first menstrual period?
10. Do you have monthly menstrual cycles?
11. How many menstrual cycles have you had in your last year?
12. Have you ever had a stress factor?

Source: From Weiss Kelly, A. K., Hect, S., & Council on Sports Medicine and Fitness. (2016). The female athlete triad. *Pediatrics, 138*, 10.1542/peds.2016.0922.

If this patient was male (instead of female), how would that change management and/or treatment?

The International Olympic Committee has proposed changing the name to relative energy deficiency in sports (RED-S) since males can also be affected. RED-S also encompasses endocrine, metabolic, hematologic, growth and development, cardiovascular, gastrointestinal, and immunological effects of energy deficiencies.

REFERENCES AND RESOURCES

American College of Obstetricians and Gynecologists. (2017). Committee Opinion No. 702. Female athlete triad. *Obstetrics & Gynecology, 129,* 3160–3167.

American College of Obstetricians and Gynecologists. (2015). Committee Opinion No. 651. Menstruation in girls and adolescents: Using the menstrual cycle as a vital sign. *Obstetrics & Gynecology, 126,* e143–146.

Bennell, K., White, S., & Crossley, K. (1999). The oral contraceptive pill: A revolution for sportswomen? *British Journal Sports Medicine, 33,* 321–328.

Campbell, K., & Peebles, R. (2014). Eating disorders in children and adolescents: State of the art review. *Pediatrics, 134,* 582–592.

Nazem, T. G., & Ackerman K. E. (2012). The female athlete triad. *Sports Health, 4,* 302–311.

Weiss Kelly, A. K., Hecht, S., & Council on Sports Medicine and Fitness. (2016). The female athlete triad. *Pediatrics, 138,* 10.1542/peds.2016.0922.

Case 5.3 Menstrual Cramps

RESOLUTION

What is the most likely differential diagnosis and why?
Primary dysmenorrhea:
Primary dysmenorrhea is defined as painful menstruation in the absence of pelvic pathology (American College of Obstetricians and Gynecologists [ACOG], 2015). Khaleesi is within the age range (14–18 years old) where symptoms of primary dysmenorrhea are most prevalent (Osayande & Mehulic, 2014). Diagnosis is often based on clinical history; Khaleesi's history of lower abdominal pain and cramps is consistent with the timing of the menstrual cycle.

Which diagnostic or imaging studies should be considered to assist with or confirm the diagnosis?
Although Khaleesi denies sexual activity, it would be prudent to do a urine pregnancy test to rule out pregnancy, missed or threatened abortion, and offer tests for sexually transmitted infection (STI) screening. She also should have a CBC with differential checked with the history of frequent periods and therefore risk for anemia. In the absence of symptoms of STIs, a pelvic exam is not necessary (Bowers, 2018).

What questions would you ask Khaleesi about her menstrual cycle?

- *What was her age at menarche?* During the first 1–2 years following menarche, cycles are highly irregular and anovulatory. Once ovulation starts to occur, the amount of prostaglandin responsible for the symptoms associated with primary dysmenorrhea increases (ACOG, 2018; Bowers, 2018; Moriarty Daley & Fender, 2011).
- *What are her number of days of bleeding and the number of hygienic products used in 24 hours?* Consider a workup for bleeding disorders or secondary causes if:
  - Bleeding lasts more than 7 days.
  - Bleeding soaks through one or more tampons or pads every hour for several hours in a row.
  - Patient will wear more than one pad at a time to control menstrual flow.
  - Patient needs to change pads or tampons during the night.
  - Patient reports passing blood clots that are as big as a quarter or larger (ACOG, 2016).

The Family Nurse Practitioner: Clinical Case Studies, Second Edition. Edited by Leslie Neal-Boylan.
© 2021 John Wiley & Sons Ltd. Published 2021 by John Wiley & Sons Ltd.

- *Ask her to describe her symptoms.* Complaints of lower abdominal, back, and/or thigh pain at the onset of menstruation is commonly reported with primary dysmenorrhea. Associated symptoms may also include nausea, vomiting, diarrhea, fatigue, and headache (Barassi et al., 2018; Osayande & Mehulic, 2014). If breast tenderness or bloating is reported, also consider a diagnosis of premenstrual syndrome (PMS).
- *Ask Khaleesi when she experiences the onset of pain.* Symptoms of primary dysmenorrhea usually peak in the first 48 hours of menstrual flow, associated with the highest level of prostaglandins. Consider PMS if Khaleesi reports symptoms of pain and discomfort in the luteal phase: days 14 through 28 of the menstrual cycle.

What additional information/questions are needed?

- *Ask Khaleesi how often she participates in sexual activity and whether it is with males, females, or both. Ask whether she uses condoms 100% of the time.* Obtain more detailed information about sexual activity to help to determine the risks of sexually transmitted infections (STIs) and pregnancy. Review signs and symptoms of STIs or pelvic inflammatory disease (PID) such as fever, abnormal vaginal discharge, or pelvic pain (Osayande & Mehulic, 2014).
- *Ask Khaleesi if she has tried anything for her cramps.* If a patient is already using nonsteroidal anti-inflammatory drugs (NSAIDs) or oral contraceptive pills (OCPs) without relief of symptoms, consider an underlying pathology with a diagnosis of secondary dysmenorrhea (Barassi et al., 2018).
- *Has she always had cramps or is this a more recent change?* If an adolescent presents with menstrual pain before the age of 14 or first experiences menstrual pain after the age of 19, consider causes of secondary dysmenorrhea (Moriarty Daley & Fender, 2011).
- *Is there a family history of endometriosis?* Endometriosis is the most common cause of secondary dysmenorrhea, and should be considered with a history of menorrhagia, intermenstrual bleeding, dyspareunia, pain that occurs mid-cycle or is acyclic, post-coital bleeding, or infertility (Bowers, 2018; Osayande & Mehulic, 2014). Endometriosis in a first-degree relative, or relatives with more severe disease, would warrant early screening for endometriosis (Bowers, 2018; Zannoni et al., 2014).
- *Does she have a history of diarrhea, constipation, generalized abdominal pain, or passing gas?* Information can help rule out gastrointestinal disorders such as irritable bowel syndrome, lactose intolerance, constipation, and inflammatory bowel disease (Moriarty Daley & Fender, 2011).
- *Does she have a history of psychosocial problems?* A positive history of cigarette smoking, trauma, abuse, anxiety, depression, or other somatic complaints has been associated with symptoms of dysmenorrhea (ACOG, 2015; Moriarty Daley & Fender, 2011).

What is the plan of treatment?

NSAID therapy is the first-line empiric treatment to disrupt cyclooxygenase-mediated prostaglandin production (ACOG, 2015; Bowers, 2018). Treatment can be started before menstruation, with the onset of symptoms, or with the beginning of menstruation. Ideally, medications should be taken 1–2 days prior to the anticipated onset of menses, and continued on a fixed schedule for 2–3 days (ACOG, 2015; Barassi et al., 2018; Bowers, 2018; Osayande & Mehulic, 2014). Ensure that the patient is taking an adequate dose, as subtherapeutic treatment is sometimes reported (Bowers, 2018). Taking NSAIDS with food and increasing fluid intake may help with GI and renal adverse affects (ACOG, 2015).

NSAID treatment demonstrates effectiveness confirmed over placebo of all NSAIDs tested in a 2015 Cochrane Review (ACOG, 2015; Marjoribanks, Ayeleke, Farquhar, & Proctor, 2015). When NSAIDs were compared with each other, most studies found no evidence of a difference between them. See Table 5.4.1 for dosing and schedule of commonly prescribed NSAIDs for dysmenorrhea.

Table 5.4.1. Nonsteroidal Anti-Inflammatory Drugs Used in the Treatment of Primary Dysmenorrhea.

Drug	Dosage	Follow-Up Dosing
Celecoxib (Celebrex) *For females older than 18*	400 mg initially	200 mg every 12 hours
Ibuprofen (Advil, Motrin)	200 to 600 mg every 6 hours	200 to 600 mg every 6 hours
	Alternative: 800 mg initially	*Alternative: 800 mg every 8 hours*
Mefenamic acid	500 mg initially	250 mg every 6 hours
Naproxen	440 to 550 mg initially	220 to 275 mg every 12 hours

Source: Marjoribanks, J., Ayeleke, R. O., Farquhar, C., & Proctor, M. (2015). Nonsteroidal anti-inflammatory drugs for dysmenorrhoea. *Cochrane Database of Systematic Reviews, 2015*(7), CD001751. doi:10.1002/14651858.CD001751.pub3 (ACOG, 2015; Osayande & Mehulic, 2014).

After starting a specific NSAID, wait 2–3 cycles before switching medications if symptoms are not alleviated. Failure of NSAID treatments should not be determined unless they have been tried for longer than 3–6 months (ACOG 2015; Moriarty Daley & Fender, 2011).

In addition to the use of NSAIDs, ACOG (2015) recommends hormonal contraception as an adjunct to NSAIDs to inhibit ovulation, thereby reducing prostaglandin release. Contraceptive counseling should be provided and decisions should be patient driven (ACOG, 2015; Bowers, 2018). Once started, the contraceptive method should be used for 3–4 months before considering treatment failure.

Are there other options?

Approximately 10–25% of patients do not respond to NSAID and hormonal contraception therapy. Limited evidence-based research exists for alternative therapies (Barassi et al., 2018; Osayande & Mehulic, 2014). With low risk of harm and low cost of topical heat therapy and exercise, and the overall health benefits of exercise, ACOG (2015) encourages these two alternative options. Other examples of therapies include transcutaneous electric nerve stimulation (TENS), smoking cessation (ACOG, 2015), and acupuncture (Zhang et al., 2018). Neuromuscular therapy may ensure longer duration of NSAID analgesia (Barassi et al., 2018), and laparoscopic presacral neurectomy, and transdermal nitroglycerin have also been researched as alternative therapies (Moriarty Daley & Fender, 2011). Dietary modification and/or Supplementation with potential dietary supplements, include: Omega-3 fatty acids, Thiamine (vitamin B_1), magnesium, fenugreek, ginger, valerian, zataria, zinc, vitamin D. Safety and efficacy on herbal treatments is limited (ACOG, 2015).

In treatment failure, consider secondary causes of dysmenorrhea including endometriosis, adenomyoisis, myomas, congential malformations, obstructions, or ovarian cysts (Bowers, 2018). Testing may include a bimanual gynecologic exam, and/or a transvaginal or abdominal ultrasound (Bowers, 2018). Diagnostic laparoscopy may be performed in cases with a high index of suspicion of endometriosis not confirmed by imaging or severe pain nonresponsive to therapies (Zannoni et al., 2014).

Is it common for teen girls to miss school because of their periods?

Yes. Dysmenorrhea is the number-one reason for school absences and for refusal to participate in physical activity for adolescent females (Moriarty Daley & Fender, 2011). Adolescents who report severe dysmenorrhea show significantly higher absenteeism from school (Zannoni et al., 2014). It is also associated with a high rate of absenteeism from work (Barassi et al., 2018).

When should she be seen for follow-up?

Patients should be monitored for response to treatment; consider following up in 8 weeks and as needed. A menstrual diary to include descriptions of pain, medication used and its effect, and any other symptoms will be helpful in determining treatment plan (Moriarty Daley & Fender, 2011).

Follow-up appointments after initiating contraception should include review of pain symptoms, response to medications, and reviewing signs and symptoms for adverse affects of hormonal contraception, or any concerns with use or adherence to use (Steenland, Zapata, Brahmi, Marchbanks, & Curtis, 2013). Blood pressure, weight, and warning signs for thromboembolism (using the mnemonic ACHES: *a*bdominal pain, *c*hest pain, *h*eadaches, *e*ye problems, *s*evere calf or thigh pain) should also be monitored at follow-up visits.

What health education should be provided to this patient?

The American College of Obstetricians and Gynecologists (ACOG; 2015) regularly update patient information and handouts in both English and Spanish. Available at https://www.acog.org/Patients/FAQs/Dysmenorrhea-Painful-Periods

Are there technologies available to assist this patient in her care?

In addition to ACOG's website, there are many online resources available for adolescents to learn more about their menstrual cycle and symptoms. One valuable resource is kidshealth.org (Nemours Foundation, 2019), which includes audio explanations of periods, cramps, abnormal period,s and more topics, provided in both English and Spanish.

The advent of apps in healthcare is also a useable resource for teens with smartphones. Popular period tracker apps including Period Tracker, Flo, Glow, Ovia, and Clue. Awareness of data collection through apps should be expressed to adolescents (Kresge, Khrennikov, & Ramli, 2019), with emphasis on privacy settings.

REFERENCES AND RESOURCES

American College of Obstetricians and Gynecologists (2015, January). *Dysmennorrhea: Painful period*. https://www.acog.org/Patients/FAQs/Dysmenorrhea-Painful-Periods

American College of Obstetricians and Gynecologists (2016, June). *Heavy menstrual bleeding*. https://www.acog.org/Patients/FAQs/Heavy-Menstrual-Bleeding?

American College of Obstetricians and Gynecologists (2018, December). Dysmenorrhea and *endometriosis in the adolescent*. https://www.acog.org/clinical/clinical-guidance/committee-opinion/articles/2018/12/dysmenorrhea-and-endometriosis-in-the-adolescent

Bowers, R. (2018). Help teens and young women manage dysmenorrhea symptoms effectively. *Contraceptive Technology Update*, *40*(2). www.reliasmedia.com/articles/143817

Barassi, G., Bellomo, R. G., Porreca, A., Di Felice, P. A., Prosperi, L., & Saggini, R. (2018). Somato-visceral effects in the treatment of dysmenorrhea: Neuromuscular manual therapy and standard pharmacological treatment. *Journal of Alternative & Complementary Medicine*, *24*(3), 291–299. doi:10.1089/acm.2017.0182

Harel, Z. (2012). Dysmenorrhea in adolescents and young adults: An update on pharmacological treatments and management strategies. *Expert Opinion on Pharmacotherapy*, *13*(15), 2157–2170. doi:10.1517/14656566.2012.725045

Kresge, N., Khrennikov, I., & Ramli, D. (2019, January 24). Period-Tracking apps are monetizing women's extremely personal data: More than 100 million women monitor their cycles on their phones. Here come the ads. *Bloomberg Businessweek*. https://www.bloomberg.com/news/articles/2019-01-24/how-period-tracking-apps-are-monetizing-women-s-extremely-personal-data

Lauretti, G. R., Oliveira, R., Parada, F., & Mattos, A. L. (2015). The new portable transcutaneous electrical nerve stimulation device was efficacious in the control of primary dysmenorrhea cramp pain. *Neuromodulation: Journal of the International Neuromodulation Society*, *18*(6), 522–526. https://doi-org.10.1111/ner.12269

Marjoribanks, J., Ayeleke, R. O., Farquhar, C., & Proctor, M. (*2015*). Nonsteroidal anti-inflammatory drugs for dysmenorrhoea. *Cochrane Database of Systematic Reviews*, *2015*(7), CD001751. doi:10.1002/14651858.CD001751.pub3

Moriarty Daley, A., & Fender, T. (2011). Case 5.4 Menstrual cramps. In L. Neal-Boylan (Ed.), *Clinical case studies for the family nurse practitioner* (pp. 147–150). Wiley.

Nemours Foundation. (2019). All about menstruation. Retrieved from

Osayande, A. S., & Mehulic, S. (2014). Diagnosis and initial management of dysmenorrhea. *American Family Physician*, 89(5), 341–346. https://www.aafp.org/afp/2014/0301/p341.html

Steenland, M. W., Zapata, L. B., Brahmi, D., Marchbanks, P. A., & Curtis, K. M. (2013). Appropriate follow up to detect potential adverse events after initiation of select contraceptive methods: A systematic review. *Contraception*, 87(5), 611–624. doi:10.1016/j.contraception.2012.09.017

Upadhya, K. K., Santelli, J. S., Raine-Bennett, T. R., Kottke, M. J., & Grossman, D. (2017). Over-the-counter access to oral contraceptives for adolescents. *Journal of Adolescent Health*, 60(6), 634–640. https://doi.org/10.1016/j.jadohealth.2016.12.024

Zannoni, L., Giorgi, M., Spagnolo, E., Montanari, G., Villa, G., & Seracchioli, R. (2014). Dysmenorrhea, absenteeism from school, and symptoms suspicious for endometriosis in adolescents. *Journal of Pediatric and Adolescent Gynecology*, 27(5), 258–265. https://doi.org/10.1016/j.jpag.2013.11.008

Zhang, F., Sun, M., Han, S., Shen, X., Luo, Y., Zhong, D., Zhou, X., Liang, F., & Jin, R. (2018). Acupuncture for primary dysmenorrhea: An overview of systematic reviews. *Evidence-Based Complementary & Alternative Medicine (ECAM)*, 1–11. doi:10.1155/2018/8791538

Case 5.4 Missed Periods

Which diagnostic or imaging studies should be considered to assist with or confirm the diagnosis?

A urine pregnancy test should be ordered. Genny should also be offered STI testing, including HIV testing and counseling with a history of unprotected sex. A Pap smear is recommended 3 years after the onset of sexual activity or by age 21, so it is not appropriate for Genny at this time.

If the pregnancy test is positive, in the absence of symptoms, delaying the pelvic exam until a consultation with an obstetrician or at a termination appointment is appropriate. If there is a question regarding gestation, due to uncertainty with dates or irregular menstruation, referral for a pelvic exam and/or an ultrasound to determine dates is warranted (Hornberger, 2017).

If Genny's pregnancy test is negative today, she should return for a repeat test in 2–4 weeks if she has no menses (ACOG, 2017).

Why is it important to ask Genny what she feels her boyfriend would want if she were pregnant?

The perceived desire of the partner is an important influence on pregnancy (Moriarty Daley & Fender, 2011). Counseling may help Genny negotiate the use of condoms by her male partner to avoid an unintended pregnancy (Pereira, Pires, Araújo-Pedrosa, & Canavarro, 2018). In addition, engaging fathers in prenatal and infant care is essential in promoting involvement and decreasing parenting stress (Magness, 2012).

What additional questions should Genny be asked?

- "How would you feel about a positive or negative pregnancy test today?"
- "How do you think your partner would react to a positive or negative pregnancy test?"
- "Do you have any additional signs or symptoms, such as lower abdominal pain, breast tenderness, nausea, vomiting, or fatigue?"
- "Have you talked to anyone about your possible pregnancy?"
- "Is there a supportive adult with whom you could discuss a positive pregnancy test?"
- "Do you know what your 3 options are if the test is positive?"
- "What would you do if the test is positive today?"

The Family Nurse Practitioner: Clinical Case Studies, Second Edition. Edited by Leslie Neal-Boylan.
© 2021 John Wiley & Sons Ltd. Published 2021 by John Wiley & Sons Ltd.

- "How will pregnancy affect your living situation? Your education? Your employment?"
- "If the test is negative, would you like to begin a more effective contraception?"

If Genny is pregnant today, what are her options?

Educate Genny on her options regarding the pregnancy in a factual, respectful, nonjudgmental and adolescent-friendly manner. The American Academy of Pediatrics first published a policy statement on options counseling in 1989, which has continued to be reaffirmed (Hornberger, 2017). Options counseling can be done at the first visit or over several future visits. Maintain confidentiality and give Genny the results of her test alone first, then give her an opportunity to discuss her feelings, pregnancy, and contraception options without a parent or guardian present initially (ACOG, 2017; Hornberger, 2017). However, parental involvement is often necessary, both emotionally and financially, so encouragement to share positive test results and involve parents with Genny's decision is important. If parental support is not possible or likely, encourage Genny to seek involvement of another trusted adult.

Depending on the stage of pregnancy, there are 3 options: (1) continuing the pregnancy and raising the infant; (2) continuing the pregnancy to delivery and then having an adoption plan; or (3) terminating the pregnancy (Hornberger, 2017). Offer additional visits with her supportive adult, the male partner, her parents, or her partner's parents, if desired. Emphasize that the decision is time-sensitive, and options may depend on gestational age.

Should contraception be prescribed today?

Condoms and an advance prescription for emergency contraception (Plan B) should be provided at this visit. Emergency contraception should be offered if the adolescent has had unprotected sex in the past 5 days and does not desire pregnancy (Hornberger, 2017). In addition, if she has a negative pregnancy test, a prescription for hormonal contraception can be given today with clear instructions on how to start if she begins her menstrual cycle. If she desires injectionable contraception (depot medroxyprogesterone acetate (DMPA)), she should call at the onset of her period to begin injections.

Consider family history, coexisting medical conditions, and current medications when offering contraception options. Patient choice should be the primary factor in prescribing one method over another (ACOG, 2017). Contraception counseling should include reproductive goals, awareness of unprotected intercourse risks, efficacy and failure rates of different contraceptive methods, adverse effects and risks, ease of use, and additional barrier methods needed to prevent STIs (ACOG, 2017; Pereira et al., 2018). As contraceptive failures are often reported in unplanned pregnancy (such as condom rupture or forgetting to take a pill), backup methods and emergency contraception should also be discussed (Pereira et al., 2018).

Long-acting reversible contraceptives (LARCs) are the most effective form of birth control (Fernandez, 2017) and should be offered and discussed with Genny. LARC methods are easier for the patient to manage, as they do not require a daily, weekly, or monthly action by the patient (Fernandez, 2017). Initiation of implants or IUDs can occur immediately after delivery, pregnancy loss, or abortion, and in the case of a negative pregnancy test, if there is reasonable certainty that Genny is not pregnant (ACOG, 2017). "Quick start" initiation the same day can be with the implant, DMPA, and OCPs, and benefits likely exceed any risk (ACOG, 2017).

The American College of Obstetricians and Gynecologists' clinical guidance is available online at www.acog.org.

What health education should be provided to this patient?

Community resources for each pregnancy option are helpful, and are dependent on rural or urban demographic area. It is important to make sure Genny has the appropriate services, financial resources, and social support for whatever her decision may be.

For patients choosing to maintain their pregnancy, education regarding understanding pregnancy and placing them in contact with an OB/GYN is imperative. Prescribe prenatal vitamins, review health education regarding signs and symptoms of miscarriage and infection, and review when to call an OB/GYN and/or go to the emergency room early in pregnancy.

Discuss ways to increase success in preventing pregnancy and sexually transmitted infections. Offer STI/HIV testing, to include HIV, syphilis, chlamydia, and gonorrhea, and, if maintaining pregnancy, Hepatitis B (Hornberger, 2017). Screening for STIs should be done at the time of counseling or LARC insertion (Fernandez, 2017). Addressing adolescent reproductive health care needs with a combination of health and sexuality education and contraceptive-promoting interventions can decrease risk of unplanned adolescent pregnancy (Klein & Ray, 2017; Pereira et al., 2018). Consider peer teaching with active learning, examples, and visual aids to promote empowerment and patient understanding (Magness, 2012).

Are there technologies available to assist this patient in managing or understanding her menstruation?

Promote adherence to contraception through use of cell-phone or electronic reminders (ACOG, 2017). Many online websites assist the patient in identifying which contraceptive method would be best for their lifestyles. Many resources are available for pregnancy and sexual health education. Examples include ACOG's patient information site (available at https://www.acog.org/Patients) and the National Campaign to Prevent Teen and Unplanned Pregnancy (available at powertodecide.org and www.bedsider.org; National Campaign, 2019).

The advent of apps useful in health care is also a resource for teens with smartphones, including period tracker and pregnancy tracker apps; examples include Flo, Glow, Ovia, and Clue. Awareness of data collection through apps should be expressed to adolescents (Kresge, Khrennikov, & Ramli, 2019) with emphasis on privacy settings.

REFERENCES AND RESOURCES

American College of Obstetricians and Gynecologists. (2017, May). *Committee opinion: Adolescent pregnancy, contraception, and sexual activity*. Retrieved from https://www.acog.org/Clinical-Guidance-and-Publications/Committee-Opinions/Committee-on-Adolescent-Health-Care/Adolescent-Pregnancy-Contraception-and-Sexual-Activity

American College of Obstetricians and Gynecologists. (2019). The ACOG patient page. Retrieved from https://www.acog.org/Patients

Fernandez, S. (2017). Long-acting reversible contraception: A primer for the primary care pediatrician. *Pediatric Annals, 46*(3), 79–82. https://doi-org.10.3928/19382359-20170220-03

Hornberger, L. L. (2017). Diagnosis of pregnancy and providing options counseling. *Pediatrics, 140*(3), 1–9. https://doi-org.10.1542/peds.2017-2273

Klein, D. A., & Ray, M. E. (2017). Preventing unintended adolescent pregnancy. *American Family Physician, 95*(7), 422–423. Retrieved from https://www.aafp.org/afp/2017/0401/p422.html

Kresge, N., Khrennikov, I., & Ramli, D. (2019, January 24). Period-tracking apps are monetizing women's extremely personal data: More than 100 million women monitor their cycles on their phones. Here come the ads. *Bloomberg Businessweek.* Retrieved from https://www.bloomberg.com/news/articles/2019-01-24/how-period-tracking-apps-are-monetizing-women-s-extremely-personal-data

Magness, J. (2012). Adolescent pregnancy: The role of the healthcare provider. *International Journal of Childbirth Education, 27*(4), 61–64.

Moriarty Daley, A., & Fender, T. (2011). Case 5.4 Menstrual cramps. In L. Neal-Boylan (Ed.), Clinical case studies for the family nurse practitioner (pp. 147–150). Hoboken, NJ: Wiley.

National Campaign to Prevent Teen and Unplanned Pregnancy (2019). The power to decide. Retrieved from https://powertodecide.org/ and https://www.bedsider.org/

Pereira, J. I. F., Pires, R. S. A., Araújo-Pedrosa, A. F., & Canavarro, M. C. C. S. P. (2018). Reproductive and relational trajectories leading to pregnancy: Differences between adolescents and adult women who had an abortion. *European Journal of Obstetrics & Gynecology & Reproductive Biology, 224,* 181–187. https://doi-org.10.1016/j.ejogrb.2018

Case 5.5 Birth Control Decision-Making

Given the information provided, what other questions would you ask?

When deciding which contraceptive options would be the best choice for a patient, knowledge of any contraindications to specific contraceptive types is essential. Gathering a thorough past medical history and family medical history would be appropriate at this time. A family medical history related to coagulation disorders and cancer may affect any diagnostic tests or screenings the provider would choose to complete with the patient if hormonal contraceptives are being considered. Obtaining this information may be difficult with the adolescent patient or a poor historian, and may require the involvement of other family members to ensure that no relative or absolute contraindications are present prior to prescribing.

Smoking status should be considered with prescription of hormonal contraceptives, but it is not a contraindication unless the patient is 35 years old or older and smokes 15 or more cigarettes per day. This should include vaping or juuling as well. Screening for other substance use is equally important, as adolescents under the influence are more likely to participate in risky sexual behaviors, including an inability to provide consent for intercourse.

Ask the patient the regularity of her periods as well as frequency of sexual activity and last date of intercourse. She has disclosed that she uses condoms always for intercourse, but screening for proper use should also be part of the dialogue when reviewing contraceptive options. Be sure to give positive feedback as well for any contraceptive use if applicable.

It is also important for the provider to determine in mutual decision-making what the patient's goals are related to her contraceptive choices, such as shorter bleeding time, no periods, or not having to take a pill daily. Future family planning should also be assessed during contraceptive decision-making. While the adolescent patient may not have family planning in mind at the time of the visit, it is important to assess whether they are planning to ever become pregnant, to become pregnant in the near future, or to become pregnant many years from the time of the visit. It is easy to assume that the teen may want to avoid pregnancy for many years, but this assumption could lead to a bias in recommendations for contraceptive options and may affect the rapport established between the provider and patient if that teen does desire to become pregnant in the near future.

The Family Nurse Practitioner: Clinical Case Studies, Second Edition. Edited by Leslie Neal-Boylan.
© 2021 John Wiley & Sons Ltd. Published 2021 by John Wiley & Sons Ltd.

What diagnostic or screening tests would you consider running on this patient?

Minimal diagnostic and screening tests are required for the healthy adolescent patient asking to start contraceptives. Determining pregnancy status is the most important screening to complete prior to starting contraceptives, and determines when a contraceptive can be initiated. A provider can be reasonably certain that a patient is not pregnant if it has been 7 or fewer days since their last menses, they have not had intercourse since their last menses, they have been using other contraceptive methods reliably, it has been 7 or fewer days since a spontaneous or induced abortion, they are within 4 weeks postpartum, or they are fully or near fully breastfeeding with amenorrhea and less than 6 months postpartum. A urine pregnancy test can be obtained to corroborate the history provided by the patient, but timing of menses and ovulation must be taken into account and a repeat test may be required 2–4 weeks later. A beta pregnancy test would be unnecessary at this time unless the patient were to miss their next menstrual cycle.

STD testing should be encouraged and completed at the time of the visit when discussing contraceptives. A urine gonorrhea and chlamydia test is an easy, noninvasive test to diagnose more two more common STDs in adolescents. Consideration of serum testing for HIV and syphilis may also be appropriate. For this patient it would be unnecessary as she is asymptomatic, uses condoms regularly with intercourse, and does not have a high-risk sexual history of multiple partners or partners of the same sex/homosexual male partners. That being said, it is up to the patient and provider to decide which tests are most appropriate.

A pelvic exam would only be necessary in an adolescent patient who has decided to use an intrauterine device (IUD) as their form of birth control. The provider would need to be qualified in performing this procedure and complete a bimanual and cervical exam. A Pap smear is not required until the patient is 21 years old, regardless of sexual history, based on guidelines from the 2009 recommendations of the American College of Obstetricians and Gynecologists. Invasive cervical cancer has been determined to be rare in those less than 21 years old and the younger female population tends to have high rates of minor change in cytology, leading to further unnecessary and invasive testing with higher risks both immediately and in consideration of future family planning.

Obtaining bloodwork for a CBC and lipid panel is not necessary but may influence the provider and patient in deciding which method of contraception is appropriate based on side effects. For example, a CBC displaying a low hemoglobin level may lead the provider to test further for iron deficiency and determine whether a method that minimizes menstrual bleeding (duration and severity) or causes amenorrhea may be a good choice for that patient. Many combined oral contraceptive pills (OCPs) contain iron in the placebo week as well and may protect against any further deficiency. Neither would provide information that would contraindicate a specific contraceptive method.

Lauren agrees to complete a urine pregnancy screening today, which is negative, and a urine GC/CT test is sent to the lab (which returns negative). She declines bloodwork at the time of the visit.

What are the concerns at this point?

While Lauren appears to be acting responsibly regarding her own sexual health, concerns today would be risk for unintended pregnancy and transmission of sexually transmitted infections. While male latex condom use can protect against both, there is a high failure rate with typical use and as many as 18 out of 100 women using condoms as their only contraceptive will become pregnant unintentionally each year.

What is the diagnosis at this point?

Healthy, sexually active adolescent female at risk for pregnancy and/or STIs.

What types of contraceptives should be considered for Lauren?

The initial decision regarding appropriate contraceptive options is to determine whether she prefers hormonal versus nonhormonal options. With a negative personal and family history, either would be appropriate. All are safe for nulliparous females.

Nonhormonal options include male latex condoms and the long-acting reversible contraceptive (LARC) copper IUD (Paragard). Hormonal options include LARCs (Nexplenon implant, levonorgestrol (LNG) IUDs such as Mirena or Skyla), Depo-Provera (DMPA) injection, combined hormone contraceptives (OCPs, patch, and vaginal ring), progestin-only pills ("minipill"), and emergency contraceptives (Plan B or Ella). Ideally, the provider would present each option from most effective (LARCs such as the implant or IUDs) to least effective and provide education regarding administration of each method. Assessing possible barriers to each form of contraception is essential to maintain compliance and prevent unwanted pregnancies. This would be a great time to assess Lauren's comfort with invasive procedures (implant or IUD), comfort with her own body (inserting a vaginal ring), and desires for dosing frequency (not wanting to take a pill every day) or availability for follow-up visits. If she is not able to return for follow-ups at least every 3 months, DMPA injections would not be a good option for her. Exploring confidentiality and a desire to involve parents/guardians at this time will also affect which contraception method is the best fit for her. Cost may affect this decision as well, especially if parental involvement is not preferred.

How would each contraceptive option be initiated?

The "quick start" method for most contraceptives is preferred to increase adherence. Initiating the contraceptive on the day of the visit would be appropriate for most patients as long as there is reasonable certainty that pregnancy has been ruled out. Knowing the date of the start of the last menstrual period (LMP) as well as the date of last unprotected intercourse is necessary to make this determination.

- IUDs: If the patient had unprotected sexual intercourse within 5 days of the appointment, the copper IUD can be inserted as an emergency contraception option as well as for future pregnancy prevention. Pregnancy must be ruled out if it has been greater than 5 days since last unprotected intercourse and the patient is not currently menstruating. If unsure, another form of contraception can be initiated until the next menstrual cycle and the patient could then return for IUD insertion. The copper IUD does not require any back-up method after insertion. LNG IUDs require back-up contraception or abstaining from intercourse for 1 week if it has been greater than 7 days since their LMP.
- Implant (Nexplenon): The implant can be inserted on the same day as the initial visit when it is reasonably certain that the patient is not pregnant. If uncertain, benefits of inserting outweigh possible risks and the implant can still be inserted that day with a follow-up pregnancy test in 2–4 weeks. Backup contraception or abstaining from intercourse for 1 week is recommended if it has been greater than 5 days since LMP.
- DMPA (Depo-Provera) injection: The injection can be given at the time of the visit if the health care provider is reasonably certain that the patient is not pregnant. If uncertain, the injection can be given with a follow-up urine pregnancy test in 2–4 weeks. Backup contraception or abstaining from intercourse for 1 week is recommended if it has been greater than 7 days since the patient's LMP. The injection is then repeated every 13 weeks (3 months), although it can be given earlier, and for the adolescent population, appointments should be scheduled 11–12 weeks out in case of missed or delayed appointments. If it has been greater than 15 weeks between doses, reconfirmation of negative pregnancy status is required and backup contraception is recommended for 1 week following repeat injection.
- Combined hormonal contraceptives (OCPs, patch, vaginal ring): Quick start on day of visit if desired and patient is not pregnant. If uncertain, start and have patient return in 2–4 weeks for pregnancy test. Backup contraception or abstaining from intercourse is recommended if it has been 5 or more days since LMP. These methods can also be started on the first day of the next menstrual cycle, or using the "Sunday start" method, meaning the patient would begin on the Sunday after the start of their next menstrual cycle. An OCP will then need to be taken every day at the same time. The patch is applied once a week for 3 weeks, then removed for 1 week to allow for a withdrawal bleed. The vaginal ring is inserted and remains in place for 3 weeks, then is removed for 1 week prior to inserting a new ring.

- Progestin-only pill (mini-pill): Quick start on day of visit when it is reasonably certain that the patient is not pregnant. If uncertain, pills can be initiated and patient should return in 2–4 weeks to repeat pregnancy test. Backup contraception or abstaining from intercourse is recommended for 2 days if it has been greater than 5 days since LMP. The progestin-only pill must be taken at the same time each day for maximum effectiveness, and backup would be required for 2 days even if the pill is taken later than 3 hours after intended.
- Emergency contraception (Plan-B, Ella): Medication is to be taken within 5 days of unprotected intercourse. While Plan-B (levonorgestrel) is most effective 1–3 days after unprotected intercourse, Ella (Ulipristal) is more effective than Plan-B on days 3–5. Ella requires a prescription, but levonorgestrel emergency contraception can be purchased over the counter from a pharmacist.

What are some common contraindications to contraceptives?

While most contraceptive options are considered very safe, certain medical conditions can exacerbate possible adverse effects of these medications. While some are relative risks, a few are absolute contraindications in which the risks of potential adverse effects outweigh the benefits. It is important to consider when working with an adolescent with chronic medical issues that the risks of pregnancy may be greater than the risks of using contraceptives, and collaboration with their specialists is essential to ensure safe and effective treatment for that teen.

- IUDs: Anatomical abnormalities of the uterus, acute pelvic infection, known or suspected pregnancy, Wilson disease (copper IUD), undiagnosed vaginal bleeding, breast cancer (LNG-IUD), and hepatocellular adenoma or hepatoma (LNG-IUD).
- Implant (Nexplenon): Known or suspected pregnancy, severe cirrhosis, hepatocellular adenoma or hepatoma, undiagnosed vaginal bleeding, systemic lupus erythematosus with antiphospholipid antibodies, and breast cancer (known, suspected, or history of).
- DMPA (Depo-Provera): Cardiovascular disease (and risk factors), severe hypertension, ischemic heart disease or stroke, systemic lupus erythematosus with thrombocytopenia and/or antiphospholipid antibodies, undiagnosed vaginal bleeding, breast cancer, diabetes with vascular complications, severe cirrhosis, and hepatocellular adenoma or hepatoma.
- CHCs (OCPs, patch, ring): Arterial cardiovascular disease, hypertension, ischemic heart disease or stroke, known thrombophilia or thrombogenic mutations (coagulation disorders), history of deep vein thrombosis or pulmonary embolism, superficial venous thrombosis (current or history of), increased risk of thromboembolism (post-op, <21 days postpartum), complicated valvular heart disease, migraine with aura, breast cancer, complicated diabetes with vascular changes, medically treated gallbladder disease, acute viral hepatitis, history of surgery for obesity with malabsorption procedure, and drug interactions (few antiretroviral therapies, anticonvulsants, rifampin).

How should Lauren be counseled about side effects?

Possible side effects should be discussed with the patient at the initial visit as well as with each follow-up visit. When a patient experiences a side effect of a contraceptive method that they were not prepared for, this can decrease adherence or cause the patient to discontinue the method on their own, putting them at risk for unintended pregnancies.

Weight gain is often the most concerning side effect that adolescents worry about related to contraceptive use, but evidence shows that weight changes are typically not related to contraceptives with the exception of the DMPA injection. Diet and exercise counseling should be provided at all contraceptive visits when weight gain is suspected and of any concern to the patient or provider. A baseline weight should be obtained at the first contraceptive visit and monitored with each follow-up appointment.

- IUD: Irregular menstrual bleeding and/or cramping (heavy bleeding is more typical with the copper IUD, while irregular spotting is more common with the LNG-IUD and may lead to amenorrhea), infection (risk higher only in the first 21 days post-insertion), expulsion, perforation, pregnancy (ectopic or intrauterine, with both being rare).

- Progestin-related side effects with the LNG-IUD are less common due to low circulating levonorgestrel levels, but can cause acne, weight changes, hirsutism, headaches, nausea, and mood changes in females who are sensitive to hormone changes.
- Implant: Irregular menstrual bleeding, amenorrhea, headache, weight changes, acne, abdominal pain, breast tenderness, mood changes, local site reaction.
- DMPA injection: Local site reaction, irregular menstrual bleeding, amenorrhea, weight gain/increased appetite, headache, mood changes, decreased bone mineral density (reversible with discontinuation, but important to counsel regarding calcium/vitamin D intake or supplementation).
- CHCs (OCPs, patch, ring): Breast tenderness, nausea, bloating, irregular menstrual bleeding (typically resolves within first 3 months of use), local site reaction with patch, leukorrhea and vaginitis with ring.
- Progestin-only pill: Irregular menstrual bleeding, acne.
- Emergency contraceptives: Headache, abdominal pain, nausea, menstrual changes, fatigue, dizziness, breast tenderness.
- Condoms: Local site reaction/allergy to components.

What are the plans for referral and follow-up care?

Follow-up and referral is dependent on the setting of the initial contraceptive counseling visit and the provider's comfort and training with each method. If the adolescent is seen at their primary care pediatric office, contraceptive methods being prescribed by that primary care provider may be limited due to training. A referral to an adolescent gynecologist would be appropriate when more invasive contraceptive methods are being considered, such as the implant or IUD, or if a patient is not tolerating another prescribed method.

In adult medicine, routine follow-up for contraceptives is not recommended unless there are specific concerns. Working with adolescents typically requires closer, more frequent follow-up to screen for compliance and side effects, as well as assess the adolescent's satisfaction with their chosen contraceptive method. These visits also provide additional opportunities to educate the patient further on reproductive health.

What other education should Lauren be provided with related to reproductive health?

Reinforcing safe sex practices is essential during each contraceptive visit with the adolescent. She should be encouraged to continue use of condoms even with other contraceptives on board, as condoms are the only way to further protect her from STIs. Proper condom use should be reviewed with her as well during the visit to ensure as close to perfect use as possible. Reviewing how STIs are spread is imperative as well, since many teens engage in risky sexual behaviors but only use condoms for penile-vaginal penetration.

If she has not received the human papilloma virus (HPV) vaccine already, this would be an essential time to provide counseling to the patient (and parent if possible) to ensure that every step is being taken to protect her from future malignancy secondary to contracting HPV at a young age.

If the patient chooses not to discuss her choice to seek out birth control options with her mother, how would you proceed?

Adolescent confidentiality can provide for excellent rapport between a provider and teen patient, but can be a source of contention when a parent is seeking out confidential information regarding their adolescent child. The adolescent patient is more likely to share information regarding their reproductive health with the knowledge that what they disclose will remain between the provider and patient. Explaining confidentiality, including times where a breach in confidentiality would be required (disclosures of abuse, suicidal ideation, and/or homicidal ideation) to the patient at the start of each visit is important to maintaining a trusting relationship.

Reproductive health and adolescent confidentiality can be considered more complex in that the teen's ability to consent to reproductive care and contraceptives is regulated by state laws. A teen can consent to STI testing and treatment in every state. Providers should familiarize themselves with their state laws regarding consent for contraceptives and use these to guide patients to the safest, most effective way for the teen to obtain contraceptives. Open communication should be promoted between the teen and their parent/guardian.

Are there any standardized guidelines that should be used to treat this case? If so, what are they?

The Centers for Disease Control (CDC) and World Health Organization (WHO) provide many guidelines not only for the prescribing and initiation of contraceptives in the general population, but also for those with other medical conditions. The CDC also provides guidance for providers during special circumstances, such as when a patient who takes OCPs misses their pills or when a patient with an IUD is diagnosed with pelvic inflammatory disease. The American Academy of Pediatrics (AAP) has also developed a policy statement with guidance for prescribing contraceptives to teen patients.

- U.S. Medical Eligibility Criteria for Contraceptive Use (CDC, 2016)
- U.S. Selected Practice Recommendations for Contraceptive Use (CDC, 2016)
- Medical eligibility criteria for contraceptive use (WHO, 2015)
- Policy Statement: Contraceptive for Adolescents (AAP, 2014)

REFERENCES

Abma, J. C., & Martinez, G. M. (2017). Sexual activity and contraceptive practices among teenagers in the United States, 2011–2015. *National Health Statistics Report*. Retrieved June 25, 2019, from https://www.cdc.gov/nchs/data/nhsr/nhsr104.pdf

American Academy of Pediatrics. (2014). Policy statement: Contraception for adolescents. *Pediatrics*. doi:10.1542/peds.2014-2299

Aoun, J., Dines, V. A., Stovall, D. W., Mete, M., Nelson, C. B., & Gomez-Lobo, V. (2014). Effects of age, parity, and device type on complications and discontinuation of intrauterine devices. *Obstetrics & Gynecology*, *123*(3). doi:10.1097/AOG.0000000000000144

Callegari, L. S., Aiken, A. R., Dehlendorf, C., Cason, P., & Borrero, S. (2017). Addressing potential pitfalls of reproductive life planning with patient-centered counseling. *American Journal of Obstetrics and Gynecology*, *216*(2), 129–134. doi:10.1016/j.ajog.2016.10.004

Centers for Disease Control and Prevention. (2016). U.S. medical eligibility criteria for contraceptive use, 2016. *Morbidity and Mortality Weekly Report*, *65*(3). https://www.cdc.gov/mmwr/volumes/65/rr/pdfs/rr6503.pdf.

Centers for Disease Control and Prevention. (2016). U.S. selected practice recommendations for contraceptive use, 2016. *Morbidity and Mortality Weekly Report*, *65*(4). https://www.cdc.gov/mmwr/volumes/65/rr/pdfs/rr6504.pdf

Darney, P., Patel, A., Rosen, K., Shapiro, L. S., & Kaunitz, A. M. (2009). Safety and efficacy of a single-rod etonogestrel implant (Implanon): Results from 11 international clinical trials. *Fertility and Sterility*, *91*(5). doi:10.1016/j.fertnstert.2008.02.140

Diedrich, J. T., Desai, S., Zhao, Q., Secura, G., Madden, T., & Peipert, J. F. (2015). Association of short-term bleeding and cramping patterns with long-acting reversible contraceptive method satisfaction. *American Journal of Obstetrics and Gynecology*, *212*(1). doi:10.1016/j.ajog.2014.07.025

Foxx, A., Zhu, Y., Mitchel, E., Khabele, D., Griffin, M. R., & Nikpay, S. (2018). Cervical cancer screening and follow-up procedures in women age <21 years following new screening guidelines. *Journal of Adolescent Health*, *62*, 170–175. doi:10.1016/j.jadohealth.2017.08.027

Hubacher, D., Lopez, L., Steiner, M. J., & Dorflinger, L. (2009). Menstrual pattern changes from levonorgestrel subdermal implants and DMPA: Systematic review and evidence-based comparisons. *Contraception*, *80*(2), 113–118. doi:10.1016/j.contraception.2009.02.008

Jain, J., Jakimiuk, A., Bode, F., Ross, D., & Kaunitz, A. (2004). Contraceptive efficacy and safety of DMPA-SC. *Contraception*, *70*(4), 269–275. doi:10.1016/j.contraception.2004.06.011

Kavanaugh, M., Frohwirth, L., Jerman, J., Popkin, R., & Ethier, K. (2013). Long-acting reversible contraception for adolescents and young adults: Patient and provider perspectives. *Journal of Pediatric and Adolescent Gynecology*, *26*(2). doi:10.1016/j.jpag.2012.10.006

Lopez, L. M., Edelman, A., Chen, M., Otterness, C., Trussell, J., Helmerhorst, F. M., & Ramesh, S. (2016). Progestin-only contraceptives: Effects on weight. *Cochrane Database of Systematic Reviews*. doi:10.1002/14651858.CD008815.pub4

Lopez, L. M., Gallo, D. A., Gallo, M. F., Stockton, L. L., & Schultz, K. F. (2013). Skin patch and vaginal ring versus combined oral contraceptives for contraception. *Cochrane Database Systematic Reviews*. doi:10.1002/14651858.CD003552.pub4

Marcell, A. V., & Burstein, G. R. (2017). Sexual and reproductive health care services in the pediatric setting. *Pediatrics*, *140*(5). doi:10.1542/peds.2017-2858

Pfizer, Inc. (n.d.). *DEPO-PROVERA—medroxyprogesterone acetate injection, suspension*. Retrieved June 27, 2019, from http://labeling.pfizer.com/ShowLabeling.aspx?id=522

Pritt, N. M., Norris, A. H., & Berlan, E. D. (2017). Barriers and facilitators to adolescents' use of long-acting reversible contraceptives. *Journal of Pediatric and Adolescent Gynecology*, *30*(1). doi:10.1016/j.jpag.2016.07.002

Shapiro, S., & Dinger, J. (2010). Risk of venous thromboembolism among users of oral contraceptives: A review of two recently published studies. *Journal of Family Planning and Reproductive Health Care*, *36*(1), 33–38. doi:10.1783/147118910790291037

Steiner, M. J., Trussell, J., Mehta, N., Condon, S., Subramaniam, S., & Bourne, D. (2006). Communicating contraceptive effectiveness: A randomized controlled trial to inform a World Health Organization family planning handbook. *American Journal of Obstetrics and Gynecology*, *195*(1), 85–91. doi:10.1016/j.ajog.2005.12.053

U.S. FDA Prescribing Information. (2017, September). *Plan B (levonorgestrel)*. https://www.accessdata.fda.gov/drugsatfda_docs/label/2017/021045s016lbl.pdf

U.S. Food and Drug Administration (FDA) approved product information. (2018, October 5). *NEXPLANON—etonogestrel implant*. Retrieved June 27, 2019, from https://dailymed.nlm.nih.gov/dailymed/drugInfo.cfm?setid=b03a3917-9a65-45c2-bbbb-871da858ef34

U.S. Food and Drug Administration (FDA) approved product information. (2018, December 18). *NORETHINDRONE ACETATE—norethindrone tablet*. Retrieved June 27, 2019, from https://dailymed.nlm.nih.gov/dailymed/drugInfo.cfm?setid=64cb920c-36e8-4d62-9d08-3ddf3989d313

U.S. Food and Drug Administration (FDA) approved product information. (2018, June 8). *ELLA—ulipristal acetate tablet*. Retrieved June 27, 2019, from https://dailymed.nlm.nih.gov/dailymed/drugInfo.cfm?setid=052bfe45-c485-49e5-8fc4-51990b2efba4

Westhoff, C. L., Heartwell, S., Edwards, S., Zieman, M., Stuart, G., Cwiak, C., ... Robilotto, T. (2007). Oral contraceptive discontinuation: Do side effects matter? *American Journal of Obstetrics and Gynecology*, *196*(4). doi:10.1016/j.ajog.2006.12.015

World Health Organization. (2015). *Medical eligibility criteria for contraceptive use* (5th ed.). Geneva: Department of Reproductive Health and Research, World Health Organization. Retrieved June 24, 2019, from https://www.who.int/reproductivehealth/publications/family_planning/MEC-5/en/.

Case 5.6 Vaginal Discharge

Which diagnostic studies should be considered to assist with or confirm the diagnosis?

- NAAT for chlamydia/gonorrhea: diagnostic for chlamydia.
- Wet mount: pH = 3.9, Negative whiff test, WBCs present but no clue cells or trichomonads.
- Urine HCG: negative.
- HIV offered but refused this visit.
- RPR offered but refused this visit.

What is the most likely differential diagnosis and why?
Chlamydia (uncomplicated genital):
Chlamydia is often asymptomatic; however, Nora's symptoms of cloudy, mucoid discharge and intermenstrual spotting are indicative of infection.

What is the plan of treatment?
Nora will be treated with Azithromycin 1 gm orally for a single dose as recommended for treatment of uncomplicated chlamydia. Doxycycline 100 mg, BID × 7 days is an effective alternative, although compliance may be an issue.

How should this patient be counseled regarding the prevention of STIs?
Nora should be educated regarding the signs and symptoms of STIs. She should be reminded that STIs may be asymptomatic, making risk reduction and prevention essential. Discuss risk reduction including abstinence, monogamy, and condom use. Counsel Nora about correct and consistent condom use and subsequent reduction of any risk of recurrent chlamydia and/or other STIs. Remind her that this is a responsibility of both her and her partner. Counsel her about contraception options. She should be informed that hormonal contraception does not protect against STDs and HIV. Give Nora printed information about HIV testing and inform her that effective treatment for chlamydia may reduce susceptibility but not prevent transmission of HIV. Tell Nora that chlamydia is a reportable disease in all 50 states.

The Family Nurse Practitioner: Clinical Case Studies, Second Edition. Edited by Leslie Neal-Boylan.
© 2021 John Wiley & Sons Ltd. Published 2021 by John Wiley & Sons Ltd.

Is this patient at risk for HIV?

Risk for HIV exists in the presence of multiple partners and unprotected sex along with a diagnosed STI, including chlamydia.

Should this patient be retested for cure following treatment?

Nora should return for follow up testing in 3 months. The Centers for Disease Control recommends that all male or female persons with diagnosed chlamydia be rescreened in 3 months after initial treatment. This is recommended even if the patient believes that all partners have been treated. Chlamydia reinfection may occur in up to 1 in 5 individuals after treatment for initial infection.

Should this patient's partners be treated?

All partners within the past 60 days should be treated. Nora should be encouraged to tell all partners of her diagnosis to prevent reinfection of herself or others. If Nora expresses anxiety about partner treatment, explain that expedited partner therapy (EPT) is an option. (This option is state-specific, so check in your state).

REFERENCES AND RESOURCES

World Health Organization. 2016. *WHO guidelines for the treatment of chlamydia trachomatis* World Health Organization. Available from: https://www.ncbi.nlm.gov/books/NBK379707/

Papp, J. R., Schachter, J., Gaydos, C. A., & Van Der Pol, B. (2014). Recommendations for the laboratory-based detection of Chlamydia tracomatis and Neisseria gonorrhoeae–2014. *MMWR Recommendation Report*, 63,1–19.

Workowski, K. A., & Bolan, G.A. (2015). Sexually transmitted diseases treatment guidelines–2015. *MMWR Recommendation Report*, 64(RR-03), 1–137.

What concerns should be addressed at this visit and why?

1. Sexual identity: Michelle speaks clearly about her desire to present as a male. She again notes that she is not sexually active but is attracted to girls. This should be discussed in open, nonjudgmental conversation. Explain that sexual identity is not a diagnosis and that it is not necessary to be sexually active to define neither sexual orientation nor does being attracted to the same sex make one gay. Standard confidentiality practices for minor patients should be acknowledged but implications of premature disclosure of sexual identity (e.g., rejection, alienation) must be considered. Allow Michelle to set the pace of disclosure. A confidentiality agreement should be established and she must be aware of when it may be broken. This agreement commits the provider to keeping conversations private unless the adolescent is at risk of self-harm and/or harm of others. Trust is the basis for any future effective communication.
2. Anxiety/Depression: Explain the PHQ9 screening for depression and anxiety. Michelle should be aware that these screenings along with regular evaluation of safety are important concerns in adolescents with sexual identity issues. Encourage her to report any mood changes or negative thoughts to an accepting, supportive individual and seek help.

What case-specific questions should be asked addressing Michelle's desire for amenorrhea?

Ask Michelle to discuss her desire to stop having menstrual periods. Understanding her reasoning is basic to understanding any gender dysphoria. Michelle does not express opposition to her true gender assignment nor does she want "boy hormones" (testosterone). She states that she does not want to change her body but that not having a period will improve her chosen lifestyle. Listen to her concerns. She asks if there are ways to stop her period with medications. Explain that amenorrhea can be induced using continuous administration of oral contraceptive pills, progesterone-only long-acting reversible contraceptives (LARC) like depo-medroxyprogesteron acetate injections, or a levonorgestrel intrauterine device (IUD). Review the side effects, risks, and benefits of each method. Explain that possibility of long-term risks is unknown. Michelle tells you she has friends who use those methods for contraception. Encourage her to discuss the options with her mother or aunt and call with any questions.

Are any referrals needed?

A referral to a mental health professional who either specializes in, or is experienced with, gender issues is warranted. This is particularly important to help with feelings of depression, anxiety, or suicidal ideation. Michelle has described some depression and anxiety during your interview. It is also important to assist the adolescent with establishing a support system. This should include, in addition to adult family support, access to lesbian, gay, bisexual, transgender, queer (LGBTQ) groups. Michelle's rural area lacks support and inclusion groups at school or in the immediate community. Provide online sources and encourage her to look for groups outside the immediate community.

What complications exist related to the rural setting?

An LGBTQ lifestyle is less accepted in small rural areas than in urban cities. Safety is a primary concern for all LGBT people but is a greater concern in an unaccepting area where alternative lifestyles are not accepted. Access to wooded areas and firearms along with a decreased police presence should be considered. Bullying is a school concern and Michelle needs to be able to be open and report incidents to her mother or another support person. Assist and encourage Michelle to preserve family relationships and open conversation.

Are there implications for future medical care?

Comprehensive health care is necessary to promote normal adolescent development and continued physical health. An adolescent who is not yet sexually active should be educated about increased risk of STI, HIV, and HPV in the LGBTQ community.

What psychosocial challenges present with "coming out"?

Michelle tells you she started having dreams and fantasized about being a boy a few years ago. She wants to start dressing as a male and having her hair cut "like a boy." She wants to be called "Mick" instead of Michelle and prefers the pronoun "they" but has not told others yet. It is important that they develop a healthy, integrated identity; however, this will be challenged by prejudice, negative stereotypes, and in some instances lack of societal and family support. The fact that they feel, and will look, different than their peers will cause some turmoil. They have to be prepared to cope with this in a safe and healthy manner. Some adolescents turn to substance abuse to deal with negative, upsetting situations.

REFERENCES AND RESOURCES

AACAP releases practice parameter on sexual orientation, gender nonconformity, and gender identity issues in children and adolescents. (2013, August 1). *American Family Physician*, *88*(3),202–205.

Higgins, J. A., & Smith, N. K. (2016). The sexual acceptability of contraception: Reviewing the literature and building a new concept. *Journal of Sex Research*, *53*(4–5), 417–456.

Case 5.8 Knee Pain

RESOLUTION

Which diagnostic tests should be ordered in this case and why?

A CBC with differential can help indicate whether infection or malignancy is contributing to the patient's knee pain, as an elevated white blood cell (WBC) count would indicate infection. The CMP could be helpful in determining whether the liver and kidneys are functioning normally. In a case of Lyme disease, some transient elevation of liver enzymes can be found. ESR and CRP indicate inflammation and are nonspecific as to the cause of inflammation, but can help a provider determine how long inflammation has been present. An elevated rheumatoid factor and ANA can lead the provider toward a diagnosis of an autoimmune disorder, such as rheumatoid arthritis. It is important to note, however, that the ANA can be elevated in a majority of the population without significance. An LDH level indicates cell damage such as in a case of malignancy.

The ELISA with reflex Western blot test for Lyme disease can be diagnostic of Lyme disease if completed at the appropriate time after exposure to the disease. Most patients will be seropositive 6 or more weeks after exposure. If the test is done too soon, there is an increased likelihood of false negatives. If symptoms have been present for <30 days, IgM and IgG Western blot testing is performed. If symptoms have been present for >30 days, only IgG Western blot is performed. The IgM blot is considered positive if 2 or more of 3 bands are present. The IgG blot is considered positive if 5 or more bands of the 10 bands are present.

Imaging can also be helpful in determining a diagnosis for knee pain and swelling. An X-ray could assist a provider in determining whether trauma, injury, or malignancy is contributing to symptoms, and can rule out other diagnosis such as fractures, periostitis, avascular necrosis, bone tumors, and dysplasias. X-rays can also show the degree of joint effusion, or fluid accumulation in the joint, that is present. An MRI is typically completed when there is suspected injury to soft tissues, and can confirm diagnosis such as a torn cruciate or collateral ligaments, or torn meniscus.

A sample of synovial fluid, or fluid that has accumulated in the joint, can be diagnostic of the cause of the effusion. Cell counts such as an elevated WBC count would indicate an infection. A Gram stain, PCR, and culture/sensitivity can lead the provider to both a diagnosis and the most appropriate course of treatment. It is important to note that this is an invasive procedure.

The Family Nurse Practitioner: Clinical Case Studies, Second Edition. Edited by Leslie Neal-Boylan.
© 2021 John Wiley & Sons Ltd. Published 2021 by John Wiley & Sons Ltd.

Peter was sent to his local outpatient laboratory/imaging center for bloodwork and an X-ray of his knee. His WBC count was mildly elevated with a left shift toward immature cells, which can indicate an infection. The CMP displayed normal liver and kidney functions. His CRP was normal, but a moderately elevated ESR level was indicative of an infectious or autoimmune process that has been present and causing inflammation for some time. His ANA and rheumatoid factors were both negative, and LDH was within normal limits.

Peter's ELISA test was positive, so only an IgG Western blot was performed due to the presence of symptoms (fatigue, headaches) for >30 days. Seven IgG bands were detected, which is positive for Lyme disease that has been present for at least 6–8 weeks.

An X-ray of Peter's knee showed normal bone structure and spacing between bones with no fractures present, but demonstrated a significant joint effusion. An MRI or synovial fluid aspiration was not indicated at this time. An MRI may be suggested in the future if symptoms persist, and would likely be ordered and interpreted by a specialist such as an orthopedist. The same can be said regarding synovial fluid aspiration. If Peter were to become acutely ill or in need of inpatient care, synovial fluid aspiration may be warranted and an infectious disease team would be involved in this decision making.

What is the most likely differential diagnosis and why?

Based on the results of Peter's bloodwork and imaging, a diagnosis of Lyme arthritis is made. Oligoarthritis, commonly involving one large weight-bearing joint, is the most common late manifestation of disseminated Lyme disease. Lyme disease is an infection caused by the bacteria *Borrelia burgdorferi* that is transmitted to humans via a bite from a deer tick. The highest prevalence of Lyme disease is in the Northeast and Mid-Atlantic regions of the United States, and bites can be contracted from spending time in wooded areas. The tick must be attached for greater than 24 hours to transmit the infection. Because of the deer tick's small size and lack of pain associated with a bite, patients are often unable to recall the bite itself, as is the case with Peter. The most common initial sign of Lyme disease is the presence of the erythema migrans (EM), or "bull's-eye" rash at the site of the bite. Based on Peter's history, the development of an EM rash may have occurred in a place with less visibility, such as on the scalp under hair or on the buttocks.

What is the plan of treatment?

In Peter's case, the focus should be on both treating the infection and symptom management. Antibiotics are indicated for treatment of Lyme disease, with Doxycycline being the drug of choice. Based on Peter's weight and age, as well as his diagnosis of late (versus early) disseminated Lyme disease, he would be instructed to start Doxycycline 100 mg by mouth twice daily for 28 days. Musculoskeletal symptoms would be expected to resolve within 1–3 months of antibiotic therapy, and approximately 90% of patients see resolution with one course of antibiotics. More severe symptoms could result in hospitalization and IV antibiotic administration. Symptom management is often obtained through the use of nonsteroidal anti-inflammatory drugs (NSAIDs) to address both pain and inflammation, and should be given with food to avoid gastrointestinal side effects.

What are the plans for referral and follow-up care?

Early signs of Lyme disease can be treated and followed by the primary care provider. Involvement with specialists is sometimes warranted to assist in managing symptoms and treatment options in more progressive cases. In this case, referral to an orthopedist and infectious disease specialist could be beneficial for the patient to ensure that the infection is adequately treated and long-term complications are avoided. A referral would be especially appropriate if symptoms are persisting past the initial 28-day course of Doxycycline.

What health education should be provided to this patient?

Initially, education for this patient and family should focus on diagnosis and treatment options. The patient should receive thorough instructions regarding Doxycycline administration and the importance of completing the full course of antibiotics, as well as common side effects such as esophagitis and allergic reactions. A key part of educating patients and families about tick-borne illnesses lies in prevention. Minimizing exposure to ticks, especially during warmer months, is an important step in preventing tick-borne illnesses. Centers for Disease Control and Prevention (CDC) recommendations should be reviewed with patients, including avoiding wooded areas with high grass, wearing insect repellent, wearing long sleeves/long pants in wooded areas with socks pulled over pant legs, and completing comprehensive tick checks on yourself, children, and pets after outdoor exposure, with careful examination of commonly missed places such as folds.

What demographic characteristics might affect this case?

The patient's ethnicity and gender do not affect this case. The age of the patient does affect treatment options. The education level of the patient should be taken into consideration no matter the diagnosis when it comes to providing appropriate education and materials.

The geographic location of the patient and family should be taken into account when considering a differential diagnosis including tick-borne illnesses. It is always important to ask about travel, especially in this case, where the patient lives in an urban setting (New York City) but was living in a rural setting working in an outdoor camp (Connecticut).

While not present in this particular case, studies have found larger-scale health disparities associated with Lyme disease in the United States. Areas of temporarily or permanently vacant homes (where rodents and other small mammals for tick species live) show increases in rates of infection among humans. Another possible factor is overgrown greening and lack of pest control. Another contrasting study showed evidence of reverse health disparity with Lyme disease, where the incidence was highest in counties with more socioeconomically advantaged populations and was positively associated with population with a bachelor's degree or higher: the contrasting health disparities in this study remain unclear (Springer & Johnson, 2018).

Are there any standardized guidelines that should be used to treat this case? If so, what are they?

The American Academy of Pediatrics (AAP) Red Book contains up-to-date guidelines for diagnosing and treating infectious diseases, including Lyme disease. The CDC also provides diagnosis and treatment guidelines for health care providers, as well as education for the general population.

Is there any other information that would be helpful in determining a diagnosis?

A comprehensive history, exam, and laboratory testing is most helpful in determining a diagnosis. Some information that could help direct a provider toward a clear diagnosis would be obtaining more information about Peter's time spent in the woods and whether he was performing tick checks, as well as a thorough review of systems and assessment of his pain, including what time of day and what activities exacerbate his knee pain.

If this patient were 6 years old, would it change how he would be tested and treated?

In a 6-year-old patient presenting with acute monoarticular arthritis, as with a patient of any age, testing is dependent on the severity and quality of symptoms. Serum laboratory screening would likely be ordered assessing for the same differential diagnosis to help determine the cause (infectious, injury, autoimmune, or malignancy) of the swelling and pain. Consideration of the child's developmental status would be important when considering imaging such as an MRI, where the child would have to remain still for an extended period of time. Synovial fluid testing is an invasive procedure that would possibly require sedation in a younger child, and would likely only be performed if the child were inpatient and if that information were pertinent to determining a diagnosis.

If the child in the case were a 6-year-old who tested seropositive for Lyme disease, the antibiotic of choice is Amoxicillin due to concerns of tooth staining with Doxycycline use in young children. Children under 8 years old require Amoxicillin 50 mg/kg/day divided 3 times a day for treatment of Lyme disease, with the duration of the course of antibiotics depending on their symptoms. Musculoskeletal symptoms such as arthritis still require a 28-day course of antibiotics.

At what point would inpatient treatment be more appropriate than outpatient for this patient?

Inpatient treatment would be appropriate for this patient if the teen were experience more severe symptoms, such as prolonged high fevers (>104° F for >3 days) or inability to bear weight on the affected leg. A child with this severity of symptoms may require IV antibiotics as treatment as well, as more invasive testing (synovial fluid, lumbar puncture) to determine whether Lyme disease is the correct and only diagnosis causing symptoms for this patient.

REFERENCES AND RESOURCES

Agodi, A., Barchitta, M., Trigilia, C., Barone, P., Marino, S., Garozzo, R., . . . Cataldo, A. D. (2013). Neutrophil counts distinguish between malignancy and arthritis in children with musculoskeletal pain: A case–control study. *BMC Pediatrics, 13*(1). doi:10.1186/1471-2431-13-15

Bockenstedt, L. K., & Wormser, G. P. (2014). Unraveling Lyme disease. *Arthritis & Rheumatology, 66*(9), 2313–2323. doi:10.1002/art.38756

Centers for Disease Control. (2018, December 21). Preventing tick bites on people | Lyme disease. Retrieved June 17, 2019, from https://www.cdc.gov/lyme/prev/on_people.html

Cruz, A. I., Aversano, F. J., Seeley, M. A., Sankar, W. N., & Baldwin, K. D. (2017). Pediatric Lyme arthritis of the hip. *Journal of Pediatric Orthopaedics, 37*(5), 355–361. doi:10.1097/bpo.0000000000000664

Daikh, B. E., Emerson, F. E., Smith, R. P., Lucas, F. L., & McCarthy, C. A. (2013). Lyme arthritis: A comparison of presentation, synovial fluid analysis, and treatment course in children and adults. *Arthritis Care & Research, 65*(12), 1986–1990. doi:10.1002/acr.22086

Gerber, M. A., Shapiro, E. D., Burke, G. S., Parcells, V.J., & Bell, G. L., for the Pediatric Lyme Disease Study Group. (1996). Lyme disease in children in southeastern Connecticut. *New England Journal of Medicine, 335*(17), 1270.

Kimberlin, D. W., Brady, M. T., Jackson, M., & Long, S. S. (2018). *Red Book: 2018 report of the Committee on Infectious Diseases, American Academy of Pediatrics* (31st ed.). Itasca, IL: American Academy of Pediatrics.

Reisen, W. K. (2010). Landscape epidemiology of vector-borne disease. *Annual Review of Entomology, 55*, 461–483. pmid 193737082.

Springer, Y. P., & Johnson, P. T. J. (2018). Large-scale health disparities associated with Lyme disease and human monocytic ehrlichiosis in the United States, 2007–2013. *PLoS ONE, 13*(9), e0204609. https://doi.org/10.1371/journal.pone.0204609

Steere, A., Levin, R., Molloy, P., Kalish, R., Abraham, J., 3rd, Liu, N., & Schmid, C. (1994). Treatment of Lyme arthritis. *Arthritis & Rheumatology, 37*(6), 878.

Thiers, B. (2006). Hematogenous dissemination in early Lyme disease. *Yearbook of Dermatology and Dermatologic Surgery, 2006*, 114. doi:10.1016/s0093-3619(08)70071-6

Thompson, A., Mannix, R., & Bachur, R. (2009). Acute pediatric monoarticular arthritis: Distinguishing Lyme arthritis from other etiologies. *Pediatrics, 123*(3), 959–965. doi:10.1542/peds.2008-1511

Wallendal, M. (1996). The discriminating value of serum lactate dehydrogenase levels in children with malignant neoplasms presenting as joint pain. *Archives of Pediatrics & Adolescent Medicine, 150*(1), 70. doi:10.1001/archpedi.1996.02170260074012

Wormser, G. P., Dattwyler, R. J., Shapiro, E. D., Halperin, J. J., Steere, A. C., Klempner, M. S., . . . Nadelman, R. B. (2006). The clinical assessment, treatment, and prevention of Lyme disease, human granulocytic anaplasmosis, and babesiosis: Clinical practice guidelines by the Infectious Diseases Society of America. *Clinical Infectious Diseases,43*(9), 1089–1134. doi:10.1086/508667

Case 6.1 Preconception Planning

What health recommendations should be made for Delilah in order to help her prepare for pregnancy?

- Delilah's BMI is 30.5, which is considered obese. Obesity is associated with increased rates of infertility, along with a multitude of other chronic health conditions. Counseling on weight loss, healthy diet, and increasing physical activity levels would be appropriate.
- Smoking and alcohol use during pregnancy are associated with a number of risks, including premature birth, spontaneous abortion (miscarriage), stillbirth, and intrauterine growth retardation. Smoking cessation counseling as well as counseling on reducing/eliminating alcohol consumption prior to trying to conceive is of utmost importance at this visit. Patients are often more motivated to discuss smoking and alcohol cessation when thinking about conceiving or becoming pregnant.
- Delilah's sleep habits are poor due to her work schedule; helping her find a way to develop a more regular sleep routine would be beneficial to her overall health. Additionally, limiting caffeine intake is recommended when trying to conceive and during pregnancy.
- Ensuring that Delilah's asthma remains well controlled prior to pregnancy is important; the use of inhaled steroids is not contraindicated during pregnancy.
- Due to her job, a detailed travel history should be obtained and risks associated with Zika exposure should be reviewed.
- Depression and anxiety are common conditions in women of childbearing age and untreated depression during pregnancy is associated with poorer maternal and child outcomes. Screening for depression and anxiety during the preconception visit is recommended so, if necessary, treatment can be started and adjusted prior to conceiving.
- Assessing risk for sexually transmitted infections is also recommended. If any risk exists, STI screening should be completed. Screening for HIV is recommended in all pregnant women.
- Reviewing Delilah's immunization history and ensuring up-to-date vaccinations and/or evidence of immunity to tetanus, diphtheria, pertussis, varicella, measles, mumps, and rubella is an important part of preconception care.

The Family Nurse Practitioner: Clinical Case Studies, Second Edition. Edited by Leslie Neal-Boylan.
© 2021 John Wiley & Sons Ltd. Published 2021 by John Wiley & Sons Ltd.

What laboratory/diagnostic testing is recommended?

HIV screening is recommended for all women planning pregnancy. Screening for tuberculosis (TB) may be recommended, depending on whether Delilah travels to regions with a high prevalence of TB. Delilah is due for her Pap smear, which can be completed today. Routine HPV screening is not recommended in women under the age of 30. Screening for diabetes with a fasting blood sugar or hemoglobin A1c is warranted based on her mother's history.

How should Delilah's medication list be adjusted? Are any of the medications teratogenic? Are there any medications/vitamins or supplements she should start taking?

None of Delilah's current prescription medications are teratogenic. It is important that she continue on her asthma controller medication to ensure adequate asthma control. Delilah should be counseled that when she is pregnant she should avoid products containing ibuprofen; acetaminophen-based products are fine. She does not have to change this until she is actively trying to become pregnant.

In preparation for pregnancy it is recommended that Delilah start taking a daily folic acid supplement to help prevent neural tube defects. A supplement with 0.4 mg of folic acid per day is adequate for most women. A daily prenatal vitamin would also be recommended. The folic acid requirement is often found within the prenatal vitamin.

When should she stop her birth control pills?

Oral contraceptive (birth control) pills are considered an immediately reversible form of contraception. Therefore, it is possible for Delilah to become pregnant immediately after stopping the pill. If she and her husband would like to conceive in 6 months, it would be recommended that she remain on her birth control pill until that time.

How should she be counseled about seeing a fertility specialist? When would this be recommended?

The risk of infertility increases with age. In women under the age of 35, evaluation by a fertility specialist is not recommended until they have been actively trying to conceive for 12 months.

Would anything be different if Delilah were 38 instead of 28?

Once over the age of 35, evaluation with a fertility specialist is recommended after 6 months of actively trying to conceive.

REFERENCES AND RESOURCES

Frieder, A., Dunlop, A. L., Culpepper, L., & Bernstein, P. S. (2008). The clinical content of preconception care: Women with psychiatric conditions. *American Journal of Obstetrics and Gynecology, 199*(6), S328–S332.

Moos, M. K., Dunlop, A. L., Jack, B. W., Nelson, L., Coonrod, D. V., Long, R., . . . Gardiner, P. M. (2008). Healthier women, healthier reproductive outcomes: Recommendations for the routine care of all women of reproductive age. *American Journal of Obstetrics and Gynecology, 199*(6 Suppl. 2), S280–S289.

Case 6.2 Bleeding in the First Trimester of Pregnancy

RESOLUTION

What is the most likely differential diagnosis in this case?
Spontaneous inevitable abortion.

Which diagnostic tests are required in this case and why?
CBC with differential: A CBC with differential is necessary to determine baseline level and/or need for emergent consultation if there is a significant hemorrhage or to rule out rupture of an ectopic pregnancy.

Blood type with Rhesus type and antibody screen: Blood type with Rhesus type and antibody screen may be considered for this patient. Although not diagnostic, many patients have Rh sensitization as the reason for recurrent spontaneous abortions.

Beta hCG: Beta hCG is a necessary test for this patient to determine if Tasha is pregnant. One of the first considerations is to determine if the vaginal bleeding is due to an obstetrical nonobstetrical cause. A beta hCG will help confirm a diagnosis of miscarriage and is required for management of this patient in determining baseline data and trending data with serial beta hCG testing for follow-up. Normal beta hCG levels double every 1–2 days in early pregnancy; slow-rising levels or lower-than-expected levels help confirm a diagnosis of spontaneous miscarriage.

Progesterone level: A progesterone level can help confirm the diagnosis of a miscarriage. Values less than 5 ng/ml indicate abnormal or nonviable pregnancy.

Doppler fetal heart tones: Heart tones can be considered in a fetus that is 10 weeks gestational age or greater and can confirm a pregnancy if fetal heart tones are heard. In this patient, who is having a miscarriage, fetal heart tones cannot be heard so this is not useful as a diagnostic tool.

Transvaginal ultrasound: A transvaginal ultrasound is warranted in this case to help determine the diagnosis and will guide the management of this patient. A transvaginal ultrasound will determine if there is an intrauterine versus extrauterine pregnancy, can confirm fetal heartbeats (which is diagnostic), and can provide an estimated due date and gestational age. In addition, a diagnosis can be made regarding the type of spontaneous abortion: complete, threatened, missed, or incomplete.

Abdominal ultrasound: An abdominal ultrasound is often a useful diagnostic tool; however, in early pregnancy, the products of conception are frequently located in the uterus, which is tucked behind the symphysis pubis, making it difficult to fully complete an abdominal ultrasound. In pregnancy, abdominal ultrasounds are most useful in the second and third trimesters.

The Family Nurse Practitioner: Clinical Case Studies, Second Edition. Edited by Leslie Neal-Boylan.
© 2021 John Wiley & Sons Ltd. Published 2021 by John Wiley & Sons Ltd.

What are the concerns at this point?

The patient presents with excessive vaginal bleeding so the primary concern should be of an acute hemorrhage and ectopic pregnancy. After the emergency evaluation, the focus should be on diagnosing a spontaneous inevitable abortion.

What is the plan of treatment?

An inevitable abortion will require management to ensure complete evacuation of the products of conception. Most women will spontaneously pass the products of conception and expectant management is an acceptable treatment.

Expectant management is a recommended treatment if the pregnancy is less than 12 weeks gestational age, the patient is hemodynamically stable, and there are no signs of infection. Expectant management allows the patient to continue and naturally pass products of conception outside the clinical/hospital setting. Patients should be educated to monitor for excessive bleeding or saturation of a sanitary pad every hour or more frequently. They should monitor for fever and report fevers greater than 100.4°F to the health care provider. Pain and cramping are normal expectations, especially during the passing of tissues. The patient can take over-the-counter ibuprofen 600 mg every 6 hours. If expectant management is unsuccessful after 4 weeks, then medical or surgical management is recommended.

Surgical evacuation should be performed on patients who are hemodynamically unstable or have additional complications. The treatment plan should include surgical evacuation. Surgical evacuation is done with dilatation and curettage (D&C). Surgical management has been shown to have high success rates for evacuation of the products of conception; however, there are increased risks to surgical procedures

What are the plans for follow-up care?

Beta hCG testing: Beta hCG levels should return to normal within 2–6 weeks after the evacuation of the products of conception. For patients who have had expectant management or medical management, weekly hCG levels should be drawn until the level is undetected.

Counseling: Many patients may require counseling after a spontaneous abortion. Regardless of whether the pregnancy was planned or unplanned, many patients will grieve for the loss and may need some support.

Family planning: Talk with the patient regarding the need for family planning and the need for safe sexual practices while in the perimenopausal state. The perimenopausal period can last a few years, during which the patient can become pregnant. Contraception should begin as soon as the abortion is complete.

Are there any standardized guidelines that should be used to treat this case? If so, what are they?

The American College of Emergency Medicine has a clinical policy on the evaluation and management of patient in early pregnancy (https://www.sciencedirect.com/sdfe/pdf/download/eid/1-s2.0-S0196064412004064/first-page-pdf).

The American College of Obstetricians and Gynecologist has a practice bulletin on the management of spontaneous abortions (https://www.acog.org/Clinical-Guidance-and-Publications/Practice-Bulletins/Committee-on-Practice-Bulletins-Gynecology/Early-Pregnancy-Loss).

REFERENCES AND RESOURCES

American College of Obstetricians and Gynecologists. (2015). Practice bulletin number 100: Early pregnancy loss. *Obstetrics and Gynecology*, *125*(5), 1258. https://www.acog.org/Clinical-Guidance-and-Publications/Practice-Bulletins/Committee-on-Practice-Bulletins-Gynecology/Early-Pregnancy-Loss

Hahn, S. A., Lavonas, E. J., Mace, S. E., Napoli, A. M., & Fesmire, F. M. (2012). Clinical policy: Critical issues in the initial evaluation and management of patients presenting to the emergency department in early pregnancy. *Annals of Emergency Medicine*, *60*(3), 381–390.

King, T. L., Brucker, M. C., Kriebs, J. M., & Fahey, J. O. (2013). Varney's midwifery (5th ed.). Jones & Bartlett.

Case 6.3 Night Sweats

RESOLUTION

What are the top three differential diagnoses to consider for Susan and why?

Menopause-related symptoms:

Susan is experiencing several of the most common symptoms (e.g., hot flashes, night sweats, sleep disturbances, weight gain, altered sexual function) related to menopause transition as well as several associated symptoms (e.g., altered mood, hair thinning, memory changes) (see Table 6.3.1) (Alexander, Jakubisin Konicki, Barandouzi, et al., in press; Baber, Panay & Fenton, 2016; North American Menopause Society [NAMS], 2014). This diagnosis is usually made based on the history and physical examination. Selected diagnostic studies may be warranted to rule out comorbid conditions that may affect Susan's symptom severity and the management plan (Alexander, Jakubisin Konicki, Barandouzi, et al., in press; Baber et al., 2016; NAMS, 2014).

Endocrine disorder:

An endocrine disorder, especially hypothyroidism, must also be considered. Hypothyroidism has many common presenting symptoms that overlap with symptoms of the menopause transition (North American Menopause Society [NAMS], 2014). For example, Susan has described hair loss, fatigue, reduced libido, weight gain, irritability, memory loss, altered menstrual cycles, and reduced libido. These symptoms are all associated with both menopause and hypothyroidism (Garber et al., 2012; NAMS, 2014). She has not described cold temperature intolerance, weakness, constipation, hair texture changes, skin texture changes (dry and rough), or muscle aches, which are other symptoms associated with hypothyroidism (Garber et al., 2012). Additionally, she has described symptoms that are not commonly associated with hypothyroidism but that are commonly associated with the transition to post-menopause, such as hot flashes, night sweats, and sleep disturbances (Alexander et al., in press; NAMS, 2014). Given the overlap in symptoms and the potential for untreated hypothyroidism to exacerbate symptoms of the transition to post-menopause, it would be prudent to check Susan's TSH level.

Like hypothyroidism, a sexual desire disorder is an important comorbid diagnosis to consider for Susan. Reduced libido is common among midlife women; however, a specific sexual desire disorder can also be present. The management of these 2 problems differs, so it is important to distinguish exactly what Susan is experiencing. The most common sexual desire disorder among women is female sexual interest/arousal disorder, formerly known as hypoactive sexual desire disorder, which affects approximately 43% of women (American College of Obstetrics and Gynecology [ACOG],

The Family Nurse Practitioner: Clinical Case Studies, Second Edition. Edited by Leslie Neal-Boylan.
© 2021 John Wiley & Sons Ltd. Published 2021 by John Wiley & Sons Ltd.

Table 6.3.1. Symptoms Associated with the Menopause Transition.

System	Symptoms
Central nervous system	Anxiety/nervousness, cognitive changes, depression, dizziness, fatigue, forgetfulness, formication, headache, hot flashes/flushes, insomnia, irritability/ mood disturbances/"rage," night sweats, poor concentration, sleep disturbances, paresthesia
Eyes	Dry eyes
Cardiovascular	Palpitations
Breast	Mastalgia
Gynecologic and sexual	Dyspareunia, irregular menstrual bleeding, recurrent vaginitis, reduced libido, vaginal atrophy, vaginal dryness, vaginal/vulvar irritation, vaginal/vulvar pruritus
Musculoskeletal	Arthralgia, asthenia, myalgia
Urinary	Dysuria, genitourinary burning, recurrent cystitis, nocturia, stress urinary incontinence[*], urinary frequency, urinary urgency
Skin and hair	Acne, dry skin and hair, hirsutism/virilization, skin dryness/atrophy, thinning hair, odor (increased perspiration)

*Data are inconclusive.
Source: From: Alexander et al. (in press); Baber et al. (2016); North American Menopause Society [NAMS] (2014).

2019; Shifren, Monz, Russo, Segreti & Johannes, 2008). Female sexual interest and arousal disorder is a lack of or decrease in at least three areas involving sexual activity interest, thoughts, responsiveness, excitement or pleasure, arousal, or sensations associated with sexual activity for a minimum of 6 months that has resulted in personal distress. This diagnosis is only met when there is no other non-sexual disorder to explain the symptoms (ACOG, 2019). While Susan described missing her previous level of desire for sex, she does enjoy sex when it happens; and she does not describe significant distress, noting that it is a "bummer" and that she misses wanting sex like she used to. It is also unlikely that Susan is experiencing female sexual interest and arousal disorder as she does not avoid sexual contact with her partner; conversely, she has noted that she misses their usual level of sexual activity.

Depression:
Depression is less likely for Susan due to the array of symptoms that she is not experiencing and that are required to make a diagnosis of depression. The 5th edition of the *American Psychiatric Association Diagnostic and Statistical Manual of Mental Disorders (DSM-5)* specifies criteria for the diagnosis of depression (American Psychiatric Association [APA], 2013). *DSM-5* states that patients must experience symptoms for at least 2 weeks, including a change in functioning with either depressed mood or a loss of interest in things that they used to enjoy. Additionally, there must be at least 7 other symptoms, which can include depressed mood or loss of interest in enjoyable activities/anhedonia, as well as substantive appetite and weight changes, sleep disturbances, suicidal thoughts or ideation, feeling worthless or excessively guilty, fatigue, cognitive changes (forgetfulness, difficulty concentrating), or psychomotor changes (retardation or agitation) (APA, 2013). When considering depression it is important to note that Susan does not describe enough symptoms to meet the *DSM-5* criteria for depression. However, it is also important to recognize that depression often does affect women at midlife and may exacerbate symptoms of the menopause transition (Green, Key, & McCabe, 2015; Natari, Clavarino, McGuire, Dingle, & Hollingworth, 2018; NAMS, 2014; Weber, Maki, & McDermott, 2014).

Other:
Other even less likely differentials might include TB, untreated DM or HTN, and other psychiatric disorders. None of these diagnoses carry enough overlapping symptoms with those described by Susan and commonly associated with the transition to post-menopause to make them likely as her primary diagnosis. DM and HTN could exacerbate her menopause-related symptoms. However, she does not have an elevated BP on examination, and she does not have symptoms suggestive of DM. TB is the least likely of all because the only overlapping symptom is night sweats.

Which diagnostic tests are required for managing Susan's condition and why?

Diagnostic testing is not needed to diagnose the menopause transition except for ruling out comorbid conditions or identifying medical problems that may exacerbate the woman's menopause transition symptoms and thus affect the plan of care.

1. *FSH, estrogen, and LH levels:* Hormone levels are not tested to determine menopausal status (NAMS, 2014). Hormone levels are very volatile during the perimenopausal years, rendering testing at any one point in time useless (NAMS, 2014). The goal of treatment is symptom management, and hormone levels are not used to monitor efficacy. Thus knowledge of specific hormone levels is unnecessary. Additionally, if hormone levels are tested, the information may falsely suggest that the woman is postmenopausal when she is actually perimenopausal and could still ovulate and become pregnant.
2. *TSH level:* Testing TSH may be useful to determine if Susan also has a thyroid problem. It will not aid in diagnosing the menopause transition but may guide care, as an untreated thyroid disorder can exacerbate symptoms of the menopause transition.
3. *Fasting lipid panel and fasting blood sugar level:* While it may be reasonable to order a fasting lipid panel for Susan if she has not had one recently, it will not forward the diagnosis of her symptoms. Testing a fasting blood sugar level may be useful in identifying if Susan also has DM. This also will not aid in diagnosing the menopause transition but may guide care, as untreated DM can exacerbate symptoms of the menopause transition and may alter the selection of pharmacotherapeutics.
4. *CBC, BUN/creatinine, eGFR:* These tests are not needed for diagnosing the menopause transition. Knowing Susan's kidney function status may be useful when determining whether to use pharmacotherapeutics to manage her symptoms.
5. *LFTs:* These tests are not needed for diagnosing the menopause transition. Knowing Susan's liver function status may be useful when determining whether to use pharmacotherapeutics to manage her symptoms.
6. *Beck Depression Inventory (BDI):* Administering the BDI may be useful to determine if Susan also has depression. It will not aid in diagnosing the menopause transition, but it may guide care, as untreated depression can exacerbate menopause transition symptoms and may alter the selection of pharmacotherapeutics.
7. *PPD/Quantiferon gold:* If Susan had a history suggesting exposure to TB, it would be prudent to check PPD or quantiferon gold because she is experiencing night sweats. However, most of her history suggests an alternate diagnosis; for example, she is gaining, rather than losing weight and she has no cough or other symptoms suggestive of TB. Thus, it is unlikely that testing for TB will provide useful clinical information.
8. *DXA:* It is too early to order a routine DXA for Susan (Cosman et al., 2014). Guidelines recommend evaluating all postmenopausal women at age 65 unless they have specific additional risk factors (Cosman et al., 2014). DXA test results will not aid in the diagnosis of her symptoms.
9. *Colonoscopy:* The American Cancer Society recommends that all adults receive colon cancer screening at age 50 or earlier depending on personal history (Wolf et al., 2018). Colonoscopy, however, will not aid in the diagnosis of her symptoms.

What are the concerns at this point?

Susan has a history of gestational hypertension with her second pregnancy. There is a twofold risk for the development of cardiovascular disease in women with a history of hypertensive disorders of pregnancy (HDP) (Timpka et al., 2018). Susan will benefit from lifestyle measures that focus on promotion of heart- healthy behaviors and monitoring for cardiovascular disease.

What is the plan of treatment options to be discussed with Susan?

Most of Susan's symptoms are related to her hot flashes. Vasomotor symptoms cause sleep disruptions, which in turn affect mood, energy level, memory, and cognitive processes. Once the hot flashes are controlled and sleep is restored, the associated symptoms usually will resolve (NAMS, 2007). A stepped approach is recommended for managing vasomotor symptoms associated with the menopause transition (Alexander et al., in press; Daley, Stokes-Lampard, Thomas, & MacArthur, 2014). Start by advising Susan about lifestyle and environmental changes that can reduce her symptoms, then explore complementary and alternative medicine therapies (CAM) that might help her, and, finally, prescribe medications if needed.

Susan likely would benefit from increasing her routine aerobic activity. Her goal should be at least 1 hour each day, but even small increases may be beneficial (Baber et al., 2016; NAMS, 2014). Aerobic exercise helps to decrease hot flash severity and frequency by improving the body's ability to maintain temperature regulation (Thompson, Church, & Blair, 2008). Regular exercise also improves sleep quality, memory, and quality of life; decreases depression; reduces cardiac disease risk; and helps to maintain normal blood glucose levels and weight in midlife women (Thompson et al., 2008).

Susan also needs to be counseled to avoid hot flash triggers such as caffeine (any type —cold, hot, solid, liquid—can trigger flashes), concentrated sugar, alcohol, and food additives such as sodium nitrates, sulfites, and monosodium gluconate. Reducing or avoiding use of these substances can reduce both frequency and severity of her vasomotor symptoms (NAMS, 2014). Increasing her consumption of ice water may help to stabilize her core temperature and reduce hot flashes (ACOG, 2016).

Susan can further reduce her symptoms by wearing breathable fabrics like cottons that allow for greater air movement and avoiding synthetics and tight clothing. Wearing layers that can easily be removed when she feels hot and avoiding high necklines and turtleneck shirts may reduce her symptoms and embarrassment at work. Using breathable fabrics for her pajamas, sheets, and blankets is important as well. Using a fan to circulate the air and keeping the room temperature at a moderately cool level may also reduce hot flashes (Alexander et al., in press; NAMS, 2014).

Several CAM therapies such as relaxation and deep breathing exercises, acupuncture, and selected botanical or herbal preparations may be useful in reducing vasomotor symptoms caused by the menopause transition. Stress and anxiety are triggers for hot flashes (Alexander et al., 2004), so it stands to reason that relaxation and stress-reducing practices, like yoga, prayer, and talking over problems, can decrease hot flashes (NAMS, 2014). Susan can be taught to do paced deep breathing (like yoga breathing: breathe in deeply over a count of 5, hold the breath for a count of 7, then exhale over a count of 9) to reduce hot flashes when they occur or to reduce her stress in general (Freedman & Woodward, 1992; Freedman, Woodward, Brown, Javaid, & Pandy, 1995). Acupuncture is another CAM therapy that provides stress relief. Evidence suggests that there are some beneficial effects of acupuncture in the treatment of menopause-related symptoms of sleep disorders and vasomotor symptoms (Befus et al., 2018; Chiu et al., 2015; NAMS, 2014; Nedeljkovic et al., 2014). Susan could try acupuncture if she is interested; it is a well-accepted and safe practice that promotes relaxation.

Many women are interested in trying botanical and herbal preparations to manage their menopause transition symptoms. Several preparations are commonly used, including black cohosh, dong quai, various isoflavones (i.e., soy extracts, red clover, soy supplementation), oil of evening primrose, and ginseng (Ahsan & Mallick, 2017; Messina, 2014). Black cohosh is usually well tolerated and has the most evidence supporting its use. It may have some estrogenic activity (NAMS, 2014), so if Susan decides to try this she will need to be monitored for endometrial overgrowth. She also needs to be warned to watch for signs of liver problems, as case reports have identified hepatitis and liver toxicity in some women (Mahady et al., 2008).

Pharmacotherapeutics: Both nonhormonal and hormonal prescription options are available to help Susan if she is still experiencing moderate to severe symptoms (see Table 6.3.2). Many women wish to avoid the use of hormones, so Susan needs to be carefully questioned about her specific preferences. Additionally, because every medication has contraindications, Susan's medical, family, and personal history must be carefully reviewed to assure that any specific medication being considered

Table 6.3.2. Prescription Options* for Managing Vasomotor Symptoms Associated with Menopause Transition.

Medication Class	Example(s)	General Cautions and Contraindications	Comments
Anticonvulsants	Gabapentin (Neurontin)	Do not take within 2 hours of antacids. CNS depression potentiated by alcohol.	Avoid discontinuing abruptly. Titrate dose up slowly to reduce somnolence.
Anti-hypertensives	Bellergal Clonidine Methyldopa	Tricyclic antidepressants antagonize clonidine. CNS depressants are potentiated by clonidine.	Clonidine is available as a patch. SSRIs/SNRIs and gabapentin have higher efficacy than clonidine. Avoid abruptly discontinuing clonidine. Bellergal and methyldopa are not recommended because of toxicity.
Breast cancer agent (progestin)	Megestrol (Megace)	Use caution in patients with diabetes or a history of a thromboembolic disorder.	May increase requirements for insulin.
Selective serotonin reuptake inhibitors (SSRIs)/ serotonin norepinephrine reuptake inhibitors (SNRIs)	Desvenlafaxine (Pristiq) Fluoxetine (Prozac) Paroxetine (Paxil, Paxil CR) Venlafaxine (Effexor XR)	Avoid use with thioridazine or monoamine oxidase inhibitors. Use caution in patients taking warfarin. Warn patients to avoid using with alcohol. Use caution in patients with diabetes, diseases that alter metabolism, and heart disease.	Avoid discontinuing abruptly. Monitor weight regularly (fluoxetine).
Estrogen**	Conjugated estrogens and conjugated estrogens, B (Cenestin, Enjuvia, Premarin) Estradiol (Alora, Climara, Divigel, Elestrin, Esclim, Estraderm, Estrasorb, Estro-Gel, Evamist, Menostar, Vivelle, Vivelle-Dot) Estradiol acetate (Femtrace, Femring) Estradiol hemihydrate (Vagifem) Esterified estrogens (Menest) Estropipate (Ogen, Ortho-est) Micronized estradiol (Estrace, Estring)	Do not use in patients with unexplained vaginal bleeding. Do not use in patients with cardiovascular disease, liver disease, breast cancer, estrogen-dependent cancer, pregnancy, or thromboembolism.	Available in multiple delivery forms: oral pill; transdermal patch, mousse, cream, gel, spray; injectable; vaginal cream, tablet, ring. Also available in combination with progestogens or methyltestosterone in varied forms. Use the lowest dose that controls symptoms for the shortest period of time possible. Wean off with slowly decreasing doses.

*Consult a prescribing reference to obtain complete information regarding doses, cautions, contraindications, and side effects. The use of nonhormonal medications to manage vasomotor symptoms associated with the menopause transition is off label. Nonhormonal medications are less effective than estrogen for managing vasomotor symptoms.

**Progestogen is used to prevent endometrial hyperplasia and endometrial cancer for any woman who is taking estrogen and has her uterus.

Source: Alexander et al. (in press); North American Menopause Society [NAMS] (2014, 2018); Ahsan and Mallick (2017); Messina (2014); ePocrates. *Computerized pharmacology and prescribing reference.* Updated daily. Available at: www.epocrates.com (accessed August 29, 2019).

is an appropriate option for her. Similarly, common side effects from specific medications must be reviewed to determine if they would help or further increase any of Susan's symptoms. For example, selective serotonin reuptake inhibitors (SSRIs) and serotonin norepinephrine reuptake inhibitors (SNRIs) are known to commonly cause sexual disturbances and anorgasmia. In Susan's case it may be prudent to avoid use of this class of medication since she is already experiencing vaginal dryness, reduced libido, and increased time to orgasm. Systemic estrogen therapy will reduce hot flash frequency and severity as well as improve vaginal dryness, among a number of other symptoms. This medication option is reasonable for Susan as she has none of the contraindications that might preclude its use (e.g., no breast cancer, no unexplained bleeding, no heart disease, no inherited or personal history of thromboembolic disease).

Hormone therapy (HT) is the most effective agent for managing vasomotor symptoms as well as multiple other symptoms associated with the menopause transition (Baber et al., 2016; NAMS, 2015, 2018). For a woman with her uterus in place, such as Susan, estrogen is taken daily and progesterone is either taken daily to impede endometrial lining buildup or monthly to cause sloughing of the endometrial lining resulting in a withdrawal of bleed. Progesterone is used to prevent the development of endometrial hyperplasia and endometrial cancer (Baber et al., 2016; NAMS, 2015, 2018).

The combined data from multiple studies, including the Women's Health Initiative (WHI), have indicated that HT is safe for women less than 60 years of age and within 10 years of menopause to take for 3–5 years when initiated around the time of transition to postmenopause (NAMS, 2018). After 3–5 years of use the risks for developing breast cancer and heart disease may increase. Indeed, most national and international organizations recommend the use of HT for managing symptoms associated with the menopause transition at the lowest dose that effectively controls symptoms and for the shortest time period possible. Women should have regular health screenings, such as mammograms and blood pressure measurements, while taking HT.

What are the recommendations for referral and follow-up care?

Referrals are not likely to be needed for Susan unless her symptoms are resistant to usual management options. If this occurs, then referral to a menopause specialist is warranted.

A gynecologic exam is not required to initiate HT. Routine follow-up is important with annual bimanual exams, clinical breast exams, and mammography. Follow-up specific to initiating HT or another medication for symptom management is intended to monitor efficacy while also identifying early any untoward side effects or sequelae. HT takes up to 6 weeks to reach full efficacy. Thus an appointment around 6 weeks after initiation is reasonable to determine whether the initial dose is appropriate and effective and to evaluate for bleeding, increased blood pressure, or other side effects.

The North American Menopause Society (2018) recommends starting at a low dose and increasing using small increments if symptom management is not achieved. Once symptoms are stabilized, annual reevaluation of the need for therapy and the present dose is recommended (NAMS, 2018). For Susan, a return appointment at about 6 weeks and again at 1 year is appropriate if she is not having concerning side effects and if her symptoms are manageable. At 1 year it might be reasonable to try skipping some days of therapy or reducing the dose even further to see if her symptoms increase or if she is tolerant to a small increase in symptoms. If not, then return to the prior dose; and if so, then consider reducing the dose further or remain at the lowered dose and reassess in another year.

If Susan's symptoms are not well controlled, or if her libido does not respond to estrogen plus progestin therapy despite an adequate dose, it may be reasonable to add methyltestosterone. Although off-label for sexual benefit, this treatment is approved for women who have resistant vasomotor symptoms and has been shown to improve libido and sexual experiences for women (NAMS, 2018).

What health education should be provided for Susan?

Susan needs to be counseled about sexual health and vaginal dryness. HT can take up to 6 weeks to become effective and SSRIs/SNRIs will not help with vaginal dryness. Susan may need to use vaginal lubricants or vaginal estrogen therapy either until the full effect of systemic HT is realized or for the duration of therapy with SSRI/SNRIs and beyond.

In addition, Susan needs to have counseling about midlife health risks such as osteoporosis and heart disease. If she takes HT it will help protect her from bone loss. She will also need to ensure that she is getting an adequate daily intake of calcium (1200–1500 mg) and vitamin D (800–1000 IU); has regular exercise that includes aerobic, resistive, and weight- bearing activities; avoids smoking or excessive use of alcohol or caffeine; and has regular DXA screening tests when appropriate. If she elects to use a nonhormonal medication or when she stops taking the HT she may also require medication to prevent or treat osteoporosis.

Regular exercise will also help her to prevent heart disease. Given her history of HDP she has an increase risk for heart disease. This risk further increases dramatically after menopause and may even exceed the risks carried by men. Susan needs to have regular lipid panel screening tests, follow a heart- healthy diet, and maintain a normal weight to identify problems early and keep her risk factors as low as possible.

What if Susan also had diabetes or hypertension?

If Susan had diabetes or hypertension a transdermal delivery method for HT might be preferable to oral. This is because oral HT can alter blood sugar levels and is processed in the liver with a first-pass effect. These combined effects can create medication interactions that potentially interfere with diabetes and hypertension management. These effects are reduced with transdermal therapy. There is little to no liver first- pass effect with transdermal therapy; and since the delivery is via the skin, hormone levels may be steadier, possibly reducing the effects on glucose levels.

What if Susan were over age 65?

The WHI study evaluated the use of HT, either estrogen plus progesterone or estrogen alone; the estrogen plus protesterone portion of the study terminated early due to a concern that the risks of use outweighed the benefits. Subanalyses of the WHI and new data from the past 10 years demonstrated that there is an important effect related to when HT is started. There is variability by both age and time since menopause of HRT on organ systems (Baber et al., 2016). The risks seen in the larger study were not present in younger women (< 60 years of age) when the data were analyzed according to 10-year aged cohorts (i.e., 50–59, 60–69, 70–79) (Chlebowski et al., 2009; Hsia et al., 2006; Rossouw et al., 2007). Thus, if Susan were 65 or greater than 10 years from menopause and presented with similar symptoms, HT would not be a great option for her. Instead, Susan might do better with gabapentin or one of the SSRIs/SNRIs, despite the possible sexual side effects.

Does Susan's psychosocial history affect the management recommendations?

Several aspects of Susan's psychosocial history can be important when developing a management plan with her. If Susan had depression in addition to experiencing symptoms associated with the menopause transition, she might benefit from the use of an antidepressant agent, despite the possible risks for reduced sexual functioning. Consideration of Susan's insurance medication coverage is also important when selecting an agent. Several generic medications are available among both the hormonal and nonhormonal prescription options. This is taken into account when prescribing an agent for Susan so that the cost of therapy does not become a barrier to her ability to use the therapy she has selected. Additionally, Susan's preference for prescription therapy versus CAM therapy is important. If Susan does not think HT is safe, then she may have increased anxiety if she uses it, or she might take the prescription and never fill it. An open discussion that provides her with ample opportunity to share her concerns and considerations and that provides factual information including both benefits and risks is needed to individualize therapy for Susan and develop an acceptable and beneficial management plan.

Are there any standardized guidelines that should be used when developing a management plan with Susan? If so, what are they?

The combined data from multiple studies, including the WHI study, suggest that HT is safe for healthy women to take for at least 5 years when initiated before the age of 60 (Baber et al., 2016;

Hsia et al., 2006; NAMS, 2014, 2018; Rossouw et al., 2007). Further, the research indicates that combined HT started in those < 60 years of age early in this window of opportunity may confer some cardioprotection (Baber et al., 2016). After 5 years of use, the individual risk profile of the woman must be evaluated, as the risks for developing breast cancer and heart disease may increase. Thus, most national organizations and the US Food and Drug Administration recommend the use of HT only for managing symptoms associated with menopause at the lowest dose that effectively controls symptoms and for the shortest time possible (Baber et al., 2016; NAMS, 2014, 2018). Regular health screenings are also recommended while any woman is taking HT, so Susan should be counseled to have an annual mammogram, regular blood pressure screenings, and to report any signs or symptoms of heart disease or any breast changes.

REFERENCES AND RESOURCES

Ahsan, M., & Mallick, A. K. (2017). The effect of soy isoflavones on the menopause rating scale scoring in perimenopausal and postmenopausal women: A pilot study. *Journal of Clinical and Diagnostic Research: JCDR*, *11*(9), FC13.

Alexander, I. M., Jakubisin Konicki, A., Barandouzi, Z. A., et al. (in press). Chapter 14: Menopause. In F. Likis & K. Schuiling (Eds.), *Women's gynecologic health* (4th ed.). Sudbury, MA: Jones & Bartlett Learning.

Alexander, I. M., Ruff, C., Rousseau, M. E., White, K., Motter, S., McKie, C., & Clarke, P. (2004, August). *Experiences and perceptions of menopause and midlife health and self-management strategies identified by black women.* Department of Health and Human Services (DHHS) Conference: Women of Color Taking Action for a Healthier Life: Progress, Partnerships and Possibilities, Washington, DC.

American College of Obstetrics and Gynecology. (2016). Practice bulletin no. 141: Management of menopausal symptoms: Correction. *Obstetrics & Gynecology*, *127*(1), 166. doi:10.1097/AOG.0000000000001230

American College of Obstetrics & Gynecology. (2019). Practice bulletin clinical management guidelines for obstetrician–gynecologists, number 213: Female sexual dysfunction. *Obstetrics & Gynecology*, *134*(1), e1–e18. doi:10.1097/AOG.0000000000003324

American Psychiatric Association. (2013). Diagnostic and statistical manual of mental disorders (5th ed.). Washington, DC: American Psychiatric Association.

Baber, R. J., Panay, N., & Fenton, A. (2016). 2016 IMS recommendations on women's midlife health and menopause hormone therapy. *Climacteric*, *19*(2), 109–150. doi:10.3109/13697137.2015.1129166.

Befus, D., Coeytaux, R. R., Goldstein, K. M., McDuffie, J. R., Shepherd-Banigan, M., Goode, A. P., . . . Williams, J. W. Jr. (2018). Management of menopause symptoms with acupuncture: An umbrella systematic review and meta-analysis. *Journal of Alternative and Complementary Medicine*, *24*(4), 314. doi:10.1089/acm.2016.0408

Chiu, H. Y., Pan, C. H., Shyu, Y. K., Han, B. C., & Tsai, P. S. (2015). Effects of acupuncture on menopause-related symptoms and quality of life in women in natural menopause: A meta-analysis of randomized controlled trials. *Menopause*, *22*(2), 234–244.

Chlebowski, R. T., Kuller, L. H., Prentice, R. L., Stefanick, M. L., Manson, J. E., Gass, M., . . . Anderson, G., for the WHI Investigators. (2009). Breast cancer after use of estrogen plus progestin in postmenopausal women. *New England Journal of Medicine*, *360*(6), 573–587.

Cosman, F., de Beur, S. J., LeBoff, M. S., Lewiecki, E. M., Tanner, B., Randall, S., & Lindsay, R. (2014). Clinician's guide to prevention and treatment of osteoporosis. *Osteoporosis International, Online* (August 2014), 1–25. Accessed July 30, 2019. Available at file:///C:/Users/ima00001/Downloads/Clinicians-Guide.pdf

Daley, A., Stokes-Lampard, H., Thomas, A., & MacArthur, C. (2014). Exercise for vasomotor symptoms. *Cochrane Database of Systematic Reviews*, *11*, CD006108. doi:10.1002/14651858.CD006108.pub4

Freedman, R. R., & Woodward, S. (1992). Behavioral treatment of menopausal hot flashes: Evaluation by ambulatory monitoring. *American Journal of Obstetrics and Gynecology*, *167*, 436–439.

Freedman, R. R., Woodward, S., Brown, B., Javaid, J. I., & Pandy, G. N. (1995). Biochemical and thermoregulatory effects of treatment for menopausal hot flashes. *Menopause*, *2*, 211–218.

Garber, J. R., Cobin, R. H., Gharib, H., Hennessey, J. V., Klein, I., Mechanick, J. I., . . . Woeber, K. A. (2012). Clinical practice guidelines for hypothyroidism in adults: Cosponsored by the American Association of Clinical Endocrinologists and the American Thyroid Association. *Endocrine Practice: Official Journal of the American College of Endocrinology and the American Association of Clinical Endocrinologists*, *18*(6), 988. doi:10.4158/EP12280.GL

Green, S. M., Key, B. L., & McCabe, R. E. (2015). Cognitive-behavioral, behavioral, and mindfulness-based therapies for menopausal depression: A review. *Maturitas, 80*(1), 37–47.

Hsia, J., Langer, R. D., Manson, J. E., Kuller, L., Johnson, K. C., Hendrix, S. L., . . . Prentice, R., for the Women's Health Initiative Investigators. (2006). Conjugated equine estrogens and coronary heart disease: The Women's Health Initiative. Archives of Internal Medicine, *166*(3), 357–365.

Mahady, G. B., Low Dog, T., Barrett, M. L., Chavez, M. L., Gardiner, P., Ko, R., . . . Sarma, D. N. (2008). United States pharmacopeia review of the black cohosh case reports of hepatotoxicity. *Menopause, 15*(4 Pt 1), 628–638.

Messina, M. (2014). Soy foods, isoflavones, and the health of postmenopausal women. *American Journal of Clinical Nutrition, 100*(Suppl 1), 423S–430S.

Natari, R. B., Clavarino, A. M., McGuire, T. M., Dingle, K. D., & Hollingworth, S. A. (2018). The bidirectional relationship between vasomotor symptoms and depression across the menopausal transition: A systematic review of longitudinal studies. *Menopause, 25*(1), 109–120.

Nedeljkovic, M., Tian, L., Ji, P., Déglon-Fischer A., Stute P., Ocon E., . . . Ausfeld-Hafter, B. (2014). Effects of acupuncture and Chinese herbal medicine (Zhi Mu 14) on hot flushes and quality of life in postmenopausal women: Results of a four-arm randomized controlled pilot trial. *Menopause, 21*(1), 15–24.

North American Menopause Society . (2014). Menopause practice: A clinician's guide (5th ed.). Mayfield Heights, OH: North American Menopause Society.

North American Menopause Society. (2018). The 2017 hormone therapy position statement of the North American Menopause Society. *Menopause, 25*(11), 1362–1387. doi:10.1097/GME.0000000000001241

Rossouw, J. E., Prentice, R. L., Manson, J. E., Wu, L., Barad, D., Barnabei, V. M., . . . Stefanick, M. L. (2007). Postmenopausal hormone therapy and risk of cardiovascular disease by age and years since menopause. *Journal of the American Medical Association, 297*(13), 1465–1477.

Shifren, L. J., Monz, U. B., Russo, A. P., Segreti, B. A., & Johannes, B. C. (2008). Sexual problems and distress in United States women: Prevalence and correlates. *Obstetrics & Gynecology, 112*(5), 970–978. doi:10.1097/AOG.0b013e3181898cdb

Timpka, S., Fraser, A., Schyman, T., Stuart, J. J., Åsvold, B. O., Mogren, I., . . . Rich-Edwards, J. W. (2018). The value of pregnancy complication history for 10-year cardiovascular disease risk prediction in middle-aged women. *European Journal of Epidemiology, 33*(10), 1003–1010.

Thompson, A. M., Church, T. S., & Blair, S. N. (2008, March 13). Effect of different doses of physical activity on quality of life in overweight, sedentary, postmenopausal women (presentation, abstract). Paper presented at the American Health Association Nutrition, Physical Activity and Metabolism Conference and 48th Annual Cardiovascular Disease Epidemiology and Prevention Conference, Colorado Springs, CO.

Weber, M. T., Maki, P. M., & McDermott, M. P. (2014). Cognition and mood in perimenopause: A systematic review and meta-analysis. *Journal of Steroid Biochemistry and Molecular Biology, 142*, 90–98.

Wolf, A. M. D., Fontham, E. T. H., Church, T. R., Flowers, C. R., Guerra, C. E., Lamonte, S. J., . . . Smith, R. A. (2018). Colorectal cancer screening for average-risk adults: 2018 guideline update from the American cancer society. *CA: A Cancer Journal for Clinicians, 68*(4), 250–281. doi:10.3322/caac.21457

RESOLUTION

What is the most likely differential diagnosis in this case?

Pelvic inflammatory disease (PID).

Which diagnostic tests are required in this case and why?

CBC: A CBC is not needed for the diagnosis of PID; however, a CBC would be useful to know if the white blood count is elevated.

Nucleic acid amplification tests: NAAT testing should be done to test for *Neisseria gonorrhea* and *Chlamydia trachomatis*. *Neisseria gonorrhea* and *Chlamydia trachomatis* are the two most common sexually transmitted infections (STIs) associated with PID. A positive test supports the diagnosis of PID; however, a negative test does not rule out PID, as other bacteria can cause PID, such as anaerobes, *G. vaginalis*, enteric Gram-negative rods, and *Streptococcus agalactiae*.

Beta hCG: Beta hCG is a necessary test for this patient to determine if she is pregnant and to rule out an ectopic pregnancy.

HIV: HIV is not diagnostic for PID; however, this test should be included in the general management of a patient who presents with a history of multiple sex partners and recent sexually transmitted infections.

Wet mount: A wet wound examination of vaginal secretions with saline may show an abundance of white blood cells and can help confirm the PID diagnosis.

Treponema pallidum: Treponema pallidum is not diagnostic for PID; however, this test should be included in the general management of a patient who presents with a history of STIs to rule out other possible STIs.

Transvaginal ultrasound: A transvaginal ultrasound can be performed to confirm the diagnosis. Imaging should be considered if there is concern about a tubo-ovarian abscess. Imaging may demonstrate thickening and fluid-filled Fallopian tubes.

What is the plan of treatment?

Outpatient treatment is an acceptable option for patients with mild to moderate PID, who tolerate oral antibiotics and can adhere to the prescribed course of therapy. Patients will require hospitalizations if they have severe PID or complications such as pregnancy or tubo-ovarian abscess, are unable to follow or tolerate oral medication, or fail to respond to outpatient treatment within 72 hours.

The Family Nurse Practitioner: Clinical Case Studies, Second Edition. Edited by Leslie Neal-Boylan.
© 2021 John Wiley & Sons Ltd. Published 2021 by John Wiley & Sons Ltd.

Oral Treatment	IV Treatment
Ceftriaxone 250 mg IM in a single dose	Cefotetan 2 g IV every 12 hours
Or	**Or**
Cefoxitin 2 g IM in a single dose and Probenecid, 1 g orally administered concurrently in a single dose	Cefoxitin 2 g IV every 6 hours
Or	**PLUS**
Another parenteral third-generation cephalosporin	Doxycycline 100 mg orally or IV every 12 hours
PLUS	
Doxycycline 100 mg orally twice a day for 14 days	
(WITH or WITHOUT)	
Metronidazole 500 mg orally twice a day for 14 days	

Source: Workowski and Bolan (2015).

What are the plans for follow-up care?

For patients with outpatient treatment, follow-up should occur within 48–72 hours to ensure effective treatment and improvement of symptoms. If the patient is improving, they can continue with outpatient treatment; for patients with worsening symptoms or minimal improvement, hospitalization with intravenous therapy should be considered.

Repeat testing for gonorrhea and chlamydia should occur within 3–6 months for patients with previously positive results.

What health education should be provided to this patient?

The patient should adhere to pelvic rest until therapy is completed and symptoms are resolved. Pelvic rest includes abstaining from vaginal intercourse and avoiding inserting anything into the vagina such as tampons or douching.

Shanae should be taught safe sexual practices. Although Shanae is using oral contraception, she is still at risk for STIs.

Shanae's male sexual partners should be treated for gonorrhea and chlamydia if they have had sexual intercourse with her within the past 60 days prior to her clinical symptoms. Shanea should abstain from sexual intercourse until her sexual partner has been treated.

Are there any standardized guidelines that should be used to treat this case? If so, what are they?

The Centers for Disease Control has detailed information on the treatment of PID (https://www.cdc.gov/mmwr/preview/mmwrhtml/rr6403a1.htm).

REFERENCES AND RESOURCES

Workowski, K. A., & Bolan, G. A. (2015). Sexually transmitted diseases treatment guidelines, 2015. *Morbidity and Mortality Weekly Report. Recommendations and Reports*, 64(RR-03), 1. https://www.cdc.gov/mmwr/preview/mmwrhtml/rr6403a1.htm

Case 6.5 Vaginal Itching

Which diagnostic or imaging studies should be considered to assist with or confirm the diagnosis?

A wet mount, including KOH and whiff test, would be indicated. Martha's multiple partners warrant a check for sexually transmitted infections (STIs). Martha should be asked about these tests before they are done. The testing for STIs (gonorrhea and chlamydia) may be done via a urine sample or through cultures during the pelvic exam. Recurrent infections would warrant HIV testing. A urinalysis would be indicated to rule out signs of a urinary tract infection given her complaint of burning with urination. A Pap smear is not indicated, given that her last Pap smear was 2 years ago and was normal.

If a wet mount were performed, what findings would be expected for the following diagnoses?

See Table 6.5.1.

What is the most likely differential diagnosis and why?

See Table 6.5.2.

Candidiasis

The symptom of itching, the curd-like white discharge, the burning with urination, and the dyspareunia support this diagnosis. The vaginal swelling also contributes to the diagnosis. Martha's recent antibiotic use increases her risk for this diagnosis.

What is the plan of treatment?

Both topical and oral treatment options are available. When deciding between topical and oral preparations clinicians should consider patient preference and cost, as well as the following:

- Topical agents are generally used for between 1 and 7 days depending on the formulation. They can provide more immediate relief due to their local action and many are available over the counter (OTC). However, topical agents can potentially cause local hypersensitivity reactions resulting in increased itching or burning.

The Family Nurse Practitioner: Clinical Case Studies, Second Edition. Edited by Leslie Neal-Boylan.
© 2021 John Wiley & Sons Ltd. Published 2021 by John Wiley & Sons Ltd.

Table 6.5.1. Wet Mount Findings.

Diagnosis	pH	Saline Prep	KOH Prep
Bacterial vaginosis	>4.5	>20% clue cells	+ whiff test
Candidiasis	Normal (3.8–4.2)	Possible visualization of hyphae/buds on saline prep, more visible on KOH prep	Hyphae/pseudohyphae, buds or spores Negative whiff test
Trichomonas	>4.5	Mobile protozoa with flagella, increased WBCs	Sometimes + whiff (not always)

Table 6.5.2. Differential Diagnosis.

Condition	Signs and Symptoms
Trichomonas	Foul-smelling discharge, usually a fishy odor; vaginal burning sensation; possible postcoital bleeding; itching; dysuria, dyspareunia; may be asymptomatic.
Bacterial vaginosis	Fishy vaginal odor; thin white or gray discharge; postcoital burning; possible itching; may be asymptomatic.
Chlamydia	Possibly mucopurulent discharge; pelvic pain; dysuria, spotting, and altered menstruation; postcoital bleeding; may be asymptomatic. Male: Dysuria, cloudy and thick penile discharge; may be asymptomatic.
Gonorrhea	Asymptomatic early; leukorrhea; suprapubic pain, dysuria, dyspareunia, pharyngitis; labial pain and swelling. Later: purulent discharge, rectal pain and discharge; nausea, vomiting, fever; arthralgias and joint swelling; genital lesions and swelling. Male: Dysuria, pharyngitis, white penile discharge that progresses to yellow-green, epididymitis, and proctitis; may be asymptomatic.
Herpes genitalis	First episode: Lesions; malaise, fever, dyspareunia, arthralgias and myalgias, fever, and lymphadenopathy. Recurrent episodes: Less symptomatic, usually have prodrome of itching, burning, or tingling.
Urinary tract infection	Dysuria, urinary frequency, urinary urgency, suprapubic pressure/discomfort, mild low back discomfort.

- Oral agents have convenient dosing (typically just 1 pill taken once) and are less messy and cumbersome than topical agents. However, they can have systemic side effects and interact with other medications.

Topical agents:

- Butoconazole cream (prescription)
- Terconazole cream or suppositories (prescription)
- Clotrimazole cream (OTC)
- Miconazole cream or suppositories (OTC)
- Tioconazole ointment (OTC)

First-line oral agent:

- Fluconazole 150mg table ×1

What education should be provided to Martha at this visit?

Instruction regarding how to avoid recurrent candida infections and how to avoid STIs will be paramount during the visit. Martha should avoid intercourse until her symptoms resolve. Important points to discuss around the prevention of future vaginal infections include: avoiding douching, feminine deodorants, and heavily scented soaps or detergents; removing damp or wet clothing immediately (for instance, after swimming or exercise) and wearing loose, breathable clothing when possible.

Are any referrals needed?

No referrals are needed unless Martha has an intractable case; she does not require follow-up unless this infection is unresponsive.

Is the family history of diabetes relevant to this case?

Martha has a family history of diabetes mellitus, so it is worthwhile testing her for DM and monitoring her for prediabetes. Vaginal candidiasis, especially frequent infections, can be a warning sign of diabetes.

How can the clinician support the patient regarding her confusion with her sexual preferences?

The clinician can work to develop a rapport with Martha and gain her trust so that Martha feels comfortable sharing her feelings. The clinician should avoid making assumptions or judgments, use neutral and inclusive terms/vocabulary, normalize any questions being asked ("I ask all of my patients these questions"), and provide factual information and resources.

REFERENCES AND RESOURCES

Hawkins, J. W., Roberto-Nichols, D. M., & Stanley-Haney, J. L. (2015). Guidelines for nurse practitioners in gynecologic settings (11th ed.). New York: Springer.

Paladine, H. L., & Desai, U. A. (2018). Vaginitis: Diagnosis and treatment. *American Family Physician, 97*(5), 321–329.

NOTE: The author would like to thank Leslie Neal-Boylan, PhD, APRN, CRRN, FAAN, FARN for her contribution to this case in the first edition of this book.

Case 6.6 Redness and Swelling in the Breast

Which diagnostic tests should be considered?

In a young symptomatic patient like Jill (pain, edema of the skin, and fluctuant mass), an ultrasound of the breast should be the first investigative study. Young women have breast tissue that is much denser than in older women and this can make it harder to detect an abnormality using mammography. Ultrasound is a noninvasive way of determining if a mass is solid or fluid filled and if aspiration of the fluid is necessary; this will help in guiding the needle during aspiration. Jill also has experienced chills and a fever, so a CBC with differential and a culture for bacterial identification and sensitivities of antibiotics should be done at the time of the breast aspiration.

Which differential diagnoses should be considered?

Mastitis, cellulitis, nonpuerperal breast abscess, periductal mastitis inflammatory breast cancer

Which is the most likely differential diagnosis and why?

Nonpuerperal breast abscess:

Jill is G0P0; she underwent nipple piercings 3 months ago while vacationing in the Caribbean. She noticed redness on the right breast 4 days ago accompanied by swelling, pain, erythema, drainage, and fever. Nipple piercing has become common and there is little regulation of the studios where piercing is done. Complications from the procedure may include breast infection, allergic reactions to the jewelry that is used, and scarring. The channels of the piercing may take a long time to heal, increasing the risk for infections. The onset of breast infection following nipple piercing can occur days to months after the event. Other risk factors for development of nonpuerperal breast abscesses in addition to nipple piercings are nicotine use: the breast concentrates cotinine, a derivative of nicotine, in the subareolar ducts; this in turn damages the subareolar ducts, leading to tissue necrosis and subsequent infection, diabetes (DM), and periductal mastitis, a condition that causes inflamed ducts that can rupture and lead to abscess formation (Dixon, 2017).

The culture from the ultrasound-guided aspiration of Jill's abscess grew out Streptococcus Group B. The literature shows that the most common organisms associated with nipple piercing are Mycobacterium, Gram-negative Staphylococcus, and Streptococcus Group B. In contrast to

The Family Nurse Practitioner: Clinical Case Studies, Second Edition. Edited by Leslie Neal-Boylan.
© 2021 John Wiley & Sons Ltd. Published 2021 by John Wiley & Sons Ltd.

patients who have breast abscesses not associated with nipple piercings, in this setting the bacteria more commonly found are *Staphylococcus aureus* (with an increasing association with methicillin-resistant *Staphylococcus aureus*), *Pseudomonas aeruginosa*, and *Proteus mirabilis* (Dixon, 2017).

What is the plan of treatment?

Traditional first-line treatment of both puerperal and nonpuerperal breast abscesses had previously consisted of incision and drainage of the breast coupled with antibiotic therapy; however, several studies have reported clinical success treating breast abscesses with diagnostic ultrasound followed by needle aspiration and antibiotic therapy with close clinical follow-up.

Aspiration has supplanted surgical incision and drainage as first-line management of both puerperal and nonpuerperal abscesses in many clinical situations (Geiss, Golshan, Flaherty & Birdwell, 2014). Fluid obtained from the aspiration is sent to the lab for microbiology to identify the causative organism and tested for bacterial sensitivities. The most commonly found organisms in soft tissue infections of the breast are Staphylococcus species and Streptococcus species. Effective antibiotics to be used to treat the infection (in the absence of risk factors for MRSA) would be Dicloxacillin 500 mg 4 times daily × 7–10 days, Cephalexin 500 mg 4 times daily × 7–10 days, or Clindamycin 300 to 400 mg 3 times daily × 7–10 days. In the setting of infection with risk factors for MRSA (recent hospitalization, residing in a long-term-care facility, recent surgery, hemodialysis, or HIV infection), Trimethoprim-Sulfamethoxazole DS 1 tablet every 12 hours × 10 days or Clindamycin 300–450 mg 4 times daily × 7–10 days (Dixon, 2017).

What is the plan for follow-up?

The patient should return in 2–3 days for a follow-up ultrasound to check for reaccumulation of the fluid and may need a second aspiration. If a second aspiration is needed, see the patient again in 2–3 days for another follow-up ultrasound. If there is no further need for ultrasound and aspiration, then the patient may follow up when the antibiotics are completed. Patients should have annual clinical breast exams by the primary care provider beginning at age 25 and have an annual mammogram alternating with breast MRI 10 years before the onset of breast cancer in any family members. Jill should have an MRI at age 33 due to a breast cancer diagnosis in her paternal grandmother at age 43. This relative was a known BRCA 2 mutation carrier.

Would the work-up or treatment be different if this patient were a man?

Men also can develop these abscesses from piercings or from gynecomastia that can cause blockage in the ducts. The evaluation and treatment plan would be the same.

Are any referrals needed?

A referral to a breast surgeon should be made if the patient fails to improve after aspiration and treatment with antibiotics or if the patient improves but symptoms recur after a few months. The ducts may stay obstructed and require surgical resection for successful resolution of the problem.

What health education is important for this patient?

Jill should be instructed in the following:

Take antibiotics as directed; complete the entire course of medication.

Report symptoms: Temp > 101, increase in drainage, redness, pain, or swelling.

Manage pain with warm compresses to the area 2–3 times per day, take pain medication as directed, and wear a supportive bra.

Cellulitis should improve within 48 hours after starting the antibiotics. If the clinician has outlined the area of redness on the breast, the patient should call if the redness progresses beyond the outline. The patent should not reinsert the nipple jewelry and should try to stop smoking.

REFERENCES AND RESOURCES

Crico. (2014). Breast care management algorithm: *A decision support tool.* www.rmf.harvard.edu/guidebreasts

Fahmi, M., Schwarz, E. I., Stadimann, S., Singer, G., Hauser, N., & Kubik-Huch, R. A. (2012). Breast abscesses: Diagnosis, treatment and outcome. *Breast Care, 7*(1), 32–38.

Dixon, J. M. (2017). Nonlactational mastitis in adults. *UpToDate.* Retrieved from www.uptodate.com

Giess, C.S., Golshan, M., Flaherty, K., & Birdwell, R. (2014). Clinical experience with aspiration of breast abscesses based on size and etiology at an academic medical center. *Journal of Clinical Oncology, 42*(9), 513–521.

Leibman, A. J., Misra, M., & Castaldi, M. (2011). Breast abscess after nipple piercing. *Journal of Ultrasound in Medicine, 30*(9).

RESOLUTION

What is the most likely differential diagnosis in this case and why?
Sexual assault:
Although Aiyata does not disclose a sexual assault, one should be suspected in her case. Consuming alcohol to the point in which the individual becomes impaired and cannot consent to intercourse leads to a strong suspicion of assault. In addition, the male friend gave her the drinks and her behaviors after drinking these drinks impaired her memory. A drug-facilitated sexual assault should be suspected.

Which diagnostic tests are required in this case and why?
CBC with differential: CBC testing may be useful in a patient who is bleeding to determine HGB and HCT and to determine whether the patient is anemic.

   Metabolic panel: Metabolic labs should be performed to obtain baseline levels if the patient is going to beginning HIV post-exposure prophylaxis (PEP). While taking HIV PEP, some patients can develop abnormal kidney function as evidenced by the BUN and creatinine, so baseline data will help to monitor patients.

   LFTs: LFTs to obtain baseline levels should be performed if the patient is going to begin HIV PEP. Some patients can develop abnormal LFTs while taking HIV PEP.

   Toxicology: Routine toxicology is not recommended for sexual assault patients unless a drug-facilitated assault is suspected. In this patient, given the memory loss and history of drinks, a drug-facilitated assault is suspected, so toxicology testing should be performed. Many hospital laboratories are not equipped to perform the specific testing to detect the presence of date rape drugs. You may need to refer to specialized laboratories for toxicology testing in cases of suspected drug-facilitated sexual assault.

   HCG: HCG is an essential test that should be performed to establish whether the patient is pregnant. A positive pregnancy test result will require changes to the treatment plan and medications.

   HIV: HIV testing should be performed on patients who have been sexually assaulted, especially in cases where the assault is at high risk for HIV and the patient is going to begin HIV PEP. HIV testing will provide the baseline HIV status. HIV testing is a sensitive topic for many patients so the patient should have access to proper counseling in cases of positive results.

The Family Nurse Practitioner: Clinical Case Studies, Second Edition. Edited by Leslie Neal-Boylan.
© 2021 John Wiley & Sons Ltd. Published 2021 by John Wiley & Sons Ltd.

Urinalysis: Routine urinalysis may be considered; however, since the dysuria this patient reported was most likely due to trauma and not to a UTI, a urinalysis in this case would not be diagnostic.

Urine NAAT: Urine NAAT is recommended for testing for gonorrhea, chlamydia, and trichomonas.

CT scan of neck: A CT of the neck should be a priority diagnostic test for this patient. The patient has positive signs and symptoms of possible strangulation. Her lateral neck is tender to palpation, there are dark red ecchymosed areas on the right side of the neck, and subconjunctival hemorrhages. All of these can be physical signs of strangulation. In addition, this patient has poor memory recall, which may also result from strangulation and hypoperfusion. A CT scan of the neck is warranted to determine any soft tissue injury to the trachea or neck ligatures.

What are the concerns at this point?

The initial concern is that this patient has been sexually assaulted and that a drug-facilitated assault is suspected with injuries.

What is the plan of treatment?

Caring for patients who have been sexually assaulted requires three aspects of care: (1) medical evaluation, (2) psychological evaluation, and (3) forensic evaluation. The medical evaluation process includes general medical care and treatment for the prevention of sexually transmitted infections and pregnancy. Assessments should first always address life-threatening, serious, or time-sensitive needs. All patients should be assessed for injuries. Injuries can present at different time periods after an assault. Although strangulation was not disclosed, the patient presented with several red flags indicating possible strangulation, which can be a life-threatening injury. If strangulation is suspected, the patient should be specifically asked about strangulation to determine if she has any memories that may help guide the assessment and treatment plan. This patient should have a CT scan of the neck to determine if there are any soft tissue injuries to the neck. Unless this patient declines, she should receive post-exposure prophylaxis treatment for sexually transmitted infections, HIV, and pregnancy.

What are the plans for referral and follow-up care?

All patients who disclose or for whom sexual assault is suspected should be referred for or offered a medical forensic examination with evidence collection. Patients should be referred to any health care facility that has sexual assault response teams (SARTs) or sexual assault nurse examiners (SANEs). SARTs and SANEs provide expert-level care, including medical forensic examination. The purpose of a medical forensic exam with evidence collection is to provide law enforcement with details and evidence from the assault. A medical forensic examination with evidence collection is a lengthy process that includes consent, medical forensic interview, documentation, and a lengthy evidence collection process. If patients decline the medical forensic examination, they should be informed of the risks and benefits of a prompt evaluation and their right to obtain one in the future according to local jurisdictional practices.

Sexual assault can have significant psychological impact on patients. All patients should be referred to local rape crisis counselors. Many local rape crisis centers have advocates and resources that support sexually assaulted patients throughout the recovery process. They help address immediate and long-term safety issues and the mental and emotional health needs of the patient.

Many patients who have been sexually assaulted will begin several types of prophylactic medications. Patients will need follow-up testing for HIV and STIs and blood monitoring if the patient is taking HIV PEP.

All patients should be assessed for safety. In many cases of sexual assault, the assailant is known to the individual and there is genuine concern for safety. Make referrals to law enforcement or social work to help navigate concerns for safety or in cases where there is a need for restraining orders.

Mandatory reporting of patients who have been sexually assaulted differs from state to state. It is important to know your local mandatory reporting requirements and the agencies to which you report.

What health education should be provided to this patient?

Education for this patient should include the importance of follow-up care and completing the course of HIV PEP medications. Many patients will receive the one-time post-exposure medications in the health care setting. HIV PEP requires completion of a 28-day course to be effective. Adherence to the 28-day course is often poor for sexually assaulted patients. Patients need be educated on the importance of completing HIV PEP medications and follow up with health care providers for additional bloodwork and testing.

Are there any standardized guidelines that should be used to assess or treat this case?

The United States Department of Justice Office on Violence Against Women has made publicly available the National Protocol for Sexual Assault Medical Forensic Examinations (https://www.ncjrs.gov/pdffiles1/ovw/241903.pdf). This guideline details a comprehensive approach in considering the medical, psychosocial, and forensic considerations when caring for patients who have been sexually assaulted.

REFERENCES AND RESOURCES

Centers for Disease Control and Prevention, U.S. Department of Health and Human Services. (2016). Updated guidelines for antiretroviral postexposure prophylaxis after sexual, injection drug use, or other nonoccupational exposure to HI –United States. *2016 nPEP Guidelines Update,* 1–91. Retrieved from https://www.cdc.gov/hiv/pdf/programresources/cdc-hiv-npep-guidelines.pdf

Scannell, M., Kim, T., & Guthrie, B. J. (2018). A meta-analysis of HIV post exposure prophylaxis among sexually assaulted patients in the United States. *Journal of the Association of Nurses in AIDS Care*, 29(1), 60–69.

U.S. Department of Justice (DOJ), Office on Violence Against Women. (2013). *A national protocol for sexual assault medical forensic examinations: Adults/adolescents* (2nd ed.). Retrieved from https://www.ncjrs.gov/pdffiles1/ovw/241903.pdf

Case 6.8 Abdominal Pain

RESOLUTION

What is the most likely differential diagnosis and why?

Rachel has cholecystitis. The positive Murphy's sign with RUQ pain and nausea support the diagnosis. Her fatty diet clearly contributes to her condition, even though she denies any associated pattern with food. The abdominal ultrasound, usually diagnostic, was inconclusive in this case but the HIDA scan confirmed the diagnosis of cholecystitis.

Which diagnostic tests are required in this case and why?

In addition to urine testing, Rachel should have had a comprehensive metabolic panel, hepatic function panel, lipase and amylase, and CBC. The CBC shows a left shift. Once her fasting blood sugar was noted to be 45 mg/dL, a fasting insulin level, c-peptide, and oral glucose tolerance test (OGTT) should have been ordered. Her first insulin level was 43 uIU/mL (normal ≤ 17), and her c-peptide was 5.1 (normal = 0.8–3.1 ng/mL). These levels are suspicious for an insulinoma. A gastric tumor must also be ruled out as Rachel has abdominal pain. Therefore, a gastrin level was obtained, which was normal. Rachel told the clinician that she had not eaten when the test was done. It was necessary to repeat this to be sure that Rachel fasted, and the best way to do this was to have these labs repeated just prior to beginning the OGTT, which would also support or refute a diagnosis of an insulinoma. Rachel's fasting levels, including the OGTT, turned out to be normal, and both an insulin tumor and a gastric tumor were ruled out.

The abdominal pain required an abdominal ultrasound to confirm or rule out cholecystitis or gallstones. If the results of the ultrasound are unclear, a **cholescintigraphy (hepatic iminodiacetic acid [HIDA] scan can confirm the diagnosis.** When Rachel mentioned the new-onset headache, the nurse practitioner performed a focused neurological assessment and suggested that Rachel make an appointment with an ophthalmologist for visual screening and instructed her in the appropriate use of analgesics. She was told to call 911 or go to the emergency room if her vision or headaches got worse. Imaging is not indicated at this time.Rachel returns in 2 weeks and states she is following a low-fat diet per your recommendations and her abdominal pain feels slightly better. Now, she denies any headaches, nausea, and dizziness. On exam, she has RUQ TTP and a positive Murphy's sign.

The Family Nurse Practitioner: Clinical Case Studies, Second Edition. Edited by Leslie Neal-Boylan.
© 2021 John Wiley & Sons Ltd. Published 2021 by John Wiley & Sons Ltd.

What is the plan of treatment?

Rachel should be referred to a medical social worker who can advise her about transportation to future medical appointments and elsewhere in her community.

Rachel should be asked to return to the clinic to review her diet progress. It is advisable to recommend that Rachel stop smoking for the sake of herself and her baby.

Are any referrals needed?

A referral may be needed to a gastroenterologist to further assess the cholecystitis and to establish a baseline for the condition of the gallbladder as surgical options are considered.

Does the patient's home situation influence the plan?

Rachel's home life does play a role in her care. She has trouble getting her in-laws to support her need for transportation or her boyfriend to support her need for socialization. The clinician should coach her and provide support to assist her in helping her in-laws and boyfriend to understand that she needs transportation for her health needs and those of her baby and also to help her make friends in her new location. Rachel is at risk for depression and the consequences of social isolation. This could then put her at high risk for child abuse. The clinician should also offer to speak with the family. It is important that the clinician act as a confidante and support for Rachel while being careful not to malign her family.

Are there any standardized guidelines that should be used to treat this case?

The American College of Gastroenterology is a good resource. UptoDate is also a useful resource for current information.

REFERENCES AND RESOURCES

Siddiqui, A. A. (2018). Gallbladder and bile duct disorders. In R. S. Porter, J. L. Kaplan, R. B. Lynn, & M. T. Reddy (Eds.), *The Merck manual of diagnosis and therapy* (pp. 215–216). Kenilworth, NJ: Merck Sharp & Dohme Corp.

Case 6.9 Urinary Frequency

What is the most likely differential diagnosis and why?

Acute cystitis or a UTI:

A UTI is characterized by difficulty with voiding and a positive urine culture. The patient is usually afebrile. Urgency, frequency, and pain with voiding are common, as is some pain following sexual activity. Some women experience hematuria, as well. A new partner for Susan is a risk factor for a UTI.

Interstitial cystitis is a diagnosis of exclusion and a negative urine culture is an essential part of the diagnosis. Other causes of urinary urgency must first be ruled out. Pyelonephritis is characterized by flank pain in addition to dysuria, urgency, frequency, and a positive urine culture. Fever and chills are typically present. If the clinician is in doubt about Susan having pyelonephritis, a CBC could be added to the workup, as it will show definite leukocytosis. For this case, none of the other diagnostic tests that are listed are necessary at this time. However, if Susan's symptoms get worse, a renal scan to look for hydronephrosis might be warranted.

Which diagnostic studies should be considered to assist with or confirm the diagnosis?

The clinician checks a urine dipstick while Susan is in the office. The results are negative except for positive leukocytes and positive nitrites. A rapid HCG is performed. If Susan is not pregnant, the clinician can simply treat her without sending out for a complete urinalysis and culture and sensitivity. The pelvic exam was helpful in Susan's case to rule out PID or vulvovaginitis. Susan has a family history of diabetes mellitus, so a fasting blood sugar should also be included in her workup. People with DM are often prone to UTIs.

What is the plan of treatment?

In Susan's case, the UTI is uncomplicated and could therefore be treated with a short course of antibiotics. Nitrofurantoin (check a creatinine clearance before using) or Bactrim are good choices. It is important to check your region for antibiotic resistance. Phenazopyridine obtained over the counter can help relieve pain with urination, but the patient should be warned that the medication will stain clothes orange. Susan should be encouraged to push fluids until she feels better and in the future to help prevent UTIs. If Susan's tests were negative for a UTI and there is no other apparent reason for her suprapubic pain, then she should have a workup for abdominal pain.

The Family Nurse Practitioner: Clinical Case Studies, Second Edition. Edited by Leslie Neal-Boylan.
© 2021 John Wiley & Sons Ltd. Published 2021 by John Wiley & Sons Ltd.

What is the plan for referrals and follow-up?

No referrals are need at this time, but a referral to a urologist might be in order if the patient has recurrent episodes or is found to have a stone.

Would the diagnosis change if the patient had fever and flank pain?

Pyelonephritis should be suspected if the patent develops fever or flank pain. Asymptomatic bacteriuria should not be treated unless the patient is pregnant, an older adult, has diabetes mellitus, has an indwelling catheter, or is at risk for complications.

Would the most likely diagnosis change if the patient were male?

If the patient were male, the likelihood of a UTI is less and is of more concern when it happens. It is important to determine the etiology of the symptoms in a male to help determine a plan of treatment. Prostatitis, epididymitis, and sexually transmitted infection are possible causes of urinary symptoms in men. A urinalysis and culture should be ordered.

What is an important symptom to consider in an older adult?

An older adult may not have any symptoms other than delirium. New onset of confusion should trigger lab testing for a UTI.

What if Susan were pregnant?

At approximately 12 weeks' gestation, the pregnant woman should be evaluated for a UTI to prevent low-birth-weight infants and poor delivery outcomes. A urinalysis and urine culture should be ordered. Avoid Bactrim and sulfa drugs if the patient is pregnant.

REFERENCES AND RESOURCES

Imam, T. I. (2018). Bacterial urinary infections. In R. S. Porter, J. L. Kaplan, R. B. Lynn, & M. T. Reddy (Eds.), *The Merck manual of diagnosis and therapy* (pp. 2176–2180). Kenilworth, NJ: Merck Sharp & Dohme Corp.

Gupta, K., Hooton, T. M., Naber, K. G., Wullt, B., Colgan, R., Miller, L. G., . . . Soper, D. E. (2011). International clinical practice guidelines for the treatment of acute uncomplicated cystitis and pyelonephritis in women: A 2010 update by the Infectious Diseases Society of America and the European Society for Microbiology and Infectious Diseases. *Clinical Infectious Diseases, 52,* e103–e120. doi:10.1093/cid/ciq257

RESOLUTION

What is the most likely differential diagnosis and why?
Migraine with aura:

Because these are new-onset headaches and also because Sophia's family history is significant for an uncle with a brain tumor, it is important to rule out other causes of her headaches, such as a brain tumor or aneurysm. Sophia's headaches appear to have an aura, because she has noticed "spots" in front of her eyes just before onset. Cluster headaches are more common in men, tend to occur over one side of the head or one eye, are excruciating and often explosive, and may also involve ipsilateral eye tearing. Patients tend to describe tension headaches as being bandlike and will motion to the temporal areas of the head bilaterally when describing the location of the pain. The headaches usually go away with rest or diversionary activities. Meningeal irritation tends to cause neck stiffness and fever as well as headache, and Brudzinski and Kernig signs tend to be positive. Sophia is too young to have temporal arteritis, a condition that is typically associated with polymyalgia rheumatica (PMR), a disease of adults over age 50 that presents with shoulder and hip girdle pain. Patients with temporal arteritis tend to have headache, possible jaw claudication, scalp or facial tenderness, and possibly diplopia. Patients who are suspected of having PMR or temporal arteritis should have an ESR done. Typically, the ESR will be very high (over 50) in these cases. High doses of prednisone are typically given to treat both conditions, and a rheumatologist should be consulted as part of the treatment plan.

Sophia might have a psychogenic headache but her history does not support this condition. That type of headache is more often bilateral and does not follow any particular pattern. Sophia's headaches are throbbing, unilateral, accompanied by nausea, preceded by an aura, and disappear with sleep. These migraines typically occur in women aged 30 to 50 years, and they often run in families.

There are various migraine triggers, such as hormonal changes (many women have premenstrual migraines), missed meals, certain foods such as chocolate or red wine, weather changes, stress or tension, birth control pills, nitrates, monosodium glutamate, tyramine, caffeine, vasodilation from any source, lack of sleep, glaring or flickering lights, aspartame, smoking, and alcohol use.

The Family Nurse Practitioner: Clinical Case Studies, Second Edition. Edited by Leslie Neal-Boylan.
© 2021 John Wiley & Sons Ltd. Published 2021 by John Wiley & Sons Ltd.

Are there tools that can be used to help assess this headache? If so, name two.

1. ID Migraine (Rapoport & Bigal, 2004):
During the past 3 months, did you have the following with your headaches?
*   You felt nauseated or sick to your stomach.
*   Light bothered you (a lot more than when you do not have headaches).
*   Your headaches limited your ability to work, study, or do what you needed to do for at least 1 day.
The ID Migraine screen is positive if 2 of the 3 items are answered in the affirmative.
2. The brief headache screen (Maizels & Burchette, 2003):
*   How often do you get severe headaches (i.e., without treatment, it is difficult to function)?
*   How often do you get other (milder) headaches?
*   How often do you take headache relievers or pain pills?
*   Has there been any recent change in your headaches?

Which diagnostic studies should be considered?

An MRI scan is appropriate, and a CBC with differential would be helpful to rule out infection and anemia as causes of the headaches. Whether to use contrast media with the MRI depends on the specific indications. If imaging the blood vessels, a CTA or MRA should supplement the MRI or CT scan and requires IV contrast. For a sudden, severe headache, get a CT scan of the head without contrast or possibly a CT with contrast. If the patient has a new-onset headache with optic disc edema, initially an MRI of the head with and without contrast are appropriate, as is a CT scan without contrast. Red flags, such as head trauma, a headache that worsens with activity, cancer, immunosuppression, an immunocompromised status, pregnancy, or age over 50 years, require other or additional imaging.

SNOOP (up to date) can be used to remember red flags:

*   Systemic symptoms
*   Neurologic symptoms
*   Onset (new, especially if new over age 50 years, or sudden)
*   Other associated conditions
*   Previous headache history with progression or change

What is the plan of treatment?

Migraine treatment can target suppressive therapy if the patient has several migraines in 1 week, abortive therapy (at the time of onset) or post migraine. Examples of suppressive therapy include NSAIDs, acetaminophen, SSRIs, valproate or topiramate, propranolol or metoprolol or timolol, and amitriptyline and venlafaxine. Abortive therapies include metoclopramide (an antiemetic), triptans, and ergotamines. If the patient is vomiting, add an antiemetic medicine. CGRP antagonists such as erenumab are not used first line but might be used in patients who are disabled by their migraine headaches or cannot tolerate other medicines. Sophia is of child-bearing age, so we might consider verapamil or flunarizine. Do not give her valproate or topiramate if she is or might become pregnant. It is important to carefully consider the medication options along with Sophia's individual needs and characteristics. Starting with a low dose and titrating upward is best practice. Do not give opioids or barbiturates to treat migraine.

If appropriate, consider a CT or MRI scan first to rule out other causes. Advising the patient to keep a headache diary in order to avoid triggers, as well as to retreat to a dark quiet room at the onset of the migraine, would also be helpful. Sophia should be seen for follow-up after 1 week to titrate the medicine as necessary and to review test and lab results.

Are any referrals or follow-up needed?

If the CT or MRI scan is abnormal or Sophia exhibits neurological deficits, she should be sent to the emergency department to see a neurologist. If Sophia were older and temporal arteritis was suspected, she would be referred immediately for an ophthalmologic consult to prevent vision loss.

Does the patient's psychosocial history impact how she might be treated?

Sophia's level of stress probably does impact her migraines; counseling regarding stress reduction and relaxation exercises may be helpful.

Is the patient's blood pressure the cause or the result of her headache?

Sophia's blood pressure may be a result of her headache pain. However, follow-up when she is not in pain is warranted to evaluate her for hypertension.

Would the treatment change if the patient were a smoker or on birth control pills?

If Sophia were a smoker or on birth control pills, she would be encouraged to stop smoking (for overall health and because smoking is a migraine trigger). Birth control pills can be a trigger for migraine, and patients with a migraine with aura should discontinue or not start birth control pills. Furthermore, smoking and the use of birth control pills can significantly increase the risk of deep vein thrombosis.

REFERENCE AND RESOURCE

Maizels, M., & Burchette, R. (2003). Rapid and sensitive paradigm for screening patients with headaches in primary care settings. *Headache, 43*(5), 441.

Rapoport, A. M., & Bigal, M. E. (2004). ID-migraine. *Neurological Science, 25*(Suppl 3), S258.

Case 6.11 Fatigue and Joint Pain

What is the most likely differential diagnosis and why?
Systemic lupus erythematosus (SLE):

SLE is most commonly seen in African American women with an onset typically between the ages of 20 and 30 years. However, Caucasian women and men also get SLE, and anyone can get it at a younger age. Only 10% of people with SLE have a family member with the disease. The development of autoantibodies and the presence of low complements are typical of SLE and are chiefly responsible for its symptoms. There is potential for multiorgan involvement (Petri, 2007).

The following environmental factors have been correlated with SLE, both onset and flares: ultraviolet light (UVA and UVB), echinacea, smoking, Epstein-Barr virus, silica exposure, and mercury exposure. Risk of developing SLE can be increased by the use of oral contraceptives or hormone replacement therapy. However, only HRT has been found to contribute to flares. Although the disease typically includes relapses and remissions, it can be characterized by continuous symptoms (Petri, 2007).

The American College of Rheumatology (ACR) is the most commonly used source for diagnosis of SLE. The patient must meet 4 of the following 11 criteria to be diagnosed with SLE:

- Malar rash
- Discoid rash
- Photosensitivity
- Oral ulcers
- Arthritis
- Serositis
- Renal disorder
- Hematologic disorder
- Neurologic disorder
- Immunologic disorder
- Positive ANA

Differential diagnoses (or co-diagnoses with SLE) include Sjögren's syndrome (dry eyes, dry mouth), fibromyalgia (muscle tender points), multiple areas of inflammation of cartilage (polychondritis),

---

The Family Nurse Practitioner: Clinical Case Studies, Second Edition. Edited by Leslie Neal-Boylan.
© 2021 John Wiley & Sons Ltd. Published 2021 by John Wiley & Sons Ltd.

and involvement of the eyes (such as scleritis). Elevated liver enzymes are not unusual. Patients with SLE may have cognitive changes, seizures, and stroke; and many have antiphospholipid syndrome (APL). APL can affect a woman's ability to deliver healthy normal children. Nephritis is another possible sequela but is often asymptomatic.

Aliyah has a malar rash (spares the nasolabial folds), livedo reticularis, nail fold capillary loops (all are very indicative of SLE), alopecia, nasal and oral ulcers, fever, weight loss, fatigue, lymphadenopathy, and polyarthritis.

Which diagnostic studies should be considered to assist with or confirm the diagnosis?

A CBC with differential will help determine if the patient has anemia or chronic disease, leukopenia, lymphopenia, or thrombocytopenia, which are all possible with systemic lupus erythematosus (SLE). An increased ESR and/or CRP will indicate active inflammation, but neither informs the clinician regarding disease or flare severity. Lipids may be abnormal due to renal dysfunction or prednisone use. In addition, the CK level may indicate myositis and the homocysteine level can be indicative of atherosclerosis or renal dysfunction. The ANA is positive in most patients with SLE. However, healthy persons can have a positive ANA. The ANA titer is most helpful because it indicates the presence of connective tissue disease. A titer of 1:640 or higher is indicative. If the ANA is positive, then perform the dsDNA, anti-Sm, Ro/SSA, La/SSB and U1 ribonucleoprotein (RNP) tests. Some labs reflex automatically from a positive ANA to these tests. The anti-DS DNA and anti-SM (Smith) tests are highly specific but not necessarily highly sensitive for SLE. Antiphospholipid (APL) antibodies (lupus anticoagulant, anti-Beta 2 glycoprotein-1) are present in half of patients with SLE at some point in the course of the disease. These antibodies are associated with an increased risk of blood clots and pregnancy losses. Anti-Ro/SSA and anti-La/SSB may be present in a patient with SLE but are more specific for Sjogren's syndrome. Anti-U1 RNP occurs in about a quarter of patients with SLE but is often present if the patient has a mixed connective disease condition. Decreased C3 and C4, while unspecific, are often present and can help signal a flare. X-rays of the hands and wrists will not show erosion as in rheumatoid arthritis. Ultrasound can detect synovitis or swelling that is not visible on examination. Other imaging should be chosen based on patient systems and the body system that is under suspicion for involvement, such as renal, pulmonary, cardiac, abdomen, or brain. Aliyah complained of a cough so a chest X-ray might be appropriate at this time.

An elevated serum creatinine, BUN, and/or proteinuria can be indicative of renal dysfunction. A renal biopsy is required to investigate this further. The urine should be examined for hematuria and red blood cell casts (Petri, 2007).

If the ANA is negative but the clinician suspects SLE, then perform a rheumatoid factor test and check for anti-CCP antibodies. This will help exclude or include rheumatoid arthritis as the diagnosis. If the history indicates a possibility of infection, check for infections such as parvovirus, hepatitis B and C, tick-borne illnesses, or other infections.

What is the plan of treatment?

Aliyah should be instructed to get exercise, rest, eat nutritiously, protect the skin from the sun, and stop smoking. Patients with SLE frequently have low vitamin D levels so levels should be monitored and treated as appropriate. If she had hypertension or abnormal lipids, those should be well managed to avoid atherosclerosis and renal dysfunction. Aliyah should receive influenza and pneumonia vaccines to protect her from opportunistic infections. Her bone density should be monitored, especially if steroids are used to help control flares. Topical glucocorticoids are typically used to help cutaneous lupus. However, a referral to a dermatologist is sensible if the patient has cutaneous symptoms.

SLE is initially treated with NSAIDs. These should be accompanied by a proton pump inhibitor to protect the gastrointestinal tract. However, a patient with Aliyah's symptoms would probably be started on Plaquenil (hydroxychloroquine), as it slows progression of the disease and helps symptoms. It is usually given at doses of 200–400 mg daily. It can cause retinal damage, so it is important for the patient to have a baseline and annual eye examination by an ophthalmologist. Prednisone is often used to control flares and methotrexate is used to supplement Plaquenil. Biologic immunosuppressive treatments, such as rituximab or cyclosporine, or azathioprine may be ordered by the rheumatologist.

What is the plan for referrals and follow-up?

Patients who are diagnosed with SLE or discoid lupus should be referred to a rheumatologist. However, it is not always possible to get patients in to see the rheumatologist right away. In the meantime, the rheumatologist can be consulted by telephone and the patient can be started on NSAIDs or Plaquenil. The patient should follow up with primary care for her general health care needs; however, follow-up pertaining to the SLE will most likely occur with the rheumatologist.

Are there other manifestations of this disease?

If discoid lupus skin lesions are suspected, it is important to order a skin biopsy. Nerve conduction studies and biopsies can help identify vasculitis and myositis.

Would it change the diagnosis or impact the prognosis or treatment if the patient were taking minocycline? What if the patient had a parvovirus?

Minocycline along with tumor necrosis factor alpha inhibitors can cause drug-induced lupus. Symptoms should resolve after removing the causal agent. Parvovirus, HIV, hepatitis, and malignancy can also cause lupus-like symptoms (Petri, 2007).

What are the potential complications of this disease?

Organ damage may occur as a result of the disease itself, prolonged steroid treatment, interstitial pulmonary fibrosis, renal complications, and atherosclerosis. Other complications include pleuritic pain, pleural effusions, pericarditis, pulmonary hypertension, and esophageal abnormalities (Petri, 2007).

REFERENCES AND RESOURCES

Belmont, H. M. (2013). Treatment of systemic lupus erythematosus—2013 update. *Bulletin for the Hospital of Joint Diseases, 71*, 208.

Bertsias, G., Ioannidis, J. P., Boletis, J., Bombardieri, S., Cervera, R., Dostal, C., Font, J., . . . Task Force of the EULAR Standing Committee for International Clinical Studies Including Therapeutics. (2008). EULAR recommendations for the management of systemic lupus erythematosus. Report of a Task Force of the EULAR Standing Committee for International Clinical Studies Including Therapeutics. *Annals of Rheumatic Diseases, 67*,195.

Gladman, D. D., Pisetsky, D. S., & Curtis, M. R. (2018). Systemic lupus erythematosus. *UpToDate*.

Gordon, C., Amissah-Arthur, M. B., Gayed, M., Brown, S., Bruce, I. N., D'Cruz, D., . . . Isenberg, D., for the British Society for Rheumatology Standards, Audit and Guidelines Working Group. (2018). The British Society for Rheumatology guideline for the management of systemic lupus erythematosus in adults. *Rheumatology (Oxford), 57*,e1–e45.

Hochberg, M. C. (1997). Updating the American College of Rheumatology revised criteria for the classification of systemic lupus erythematosus (letter). *Arthritis & Rheumatology, 40*, 1725.

Petri, M. (2007). Monitoring systemic lupus erythematosus in standard clinical care. *Best Practice & Research in Clinical Rheumatology, 21*(4), 687–697.

Petri, M., Orbai, A. M., Alarcón, G. S., Gordon, C., Merrill, J. T., Fortin, P. R., . . . Magder, L. S. (2012). Derivation and validation of the Systemic Lupus International Collaborating Clinics classification criteria for systemic lupus erythematosus. *Arthritis & Rheumatology, 64*, 2677–2686.

Pons-Estel, B. A., Bonfa, E., Soriano, E. R., Cardiel, M. H., Izcovich, A., Popoff, F., . . . Alarcón, G. S., on behalf of the Grupo Americano de Estudio del Lupus (GLADEL) and Pan-American League of Associations of Rheumatology (PANLAR). (2018). First Latin American clinical practice guidelines for the treatment of systemic lupus erythematosus: Latin American Group for the Study of Lupus (GLADEL, Grupo Latino Americano de Estudio del Lupus)-Pan-American League of Associations of Rheumatology (PANLAR). *Annals of Rheumatic Diseases 77*, 1549–1557.

Tan, E. M., Cohen, A. S., Fries, J. F., Masi, A. T., McShane, D. J., . . . Winchester, R. J.. (1982). The 1982 revised criteria for the classification of systemic lupus erythematosus. *Arthritis & Rheumatology*, *25*, 1271–1277.

Toloza, S. M., Cole, D. E., Gladman, D. D., Ibañez, D., & Urowitz, M. B.. (2010). Vitamin D insufficiency in a large female SLE cohort. *Lupus 19*, 13–19.

van Vollenhoven, R. F., Mosca, M., Bertsias, G., Isenberg, D., Kuhn, A., Lerstrøm, K., . . . Schneier, M.. (2014). Treat-to-target in systemic lupus erythematosus: Recommendations from an international task force. *Annals of Rheumatic Diseases*, *73*, 958–967.

Wallace, D. J. (2008). Improving the prognosis of SLE without prescribing lupus drugs and the primary care paradox. *Lupus*, *17*, 91.

Wallace, D. J., Pisetsky, D. S., Schur, P. H., & Curtis, M. R. (2019). Systemic lupus Eeythematosus treatment. *UpToDate*.

RESOLUTION

What is the most likely differential diagnosis and why?
Fibromyalgia (FM):
The following data support this diagnosis: Widespread pain for longer than 3 months, occurring bilaterally and above and below the waist. Patients with FM also typically have sleep disorders, depression and/or anxiety, stressful or dysfunctional childhoods and current lifestyles, and fatigue. People with FM often have burning pain and perceive that they have joint swelling but do not have it on examination. The inability to concentrate is not uncommon, and these patients often have a coexisting problem such as irritable bowel syndrome, chronic fatigue, or another systemic disease.

Which diagnostic studies should be considered to assist with or confirm the diagnosis?
Zelda has widespread pain for more than 3 months. If the history or exam raised suspicion for other illnesses, then labwork, such as ESR, rheumatoid factor, and anti-CCP and an ANA should be pursued to rule out these illnesses. However, other than a suspicion of pregnancy, Zelda does not have any symptoms that would suggest any of these other diseases. She should have an HCG to rule out pregnancy. Therefore, she should not undergo unnecessary testing. If she has not been tested recently for thyroid disease, a TSH should be considered, although fatigue seems to be her only relevant symptom.

What is the plan of treatment?
Zelda should be encouraged to lose weight, to eat more fruits and vegetables, to exercise, and to reduce her stress level. Aquatic therapy can be useful. She will probably benefit from counseling to help her through this period of stress. However, her insurance may not cover it. Cognitive behavioral therapy (CBT) often helps, as can hypnotherapy. Encouraging her to engage in pleasurable activities, both alone and with her children, will help distract her from her difficulties and from her symptoms. Zelda should be taught sleep hygiene activities so she can improve her sleep without sleeping aids, if possible. If a sleeping aid is necessary, use a nonbenzodiazepine and consider a sleep study to fully evaluate the quality of sleep.

The Family Nurse Practitioner: Clinical Case Studies, Second Edition. Edited by Leslie Neal-Boylan.
© 2021 John Wiley & Sons Ltd. Published 2021 by John Wiley & Sons Ltd.

Antidepressants can help both the symptoms of FM and the depression Zelda has been experiencing. Cymbalta (Duloxetine), 30–60 mg, is a good option as it helps both physical pain and depression. However, a less expensive alternative that works quite well is the use of amitriptyline (10–15 mg) at bedtime to help with anxiety and sleep alone or in combination with an SSRI taken in the morning. Effexor (venlafaxine), like Cymbalta, 150–225 mg daily, combines norepinephrine and epinephrine, which help decrease all of the symptoms of FM. Anxiolytics may be pursued as adjunct therapy if the patient is anxious, but should be pursued carefully and only for as long as needed.

For a patient who has hyperalgesia or allodynia to a severe degree, Neurontin (gabapentin) or Topamax (topiramate) titrated up at weekly intervals can help. Lyrica or pregabalin started at 75 mg daily and increased, if needed, to 150 mg twice each day, will make the patient sleepy and also help relieve symptoms. Savella (Milnacipran) is an alternative to Lyrica. The patient must get used to the drug, as daytime sleepiness can be initially a significant problem. Topical capsaicin can help relieve burning pain.

Patients with FM should <u>not</u> be given opioid medications or NSAIDs to treat the condition, as these have been shown to not help and may worsen symptoms in the long run. Monosodium glutamate and aspartame can also worsen symptoms.

What is the plan for referrals and follow-up?

A referral to a rheumatologist may be considered if the case is not straightforward or if there are confounding factors or symptoms that warrant suspicion of a connective tissue or inflammatory disorder. A referral to an orthopedist may be warranted if the patient is found to have joint pain or swelling with LROM on examination. Follow-up care should be provided as necessary to monitor the effects of new medications and other treatment. The patient needs opportunities to be heard and reassured that the provider listens, understands, empathizes with her, and takes her concerns seriously.

REFERENCE AND RESOURCE

American College of Rheumatology, www.rheumatology.org

Biundo, J. J. (2018). Fibromylagia. In R. S. Porter, J. L. Kaplan, R. B. Lynn, & M. T. Reddy (Eds.), The Merck manual of diagnosis and therapy (p. 269). Kenilworth, NJ: Merck Sharp & Dohme Corp.

RESOLUTION

What is the most likely differential diagnosis and why?

Hyperthyroidism:

Iris's symptoms of palpitations, tachycardia, insomnia, impaired concentration, fatigue, heat intolerance, weight loss, and irregular menses all support the diagnosis of hyperthyroidism. Additionally, the exam finding of soft, shiny hair, hyperreflexia, goiter, and thyroid bruit also support the diagnosis. However, Iris does not yet have some symptoms she might acquire without treatment, such as exophthalmos, lid lag, tremors, and atrial fibrillation. There are many causes of hyperthyroidism, but Graves' disease is the most common.

Hypothyroidism would cause other symptoms, such as oversleeping, weight gain, dryness of the skin, hair, or nails, cold intolerance, and dyspnea. The TSH would be high, and the free T4 may be low or normal.

Iris could be pregnant, or she could be going through perimenopause. Lab workup should include an HCG and an FSH. A CBC and a CMP will be helpful to rule out additional causes of her symptoms, such as infection, and to provide a baseline prior to treatment. Thyroid disease often affects LDL and HDL levels, so fasting lipid levels should be obtained. Iris may be anxious aside from the thyrotoxicosis, although her history does not appear to support that diagnosis; but screening for depression and anxiety is always helpful.

Which diagnostic tests are required in this case and why?

A low TSH and elevated T3 and T4 would confirm hyperthyroidism or thyrotoxicosis. The ANA may also be elevated, although the patient does not have systemic lupus erythematosus (if Iris is taking biotin, this could affect laboratory results). Subclinical hyperthyroidism would be indicated by a low TSH and normal free T3 and T4. However, there are other possible causes of these results, including illness unrelated to thyroid disease. If in doubt, retest the patient in 1 or 2 months. If the diagnosis indicates hyperthyroidism but it is not completely clear, such as with Iris, TRab, RAI, or ultrasound can be done to confirm the diagnosis. TRab confirms the diagnosis of Graves' disease. RAI or ultrasound should be performed if TRab is negative. However, if Iris were pregnant, she

---

The Family Nurse Practitioner: Clinical Case Studies, Second Edition. Edited by Leslie Neal-Boylan.
© 2021 John Wiley & Sons Ltd. Published 2021 by John Wiley & Sons Ltd.

could not have the RAI test. Iris does not have a thyroid nodule. If she did, provided she was not pregnant, RAI should be performed.

What is the plan of treatment?

First determine if Iris is pregnant. The choice of drug treatment will depend on whether she is pregnant. Iris could be given some propranolol or other beta blocker to temporarily relieve her symptoms of nervousness, tachycardia, diaphoresis, and palpitations. Atenolol or Metoprolol may work better for Iris if she has contraindications to propranolol. Beta blockers are often the initial drug therapy. However, RAI may be initial therapy. The goal is to achieve euthyroidism before surgery if surgery is needed. Beyond beta blockers, there is no consensus as to the best way to treat hyperthyroidism. Antithyroid drugs, such as Methimazole or PTU, may be used before surgical or radioactive iodine intervention. Methimazoile is the drug of choice, with Propylthiouracil (PTU) used only if patient cannot tolerate Methimazole or is pregnant. As symptoms of hyperthyroidism decrease and the free T4 nears the normal range, drug dosages are reduced. Radioactive iodine is a very common method for destroying the thyroid, and this treatment does not increase the risk for thyroid cancer or other cancers. Methimazole should be stopped for at least 4 days if the patient is to be started on radioactive iodine treatment. Iris smokes, so she runs the risk of increased likelihood of eye problems after iodine treatment. Follow-up with TSH and free T4 is critical, as the procedure may render the patient hypothyroid requiring thyroid replacement therapy. Thyroid surgery is another option for treatment. These three primary therapeutic options should be discussed with the patient so the best option for the individual patient is chosen. The extent of the disease (mild, moderate, or severe), eye orbit involvement, pregnancy or lactation, age, the extent of symptoms, and general health should all impact the choice of treatment.

Iris will need frequent follow-up as treatment progresses to monitor symptoms and lab results and to check for complications of the disease. Most likely, Iris will need synthetic or natural thyroid replacement following the destruction of the thyroid gland. Table 6.13.1 is included to help show the differences between hypo- and hyperthyroidism.

What is a likely diagnosis if this patient returns with severe tachycardia, confusion, vomiting, diarrhea, high fever, and dehydration?

If this patient returns with all of these symptoms, suspect thyroid storm. This condition typically requires hospitalization. Methimazole or propranolol is given. Steroids are often used and then tapered as the symptoms improve.

What if this patient's lab results return and the TSH is low with normal results for free T4 and T3?

If this patient's lab results return and the TSH is low with normal results for free T4 and T3, then the patient most likely has subclinical hyperthyroidism. However, the patient would be asymptomatic and does not need treatment.

Would the plan be any different if Iris were unemployed?

It will be important to find out if Iris is a self-pay patient and to determine her financial status before ordering a lot of tests. It will be especially important to consider whether you can stage testing so cost does not become an undue burden for Iris. Medicine may also be costly for Iris. Referral to a medical social worker might be helpful.

Are there any standardized guidelines that should be used to assess and treat this case?

The American Association of Clinical Endocrinologists has guidelines that can help the clinician make diagnostic and treatment plan choices (http://www.aace.com/).

Table 6.13.1. Comparison of Hypo- and Hyperthyroidism.

Hypothyroidism	Hyperthyroidism
Can be caused by a rare pituitary gland tumor.	Graves disease is most common; caused by IgG (binds to TSH), initiates production and release of thyroid hormone.
Typical presentation: The body cannot make enough thyroid hormone. The body produces less body heat and consumes less oxygen.	
Other causes: Hashimoto's, surgical removal of the thyroid gland, post Graves' disease (after treatment), thyroid irradiation.	Other causes: Toxic adenoma, toxic multinodular goiter, painful subacute or silent thyroiditis, iodine-induced hyperthyroid (amiodarone treatment), oversecretion of pituitary TSH, excess endogenous thyroid hormone production.
TSH is up. Free T4 is down. High lipids. Low sodium.	TSH is low. Free T4 is elevated.
	Radionucleotide uptake and scan with iodine to determine if it is secondary to Graves' disease, thyroid nodule. or thyroiditis.
	Hyperactivity of thyroid: Increased uptake on RAI.
	Nodules: Limited areas of uptake on RAI and surrounding hypoactivity.
	Subacute thyroiditis: RAI uptake is patchy and decreased overall.
Treatment: Check pituitary function.	Treatment: Radioactive iodine (if not pregnant).
Give thyroid hormone (lower dosage for elderly). Initial dose (for anyone): 125–150 mcg (0.10–0.15 mg/d). Dose depends on age, weight, cardiac status, duration, and severity of disease. Titrate after 6 weeks and following any change in dose.	Postpone pregnancy for 6 months after scan. Do not use during lactation. PTU may be used to treat condition (prevents conversion of T4 to active T3).
Use TSH to gauge dose and monitor treatment.	Give PTU BID for 7 days (can use in pregnancy) or may use Tapazole daily. Side effect of PTU is agranulocytosis.
	Post ablation: Follow up 6 weeks after treatment and regularly until evidence of early hypothyroidism (based on TSH); then start treatment for hypothyroidism.

REFERENCES AND RESOURCES

Barbesino, G., & Tomer, Y. (2013). Clinical utility of TSH receptor antibodies. *Journal of Clinical Endocrinology Metabolism, 98*, 2247.

Hershman, J. M. (2018). Thyroid disorders. In R. S. Porter, J. L. Kaplan, R. B. Lynn, & M. T. Reddy (Eds.), *The Merck manual of diagnosis and therapy* (pp. 1346–1349). Kenilworth, NJ: Merck Sharp & Dohme Corp.

Ross, D. S. (2019, May). Diagnosis of hyperthyroidism. *UpToDate.*

Case 7.1 Fatigue

RESOLUTION

Which diagnostic studies should be considered to assist with or confirm the diagnosis?

In order to get a better picture of Fred's status and the reason for his symptoms, it is appropriate to order a CBC, comprehensive metabolic panel, lipid profile, urinalysis with micro albumin and microanalysis, and serum testosterone levels. The CBC will rule out systemic illness and give a picture of general health. The comprehensive metabolic panel and Hemoglobin A1C will assess Fred's diabetes control, kidney and liver function, and fluid status. The lipid profile will evaluate the status of his hyperlipidemia, while the urine studies will evaluate several aspects of Fred's diabetes control. The serum total and free testosterone levels will evaluate for hypogonadism and may indicate secondary hypogonadism. However, total testosterone is less sensitive in older men. FSH and LH help differentiate primary from secondary hypogonadism. If the gonadotropin level is high, the patient has primary hypogonadism. However, given Fred's age, primary hypogonadism should have been apparent long ago and is not the cause of his symptoms. A prolactin level will screen for a pituitary adenoma and transferrin saturation will screen for hemochromatosis. However, a patient over 60 years of age with this profile is unlikely to have a brain mass so imaging is usually unnecessary.

Relevant test results for Fred include a free testosterone level of 128 ng/dL. Normal levels for a young adult male are 300–1000 ng/dL. In men older than 60 years with signs or symptoms of androgen deficiency, a total testosterone level below 200 ng/dL is almost always clinically significant.

What is the most likely differential diagnosis and why?

Secondary hypogonadism:

Given the objective report of clinically significant low testosterone, we can conclude that Fred has secondary hypogonadism. This explains his decreased sexual function, along with his lowered concentration and impaired mood.

However, looking further into the constellation of Fred's symptoms and conditions, it becomes evident that there is interplay of many factors. Fred's uncontrolled diabetes is a wild card, as it can also contribute to his decline in sexual function. The problem is autonomic neuropathy that results from failure of the small vessels that lead to vasodilation. In addition, it is known that obesity leads to lower free and total testosterone levels. Adding in Fred's probable depressive syndrome completes

The Family Nurse Practitioner: Clinical Case Studies, Second Edition. Edited by Leslie Neal-Boylan.
© 2021 John Wiley & Sons Ltd. Published 2021 by John Wiley & Sons Ltd.

the clinical picture that shows many overlaps in symptoms. However, an objective diagnosis of hypogonadism can be confidently made considering the laboratory results. Diagnosis is made via evaluation of serum testosterone levels.

It is known that blood concentrations of testosterone and prehormones are significantly lower in older men than younger men, as they begin a gradual decline at midlife. In aging men who have not always had symptoms, hypogonadism is referred to as secondary, since the problem is not a primary dysfunction of the testes. Signs and symptoms of secondary hypogonadism due to aging include decreased muscle mass and strength, decreased bone mass, decreased libido (desire), erectile dysfunction, impaired mood, and impaired sense of well-being.

The diagnosis of male sexual dysfunction can include any or all of the following categories: (1) decreased libido, (2) erectile dysfunction, (3) ejaculatory insufficiency, or (4) impaired orgasm. Fred reports both decreased libido and erectile dysfunction, which can have several different etiologies. Decreased libido can occur due to psychogenic factors, medications, androgen deficiency, substance use or abuse, or central nervous system disease. Erectile dysfunction can occur due to psychogenic factors, medications, endocrine disorders, aging, or systemic illness. Diagnosis is generally made on subjective reporting, and treatment is symptom based.

Fred reports being on antidepressants in the past, which alludes to a previous diagnosis of depressive disorder. Today, Fred's report of altered mood, fatigue, sexual dysfunction, poor concentration, substance use, and personal stressors all suggest the possibility of a depressive syndrome. In cases of secondary hypogonadism initiated by a systemic illness, it is important to retest FSH and LH 4 to 6 weeks after the illness has resolved.

What is the plan of treatment?

As an initial approach to Fred's low testosterone, an appropriate treatment is testosterone therapy. There are several different administration modalities, including intramuscular (IM) injections, skin patches, and transdermal gel preparations. IM injection is widely used and is an appropriate choice for Fred. The testosterone transdermal patch delivers 4 mg of testosterone daily but has a high incidence of skin irritation. There are other patch preparations that are larger and cause less irritation, but they may have a tendency to fall off with activity. The transdermal testosterone gel is widely used and the dosage is 5–10 mg of 1% testosterone gel applied daily. It causes little skin irritation, though there is a possibility for transfer through direct skin contact. There are also transdermal axillary solutions, buccal lozenges, a nasal spray, and subcutaneous implants. Since Fred has difficulty with daily medication compliance, bringing him to the clinic for routine injections is a wise choice.

In adjunct to testosterone therapy, Fred should be educated about medication compliance. Explaining to him the importance of diabetes control and the interplay of his numerous symptoms may be an effective approach.

What is the plan for referrals and follow-up?

Education about diet and exercise should be reinforced; and, if he is willing, he should be given a referral for nutritional counseling. Since Fred will be coming to the office for routine injections to start, there will be opportunities to reassess his symptoms. There will also be an opportunity to assess whether Fred or his spouse should be instructed in injection administration. Follow-up intervals should occur between every 4 months in the first year and every 6 months thereafter to evaluate progress, symptoms, and blood levels. Labs should include hematocrit, PSA, and testosterone. If the hematocrit increases, a reduction in the testosterone therapy should be considered. PSA levels should be monitored carefully. Digital rectal exams should also be performed. Therapy could continue for as long as 3–4 years.

What would be relative and absolute contraindications to the treatment plan of testosterone therapy?

Testosterone therapy is absolutely contraindicated in those with carcinoma of the prostate or of the male breast, as these cancers require androgens for proliferation. Testosterone therapy should be used with caution in older men with enlarged prostates, with urinary symptoms, or elevated hematocrit.

Are there standardized guidelines that would help in this case?

The American Association of Clinical Endocrinologists Medical Guidelines for Clinical Practice for the Evaluation and Treatment of Hypogonadism in Adult Male Patients—2002 update (http://www.aace.com/sites/default/files/2019-06/hypo-gonadism.pdf" http://www.aace.com/sites/default/files/2019-06/hypo-gonadism.pdf), as well as an Endocrine Society Clinical Practice Guideline (Bhasin et al., 2018).

REFERENCES AND RESOURCES

AACE Hypogonadism Task Force. (2002). American Association of Clinical Endocrinologists medical guidelines for clinical practice for the evaluation and treatment of hypogonadism in adult male patients—2002 update. *Endocrine Practice, 8*, 439–456.

Bhasin, S., Brito, J. P., Cunningham, G. R., Hayes, F. J., Hodis, H. N., Matsumoto, A. M., … Yialamas, M. A. (2018). Testosterone therapy in men with hypogonadism: An Endocrine Society clinical practice guideline. *Journal of Clinical Endocrinology & Metabolism, 103*(5), 1715–1744. https://doi.org/10.1210/jc.2018-00229

Hirsch, I. H. (2018). Male hypogonadism. In R. S. Porter, J. L. Kaplan, R. B. Lynn, & M. T. Reddy (Eds.), The *Merck manual of diagnosis and therapy* (pp. 2128–2132). Kenilworth, NJ: Merck Sharp & Dohme Corp.

NOTE: The author would like to acknowledge the contributions of Geraldine F. Marrocco, EdD, APRN, CNS, ANP-BC and Amanda La Manna, RN, ANP to this case in the first edition of this book.

Case 7.2 Testicular Pain

RESOLUTION

What is the most likely differential diagnosis and why?
<u>Epididymitis:</u>
As testicular torsion and testicular mass were ruled out via ultrasound and there was no report of trauma, the differential can be narrowed down to a sexually transmitted infection (STI) or epididymitis. There was no urethral discharge on exam. Coupled with the patient's report of monogamy, this suggests that the cause of the pain is not an STI. The negative urine tests for gonorrhea and chlamydia confirmed this. The acute pain and positive Phren's sign on exam point strongly toward epididymitis. Commonly, the cremasteric reflex is negative in testicular torsion.

Epididymitis is a bacterial infection and inflammation of the epididymis, which is the tube connecting the testicle with the vas deferens. It is the most common cause of acute scrotal pain in all age groups, though it is most common among sexually active men younger than 35. In the younger age group, the infection is most often due to *Chlamydia trachomatis* or *Neisseria gonorrheae*. In men who have anal intercourse, epididymitis can be caused by *Escherichia coli*. In older men, the cause is often a urinary tract infection. On exam, the affected testis will transilluminate, and there will be a positive Phren's sign.

While some sexually transmitted infections can lead to epididymitis, it is possible for some infections to affect the ductus deferens and/or the testicles. Those included are chlamydial infection, gonorrheal infection, and syphilis infection.

Testicular torsion should be suspected whenever a man complains of scrotal pain, as it is an emergent condition that can, if left untreated, lead to ischemia of the affected testis. It presents acutely as a firm, tender mass, often associated with nausea and vomiting. The cremasteric reflex is typically negative and one testis often rides high (bell clapper deformity). Testicular torsion can occur at any age but occurs more often in men younger than 25 years of age. No exam finding can completely rule out testicular torsion. Therefore, it must be ruled out via a Doppler study due to its emergent nature. A Doppler study will reveal decreased blood flow to the testis in a case of torsion.

Testicular malignancy is most prevalent in young men ages 15–35 years. Symptoms include a hard, heavy, firm, nontender mass. There will often be scrotal swelling in the affected testis, and some testicular tumors will cause discomfort or pain. Upon exam, the affected testis where the mass is located will not transilluminate.

The Family Nurse Practitioner: Clinical Case Studies, Second Edition. Edited by Leslie Neal-Boylan.
© 2021 John Wiley & Sons Ltd. Published 2021 by John Wiley & Sons Ltd.

Though uncommon, testicular trauma should be a consideration when presented with a case of scrotal pain. Usually the affected individual will identify a recent injury or trauma. Classifications of disorders due to trauma include blunt trauma, penetrating trauma, degloving trauma, and testicular rupture.

Diagnostic testing: To rule out the emergent condition of testicular torsion, it is appropriate to obtain a stat Doppler scrotal ultrasound. In addition, it is appropriate to order obtain a urine sample for a urinalysis, culture, and sensitivity to evaluate for infection and gonorrhea and chlamydia.

The results of the Doppler indicated that there was no testicular torsion. A pulse Doppler and a color Doppler were performed, revealing both testicles to be normal in size and to have a homogenous echotexture. The right testicle measured $4.4 \times 2.2 \times 2.4$ cm, and the left testicle measured 2.98×2.0 cm. There was no intratesticular or extratesticular mass present. No abnormal fluid was noted in bilateral scrotal sacs, and there was no evidence of testicular torsion. The urine tests were negative.

What is the plan of treatment?

Without knowing the offending bacterial organism, empiric treatment of the infection is appropriate at this stage. Levofloxacin 500 mg orally daily for 10 days or ofloxacin 300 mg twice a day for 10 days are the most appropriate treatment choices. Bactrim DS twice a day for 10 days is an alternative. If this patient were under age 35, ceftriaxone 250 mg IM (1 dose) plus doxycycline 100 mg twice a day for 10 days would be the first choice of treatment to cover possible gonorrhea or chlamydia. Azithromycin 1 gram orally is an alternative.

To address the patient's acute pain, an NSAID, application of ice, and elevation of the scrotum are recommended. Opioids are not recommended. Sitz baths may also provide relief.

The patient being treated for epididymitis should be brought back in 2 weeks to evaluate the success of treatment. If treatment is successful in symptom reduction, the antibiotics should be completed. If symptoms still persist, the patient should be further evaluated by a specialist.

Are there any referrals or follow-up care needed?

In cases of recurrent infection or failure to respond to treatment, it would be appropriate to consult with or refer the patient to a urologist.

REFERENCES AND RESOURCES

Eyre, R. C. (2019, May). Evaluation of acute scrotal pain in adults. *UpToDate.*

Shenot, P. J. (2018). Penile and scrotal disorders. In R. S. Porter, J. L. Kaplan, R. B. Lynn, & M. T. Reddy (Eds.), *The Merck manual of diagnosis and therapy* (pp. 2141–2142). Kenilworth, NJ: Merck Sharp & Dohme Corp.

Trojian, T. H., Lishnak, T. S., & Helman, D. (2009). Epididymitis and orchitis: An overview. *American Family Physician, 79,* 583.

NOTE: The author would like to acknowledge Geraldine F. Marrocco, EdD, APRN, CNS, ANP-BC, who wrote the original version of this case in the first edition of this book.

Case 7.3 Prostate Changes

What tool might be useful to evaluate Stanley's symptoms?

The American Urological Association symptom index is used to identify the severity and possible impact the symptoms are having on the patient's quality of life. The tool has 7 questions addressing frequency, nocturia, weak urinary stream, hesitancy, intermittence, incomplete emptying, and urgency, each of which is scored on a scale of 0 (not present) to 5 (almost always present). Symptoms are classified as mild (total score 0 to 7), moderate (total score 8 to 19), or severe (total score 20 to 35). The AUA symptom index tool is a validated, self-administered questionnaire used to assess the severity of the symptoms (O'Leary, 2005). Stanley had an AUA index score of 8.

What are the top three differential diagnoses in this case and why?

Stanley is having lower urinary tract symptoms (LUTS), including urgency, nocturia, frequency, urge incontinence, and weak stream. The symptoms indicate that he has both obstructive and irritative symptoms (Sarma & Wei, 2012). The patient's presentation (obstructive and irritative symptoms), his age (>60 years), and his race (African American) suggest the following top three differentials.

Benign prostatic hyperplasia (BPH):

BPH is an enlargement of the prostate gland that is common in older men. It can negatively impact the quality of life. Autopsy studies have shown the prevalence of BPH worldwide to be up to 60% in men over the age of 60 years, reaching up 80% of men by age 80 (McVary, 2006). Some studies have indicated that Black men experience more moderate to severe symptoms compared to White men. Nonmodifiable risk factors for BPH include age, race, genetic susceptibility, and family history of cancer. Modifiable risk factors include metabolic syndrome, beverage consumption, physical inactivity, and alcohol consumption. The enlargement of the prostate can lead to benign prostatic obstruction and bladder outlet obstruction. The most common symptoms are the lower urinary symptoms: LUTS, including frequency, nocturia, urgency, and urinary incontinence, or voiding symptoms, including slow urinary stream, hesitancy, straining, and terminal dribbling. Patients with BPH might also have hematuria; an in-office digital rectal examination can detect an enlarged prostate (McVary, 2006). The LUTS and digital rectal exam findings might be associated with an increased PSA level.

The Family Nurse Practitioner: Clinical Case Studies, Second Edition. Edited by Leslie Neal-Boylan.
© 2021 John Wiley & Sons Ltd. Published 2021 by John Wiley & Sons Ltd.

Prostate cancer:

Prostate cancer is the most common solid cancer in men, and the third most common cause of cancer-related deaths in 2017. It is most common in Blacks. The PSA test, together with the digital exam and other patient variables including ethnicity, age, and family, would warrant additional follow-up. A biopsy would be needed to confirm a cancer diagnosis. In this patient, the PSA is elevated at 4.6ng/DL; however, the digital rectal exam showed a smooth non-nodular enlarged prostate. The patient presentation and physical exam findings are more in line with BPH than prostate cancer.

Urinary tract infection:

This a reasonable differential as he presented with LUTS. Urinary tract infections are relatively rare in men under the age of 60 years but increase significantly thereafter due to prostate-related issues. Patients usually present with dysuria and urethritis. A UTI can be confirmed or ruled out by a urinalysis. A urinalysis would show white blood cells and blood in the urine (Dean & Lee, 2019). If that was the case, urine would be sent for culture and sensitivity identify the bacteria, and the drug it is sensitive to.

Which diagnostic tests are required in this case and why?

A prostate-specific antigen testing is indicated because the symptoms of prostate cancer are indistinguishable from those of benign prostatic hypertrophy. A PSA test should be done after shared decision-making. An elevated PSA together with prostate positive physical exam findings will warrant further workup. An elevated PSA with hematuria, asymmetrical nodular prostate, and LUTS would need to be followed up for possible prostate cancer. PSA levels can also be elevated in BPH, infections, and post instrumentation. Stanley's PSA was 4.6ng/DL. Normal PSA for a man > 60 years < 70 years should be < 4.5ng/DL (Carter et al., 2013). The PSA test is controversial as a prostate cancer screening tool as there are too many false positives.

Urine for urinalysis is needed to rule out a urinary tract infection, with reflex culture and sensitivity if positive. This patient had LUTS without hematuria or other signs of infection. If urinalysis did not show any white blood cells, indicating he did not have a UTI, a culture and sensitivity would not be necessary.

Bladder scan post void residual: This can be useful, especially in men who have symptoms of obstruction or suspected neurogenic involvement. This can also be useful prior to initiation of treatment. There is no consensus on what is normal PVR; definition on urinary retention in men has ranged from 100 mls to 1000 mls (Kaplan et al., 2008), with most urologists being concerned by a PVR of > 100–200 mls. A high PVR is a possible indicator for BPH, as it is associated with an increased risk for infection (Oeleke et al., 2013). The amount of PVR is not associated with the severity of BPH, and is not a predictor of surgical outcome. Even though there is no consensus on the amount, Stanley does have a PVR of 100 cc, signaling some type of urinary retention.

What are the concerns at this point?

The lower urinary symptoms are distressing and can lead to a decreased quality of life. Since Stanley has some retentive symptoms, there is a concern regarding the severity of the symptoms, for if not addressed promptly they can lead to possibly irreversible damage to the kidneys, and severe infection that could become life threatening.

What is the likely diagnosis?

BPH: This patient has LUTS, an enlarged prostate, a PVR of 100 mls, and an elevated PSA without hematuria or prostate nodules, making it likely that he has BPH with moderate symptoms.

What is the plan of treatment?

Stanley has BPH with moderate symptoms. The treatment is largely dependent on how bothersome the symptoms are to him. For those with mild symptoms, the treatment can be watchful waiting with reassurance. Stanley has LUTS with nonsuspicious prostate enlargement. With an

AUA index score of 8, he is in the moderate category. Shared decision making is important in deciding the way forward. If he is unsure of medications, lifestyle modifications and behavior modification will be recommended. The goals for treatment are:

1. Reduce bothersome LUTs symptoms
2. Alter disease progression
3. Prevent complications

(McConnell et al., 2003).

Lifestyle modifications: Lifestyle modifications are the initial recommended treatment for patients with bothersome symptoms. The patient will be encouraged to restrict fluid at night, or, when going out, instructed on double-voiding techniques to empty the bladder, avoidance of alcohol (he drinks 2 shots of cognac a night), regular physical activity, and avoidance of coffee and other highly seasoned or irritating foods. The lifestyle modifications can improve LUTS and can prevent disease progression; discontinue possibly offending meds, for example, Benadryl (Oelke et al., 2013, Pao-Hwa & Freedland, 2015).

Medications: The AUA symptom index classifies Stanley as having moderately distressing symptoms. He came to seek out treatment because of his discomfort. The symptoms are impacting his quality of life. Because of the severity of his symptoms he could decide to start with medications. Alpa-1-adrenegic antagonist monotherapy is the recommended treatment for moderate symptoms. Alpha-1-adrenegic antagonists relax smooth muscles in the bladder neck, prostate capsule, and the urethra. Currently approved alpha-1-adrenergic antagonists include terazosin, doxazosin, tamsulosin, alfuzosin, and silodosin. All these drugs have similar efficacy, so which one is prescribed might be based on cost, as well as side effects like hypotension and sexual side effects. Educate Stanley on the side effects, especially orthostatic hypotension and dizziness. Men with scheduled cataract surgery should not start on alpha-1-adrenergic antagonists until after surgery (McVary et al., 2010).

What are the plans for referral and follow-up care?
Follow up in 2–4 weeks; titrate dose up, if there has been some improvement. If there has been no improvement, refer to urology for further testing and possible combination treatment or surgery if no improvement in 1 to 2 years.

What health education should be provided to this patient?
Educate on how to take medications and possible side effects, especially orthostatic hypotension and dizziness. Take medication at night to reduce postural lightheadedness. Educate Stanley on the potential for sexual side effects and foods to avoid. Stop taking Benadryl. It might take 1 to 2 weeks before he sees improvement.

Does the patient's psychosocial history impact how you might treat him?
Avoid prescribing Silodosin, as it is more likely to cause sexual side effects.

Are there any standardized guidelines that should be used to treat this case? If so, what are they?
American Urologic Association Guidelines (McVary et al., 2010, reviewed and confirmed in 2014).

REFERENCES AND RESOURCES

Abrams, P., Chapple, C., Khoury, S., Roehrborn, C., de la Rosette, J., & International Consultation on New Developments in Prostate Cancer and Prostate Diseases. (2009). Evaluation and treatment of lower urinary tract symptoms in older men. *Journal of Urology, 181,* 1779.

Brown, C. T., Yap, T., Cromwell, D. A., Rixon, L., Steed, L., Mulligan, K., ... Emberton, M. (2007, January 6). Self-management for men with lower urinary tract symptoms: Randomised controlled trial. *BMJ, 334*(7583), 25. Epub November 21, 2006.

Carter, H. B., Albertsen, P. C., Barry, M. J., Etzioni, R., Freedland, S. J., Greene, K. L., ... Zietman, A. L. (2013). Early detection of prostate cancer: AUA Guideline. *Journal of Urology, 190*(2), 419–426.

Dean, A. J., & Lee, D. C. (2019). Bedside laboratory and microbiologic procedures. In J. R. Roberts (Ed.), Roberts and Hedges clinical procedures in emergency medicine and acute care (7th ed., Chapter 67, pp. 1442–1469. Philadelphia: Elsevier.

Kaplan, S. A., Wein, A. J., Staskin, D. R., Roehrborn, C. G., & Steers, W. D. (2008). Urinary retention and post-void residual urine in men: Separating truth from tradition. *Journal of Urology, 180*(1), 47–54.

McConnell, J., Roehrborn, C., Bautista, O., Andriole, G. L. Jr., Dixon, C. M., Kusek, J. W., ... Smith, J. A., for the Medical Therapy of Prostatic Symptoms (MTOPS) Research Group.(2003). The long-term effect of doxazosin, finasteride, and combination therapy on the clinical progression of benign prostatic hyperplasia. *New England Journal of Medicine, 349*, 2387.

McVary, K. (2006). BPH: Epidemiology and comorbidities. *American Journal of Managed Care, 12*(5 Suppl), S122.

McVary, K.T., Roehrborn, C. G., Avins, A. L., Barry, M. J., Bruskewitz, R. C., Donnell, R. F., ... Wei, J. T. (2010, validity confirmed 2014). Management of benign prostatic hyperplasia. American Urological Association. https://www.auanet.org/guidelines/benign-prostatic-hyperplasia-(bph)-guideline/benign-prostatic-hyperplasia-(2010-reviewed-and-validity-confirmed-2014)

Oelke, M., Bachmann, A., Descazeaud, A., Emberton, M., Gravas, S., Michel, M. C., ... European Association of Urology. (2013). EAU guidelines on the treatment and follow-up of non-neurogenic male lower urinary tract symptoms including benign prostatic obstruction. https://doi.org/10.1016/j.eururo.2013.03.004

O'Leary, M. P. (2005) Validity of the "bother score" in the evaluation and treatment of symptomatic benign prostatic hyperplasia. *Reviews in Urology, 7*(1), 1–10.

Sarma, A.V., & Wei, J. T. (2012). Benign prostatic hyperplasia and lower urinary tract symptoms. *The New England Journal of Medicine, 367*, 248–257. doi: 10.1056/NEJMcp1106637

Pao-Hwa, L., & Freedland, S. J. (2015). Lifestyle and LUTS: What is the correlation in men? *Current Opinion Urology, 25*(1):,1–5. doi:10.1097/MOU.0000000000000121

Wasson, J. H., Reda, D. J., Bruskewitz, R. C., Elinson, J., Keller, A. M., & Henderson, W. G. (1995). A comparison of transurethral surgery with watchful waiting for moderate symptoms of benign prostatic hyperplasia. The Veterans Affairs Cooperative Study Group on Transurethral Resection of the Prostate. *New England Journal of Medicine, 123*(1). doi:10.1056/NEJM199501123320202

Case 8.1 Substance Use Disorder (SUD)

RESOLUTION

What are the top three differential diagnoses in this case and why?

This case describes a patient who expresses the desire to stop using a substance that she and her partner have identified as responsible for contributing to negative health effects. Although there are potentially several other medical and psychiatric issues present in this complex scenario, the most pressing differentials include the following:

Opioid withdrawal:

The patient reports difficulty in stopping the use of opioids on her own and experiencing severe physical withdrawal symptoms. Withdrawal syndromes (often physical but also psychological or motivational feelings of needing a substance to feel functional) are a key feature within the widely accepted framework of addiction as a chronic, relapsing brain disease (Herron & Brennan, 2019).

Opioid use disorder:

The features of continued compulsive use (unable to stop despite efforts) despite adverse consequences (withdrawal symptoms, social problems like tardiness/job loss, school troubles) point toward this diagnosis.

Uncontrolled anxiety/depression/ADHD or other mental health disorder:

Several features in this case (e.g., a history of ADHD, a family history of alcoholism/depression/ suicide) suggest that a potential contributing factor to Chan Ming's substance use patterns may be comorbid mental health conditions. The prevalence of comorbid mental health diagnoses with substance use disorders is known to be high and, therefore, exploration of mental health diagnoses with an eye toward adequate treatment to mitigate and/or prevent substance use disorder is warranted (National Institute on Drug Abuse [NIDA], 2018).

What are the top three diagnostic tests or screens required in this case and why?

Routinely screening for alcohol, nicotine, and other drug use in general medical settings is considered an important preventive health care measure by the Substance Abuse and Mental Health Services Administration (SAMHSA; 2018). There are a variety of validated screening tools for alcohol, tobacco, and drugs that can be completed via self-report survey or administered by staff or clinicians during the office visit. Screening, Brief Intervention, and Referral to Treatment (SBIRT) is

The Family Nurse Practitioner: Clinical Case Studies, Second Edition. Edited by Leslie Neal-Boylan.
© 2021 John Wiley & Sons Ltd. Published 2021 by John Wiley & Sons Ltd.

an evidence-based approach to universal screening for substance use that can identify those patients who are most at risk for health consequences and allow for early intervention. Detailed resources for SBIRT are available at https://www.integration.samhsa.gov/clinical-practice/sbirt. In this patient's case, the patient self-identifies as needing help with opioids. The following screening tools/diagnostic criteria would be useful in this case to more accurately assess this patient:

- *Clinical Opiate Withdrawal Scale (COWS):* This 11-item scale can be administered by clinicians in inpatient or outpatient settings to determine the severity of withdrawal and assess the level of physical dependence on opioids (Wesson & Ling, 2003). Some signs and symptoms measured with this tool include pulse rate, pupil size, presence of tremor, sweating, gooseflesh, GI upset, and restlessness. This scale can be readministered over time to assess response to withdrawal treatment interventions. Management of physical withdrawal symptoms is a crucial step in maximizing a patient's capacity for further long-term treatment (Gowing, Ali, White, & Mbewe, 2017).
- Diagnostic and Statistical Manual *5th edition (*DSM-5*) criteria for opioid use disorder:* The American Psychiatric Association (APA; 2013) has identified criteria that can be used to confirm and document a diagnosis of opioid use disorder. OUD is defined as "a problematic pattern of substance use leading to clinically significant impairment or distress" manifested by presence of at least two adverse health effects related to opioid use occurring within a 12-month period. A clinician can objectively classify and determine severity (mild, moderate, severe) of OUD by applying these criteria. A checklist of the *DSM-5* criteria can be found at: https://www.ncbi.nlm.nih.gov/books/NBK535277/bin/pt2app.p35.pdf
- *Patient Health Questionnaire 9 (PHQ-9)/Generalized Anxiety Disorder 7 item (GAD-7):* Due to the risk for comorbid mental health issues in any patient who uses substances problematically, these tools serve to identify and assess common mental health conditions that, when adequately treated, may synergistically improve OUD treatment. The PHQ-9 is a valid and reliable 9-question tool that can be used in an outpatient setting to identify and classify the severity of comorbid depression (Kroenke, Spitzer, and Williams, 2001). Similarly, the GAD-7 can be used to efficiently identify anxiety disorder (Spitzer, Kroenke, Williams, and Löwe, 2006). Both scales can also be readministered over time to assess changes during therapy. Web-based versions of both tools can be found at: https://www.hiv.uw.edu/page/mental-health-screening/phq-9 and https://www.hiv.uw.edu/page/mental-health-screening/gad-7.

What are the concerns at this point?

This case presents several imminent and long-term health concerns for the family health care provider to address. The potentially life-threatening effects of opioid use disorder and comorbid mental health crises warrant immediate attention to safety issues such as overdose prevention and suicide screening. Longer-term issues may require co-management with specialists but there are several steps an astute primary care nurse practitioner (NP) can take to set the stage for optimal outcomes. The following is a list of priority concerns about this patient:

- *Opioid withdrawal:* This patient presents with both history and physical exam evidence for acute opioid withdrawal. Appropriate management including medications (see below) will address one of the family's most pressing concerns (severe withdrawal symptoms resulting in continued dangerous use) and can maximize a patient's chance for success at longer-term treatment approaches. Moreover, although withdrawal from opioids, unlike alcohol or benzodiazepines, is not associated with acute physiologic life-threats like seizures, the risk of fatal overdose from the continued use of fentanyl analogues found in the illicit drug supply is high. Therefore, every opportunity to more safely help a patient in opioid withdrawal represents a potentially life-saving health care encounter.
- *Overdose risk:* As mentioned, the use of heroin/fentanyl is extremely concerning given the U.S. opioid crisis and related overdose deaths. In 2017, the Centers for Disease Control (CDC) reported nearly 72,000 overdose deaths, of which over two-thirds were linked to opioids

(Ahmad, Rossen, Spencer, Warner & Sutton, 2018). Because of the potency and uncertainty of concentrations of illicit fentanyl in the heroin supply in the United States, opioid overdoses have dramatically increased and essentially any person who uses opioids, especially fentanyl, is at risk. Health care providers can mitigate overdose risk by providing education and access to naloxone. In a public health advisory, the U.S. Department of Health and Human Services (2018, April 5) recommends naloxone access for "patients currently taking high doses of opioids as prescribed for pain, individuals misusing prescription opioids, individuals using illicit opioids such as heroin or fentanyl, health care practitioners, family and friends of people who have an opioid use disorder, and community members who come into contact with people at risk for opioid overdose." NPs should provide education on signs of overdose and the administration of naloxone to patients and families at risk. Naloxone is available in various formulations, including an intranasal spray and intramuscular injection. Patients can receive naloxone by prescription or in many states by standing order at pharmacies or often for free at community locations. More information on naloxone for overdose prevention can be found at: www.prescribetoprevent.org.

- *Opioid use disorder treatment:* This patient's visit, for the express purpose of asking for help with her substance use, offers the NP an important opportunity to rally and coordinate services so that the patient successfully accesses formal treatment for her substance use. According to a 2018 report, only about 1 in 4 people with opioid use disorder received specialty treatment within the past year (U.S. Department of Health and Human Services, 2018, September). Providers in any health care setting should be prepared to reduce this gap by offering initiation of care or by ensuring rapid access to specialty care (i.e., a "warm handoff"; meds/counseling/ both/recovery supports).

- *Comorbid mental health issues (i.e. anxiety/depression):* As discussed, the prevalence of substance use alongside mental health conditions warrants careful examination of this patient's overall mental health. Prioritizing assessment of possible depression, including a suicide screen, is crucial as a safety concern. In addition to the screening tools mentioned earlier, NPs in general health settings should be familiar with evidence-based resources such as the Suicide Assessment Five-Step Evaluation and Triage (SAFE-T) tool developed by SAMHSA. This resource, including a Suicide Safe mobile app, can be found at: https://store.samhsa.gov/product/SAMHSA-Suicide-Safe-Mobile-App/PEP15-SAFEAPP1

What are the options for the medicinal management of acute opioid withdrawal?

Options for the medicinal management of acute opioid withdrawal include the following:

- *Methadone:* The full opioid agonist action of methadone will ameliorate opioid withdrawal symptoms. Due to the long and variable half-life of methadone (which ranges from 24 to 36 hours or longer), it can take up to 5 half-lives to reach serum steady state. Slow titration doses of methadone can be given over hours to days until COWS scores improve. Risk of overdosing during induction phase is possible and induction with methadone should be managed only by providers with experience and expertise in a qualified opioid treatment program or inpatient setting (ASAM, 2015; SAMHSA, 2018). Research has shown that most patients who go through medically supervised opioid withdrawal return to opioid use, so initiation of maintenance treatment with either methadone or buprenorphine is the preferred long-term treatment for opioid use disorder and results in significantly better morbidity and mortality than detoxification (SAMHSA, 2018). In general, methadone is restricted to federally designated addiction clinics. There is an exception, commonly referred to as the "72-hour rule," that allows non-addiction specialists to administer methadone (no take-home prescriptions or doses) for the acute management of withdrawal for a period of 72 hours only (U.S. Department of Justice, n.d.). The federal restrictions, long half-life, risk for QTc prolongation and arrhythmia (especially in combination with other medicines that prolong the QT interval), and potential for overdose make methadone a challenging medication for non-addiction specialists to manage.

- *Buprenorphine:* Buprenorphine is a partial opioid agonist that has been shown to be effective for reducing withdrawal symptoms and is safe to use in both inpatient and outpatient settings. Because of its ceiling effect, buprenorphine is less likely to be associated with respiratory depression (SAMHSA, 2018). To avoid precipitated withdrawal, buprenorphine should not be administered until 12–18 hours after the last dose of a short-acting agonist such as heroin or oxycodone, and 24–48 hours after the last dose of a long-acting agonist such as methadone (ASAM, 2015). Titrating doses (4-16 mg) are administered until withdrawal symptoms abate. NIDA has published a sample algorithm for buprenorphine induction that can be used in emergency room or other ambulatory care settings: https://www.drugabuse.gov/nidamed-medical-health-professionals/discipline-specific-resources/initiating-buprenorphine-treatment-in-emergency-department/buprenorphine-treatment-algorithm. Unlike methadone, current U.S. law allows non-addiction prescribers to become waivered by the Drug Enforcement Administration (DEA) to *prescribe* buprenorphine for opioid withdrawal as well as for longer-term maintenance (see the later section on maintenance therapy). Like methadone, buprenorphine can be also be *administered* (but not prescribed/dispensed) for 72 hours for acute withdrawal management by any prescriber even if not waivered.
- *Clonidine:* An alpha-2-adrenergic agonist has been historically used to ameliorate the sympathetic central nervous system effects of opioid withdrawal and may be helpful if opioid agonist options are not available. Limiting side effects include hypotension. Because clonidine has been found to be less effective than opioid agonists (Gowing et al., 2017), and because most patients who undergo medically supervised full withdrawal return to illicit opioid use, it is recommended that opioid agonist maintenance therapy be initiated (SAMHSA, 2018) .
- *Other symptom-specific comfort medications:* Although these medications may not be necessary for every patient (especially if using an opioid agonist or partial agonist), secondary medicines targeting specific symptoms such as antiemetics for nausea, dicyclomine for stomach cramping, loperamide for diarrhea, and over-the-counter analgesics for mild to moderate pain may be used. As with any medication, the prescriber should consider side effect risks as well as medication interactions that affect the decision to use any drug.

What are the three FDA-approved medicines for maintenance therapy for opioid use disorder (OUD) and which may be prescribed in primary care?

It is important to note that there is no single approach to treatment of substance use disorder that is perfectly suited to every patient. Providers must be committed to a patient-centered approach that considers not only the research evidence on medications but also considers the patient's values, beliefs, and preferences. The following are the three FDA-approved medications (a detailed treatment improvement protocol for the use of these medications can be found at: https://store.samhsa.gov/product/TIP-63-Medications-for-Opioid-Use-Disorder-Full-Document-Including-Executive-Summary-and-Parts-1-5-/SMA19-5063FULLDOC):

- *Buprenorphine:* High-quality research has found buprenorphine to be effective and safe (SAMHSA, 2018). Buprenorphine has been associated with improved retention in treatment, lower morbidity and mortality compared to treatment without medication, reduced overdose rates, reduced HIV risk behavior, and is effective in primary care settings (SAMHSA, 2018). Under current federal law, buprenorphine is the only *opioid-agonist* treatment for OUD that may be prescribed by primary care providers (with special training). Providers are required to take either 8 hours (MDs) or 24 hours (NPs and PAs) of training. Efforts to increase access in the United States to this life-saving drug are crucial in light of the opioid crisis. Free buprenorphine trainings can be accessed at: https://pcssnow.org/medication-assisted-treatment/. If an NP does not yet have a waiver to prescribe buprenorphine, it is important to offer information and arrange for immediate referral and follow-up to patients who desire it and may benefit from it.
- *Methadone:* Methadone has a long (almost-50-year) track record as an evidence-based, effective medicine for treatment of OUD and is used worldwide (SAMHSA, 2018). Proven benefits of

methadone treatment include improved retention in treatment, less illicit opioid use, reduced mortality, reduced crime, and reduced HIV seroconversion rates (SAMHSA, 2018). Current U.S. federal law limits the routine administration/prescribing of methadone for treatment of OUD to federally-qualified clinics or inpatient settings. Although methadone may not be prescribed for OUD in a primary care setting, all providers who take care of patients with OUD should be familiar with it. Methadone may be prescribed for treatment for the explicit indication of pain management but because of the risks and challenges outlined previously, this should ideally only be done by prescribers with specialty training and experience.

- *Naltrexone:* Naltrexone is an opioid antagonist that blocks the effect of opioids at receptor sites. The formulation of naltrexone that has been shown in research to be effective for treatment of OUD is an injectable depot extended-release naltrexone (XR-NTX). XR-NTX has been found to improve retention in treatment and reduce illicit opioid use compared to placebo (SAMHSA, 2018). Oral naltrexone has not been shown to be an effective treatment for OUD so is not recommended. Primary care providers may prescribe XR-NTX but must consider that initiation requires a patient to be fully abstinent from opioids for a period long enough (7 to 10 days after last use of short-acting opioids and 10 to 14 days after last use of long-acting opioids) to avoid precipitated withdrawal (SAMHSA, 2018). Patients must be willing to return for monthly depot injections and should be counseled about opioid blockade effects, which may complicate treatment of pain should it be necessary.

What are health promotion/health prevention/harm reduction topics that should be addressed with this patient?

In this case, in addition to addressing the primary concerns of withdrawal and OUD, the NP should strive to attend to the following issues:

- *Overdose education and naloxone provision:* With any patient at risk for opioid overdose, naloxone education should be provided to the patient and any family/friends/roommates who may be in the position to witness an overdose. If unable to dispense or provide a take-home naloxone formulation directly to the patient at the time of the visit, the NP should direct the patient/family to the nearest pharmacy/community resource that can provide it. Resources on where to obtain naloxone should be easily accessed via a web search or through a local/regional/state health department. The NP should convey harm reduction messages such as urging the patient to not use alone and to have naloxone and someone trained on its use nearby in the event of a return to opioid use.
- *Comorbid mental health:* If discovered in the screening recommended earlier, the NP should prioritize the need for urgent treatment (i.e., if suicidal ideation is present) and discuss options for treatment of comorbid mental health issues (ranging from medications to counseling across a variety of settings). Involvement of a multidisciplinary team including behavioral health specialists is ideal.
- *General health promotion/prevention:* As with any chronic health condition, the primary care NP should consider the general health needs of the patient and maintain routine screenings, immunizations, and reproductive health counseling as indicated by up-to date guidelines such as the U.S. Preventive Services Task Force (USPSTF; see www.uspreventiveservicestaskforce.org) or other professional organizations/guidelines.

What is the plan of treatment?

The plan for treatment in this case would involve an informed conversation with the patient and family about available options and preferences. Options for treatment of OUD vary widely and can be delivered in multiple settings ranging from primary care to intensive outpatient programs to inpatient to residential programs (SAMHSA, 2018). Availability of specialized treatment services vary regionally and are often limited by insurance coverage and waiting lists. SAMHSA's Behavioral Health Treatment Services Locator (https://fndtreatment.samhsa.gov) is a national resource that may help patients and providers find available treatment providers if the NP is unfamiliar with local services. A negotiated patient-centered plan might include the following components for a patient who does not require hospitalization or residential treatment:

- Praise patient and family for seeking care and provide education about OUD as a chronic health condition that is treatable.
- Ideally, induce patient on buprenorphine for withdrawal and begin maintenance therapy. Immediate initiation of buprenorphine reduces the chance a patient will delay or forego accessing care and return to use (SAMHSA, 2018).
- Provide naloxone kit or prescription and overdose education for patient/partner/friends/family.
- Consider an antidepressant if PHQ-9 or GAD-7 suggests a *DSM-5* diagnosis of anxiety or depression.
- Ideally, in an integrated care setting where behavioral health and substance use services are colocated with primary care, conduct a "warm handoff" to addiction and/or mental health counseling. If an integrated setting is not available, the NP should be familiar with community resources and refer urgently.

What are the plans for referral and follow-up care?
Referrals and follow-up for this patient should include the following:

- Ongoing pharmacotherapy treatment (if not provided by primary care provider).
- Addiction and/or mental health counseling.
- Peer recovery supports (recovery coaches) may be available in many communities. Trained recovery workers (many with lived experience) provide patients in early recovery important local support. For more details on recovery community centers and their work, see https://www.recoveryanswers.org/resource/recovery-community-centers/
- Depending on patient preferences, referral to self-help groups like AA, NA, Smart Recovery, and so on may be helpful. The SAMHSA National Helpline serves as a national centralized resource for finding local services (https://www.samhsa.gov/find-help/national-helpline).
- Close follow-up with primary care (i.e., days to weeks) to maintain therapeutic relationship and ensure stability in early recovery.
- Support groups for families dealing with OUD. The SAMHSA National Helpline can assist with these services as well. One example of a group targeting OUD specifically is Learn2Cope (https://www.learn2cope.org/).
- If OUD progresses to include injection use, referral to a syringe services program (SSP) that can provide life-saving, health-preserving harm reduction approaches even if drug use continues. Nearly three decades of quality research have shown SSPs to effectively and safely improve health outcomes such as HIV, hepatitis, and other infection rates and have not been associated with increased drug use or crime (CDC, 2019). To find local services, the North American Syringe Exchange Network maintains a listing of operating SSPs at: https://www.nasen.org/.

What health education should be provided to this patient?
Education on the following would be important in this case:

- Education on pathophysiology of OUD as chronic relapsing disorder/risks of overdose
- Risks/benefits/potential side effects/interactions of all medicines
- Naloxone for overdose prevention as above

What are demographic characteristics that might affect this case?
Demographic factors such as employment, housing stability, and insurance coverage may greatly affect access to care.

Does the patient's psychosocial history impact how you might treat him?

As discussed, the prevalence of substance use disorder with comorbid mental health disorders is high. History of trauma is also associated with higher risk for substance use disorder (SAMHSA, 2018). Sensitive consideration of these factors by the NP is important to enhance efficacy of treatment. Moreover, access to some of the more basic physical social determinants of health (i.e., housing, transportation, a safe living environment) are known to affect the ability for a person to attain their best health (CDC, 2018) and therefore must be considered closely to optimize treatment plans and ongoing care.

What if the patient lived in a rural (or urban) setting?

Several factors may create differences in the presentation and approach to OUD in a rural versus an urban setting. There may be differences in opioids used based on the illicit market supply (i.e., prescription opioids versus heroin versus fentanyl). Geographic availability of treatment services can vary widely and transportation to treatment becomes an important social factor to consider when planning treatment. NPs should become familiar with the nuances of their community's local available services.

Are there any standardized guidelines that should be used to treat this case? If so, what are they?

The following guidelines may be useful to the NP for managing care in this case:

- SAMHSA's "Medications for Opioid Use Disorder. Treatment Improvement Protocol (TIP) Series 63": Available at: https://store.samhsa.gov/product/TIP-63-Medications-for-Opioid-Use-Disorder-Full-Document-Including-Executive-Summary-and-Parts-1-5-/SMA18-5063FULLDOC
- American Society of Addiction Medicine's "National Practice Guideline for the Use of Medications in the Treatment of Addiction Involving Opioid Use." Available at: https://www.asam.org/docs/default-source/practice-support/guidelines-and-consensus-docs/asam-national-practice-guideline-supplement.pdf
- Naloxone for overdose prevention: Guidance for healthcare providers can be found at: https://prescribetoprevent.org/

What other professionals might you collaborate with to best provide comprehensive care for SUD?

A collaborative, multidisciplinary approach to treatment of OUD is ideal. The following is a list of other professionals who the NP can collaborate with to provide best care:

- Addiction specialists if available. NPs should become familiar with locally available experts or if there are accessible telemedicine services. Free general mentoring services are provided by the Providers Clinical Support System for any provider who completes buprenorphine waiver training (see: https://pcssnow.org/mentoring/).
- Mental health/psychiatry providers.
- Peer recovery coaches (see referral information above).
- Harm reduction organizations (see referral information above).

If you discovered that the patient were using substances intravenously, what other concerns/testing/treatment would you want to consider?

The use of any substance intravenously poses multiple health concerns related to enhanced drug effect (i.e., faster onset of action and high potency increases risk of opioid overdose) and infection risks. If injection use is discovered, the following is a list of potential concerns:

- Risk for skin infections (especially if needles are reused, which is common when sterile syringe services are not easily accessible or unavailable)
- Risk for bacterial endocarditis
- Risk for HIV/hepatitis and need for screening

- Education on safer injecting techniques/sterile supplies (referrals to SSPs if available or provision of safe injecting information is crucial). The Harm Reduction Coalition offers a printable manual on safe injection available at: https://harmreduction.org/drugs-and-drug-users/drug-tools/getting-off-right/
- Sexual/reproductive health counseling and provision of condoms and/or birth control as necessary
- Referrals to local services/social workers as needed for housing instability or other financial concerns such as access to health insurance
- Risk for trauma and post-traumatic stress disorder (i.e., witnessing overdoses, violence, sex work)

REFERENCES AND RESOURCES

Ahmad, F. B., Rossen, L. M., Spencer, M. R., Warner, M., & Sutton, P. (2018). *Provisional drug overdose death counts*. National Center for Health Statistics. Retrieved from:https://www.cdc.gov/nchs/nvss/vsrr/drug-overdose-data.htm

American Psychiatric Association. (2013). Opioid use disorder. In *Diagnostic and statistical manual of mental disorders* (5th ed.). Arlington, VA: American Psychiatric Publishing.

American Society of Addiction Medicine. (2015). *National practice guideline for the use of medications in the treatment of addiction involving opioid use*. Retrieved from: https://www.asam.org/docs/default-source/practice-support/guidelines-and-consensus-docs/asam-national-practice-guideline-supplement.pdf

Centers for Disease Control. (2018, January 29). *Social determinants of health: Know what affects health*. Retrieved from: https://www.cdc.gov/socialdeterminants/index.htm

Centers for Disease Control. (2019, May 23). *Syringe services programs (SSPs)*. Retrieved from: https://www.cdc.gov/ssp/index.html

Gowing, L., Ali, R., White, J. M., & Mbewe, D. (2017). Buprenorphine for managing opioid withdrawal. *Cochrane Database of Systematic Reviews, 2*, CD002025. https://doi-org.libproxy.unh.edu/10.1002/14651858.CD002025.pub5

Herron, A. J., & Brennan, T. K. (Eds.). (2019). The ASAM essentials of addiction medicine (3rd ed.). Philadelphia: Wolters Kluwer Health.

Kroenke, K., Spitzer, R. L., & Williams, J. B. (2001). The PHQ-9: Validity of a brief depression severity measure. *Journal of General Internal Medicine, 16*(9), 606–613. doi:10.1046/j.1525-1497.2001.016009606.x

National Institute on Drug Abuse. (2018, August). *Comorbidity: Substance use disorders and other mental illnesses*. Retrieved from:https://www.drugabuse.gov/publications/drugfacts/comorbidity-substance-use-disorders-other-mental-illnesses

Pew Charitable Trusts. (2019, February). *Opioid use disorder: Challenges and opportunities in rural communities*. https://www.pewtrusts.org/en/research-and-analysis/fact-sheets/2019/02/opioid-use-disorder-challenges-and-opportunities-in-rural-communities

Spitzer, R. L., Kroenke, K., Williams, J. B. W., & Löwe, B. (2006). A brief measure for assessing generalized anxiety disorder: The GAD-7. *Archives of Internal Medicine, 166*(10), 1092–1097.

Substance Abuse and Mental Health Services Administration. (2018). *Medications for opioid use disorder*. Treatment Improvement Protocol (TIP) Series 63. HHS Publication No. (SMA) 19-5063FULLDOC. Rockville, MD. https://store.samhsa.gov/system/files/tip63_fulldoc_052919_508.pdf

U.S. Department of Health and Human Services. (2018, April 5). *U.S. Surgeon General's advisory on naloxone and opioid overdose*. Washington, DC: HHS. Retrieved from: https://www.hhs.gov/surgeongeneral/priorities/opioids-and-addiction/naloxone-advisory/index.html

U.S. Department of Health and Human Services, Office of the Surgeon General. (2018, September). *Facing addiction in America: The Surgeon General's spotlight on opioids*. Washington, DC: HHS. https://addiction.surgeongeneral.gov/sites/default/files/Spotlight-on-Opioids_09192018.pdf

U.S. Department of Justice. (n.d.) *Emergency narcotic addiction treatment*. Retrieved from: https://www.deadiversion.usdoj.gov/pubs/advisories/emerg_treat.htm

Wesson, D. R., & Ling, W. (2003). The clinical opiate withdrawal scale (COWS). *Journal of Psychoactive Drugs, 35*(2), 253–259. doi:10.1080/02791072.2003.10400007

Case 8.2 Foot Ulcer

RESOLUTION

Which diagnostic or imaging studies should be considered to assist with or confirm the diagnosis?

A CBC with differential and elevated white count can indicate infection. George is a diabetic so it should be assumed that the foot ulcer is infected. The discharge and increasing discomfort also support a diagnosis of infection. An erythrocyte sedimentation rate (ESR) may also be helpful. Cultures with Gram staining can help determine the cause of the infection. Without signs of infection, a culture is not indicated. It would be helpful to get an HBA1c if George has not had one recently. The test will help determine whether George's diabetes is under control, which seems unlikely. The CMP will reveal his current blood sugar level as well as his kidney function and metabolic status. An X-ray will help diagnose osteomyelitis or gout. If osteomyelitis is highly suspected, a bone biopsy will be necessary. An MRI would be helpful if osteomyelitis is suspected and is more helpful than an X-ray.

Identify and explain three differential diagnoses.

All of the diagnoses listed in the case presentation are possible. George is a diabetic. This ulcer started with a callus, which is a very common early presentation for diabetic foot ulcers. George has a history of both peripheral vascular and peripheral arterial disease. George may also have cellulitis with or without osteomyelitis or a secondary infection because his wound has not healed. The presentation could also indicate a MRSA infection. Gout does not typically present with discharge but the great toe is the most common location for gout and the affected area typically presents with redness, warmth, and severe pain. In addition, gout usually has an acute onset. See Case 8.4 (burning leg pain) for more information. The data in this case most likely points to a diabetic ulcer or venous ulcer. The brownish tinge to the skin and the scattered varicosities are hallmark signs.

The Family Nurse Practitioner: Clinical Case Studies, Second Edition. Edited by Leslie Neal-Boylan.
© 2021 John Wiley & Sons Ltd. Published 2021 by John Wiley & Sons Ltd.

Arterial Ulcers	Venous Ulcers
Regular borders	Irregular borders
Base of yellow material or eschar	Shallow wound bed
Scant or absent granulation tissue	No eschar
Underlying structure more likely visible	No underlying structures visible
Absent or decreased pedal pulses	Positive palpable pulses
Painful	Painless
Outer sides of ankles, feet, tips of heels, toes	Below the knee; around ankle, particularly medial side
Waxy skin	Brawny skin changes
Hair loss on limb	
Cool to touch	

What is the plan of treatment?

Diabetic foot infections are serious and should be treated promptly. The choice of antibiotic depends on the extent of the infection. Diabetic ulcers are typically caused by more than one organism. Only use antibiotics if the wound is visibly infected. Antibiotic treatment should cover both Gram-positive and Gram-negative organisms, especially if the patient has recently been treated with antibiotics. If George had a recently diagnosed MRSA infection or is at high risk (regular hospitalizations or inpatient stays), he should be treated with intravenous vancomycin until the culture and sensitivity test returns. George has a worsening infection, so the best plan of treatment is to start him on IV antibiotics. After stabilization, he can be switched to antibiotics by mouth. Sometimes surgical debridement of the wound is necessary. Choose an antibiotic in consultation with a vascular surgeon and consider George's renal function.

Are there any standardized guidelines to consider?

Lipsky, B. A., Aragón-Sánchez, J., Diggle, M., Embil, J., Kono, S., Lavery, L., . . . Peters, E. J. G., on behalf of the International Working Group on the Diabetic Foot, & Peters, E. J. G. (2016). IWGDF guidance on the diagnosis and management of foot infections in persons with diabetes. *Diabetes Metabolism Research and Reviews, 32*(Suppl. 1), 45–74.

   International Diabetes Federation. (2017). *Clinical practice recommendation on the diabetic foot: A guide for health care professionals.* International Diabetes Federation.

What health education should be provided to the patient?

George will need health teaching regarding the antibiotic treatment chosen to treat his wound. If he requires debridement, he will need pre- and post-operative teaching. Otherwise, the most important instruction for George concerns getting and keeping his blood sugar under control. He will need to work with his health care providers to maintain tight control. George should also be instructed to inspect his feet daily and report calluses or open wounds, no matter how small. He should use recommend emollients to prevent dryness, scaling, and cracking. George should also report symptoms of neuropathy or nerve damage. He should be referred to a podiatrist for regular nail clipping and foot checks. His podiatrist may need to see him every 3 months.

What complicating factors specific to this case should be considered?

George has several complicating factors in his health history. He is obese and has both PAD and PVD. He is diabetic. He has hyperlipidemia, heart disease, sleep apnea, and ITP.

What collaborative assessment and care might the patient require? Include your rationale.

George needs referral to a podiatrist and wound specialist. The podiatrist will check his feet frequently, trim his toenails, and teach him how to care for his feet and about the impact of poor glucose control on his feet and skin. The wound specialist will need to evaluate the wound and weigh in on the correct antibiotic and wound treatment. An orthopedic consult will be necessary if

George has osteomyelitis or if the wound is deep enough to affect the bone. George may be hospitalized while receiving IV treatment or he may receive IV antibiotics at home by a visiting nurse. In any case, he will need follow-up care by visiting nurses.

REFERENCES AND RESOURCES

American Association of Clinical Endocrinologists: https://www.aace.com/

American Diabetes Association: www.diabetes.org

International Diabetes Federation. (2017). *Clinical practice recommendation on the diabetic foot: A guide for health care professionals*. International Diabetes Federation.

South Australian Expert Advisory Group on Antimicrobial Resistance. (2019, March 20). *Diabetic foot infections: Antibiotic management clinical guideline*. Clinical guideline no. CG304. Government of South Australia.

Case 8.3 Abdominal Pain and Weight Gain

RESOLUTION

Which diagnostic studies should be considered to assist with or confirm the diagnosis?

CBC with differential normal; hemoglobin A1c: 7.3 (elevated); chemistries normal; LFT normal; *H. pylori* stool antigen + (abnormal); TSH: 1.34; LH: 9.8 (elevated); FSH: 2.3 (low–normal: 3–20); DHEA: 244; testosterone: 88; bioavailability: 36 (elevated/high normal); HCG: negative; serum prolactin: 102 (elevated); lipids: total cholesterol: 186; triglycerides: 94; LDL: 103; HDL: 46; HIV: negative; vitamin D: 9 (low); urinalysis: normal.

To rule PCOS in or out, evaluating androgens is recommended, along with a hemoglobin A1c to evaluate insulin resistance. Hypothyroidism can be diagnosed with a TSH level. Serum prolactin and DHEA are needed to rule in or out the suspicion of hyperprolactinemia. Since Annette reports being sexually active without a form of contraception, getting an HCG is wise. Other labs for routine health maintenance include a vitamin D level, HIV test, and urinalysis. In addition to laboratory studies, a transvaginal ultrasound is needed to evaluate for the presence of ovarian abnormalities. An abdominal ultrasound can also help pinpoint the cause of the abdominal pain.

What are the most likely differential diagnoses and why?
Peptic ulcer and PCOS:

Peptic ulcers are silent in almost half the cases. Annette does not have nausea, vomiting, heartburn, or radiation of pain. However, she does have abdominal pain. The results of the transvaginal ultrasound show multiple follicles within the uterus, which are arranged in a peripheral pattern as seen in polycystic ovarian disease. She has a retroverted uterus without any abnormality and multiple cysts on the left ovary indicative of polycystic ovarian syndrome.

What is the plan of treatment?

Annette should continue to refrain from tobacco use, avoid alcohol and NSAID use, and avoid foods that cause pain. The protocol for eradicating *H. pylori* includes antibiotics and acid suppression. Antibiotic therapy works to promote ulcer healing, prevent relapse, and decrease the need for long-term acid suppression. In all cases, combination antibiotic therapy is needed due to the high rates of resistance. To suppress acid, proton pump inhibitors (PPIs) are most often used. It is important to check regional bacterial resistance to particular antibiotics before treating. An appropriate

The Family Nurse Practitioner: Clinical Case Studies, Second Edition. Edited by Leslie Neal-Boylan.
© 2021 John Wiley & Sons Ltd. Published 2021 by John Wiley & Sons Ltd.

treatment for Annette would be lansoprazole (30 mg twice daily), amoxicillin (1 g twice daily), and clarithromycin if there is no local resistance (500 mg twice daily) and metronidazole (500 mg twice a day) for 10–14 days. There are several different combination therapy suggestions ranging from 7- to 14-day treatments.

The treatment plan for Annette's PCOS should be based mostly on her symptoms. Three reasons for treatment can be considered in her case: (1) regulation of uterine bleeding and reduction in risk for endometrial hyperplasia, (2) the improvement of dermatological complaints including acne and increased dark hair growth, and (3) the correction and prevention of possible metabolic abnormalities, including DM and cardiovascular disease. To address Annette's irregular menstrual bleeding, a hormonal contraceptive method should be considered based on her individual contraceptive needs and comfort level. A common starting place is the combined oral contraceptive pill (COC), but the ring and progestin-only methods such as the implant or the hormonal IUD could also be considered.

To address Annette's complaint of acne and dark hair growth, an androgen receptor blocker could be considered as pharmacotherapy in an extreme circumstance. However, if looking for a more conservative treatment, choosing a combined contraceptive option would improve acne; and a cosmetic route could be chosen for the hair growth (such as bleaching, electrolysis, or laser removal).

The correction of any metabolic abnormalities is also of great concern, and the treatment should begin with a discussion of diet and lifestyle modifications. Many studies have shown that weight loss can lower the level of circulating androgens, thus causing the resumption of normal menstrual patterns and a reduction in insulin resistance. Since Annette's lab studies show a high hemoglobin A1c level, indicative of long-term insulin resistance, starting a hypoglycemic agent would be an acceptable adjunct therapy to lifestyle changes.

To address preventive health practices for Annette, starting her on daily calcium, vitamin D, and fish oil supplementation would also be appropriate.

Are any referrals or follow-up needed?

It is important to follow up with Annette after her treatment course to see if the *H. pylori* infection was eradicated. If the infection persists, it is appropriate to continue therapy, most likely changing antibiotics due to suspicion of resistance. If the infection is eradicated but symptoms persist for more than 4 weeks, it would be recommended that Annette be referred to a gastrointestinal specialist for endoscopic evaluation.

PCOS is a common condition that can be managed within the realm of primary care, so it is not recommended that Annette be followed by a specialist. However, to evaluate progress on the treatment options discussed today, the time frame for acceptable follow-up visits is monthly for the first 3 months and then quarterly until specific treatment goals are reached. At the follow-up visits, diet and exercise journals should be reviewed and blood tests should be done to evaluate insulin resistance (hemoglobin A1c) and androgen levels (FHS, LH, testosterone). Since this is also Annette's establishment of primary care, it is important to encourage follow-ups for routine gynecology care and other routine health maintenance.

What if the patient had a positive pregnancy test?

If Annette had a positive pregnancy test, the first step would be to establish if this was a planned and/or desired pregnancy. If the pregnancy is either unplanned or undesired, options counseling should be included to discuss keeping the pregnancy, adoption, and termination of the pregnancy. If Annette wanted to continue the pregnancy, she should be offered or referred to prenatal care. Since a common side effect of PCOS is the inability to conceive due to irregular cycles, she would have already overcome a hurdle of the condition. The treatment for irregular menstrual bleeding would be a topic to address postpartum. Metformin is category B in pregnancy, so it would be acceptable to treat the insulin resistance concomitantly with the pregnancy. Androgen receptor blockers would be contraindicated during pregnancy.

What if the patient were trying to conceive?

To treat infertility, a fair trial of treatment should be done to evaluate whether regular menstrual patterns return. If difficulty conceiving persists beyond 9 months or a year, referral to a fertility specialist is acceptable.

Are there any standardized guidelines that should be used to assess or treat this case?

European Society of Human Reproduction and Embryology. (2018). *International evidence-based guideline for the assessment and management of polycystic ovary syndrome 2018.* https://www.eshre.eu/Guidelines-and-Legal/Guidelines/Polycystic-Ovary-Syndrome

Polycystic ovarian syndrome. (2018, June). *Obstetrics & Gynecology, 131*(6), e157–e171. doi:10.1097/AOG.0000000000002656

Randel, A. (2018). H. pylori infection: ACG updates treatment recommendations. *American Family Physician, 97*(2), 135–137.

REFERENCES AND RESOURCES

Ferri, F. F. (2019). Ferri's Clinical Advisor. Philadelphia: Elsevier.

National Institutes of Health. (2019). *Health info: Peptic ulcer.* https://www.niddk.nih.gov/health-information/digestive-diseases/peptic-ulcers-stomach-ulcers/definition-facts

NOTE: The author would like to acknowledge Geraldine Marrocco, EdD, APRN, CNS, ANP-BC who write the case for the first edition of this book.

Case 8.4 Burning Leg Pain

Which diagnostic or imaging studies should be considered to assist with or confirm diagnosis?

The ankle brachial index (ABI) is a first-line diagnostic test and would be helpful in diagnosing peripheral arterial disease. If lower extremity vessels are noncompressible, the toe brachial index (TBI) is another option. Exercise ABIs may be performed if the resting ABI is normal and the patient has symptoms of intermittent claudication with walking (but in this case would not be an option since the patient is unable to walk very far). The six-minute walk test is an alternative to exercise testing to assess functional status.

Critical limb ischemia (CLI) is suspected if the patient reports leg pain when reclining (especially at night), relieved by dangling the feet, as is the case here. If critical limb ischemia is suspected and the patient has abnormal arterial pressure, the nurse practitioner (NP) should order an arterial duplex ultrasound. Since persons with peripheral artery disease (PAD) have an increased prevalence of abdominal aortic aneurysm (AAA), it is reasonable to screen for AAA with abdominal ultrasound in persons with symptomatic PAD, per the AHA/ACC.

Vascular specialists may order invasive tests such as computed tomography angiography, magnetic resonance angiography, and angiography. Because these invasive tests confer increased risk for the patient, typically they would only be ordered by a vascular specialist.

What is the most likely differential diagnosis and why?

The following risk factors support the diagnosis of PAD: hypertension, smoking history, hyperlipidemia, and diabetes. All patients with these risk factors should be assessed for PAD because of their degree of risk. The findings of dependent rubor, hairless lower extremities, diminished pedal pulses, and a punched-out appearing ulcer on the heel of the foot also support the diagnosis of PAD. Nocturnal leg pain with reclining, dependent rubor, and hairlessness are characteristic of PAD. Patients with PAD often have ulcers with regular borders that may be slow to heal. In patients who are able to walk some distance, pain in the leg muscles with walking, relieved with rest (intermittent claudication) is a hallmark of PAD. However, only 10% of patients with PAD present with

---

The Family Nurse Practitioner: Clinical Case Studies, Second Edition. Edited by Leslie Neal-Boylan.
© 2021 John Wiley & Sons Ltd. Published 2021 by John Wiley & Sons Ltd.

intermittent claudication. Approximately 40% of patients do not report leg symptoms, and approximately 50% report other types of leg pain.

With chronic venous insufficiency the whole leg aches, relieved by elevation. With venous stasis ulcers, patients typically show brawny skin changes; this is not the case here. With spinal stenosis, pain is relieved with lumbar flexion and worsens with standing. With nerve root compression, pain radiates inferiorly and worsens with sitting, standing, and walking; however, it would not cause hairlessness, dependent rubor, and diminished pedal pulses. In the case of neuropathic pain due to diabetes, symptoms progress symmetrically from the extremities superiorly. Negative symptoms include numbness and weakness; positive symptoms include tingling and pain, worse at night. Due to lack of sensation, ulcers occur over weight-bearing areas, or from abrasion with poorly fitting shoes.

What is the plan of treatment?

For behavioral therapy, the NP should work with Raymond to follow guideline-directed medical therapy (GDMT), most recently established in 2016 by the American Heart Association (AHA) and the American College of Cardiology (ACC). First-line treatment includes supervised exercise therapy; encouraging individual exercise is insufficient. In smokers, smoking cessation is also first-line therapy.

For drug therapy, AHA/ACC guidelines recommend antiplatelet therapy such as either aspirin or clopidogrel alone, or in combination with another anticoagulant, as recommended by the cardiologist. Per GDMT, statin therapy is also recommended for all patients with PAD. Also per GDMT, antihypertensive therapy should include either an ACE inhibitor (such as lisinopril) or an angiotensin receptor blocker (such as losartan to reduce the risk of myocardial infarction, stroke, heart failure, and death). For patients with diabetes and PAD, glycemic control of hemoglobin A1C below 6.5 through diet, exercise, and medication will improve microvascular and cardiovascular outcomes.

Are any referrals needed?

Since Raymond shows signs of critical limb ischemia, the NP should refer urgently to a vascular surgeon for evaluation (emergent referral for acute limb ischemia, which is not the case here). For management of Raymond's ulcer, referral to specialized wound care is indicated. As Raymond has diabetes, referral to a certified diabetes nurse educator or endocrinologist will help with glycemic control. In all cases Raymond will require a team approach.

What are the differences between arterial and venous disease?

Arterial Disease Risk Factors	Arterial Disease Treatment	Venous Disease Risk Factors	Venous Disease Treatment
Age 65 or older	Smoking cessation	Prolonged standing	Weight loss
Hypertension	Exercise	Increased body weight	Exercise
Diabetes mellitus	Improved diet	Failed muscle pump function	Compression stockings
Hyperlipidemia	Glycemic control	Trauma	Do not massage/rub legs
Smoking history	ACE/ARB	Pregnancy	For venous ulcers, Unna boot
Family history of PAD	Antiplatelet therapy	Genetic predisposition	Surgical treatment
Known atherosclerotic disease in another vascular bed	Endovascular surgery		Biopsy if nonresponsive to treatment

How should the clinician differentiate between venous ulcers and arterial ulcers?

Arterial Ulcers	Venous Ulcers
Regular borders	Irregular borders
Base of yellow material or eschar	Shallow wound bed
Scant or absent granulation tissue	No eschar
Underlying structure more likely visible	No underlying structures visible
Absent or decreased pedal pulses	Positive palpable pulses
Painful	Painless
Outer sides of ankles, feet, tips of heels, toes	Below the knee; around ankle, particularly medial side
Waxy skin	Brawny skin changes
Hair loss on limb	
Cool to touch	

REFERENCES AND RESOURCES

Gerhard-Herman, M. D., Gornik, H. L., Barrett, C., Barhes, N. R., Corriere, M. A., Drachman, D. E., . . . Walsh, M. E. (2017). *2016 AHA/ACC guideline on the management of patients with lower extremity peripheral artery disease: Executive summary. A report of the American College of Cardiology/American Heart Association Task Force on Clinical Practice Guidelines.* https://www.ahajournals.org/doi/pdf/10.1161/CIR.0000000000000470

Feldman, E. L. (2019). Screening for diabetic polyneuropathy. *UpToDate.* Retrieved October 2, 2019.

Firnhaber, J. M., & Powell, C. S. (2019). Lower extremity peripheral artery disease: Diagnosis and treatment. *American Family Physician, 99*(6).

Guttendorf, Ann. (2017). Peripheral arterial and venous insufficiency. In T. M. Buttaro, J. Trybulski, P. Polgar-Bailey, & J. Sandberg-Cook (Eds.), Primary care: A collaborative Practice (5th ed.), 599–610. St. Louis: Elsevier.

Kohlman-Trigoboff, D. (2019). Update: Diagnosis and management of peripheral arterial disease. *The Journal for Nurse Practitioners, 15*(1), 87–95.

American Heart Association. (n.d.). PAD initial symptom checklist. From *Helping your patients with peripheral artery disease: A clinician's guide.* Retrieved October 2, 2019, from http://www.ksw-gtg.com/ahapad/guide/pdfs/PADSymptomChecklist.pdf

Walker, C. M., Bunch, F. T., Cavros, N. G., & Dippel, E. J. (2015). Multidisciplinary approach to the diagnosis and management of patients with peripheral arterial disease. *Clinical Interventions in Aging, 10,* 1147.

Case 8.5 Difficulty Breathing

Which diagnostic or imaging studies should be considered to assist with or confirm the diagnosis?

- Spirometry: FEV1/FVC <.70; FEV1 50% predicted.
- Chest X-ray: Overinflation of lungs; flattened diaphragm; mild cardiomegaly.
- CBC: Slight elevation of RBCs, all others WNL.
- ABGs: pH: 7.36; PCO_2: 55; PO_2: 60; HCO_3: 29; SaO2: 89.
- ECG: Sinus tachycardia; frequent PVCs; no ischemia; right axis deviation.

What is the most likely differential diagnosis and why?

COPD:

Many community-acquired pneumonias manifest in the right lung due to the right mainstem bronchus angulation. However, given the absence of infiltrates (evidence for pneumonia) or suspicious lesions on CXR (pulmonary neoplasm), the most likely diagnosis is exacerbation of COPD. The ECG is not suspicious for coronary ischemia although it identifies changes commonly found with pulmonary hypertension, including right axis deviation, often seen with right ventricular enlargement secondary to pulmonary hypertension. The result of the ABG is concerning. Janis is close to acute respiratory failure, requiring hospitalization if the PaO_2 and SaO_2 fall below their current values. Since Janis is able to perform her metered dose inhaler therapies competently and she has noticeable improvement in her dyspnea with the administration of a nebulizer bronchodilator treatment, with adjustments in her medications, she will likely show improvement. Janis should revisit smoking cessation treatments. She is approaching the point at which home oxygen is needed (paO_2 less than 55 mmHg; SaO_2 less than or equal to 88) (Brashers, 2010).

What is the plan of treatment?

Add beclomethasone dipropionate, 42 mcg/inhalation MDI, 2 puffs 3–4 times per day, and change Janis's inhaled bronchodilator therapy to a long-acting form: salmeterol, 12 mcg (range 4.5–12). Oral glucocorticoid therapy may also improve her recovery. Serious discussion about smoking cessation and the addition of pulmonary rehabilitation should occur at the time of the visit. She should be seen again in 2–3 days for repeat spirometry and clinical assessment of her lungs.

The Family Nurse Practitioner: Clinical Case Studies, Second Edition. Edited by Leslie Neal-Boylan.
© 2021 John Wiley & Sons Ltd. Published 2021 by John Wiley & Sons Ltd.

What is the plan for follow-up care?

Janis may improve with pulmonary rehabilitation. Prescription or over-the-counter smoking cessation medication should be recommended. She should be instructed to call in the case of increased temperature, dyspnea, or chest pain. Plan to review risk factors with Janis at the next visit, and invite her husband to attend. Working with Janis to improve overall health is essential. Smoking cessation and pulmonary rehabilitation are top evidence-based treatments for COPD (Rabe et al., 2007; Rabe, 2017). Her current trajectory places her at grave risk for continued decline and early mortality.

Are any referrals needed?

Annual evaluation by a pulmonologist is recommended. Once Janis's condition has improved, she should also be referred to a cardiologist for further workup to rule out coronary artery disease (CAD). In light of this risk, an assessment of her lipids and an evaluation of her diet are recommended to examine other lifestyle modifications that might slow the development of CAD. With ECG evidence of right axis deviation, it is likely that her right ventricle may be enlarged secondary to pulmonary hypertension. This places her at risk for progression to heart failure (cor pulmonale). These serious effects of her condition require careful discussion so that she is fully aware of her risks and can make informed decisions about her future. Her husband should be invited to meet with the medical team to discuss his risks and how his continued smoking may be contributing to Janis's condition.

What additional risk factors are evident for this patient?

Janis is at great risk for coronary artery disease and lung cancer. She should also have an annual influenza vaccine, given her progression of disease. A pneumococcal vaccine is also recommended.

Are there any standardized guidelines that should be used to treat this patient?

Careful review of the progression and treatment recommendations (Rabe et al., 2007) provide evidence-based guidelines for stages of COPD. These highlight the 4 components of management, including assessment and monitoring of the disease and its progression, reduction of risk factors, management of stable disease, and exacerbations. In addition, the Agency for Healthcare Research and Quality (2008) provides guidance for acute respiratory conditions that serve as helpful targets for acute or chronic condition management.

REFERENCES AND RESOURCES

Agency for Healthcare Research and Quality (2008). *ACR Appropriateness criteria acute respiratory illness. National Guideline Clearinghouse.* http://www.guideline.gov/summary/summary.aspx?doc_id= 13678

Brashers, V. L. (2010). Alterations of pulmonary function. In K. L. McCance, S. E. Huether, V. L. Brashers, & N. S. Rote (Eds.), *Pathophysiology: The biologic bases for disease in adults and children* (6th ed., Chapter 33, pp. 1266–1309). Maryland Heights, MO: Mosby Elsevier.

Falk, J. A., Kadiev, S., Criner, G. J., Scharf, S. M., Minai, O. A., & Diaz, P. (2008). Cardiac disease in chronic obstructive pulmonary disease. *Proceedings of the American Thoracic Society, 5*, 543–548.

Global Initiative for Chronic Obstructive Lung Disease. (2019). *GOLD report.* www.gold-2019-v1.7-final-14Nov2018.WMS.pdf.

Kuzma, A. M., Meli, Y., Meldrum, C., Jellen, P., Butler-Lebair, M., Koczen-Doyle, D., Rising, P., Stavrolakes, K., & Brogan, F. (2008). Multidisciplinary care of the patient with chronic obstructive pulmonary disease. *Proceedings of the American Thoracic Society, 5*, 567–571.

Rabe, K. F. (2017). Chronic Obstructive Pulmonary Disease. *The Lancet, 389*(10082), 1931–1940.

Rabe, K. F., Hurd, S., Anqueto, A., Barnes, P. J., Buist, S. A., Calverley, P., . . . Zielinski, J. (2007). Global strategy for the diagnosis, management, and prevention of chronic obstructive pulmonary disease: GOLD executive summary. *American Journal of Respiratory Critical Care Medicine, 176*(6), 532–555. http://ajrccm. atsjournals.org/cgi/reprint/176/6/532

Sarna, L., Cooley, M. E., Brown, J. K., Chernecky, C., Elashoff, D., & Kotlerman, J. (2008). Symptom severity 1 to 4 months after thoracotomy for lung cancer. *American Journal of Critical Care, 17*, 455–467.

Case 8.6 Epigastric Pain

RESOLUTION

What is the most likely differential diagnosis and why?
Gastroesophageal reflux disease:
This diagnosis is supported by the patient's symptoms of retrosternal burning pain that occurs after meals and is exacerbated by certain foods and heavy meals. The sour taste, coughing, and regurgitation are also relevant symptoms. The fact that Meredith has achieved some relief with Maalox and Tums helps the clinician to validate that the condition is probably related to reflux. A cardiac condition or an ulcer is unlikely to result in relief from an antacid.

Which diagnostic studies should be considered to assist with or confirm the diagnosis?
Current guidelines recommend that none of these tests be performed if the patient is responsive to acid-suppressing therapy. However, Meredith's symptoms are severe, so the clinician might order an endoscopy now or after beginning therapy. Possible complications of GERD and ulcers will need to be ruled in or out by an endoscopy. If the endoscopy is normal, 24-hour pH testing might be considered. For a patient whose symptoms are not severe, the endoscopy can usually wait while the patient is monitored under conservative treatment with medication and diet changes. If the patient has not had a recent ECG or there is immediate concern that this might be cardiovascular in etiology, then she should have an ECG today. Since the guaiac was positive, a follow-up fecal immunochemical test (FIT) and/or colonoscopy should be done, especially if the patient has not had a colonoscopy done recently. The choice of the initial test should depend on her family and personal medical history. If a FIT is positive, then a colonoscopy must be done regardless of how long it has been since the last one. However, the gastroenterologist should be consulted about this and will need to arrange the colonoscopy. If the suppressive therapy is ineffective or the endoscopy rules out GERD, the clinician should rule out a cardiac condition, pulmonary problem, ulcer, hepatitis, and infection. The other tests listed in the case might then be performed. Meredith's Lipitor dose may be inadequate to treat her hyperlipidemia so lipid values should be checked if they have not been checked recently.

The Family Nurse Practitioner: Clinical Case Studies, Second Edition. Edited by Leslie Neal-Boylan.
© 2021 John Wiley & Sons Ltd. Published 2021 by John Wiley & Sons Ltd.

What is the plan of treatment?

The first-line treatment for GERD includes antacids, H2 blockers, or proton pump inhibitors (PPI) (see Table 8.6.1). PPIs are the drug of choice because H2 blockers are less effective. However, they may be used in combination with PPIs. Meredith has already tried antacids but they are only providing minimal relief. At this point, Meredith should be started on a PPI once each day (with the possibility of increasing to twice each day if once a day is insufficient to control symptoms) for 4–8 weeks to see if that helps her symptoms to resolve. If her symptoms continue or if she develops dysphagia, weight loss, anemia, or odynophagia, and she has not yet had an endoscopy, she should be sent for one. If the endoscopy reveals abnormal results, such as an ulcer or Barrett's esophagus, the patient should be referred to a gastroenterologist. She may require surgery.

Lifestyle modification (diet, weight loss, reduction or elimination of coffee intake, smoking cessation, reduction or cessation of alcohol intake, sitting up after meals and in bed at night) might be sufficient for patients with mild cases of GERD. Patients should avoid anticholinergics if possible and fatty foods and chocolate. Most people can come off of the PPI after 8–12 weeks or just change to an as-needed basis However, Meredith has some troublesome symptoms that are affecting her quality of life. These modifications should still be recommended, but she should use the PPI therapy for 8–12 weeks. If she continues to have symptoms and requires twice-daily treatment after 12 weeks, she should be placed on the lowest dose possible with awareness of the possible adverse effects of long-term use (increased risk of *Clostridium difficile* and hip fractures). Surgery may be preferable to long-term treatment. Meredith also has high blood pressure. The HCTZ 25 mg appears to be inadequate. The clinician should add an ACEI or ARB to her regimen.

What is the plan for referrals and follow-up?

Most patients are treated based on a clinical diagnosis but some may need to be referred to a gastroenterologist for further testing and treatment. However, Meredith may need referral for an endoscopy because her symptoms are severe and long lasting. She should see the gastroenterologist if 12 weeks of a PPI is insufficient to resolve her symptoms. Intractable disease may require surgical treatment via fundoplication. Meredith should monitor her blood pressure, keep a record and return for follow-up in 2 weeks. She also needs follow-up for her diet, weight loss, smoking, and alcohol reduction/cessation and to review her lipids and whether she needs an increased statin dosage.

What are the patient's risk factors for this condition?

The risk factors that Meredith has include obesity, alcohol consumption, and smoking.

What are the possible complications of this condition?

Possible complications of GERD include adenocarcinoma, Barrett's esophagus, aspiration pneumonia, severe esophagitis that results in odynophagia and dysphagia, esophageal hemorrhage, laryngitis, reflux-induced asthma, unexplained wheezing, chronic cough, dental erosions, and a feeling of a lump in the throat.

Table 8.6.1. Medications Used to Treat GERD.

Antacids: Quick Onset, Short Duration	H2 blockers: OTC Dose Is Half the Prescription Dose. Longer Onset, Longer Duration	Proton Pump Inhibitors: Take 30 Minutes before Breakfast
Tums	Cimetidine	Omeprazole (also available with sodium bicarbonate)
Baking soda	Ranitidine	Rabeprazole
Maalox	Famotidine	Lansoprazole
Mylanta	Nizatidine	Pantoprazole
Gaviscon (to buffer antacid)		Esomeprazole
		Dexlansoprazole

REFERENCES AND RESOURCES

Ferri, F. F. (2019). Gastroesophageal reflux disease. *Ferri's clinical advisor 2019* (pp. 569–571). Philadelphia: Elsevier.

Lynch, K. L. (2018). Gastroesophageal reflux disease. In R. S. Porter, J. L. Kaplan, R. B. Lynn, & M. T. Reddy (Eds.), *The Merck manual of diagnosis and therapy* (pp. 113–114). Kenilworth, NJ: Merck Sharp & Dohme Corp.

Case 8.7 Chest Pain and Dyspnea without Radiation

RESOLUTION

Which diagnostic or imaging studies should be considered to assist with or confirm the diagnosis?

Measure blood pressure for pulsus paradoxus. This is done by initially taking the BP and then retesting systolic BP during inspiration to see if it is lower with inspiratory effort. With pericardial tamponade, cardiac compression causes lowering of the systolic BP as the inspiratory mechanics increase venous return, increasing ventricular preload, placing strain on the left ventricular capacity to pump. Repeat the ECG. Arrange for the following tests: echocardiogram, CBC, electrolytes, sedimentation rate, and serial troponins (stat, 12 and 24 hours). Measuring lipids, blood glucose, electrolytes, hemoglobin, liver function tests, and TSH can help rule out other causes. The BUN, creatinine, and urinalysis can help rule out kidney disease.

What is the most likely differential diagnosis and why?

Pericarditis:

The most likely diagnosis is acute pericarditis. The chest pain, ECG findings, and pattern of symptoms, including elevated temperature, point to this diagnosis. Due to the complaints of chest pain over several days, an acute MI must be ruled out. Although the pattern of pain does not point to MI, especially since there is relief with leaning forward, this condition must still be ruled out, especially given this patient's age and family history. While troponin I elevations are common in pericarditis (Brandt, Filzmaier, & Hanrath, 2001), the combination of serial ECG changes and echocardiographic findings will generally allow diagnostic specificity. Troponin levels are not considered a negative prognostic indicator in pericarditis (Rahman & Broadley, 2014). Infectious cardiomyopathy can be ruled out with the echocardiogram. Zachary's recent history of an upper respiratory infection and his pattern of dyspnea bring this condition into the realm of possibility. Generally, the onset is abrupt; and progressive heart failure, including all chamber enlargement, jugular venous distention, and severe dyspnea, ensues. These symptoms are similar to those seen with severe pericardial effusion/tamponade.

What is the plan of treatment?

The patient should be hospitalized for further diagnostic testing and treatment. Once myocardial infarction is ruled out, Zachary should be started on an anti-inflammatory drug such as

The Family Nurse Practitioner: Clinical Case Studies, Second Edition. Edited by Leslie Neal-Boylan.
© 2021 John Wiley & Sons Ltd. Published 2021 by John Wiley & Sons Ltd.

indomethacin. Echocardiography will quantify the degree of pericardial effusion and guide further therapy. If the pericardial effusion is small, observation is indicated. If the pericardial effusion is moderate to large, pericardiocentesis or a pericardial window will be considered based on the patient's progression of symptoms. If his blood pressure remains elevated, he will need to begin an anti-hypertension regimen. You should also instruct him regarding continued regular use of ibuprofen, Ecotrin, and glucosamine.

The patient should be instructed to decrease alcohol use, improve diet, lose weight, and reduce stress. Once permitted, Zachary should increase his exercise.

What is the plan for follow-up care?
Following hospitalization, the patient should be seen in 2 weeks. A repeat echocardiograph is indicated to ensure resolution of the effusion. A careful review of Zachary's management of gout is also indicated, and serum uric acid levels should be checked (goal 5–6 mg/dL).

Are any referrals needed?
Yes, the patient needs a cardiology consultation for definitive diagnosis and treatment. Admit the patient to the hospital, order a cardiology consult, and order the following upon admission: troponin, CBC, electrolytes, and sedimentation rate.

What if this patient had recently sustained an acute myocardial infarction?
Dressler's syndrome, or post-MI pericarditis, would be the suspected diagnosis if the patient had recently sustained an acute myocardial infarction. Generally, the pericardial sac has approximately 15–30 mL of fluid between the pericardial layer and the epicardial layer to allow for smooth filling and contraction. When inflammation develops, the fluid in this layer may increase considerably, compressing the ventricular muscle and preventing filling, reducing cardiac output and raising central venous pressure. Symptoms of dyspnea and discomfort are common. If the onset of fluid accumulation occurs rapidly, severe symptoms may develop and emergent treatment by pericardiocentesis may be required.

Are there any standardized guidelines that should be used to assess/treat this case?
The Imazio, Spodick, Brucato, Trinchero, and Adler (2010) article offers excellent summaries of medical therapy for pericarditis, including a strong overview of anti-inflammatory drugs, tapering regimens if prednisone is used, and an overview of treatment patterns, incorporating the latest published standards. In addition, Choi (2010) provides a wonderful summary of lifestyle changes that help reduce the incidence of gout. These are helpful in reducing overall cardiac risk factors as well.

REFERENCES AND RESOURCES

Brandt, R. R., Filzmaier, K., & Hanrath, P. (2001). Circulating cardiac troponin I in acute pericarditis. *American Journal of Cardiology, 87,* 1326–1328.

Choi, H. K. (2010). A prescription for lifestyle change in patients with hyperuricemia and gout. *Current Opinion in Rheumatology, 22,* 165–172.

Hilaire, M. L., & Wozniak, J. R. (2010). Gout: Overview and newer therapeutic developments. *Formulary, 45,* 84–90.

Imazio, M., Spodick, D. H., Brucato, A., Trinchero, R., & Adler, Y. (2010). Controversial issues in the management of pericardial diseases. *Circulation, 121,* 916–928.

Imazio, M., Spodick, D. H., Brucato, A., Trinchero, R., Markel, G., & Adler, Y. (2010). Diagnostic issues in the clinical management of pericarditis. *The International Journal of Clinical Practice, 10,* 1–9.

Khandaker, M. H., Espinosa, R. E., Nishimura, R. A., Sinak, L. J., Hayes, S. N., Meiduni, R. M., & Oh, J. K. (2010). Pericardial disease: Diagnosis and management. *Mayo Clinic Proceedings, 85,* 572–593.

Punja, M., Mark, D. G., McCoy, J. V., Javan, R., Pines, J. M., & Brady, W. (2010). Electrocardiographic manifestations of cardiac infectious-inflammatory disorders. *American Journal of Emergency Medicine, 28,* 364–377.

Rahman, A., & Broadley, S. A. (2014). Elevated troponin: Diagnostic gold or fool's gold? *Emergency Medicine Australasia, 26,* 125–130.

Case 8.8 Chest Pain with Radiation

What is the most likely differential diagnosis and why?

Acute coronary syndrome (ACS): probable non-ST elevation myocardial infarction (NSTEMI):
The patient has a positive family history, a history of diabetes mellitus, and a long smoking history—all risk factors for ACS. The symptoms are consistent with ACS and the ECG changes are reflective of myocardial ischemia in the inferior (II, III, and aVF) lateral (V5 and V6) leads.

The sudden onset of chest pain is a hallmark sign of pulmonary embolism (PE). Oliver also demonstrates tachypnea, hypertension, and neck vein distention, all of which may be seen with PE. Pulmonary embolism is generally associated with more dyspnea and seldom presents with epigastric distress. The patient should be screened for other risk factors associated with PE, such as prolonged immobility or history of hypercoagulable state, or a history of deep vein thrombosis (DVT).
Oliver reports feeling a need to belch. Gastroesophageal reflux can often cause symptoms of chest pain or pressure. A positive smoking history and being overweight are risk factors for gastroesophageal reflux. However, the presence of ischemia on the ECG makes a diagnosis of GERD unlikely.

Which diagnostic or imaging studies should be considered to assist with or confirm the diagnosis?

Within 2 hours of arrival to care: ECG: Inferior wall myocardial ischemia; troponin: 6 ng/dL; chem panel: Na: 138 mEq/L, K: 4.2 mEq/L, Mg: 1.7 mg/dL; BUN: 20; creatinine: 0.8; serum glucose: 189 (Figure 8.8.1).

What is the plan of treatment?

Urgent transport by the EMS system to nearest interventional cardiology service is required. The ECG demonstrates myocardial ischemia and, coupled with the serious symptoms, is a medical emergency. Since Oliver is tachypneic and has chest discomfort, pulmonary embolism is likely the top differential diagnosis. However, the preponderance of history and symptoms point to acute MI. Pain onset in early morning hours is common with AMI symptoms; Oliver's pain began at 7:00 a.m. He did not report pain consistent with PE, which often is accompanied by deep vein thrombosis. In addition, PE is generally associated with more severe dyspnea and oxygen desaturation. Coronary artery catheterization will dictate the intervention and plan, with possible angioplasty

The Family Nurse Practitioner: Clinical Case Studies, Second Edition. Edited by Leslie Neal-Boylan.
© 2021 John Wiley & Sons Ltd. Published 2021 by John Wiley & Sons Ltd.

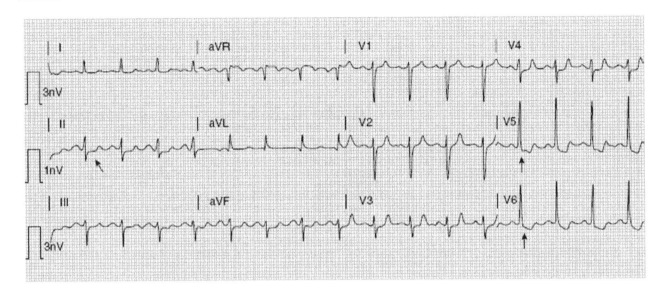

Figure 8.8.1. Oliver's ECG.

and stent placement. Calling the hospital and faxing the office ECG would allow for more rapid definitive care for this patient.

Oliver will need a number of lifestyle changes in light of his diagnosis. Management of his multiple risk factors will be attempted with the addition of medications to prevent recurrence. Lifestyle changes include the addition of exercise, smoking cessation, dietary changes to reduce his intake of saturated and trans fats, and secondary prevention measures to improve his risk profile and reduce the risk of a second cardiac event. Despite his family history, Oliver has continued a number of risky behaviors that will be very difficult to change all at once. Supportive education and reinforcement of small gains will be needed as he seeks to implement changes in his lifestyle. He and his wife need education about activating the emergency medical system, and he needs to be advised against driving independently to the office or hospital in the event of future chest pain episodes.

Are any referrals needed?
Oliver will be followed by a cardiologist. He will undergo cardiac catheterization, which will allow for assessment of his coronary artery perfusion, interventions such as angioplasty and stent placement, and ventriculography, which will provide an estimated ejection fraction. If acute MI is confirmed, the most definitive treatment will be completed. If stents are possible to stabilize the coronary lesions, they will be placed; if coronary artery bypass is required, Oliver will be hospitalized for approximately 4–5 days. If CAD is confirmed, he will be discharged on additional medications, including a beta blocker, ACE inhibitor, IIb/IIIa inhibitor, daily aspirin, and a statin. He will be referred to cardiac rehabilitation post-intervention so that he may be monitored during recovery as he increases his exercise capacity. His blood pressure will need to be controlled with an ACE inhibitor and beta-blocker, given his comorbidities of cardiovascular disease and diabetes mellitus.

Does the patient's family history impact how you might treat him?
Oliver will be placed on similar treatments as any patient following an AMI. However, his family history requires a more aggressive approach to management of lipids, hypertension, and diabetes.

What are the primary health education issues?
Smoking cessation is the top priority. Smoking is a primary risk factor. A full cholesterol panel should also be ordered and a healthy diet begun. Exercise and risk factor reduction are key elements in the educational process. Educational efforts with diabetes management should be reinforced, with tighter control of blood glucose.

What if this patient were female?

Women often present with symptoms that differ from men. Common symptoms in women include chest discomfort with radiation to the jaw, nausea, and fatigue. Radiation of pain to the back, similar to one of Oliver's symptoms, is also a primary presenting symptom in women. Women may also present with dyspnea more often than men.

What if the patient lived in a rural, isolated setting?

Anticipatory education would be strongly recommended for anyone with the family history presented in this scenario. Since Oliver had both a father and a brother who died early with cardiovascular disease—and particularly if he lived in a rural area—he should be counseled to become familiar with the emergency medical services in his area, taught to keep chewable aspirin on hand and to take one immediately with the onset of chest pressure or pain that might resemble cardiac symptoms, and be given detailed steps to take for recognition and early intervention to prevent a heart attack. Nitroglycerin PRN will be prescribed and the patient should be advised to take one sublingual tablet at the onset of chest pain and to call 911 immediately. Family members would benefit from learning CPR, especially since Oliver lives in a rural, isolated setting.

Are there any standardized guidelines that should be used to assess/treat this case?

The American Heart Association has published standards for care in both NSTEMI and STEMI; nurse practitioners should be familiar with these standards.

REFERENCES AND RESOURCES

Anderson, J. L., Adams, C. D., Antman, E. M., Bridges, C. R., Califf, R. M., Casey, D. E. Jr., . . . Wright, R. S. (2007). ACC/AHA 2007 guidelines for the management of patients with unstable angina/non-ST-elevation myocardial infarction: A report of the American College of Cardiology/American Heart Association Task Force on Practice Guidelines (Writing Committee to Revise the 2002 Guidelines for the Management of Patients With Unstable Angina/Non-ST-Elevation Myocardial Infarction) developed in collaboration with the American College of Emergency Physicians, the Society for Cardiovascular Angiography and Interventions, and the Society of Thoracic Surgeons, endorsed by the American Association of Cardiovascular and Pulmonary Rehabilitation and the Society for Academic Emergency Medicine. *Journal of the American College of Cardiology, 50,* 1–157.

Krumholz, H. M., Anderson, J. L., Bachelder, B. L., Fesmire, F. M., Fihn, S. D., Foody, J. M., . . . Nallamothu, B. K. (2008). ACC/AHA 2008 performance measures for adults with ST-elevation and non-ST-elevation myocardial infarction: A report of the American College of Cardiology/American Heart Association task force on performance measures. *Circulation, 118,* 2596–2648.

Lieberman, K. (2008). Interpreting 12-lead ECGs: A piece by piece analysis. *Nurse Practitioner, 33*(10), 28–35.

Wasylyshyn, S. M., & El-Masri, M. M. (2009). Alternative coping strategies and decision delay in seeking care for acute myocardial infarction. *Journal of CV Nursing, 24,* 151–155.

NOTE: The author would like to acknowledge the contribution of Kathy J. Booker, PhD, RN to this chapter in the first edition of this book.

Case 8.9 Persistent Cough and Joint Tenderness

RESOLUTION

Which diagnostic or imaging studies should be considered to assist with or confirm the diagnosis?

The chest X-ray showed a right upper lobe mass and diffuse right infiltrates. CBC results: Marked elevations in WBC, eosinophils, and segmented neutrophils. ABGs: pH: 7.34; PaO2: 55; PCO2: 48; HCO3: 26; SaO2: 89.

What is the most likely differential diagnosis and why?

Blastomycoses dermatitidis (BD):

BD is a fungal infection identified in the yeast form from sputum or tissue culture. It may present as a pulmonary mass or a head/neck mass. BD may mimic histoplasmosis or tuberculosis. The spores are generally inhaled and transmitted through the lymphatic system. Presenting symptoms are often similar to influenza, accompanied by a dry, hacking cough. Diagnosis requires microscopic visualization of spores from a tissue or sputum sample. In this patient, the combination of dry cough, hypoxemia, and CBC changes point to the potential for BD.

What is the plan of treatment?

Alice is admitted to the hospital for further workup and treatment of her tachypnea and hypoxemia. A pulmonary consult is ordered. Given her history, an urgent bronchoscopy is scheduled. She is started on supplemental oxygen by venti-mask at 40%.

BD infections are generally treated with amphotericin, followed by oral antifungal therapy. When fulminant fungal infections develop in the lungs, a restrictive pattern of respiratory failure is the general trajectory. As the infection spreads, inflammation and injury to alveolar tissue results in ventilation-perfusion mismatching and true shunting develop, with resultant hypoxemia. At the peak of the infection, respiratory failure may require continuous positive airway pressure or total ventilator support. Pulmonary neoplasm is a distinct possibility, especially given her history of breast cancer. However, the prodromal and admitting symptoms do not align with malignancy. Untreated, BD manifests in joint pain, which explains Alice's joint pain.

The Family Nurse Practitioner: Clinical Case Studies, Second Edition. Edited by Leslie Neal-Boylan.
© 2021 John Wiley & Sons Ltd. Published 2021 by John Wiley & Sons Ltd.

What further diagnostic tests are needed?

Bronchoscopy will allow for direct evaluation of the mass and cytology analysis of tissue or sputum sample.

What is the plan for follow-up care?

Completion of the full therapy is essential to prevent recurrence of BD. Supplemental oxygen may be necessary. Pulmonary function testing will be required to follow resumption of function. Unlike obstructive disorders associated with air trapping, restrictive pattern pulmonary disorders generally cause severe restrictions in total lung capacity, reduced tidal volumes and potentially severe hypoxemia. Amphotericin B (AmB) is toxic to the liver and kidneys and is difficult to tolerate, causing a number of side effects. Baseline renal and liver function tests should be measured prior to starting therapy. During therapy with AmB, electrolytes should be measured every 48–72 hours and renal function and liver enzymes measured at least weekly, if not more often, during therapy.

Are any referrals needed?

Alice should be followed by pulmonary medicine for at least 1 year.

Are there any standardized guidelines that should be used to assess/treat this case?

The Infectious Diseases Society of America issued a clinical practice update in 2008 (Chapman et al., 2008). This published guideline makes recommendations for treatment based on age, clinical status, and severity of symptoms. Drug therapy guidelines for pulmonary and extrapulmonary treatment include intravenous amphotericin for those with severe infections, followed by oral itraconazole. The practice guidelines also review monitoring parameters.

REFERENCES AND RESOURCES

Chapman, S. W., Dismukes, W. E., Proia, L. A., Bradsher, R. W., Pappas, P. G., Threlkeld, M. G., & Kauffman, C. A. (2008). Clinical practice guidelines for the management of blastomycosis: 2008 update by the Infectious Diseases Society of America. *Clinical Infectious Diseases*, *46*(12), 1801–1812.

Saccente, M., & Woods, G. L. (2010). Clinical and laboratory update on blastomycosis. *Clinical Microbiology Reviews*, *23*(2), 367–381.

Wheat, L. J., Freifeld, A. G., Kleiman, M. B., Baddley, J. W., McKinsey, D. S., Loyd, J. E., & Kauffman, C. A. (2007). Clinical practice guidelines for the management of patients with histoplasmosis: 2007 update by the Infectious Diseases Society of America. *Clinical Infectious Diseases*, *45*, 807–825.

NOTE: The author would like to acknowledge Kathy J. Booker, PhD, RN for her contribution to this case in the first edition of this book.

Case 8.10 Morning Headache

Which diagnostic studies should be considered to assist with or confirm the diagnosis?
ECG: The ECG shows nonspecific T wave changes; no evidence of acute ischemia. Troponin: <0.4. CBC: slightly elevated RBCs, otherwise, WNL. Electrolytes: WNL. Total cholesterol: 240; HDL: 58; LDL: 166; triglycerides: 196.

What is the most likely differential diagnosis and why?
<u>Hypertension:</u>
Morning headaches and the development of hypertension may also suggest obstructive sleep apnea. Daytime sleepiness and patterns of snoring should be explored. If either is present, Andrew should be referred for a sleep study. With this patient's strong family history of early congenital heart disease, immediate treatment of his hypertension is indicated. Close monitoring of his altered cholesterol panel values is also indicated. If he is able to improve his exercise and diet and reduces weight subsequent to these changes, cholesterol levels may improve. Since he had nonspecific T wave changes, a repeat ECG in 6 months would be important. Teaching for signs and symptoms of acute coronary syndrome is extremely important.

What is the plan of treatment?
- Start the patient on antihypertensive therapy to include a thiazide diuretic with a calcium channel blocker (CCB). Begin with lower daily dosages with increases of baseline dosages if BP targets less than 130/80 is not reached.
- URGENT—stop smoking. Prescribe nicotine substitute patch and discuss plans for smoking cessation.
- Assess pt's risk and need for aspirin supplementation using the ASCVD Risk Calculato
- Recommend low-fat, low-salt diet (DASH) high in fruits and vegetables; provide a referral to a dietitian.
- Encourage walking a minimum of 3–5 days per week. Schedule gradual increases in length and time after a 2-week initiation.

The Family Nurse Practitioner: Clinical Case Studies, Second Edition. Edited by Leslie Neal-Boylan.
© 2021 John Wiley & Sons Ltd. Published 2021 by John Wiley & Sons Ltd.

What is the plan for referrals and follow-up care?

- Return for BP check in 1 week.
- Encourage patient to monitor BP at home twice daily and keep a log.
- Encourage a log of daily walking activity with BP.
- Recheck serum cholesterol in 3 months.
- Referral for stress testing.
- Explore need for grief counseling.
- Refer to dietitian for dietary assistance.
- Refer to stop smoking clinic or web-guided smoking cessation program

What if this patient were female?

The initial treatments and counseling would be the same in females. In educating about the signs of acute coronary syndrome, women should be told about atypical symptoms including dyspnea and pain radiating to the jaw and back.

What if this patient were also diabetic?

Diabetes increases the risk of coronary artery disease (CAD), and additional teaching for glycemic control and risk factors associated with diabetes would be required. BP targets are set at a lower point (<130/80) in patients with diabetes to reduce CAD risk.

Are there any standardized guidelines that should be used to assess or treat this case?

Bakris, G., Ali, W., & Parati, G. (2019). ACC/AHA versus ESC/ESH on hypertension guidelines: JACC guideline comparison. *Journal of the American College of Cardiology, 73*(23). doi:10.1016/j.jacc.2019.03.507

REFERENCES AND RESOURCES

Bakris, G., Ali, W., & Parati, G. (2019). ACC/AHA versus ESC/ESH on hypertension guidelines: JACC guideline comparison. *Journal of the American College of Cardiology, 73*(23). doi:10.1016/j.jacc.2019.03.507

Whelton, P., & Williams, B. (2018). The 2018 European Society of Cardiology/European Society of Hypertension and 2017 American College of Cardiology/American Heart Association blood pressure guidelines more similar than different. *JAMA, 320*(17), 1749–1750. doi:10.1001/jama.2018.16755

NOTE: The author would like to acknowledge Kathy J. Booker, PhD, RN for her contribution to this case in the first edition of this book.

Case 8.11 Facial Pain

RESOLUTION

Which diagnostic studies should be considered to assist with or confirm the diagnosis?

None are necessary at this time. However, repeated sinus infections or episodes of sinusitis may warrant a CT scan of the sinuses.

What is the most likely differential diagnosis and why?

Acute sinus infection:

The headache, sinus pain and pressure, and dental pain all support this diagnosis. It is not uncommon for patients to experience blood-streaked rhinorrhea. A typical course toward the development of sinusitis includes a cold or upper respiratory infection followed by the patient feeling improved or well. However, symptoms return, and they tend to be worse and include sinus pressure and pain. A sinus infection needs time to develop and typically follows a cold, URI, or allergies, as mucus and drainage accumulates in the sinus, allowing bacteria or viruses to grow and fester.

Henry may also have allergic rhinitis, which is characterized by cobblestoning in the throat, pale boggy mucosa, clear drainage, scratchy throat, itchy eyes, and an initial presentation after age 8 years old. However, any evidence of Henry's allergies would be superseded by his sinusitis symptoms. Children may have an obvious crease in their noses called an allergic salute that is caused by constantly rubbing the nose. People with allergies may also have epistaxis and frequent throat clearing accompanied by a cough. Mouth breathing, snoring, and creases beneath the lower eyelids (Dennie lines) are sometimes also present. It is not unusual to also have sinus pressure, tenderness, and headache.

Vasomotor rhinitis is a type of nonallergic rhinitis. It is unrelated to an allergic hypersensitivity, infection, structural lesions, systemic disease, or drug use. One can also have atrophic sinusitis (from normal aging), rhinitis medicamentosa (overuse of some over-the-counter medication), or rhinitis related to the hormonal changes of pregnancy. Nonallergic rhinitis may also be caused by foreign bodies in the nose, nasal polyps, neoplasms, cocaine use, hypothyroidism, anatomic variations, and NARES (nonallergic rhinitis with eosinophilia syndrome). In NARES, there is eosinophilia in the nasal drainage, but skin and in vitro tests for allergens are negative.

The Family Nurse Practitioner: Clinical Case Studies, Second Edition. Edited by Leslie Neal-Boylan.
© 2021 John Wiley & Sons Ltd. Published 2021 by John Wiley & Sons Ltd.

Table 8.11.1. Plan of Treatment.

Illness	Pathophysiology	Signs/Symptoms	Treatment
Common cold: URI	Antigen, inflammatory response: edema, WBCs, congestion. Airborne, direct contact. Rhinovirus, coronavirus, parainfluenza virus, coxsackie, RSV. Incubation 1–5 days, virus shedding up to 3 weeks.	Mild fever possible, chills, body aches, rhinorrhea (possibly purulent), and ear congestion, HA. ≤7–10 days, peak 5 days.	Rest, fluids, analgesic, antipyretic. Atrovent nasal spray (anticholinergics), nasal spray. Afrin (watch for rebound): vasoconstriction. Dextromethorphan: Cough suppressant, may cause serotonin syndrome.
Allergic rhinitis	IgE mediated: Allergen-specific IgE after T cell release. RXN is from subsequent exposure to allergen. Early phase: Prompt, lasts 1 hour. Late: Begins in 3–6 hours, gone in 12–24 hours. Early mediated by histamine. Late mediated by chemokines, cytokines, eosinophils, basophils. Eosinophils release leukotrienes.	Sneezing, pruritus, congestion, drainage, sometimes conjunctivitis. Pale, boggy nasal mucosa, allergic shiners, nasal salute, watery eyes, cobblestoning throat and nose.	Avoidance, antihistamines (Zyrtec, Allegra, Claritin), decongestants: oral or topical (watch for rhinitis medicamentosa), intranasal steroids, antileukotrienes (Singulair), intranasal cromolyn (prevention), allergy shots (prevention).
Rhinosinusitis	Cause is usually viral URI. Sinus inflammation should resolve in <14 days. If symptoms worsen after 3–5 days or last >10 days, then probably bacterial infection. Nasal mucosa produces drainage, then congestion and swelling into sinus cavity. Hypoxia and mucus retention promote bacterial growth. *Streptococcus pneumoniae, Haemophilus influenzae, Moraxella catarrhalis.* Chronic: *Staphylococcus aureus* and anaerobic bacteria. Can also have fungal sinusitis.	>7 days of congestion, purulent rhinorrhea, PND, facial pain, pressure, ear/teeth pain, maybe cough, fever, nausea, fatigue, halitosis, impaired smell, taste. Chronic: Congestion, cough, and PND, worse at night. PE: Mucosal edema (nasal), purulent nasal secretions, sinus TTP (not specific or sensitive). Nose: Deviated septum, polyps, epistaxis, foreign bodies, tumors.	Nasal vasoconstrictors such as phenylephrine 0.25% or 0.5% (use only 3–5 days). Systemic decongestants. Nasal or systemic corticosteroids such as beclomethasone. Nasal irrigation with saline. Analgesics/antipyretics. Do not prescribe antibiotics for mild to moderate sinusitis. Most sinusitis is viral. Give antibiotics if: symptoms > 10 days, high fever, purulent nasal drainage or facial pain > 3 consecutive days or symptoms that worsen after a viral illness lasting > 5 days that improved initially First line: Augmentin (XR bid × 2 weeks) or Doxycycline Second line: Levofloxacin or moxifloxacin, clarithromycin, oral cephalosporins

What is the plan of treatment?
Treat patient for rhinosinusitis and allergic rhinitis. See Table 8.11.1.

What is the plan for referrals and follow-up treatment?
There is no need for a scheduled follow-up unless the patient reports that symptoms have persisted beyond treatment or have worsened. No referrals are needed at this time. However, a referral to an

EENT may be warranted for repeated episodes. An allergist might be worth a visit if it is deduced that allergies are the inciting causes of each episode of sinusitis.

Is the family history of migraines relevant?

Migraine headaches often appear in families. They tend to be more common in women than in men. The symptoms of migraine and sinusitis are often mistaken for each other, and each condition may be misdiagnosed as the other.

REFERENCES AND RESOURCES

Ferri, F. F. (2019). Sinusitis. *Ferri's clinical advisor 2019* (pp. 1268–1269). Philadelphia: Elsevier.

Case 8.12 Fatigue, Confusion, and Weight Loss

Which diagnostic studies should be considered to assist with or confirm the diagnosis?

CBC: Hemoglobin and hematocrit were 10.1/29.5; FBS: 149; potassium 4.8; BUN: 42; creatinine 1.44 (estimated glomerular filtration rate [GFR] was 35).

What is the most likely differential diagnosis and why?

Chronic kidney disease (CKD), stage 3:

The GFR of 35 points directly to CKD, stage 3. The low hemoglobin clearly suggests anemia, though the specific etiology is unknown. There are several mainstays of CKD management, which include blood pressure control, volume management, anemia management, and sodium/potassium management. The target blood pressure should be < 130/80 if albumin excretion is >30 mg/24 hours. Otherwise, the target blood pressure should be </= 140/90. ACE-I and ARBs are pharmacotherapy options that have been proven to be renoprotective, so switching to one of these agents for blood pressure control is wise. In addition, chlorthalidone should be added if the blood pressure remains high. Avoid loop diuretics if there is a concern about hypokalemia. Since individuals with CKD can be at risk for hyperkalemia and hypernatremia, particularly if they are also diabetic, management of sodium, phosphorous, and potassium levels is crucial. Fluid intake should be restricted if the patient has significant edema or is hyponatremic.

Maryanne also has anemia secondary to CKD, stage 3. The BUN and creatinine lab values lead us to evaluate Maryanne's kidney function. The general health of an individual's kidney is determined by the glomerular filtration rate, 35 in this case. A decrease in GFR correlates with a change in histology secondary to kidney disease. The stages of CKD are as follows:

CKD is defined as kidney damage or GFR < 60 mL/min/1.73 m² for at least 3 months with or without kidney damage. Kidney damage is defined is abnormal pathology, abnormal blood values, abnormal urine studies, or abnormal imaging.

- Stage 1: Normal or increased GFR, some evidence of kidney damage
- Stage 2: Kidney damage with mild decrease in GFR (89–60 ml/min per 1.73 m²
- Stage 3: Moderate decrease in GFR (30–59)

The Family Nurse Practitioner: Clinical Case Studies, Second Edition. Edited by Leslie Neal-Boylan.
© 2021 John Wiley & Sons Ltd. Published 2021 by John Wiley & Sons Ltd.

- Stage 3A: GFR 59–45 ml/min per 1.73m^2
- Stage 3B: GFR 44–30 ml/min per 1.73m^2
- Stage 4: Severe decrease in GFR (15–29)
- Stage 5: Kidney failure (GFR < 15 or dialysis)

The workup for anemia of CKD is initiated when the hemoglobin value is less than 12 g/dL in a post-menopausal female. Anemia of CKD can be most commonly attributed to decreased production in erythropoietin by the kidneys or to iron deficiency. Other causes of anemia of CKD include blood loss, hypothyroidism, acute and chronic inflammatory conditions, and hemoglobinopathies.

Maryanne also appears to have dementia, a condition that is characterized by a progressive decline in intellectual functioning. The functional decline tends to involve the memory, cognitive capacities, and adaptive behavior. Dementia does not involve alteration in consciousness. Dementia may start as mild cognitive impairment in its earliest stages, which refers to an isolated loss of memory without difficulty in other cognitive functions. Alzheimer's disease is the leading cause of dementia, though depression in the older adult can also present similarly. Other symptoms of depression in the older adult include hopelessness, anhedonia, and fatigue. Assessment of dementia is further evaluated with a mental status examination.

When evaluating chronic fatigue, malignancy must always be on the differential. The clinical picture often also includes severe involuntary weight loss, depression, and apathy. Laboratory studies (CBC) are paramount for ruling out a cancer.

Obstructive sleep apnea (OSA) might be considered as a differential diagnosis. It occurs when the nasopharyngeal airway patency is compromised during sleep. Risk factors include obesity, increased neck circumference, deviated septum, nasal polyps, and enlarged tonsils. Presentation includes snoring, disturbed sleep, daytime sleepiness, chronic fatigue, and personality change. The easiest way to determine whether OSA is appropriately on the differential is to have the patient observed by another during sleep to evaluate for snoring.

COPD is known as an irreversible and progressive decline in lung function due to obstruction of airflow, airway inflammation, and reduction in the expiratory flow rate. Individuals with COPD often have a history of smoking, asthma, or environmental/work exposure to irritants. COPD refers to chronic bronchitis or emphysema. Symptoms include shortness of breath, wheezing, and increased work of breathing. On examination, lung sounds can include fine or coarse crackles and wheezes. In emphysema, the AP diameter of the chest is increased, and lung sounds can be distant.

What is the plan of treatment?

To manage and further evaluate the anemia secondary to CKD, it is necessary to order further lab tests, particularly iron studies. Maryanne's hemoglobin is within the range of 9–11g/dL, so she does not need erythropoietin at this time. The iron studies to be ordered are CBC, indices, reticulocytes, serum iron, TIBC, and ferritin and rule out thalassemia. Her transferrin saturation should be >/= 20% and ferritin >100 mg/ml before starting erythropoietin therapy to avoid cardiovascular complications. If the iron studies reveal iron deficiency, Maryanne may need iron replacement. If iron studies are normal, it means that the deficiency is in fact due to the damaged kidneys producing less than normal erythropoietin. Specific changes to Maryanne's medication regimen should be as follows:

- Discontinue glucophage
- Discontinue Avandia
- Begin Actos, 30 mg daily (for glycemia control)
- Discontinue Lasix
- Begin chlorthalidone daily for hypertension
- Continue Actonel 35 mg weekly

The following lab studies should also be ordered at this time and discussed as soon as the results become available: LFTs; chemistry panel; BUN/creatinine; Hgb A1C; micro urinalysis. The nephrologist may order a CT scan of the chest, abdomen, and pelvis with contrast (if not contraindicated), a mammogram, and a transvaginal ultrasound of the uterus.

Continue statin and Zetia treatment. Normalize serum phosphate and calcium levels. Monitor salt, potassium, and fluid balance. Vitamin D supplementation may be appropriate. Maryanne may need nutritional supplementation and counseling to cope with the disease. Recommend annual influenza vaccination and a polyvalent pneumococcal vaccine. Consider vaccination with the hepatitis B series.

What is the plan for referrals and follow-up care?
Referrals should be initiated to hematology and nephrology.

Are there standardized guidelines that should be used to assess or treat this case?
International Society of Nephrology. (2013). KDIGO 2012 clinical practice guideline for the evaluation and management of chronic kidney disease. *Kidney International Supplement, 3*(1), 136–150.

REFERENCES AND RESOURCES

Ferri, F. F. (2019). Chronic kidney disease. *Ferri's clinical advisor 2019* (pp. 322–325). Philadelphia: Elsevier.
International Society of Nephrology. (2013). KDIGO 2012 clinical practice guideline for the evaluation and management of chronic kidney disease. *Kidney International Supplement, 3*(1), 136–150.

NOTE: The author would like to acknowledge Geraldine F. Marrocco , EdD, APRN, CNS, ANP-BC for her contribution to this case in the first edition of this book.

Case 8.13 Hand Numbness

RESOLUTION

What are the three most likely differential diagnoses and why?
Carpal tunnel syndrome:
Carpal tunnel syndrome (CTS) is the most likely diagnosis. Though it is more common in females than males, males may be afflicted with the condition, especially with a history of repetitive motion. In 50% of the cases, it will affect both wrists (Werner & Andary, 2011). The gradual onset of numbness, pain, and even burning are typical. Symptoms can worsen at night because individuals may sleep with a flexed wrist (McClure, 2003). It is typical for patients to describe that shaking their hand helps to relieve the numbness (Werner & Andary, 2011). This is known as the flick sign (Scanlon & Maffei, 2009). The median nerve is a mixed nerve and transmits both sensory and motor neurons. The median nerve supplies sensation to the ventral aspect of the thumb, first 2 fingers, and half of the third and to the tips of the fingers on the dorsal aspect of the same digits (Walker, 2010). Since it is a mixed nerve, it also supplies motor movement to the muscles of the thenar eminence, which abducts, flexes, adducts, and medially rotates the thumb (Walker, 2010). It first affects sensation and then motor movement. The dropping of his hammer can represent the beginning of motor weakness.

Pronator syndrome:
Pronator syndrome occurs with entrapment of the median nerve at the elbow. Pronator syndrome can mimic symptoms of CTS (Neal & Fields, 2010) and pain often occurs with repetitive motion of the forearm. It affects sensation, but not motor. Therefore, you would not see weakness or thenar atrophy. With pronator syndrome, the Tinel's and Phalen's tests are negative.

Cervical radiculopathy:
When dealing with nerve symptoms, you must always eliminate the possibility of circulation problems and determine whether the origin is from an upper motor neuron or lower motor neuron. When dealing with upper motor neuron entrapment syndromes, pain typically is not limited to the hand. According to Scanlon and Maffei (2009), if pain is located in the shoulder, upper arm, or neck, a cervical problem is suspected. With cervical radiculopathy, there may be point tenderness on vertebral palpation or percussion or pain with neck movement. Pain, weakness, or numbness or paresthesias when the C 6/7 nerve root is compressed is indicative of a spinal cord problem (Walker, 2010). Cervical problems usually present bilaterally or shift from right to left. If spinal cord injury

---

The Family Nurse Practitioner: Clinical Case Studies, Second Edition. Edited by Leslie Neal-Boylan.
© 2021 John Wiley & Sons Ltd. Published 2021 by John Wiley & Sons Ltd.

is suspected, this mandates immobilization, radiologic evaluation, and repeated neurological exams as motor symptoms may occur hours to days later (Neal & Fields, 2010).

Which diagnostic or imaging studies should be considered to assist with or confirm the diagnosis?

See Table 8.13.1.

What is the plan of treatment?

Prescribe a wrist splint for Timothy to wear at night. Advise careful use of topical and/or oral NSAIDs for pain relief. Advise avoidance of repetitive activities. Suggest a break, if possible, from his work. Consider a corticosteroid injection at this visit or in the future for pain relief. Combined treatments may be most effective.

What is the plan for referrals and follow-up?

Refer for electrodiagnostic studies. Refer for surgical evaluation in cases of severe median nerve injury. If treating with nonsurgical interventions, follow up in 4–6 weeks to assess effectiveness. Also follow up after electrodiagnostic studies to determine next steps.

What specific activities do you want to ask about?

Peripheral nerve injuries commonly occur in individuals who participate in recreational sports or specific occupational activities. Ask about repetitive motion activities, use of keyboard, hammering, knitting, and piano playing, which constantly flex the wrist. However, repetitive motion as causal for CTS is controversial.

What other important history questions must you ask so as not to miss an important differential diagnosis?

When deciding on a cause for median nerve compression, think about internal causes from a decrease in tunnel space or external causes from edema or inflammation. This will narrow down whether the nerve compression is from repetitive motion; trauma; congenital malformations; medications that can increase edema; or metabolic, infectious, or inflammatory diseases/conditions such as rheumatoid arthritis, systemic lupus erythematosus, gout or obesity.

Table 8.13.1.   Diagnostic Testing.

Complete blood count	Not necessary for diagnosis.
Chemistry profile	Not necessary for diagnosis.
Fasting plasma glucose	Yes, because of the family history and to rule out as a differential diagnosis. There is some controversy whether to obtain this lab test without suspicion of diabetes mellitus.
TSH	Yes, because of the family history and to rule out as a differential diagnosis. There is some controversy whether to obtain this lab test without suspicion of hypothyroidism.
X-ray of wrists	No.
	Conditions that you would obtain X-ray:
	History of trauma or suspicion of a tumor or bone spurs (history of a fracture or dislocation of carpal bone or distal radius and concern about malunion, wrist arthritis, or mass). Ultrasound if you suspect a structural abnormality.
Electrodiagnostic studies:	Diagnosis is usually based on history and physical exam. May treat conservatively first
Nerve conduction velocity studies (NCV)	prior to obtaining. Neal & Fields (2010) recommend obtaining NCF studies if no improvement occurs after 6 weeks after initiating conservative treatment. It is also
Electromyography (EMG)	acceptable to initiate these tests at the time of diagnosis.
MRI	Not ordered unless the following are present:
	Only in unusual cases, to rule out a mass or lesion or evaluate cervical radiculopathy.
X-ray of elbows	No, not necessary unless a history of trauma.
X-ray of neck	No, not necessary unless there is a history of trauma.

Since rheumatoid arthritis, systemic lupus erythematosus, and gout can mimic CTS, asking about pain, swelling, and erythema in other joints is important. Pain and swelling may indicate osteoarthritis. Other conditions that can cause swelling include hypothyroidism, heart failure, pregnancy, and any use of steroids. Also, conditions that can cause neuropathy, such as diabetes mellitus, should be ruled out.

Why do you inspect for thenar atrophy?

The motor aspect of the thumb is innervated by the median nerve. The abductor pollicus brevis is only innervated by the median nerve and is responsible for abduction of the thumb. The opponeus pollicus flexes, adducts, and medially rotates the thumb. With a lower motor neuron entrapment injury, the nerve innervating the muscle is compromised causing decreased movement, resulting in muscular atrophy.

Would your diagnosis change if Timothy complained of acute onset of paresthesias of the upper arm?

Yes. Acute CTS is uncommon; and, if it does occur, it is typically caused by a radial fracture or carpal injury. Other considerations for nontraumatic acute CTS can develop secondarily from infective tenosynovitis, coagulopathies, false aneurysm, gout, or rheumatoid disorders.

Why would you be concerned if Timothy's pain were past his elbows?

CTS pain may present as shooting pains radiating up to the elbow. If pain radiates past the elbow toward the shoulder or neck, consider a cervical cord problem (Scanlon & Maffei, 2009).

What significance does thumb strength have?

The motor aspect of the thumb is only innervated by the median nerve. Muscle weakness of the thumb is a strong indicator of median nerve entrapment.

What would you do if this patient were female and pregnant?

Pregnancy or any condition that increases estrogen may cause fluid retention, causing increasing pressure on the median nerve. Avoiding noxious stimuli, wrist splinting, ergonomic modification, and ultrasound treatment are the courses of treatment for pregnancy.

Are there any standardized guidelines available to be used to assess or treat this case?

The National Guideline Clearing House published the American Academy of Orthopedic Surgeons evidence-based practice guidelines for the diagnosis and treatment of carpal tunnel syndrome.

REFERENCES AND RESOURCES

American Academy of Orthopaedic Surgeons (2016). *Clinical practice guideline on the diagnosis of carpal tunnel syndrome*. https://www.guidelinecentral.com/summaries/american-academy-of-orthopaedic-surgeons-clinical-practice-guideline-on-management-of-carpal-tunnel-syndrome/#section-society

Chesterton, L. S., Blagojevic-Bucknall, M., Burton, C., Dziedzic, K. S., Davenport, G., Jowett, S. M., . . . Roddy, E. (2018). The clinical and cost-effectiveness of corticosteroid injection versus night splints for carpal tunnel syndrome (INSTINCTS trial): An open-label, parallel group, randomised controlled trial. *Lancet, 392,* 1423.

Fernández-de-Las Peñas, C., Ortega-Santiago, R., de la Llave-Rincón, A. I., Martínez-Perez, A., Díaz, H. F.-S., Martínez-Martín, J., . . . Cuadrado-Pérez, M. L. (2015). Manual physical therapy versus surgery for carpal tunnel syndrome: A randomized parallel-group trial. *Journal of Pain, 16,* 1087.

Kothari, M. J., Shefner, J. M., & Eichler, A. F. (2018). Carpal tunnel syndrome. *UpToDate.*

McClure, P. (2003). Evidence-based practice: An example related to the use of splinting in a patient with carpal tunnel syndrome. *Journal of Hand Therapy, 16,* 256.

Muller, M., Tsui, D., Schnurr, R., Biddulph-Deisroth, L., Hard, J., & MacDermid, J. C. (2004). Effectiveness of hand therapy interventions in primary management of carpal tunnel syndrome: A systematic review. *Journal of Hand Therapy, 17*, 210.

Neal, S. L., & Fields, K. B. (2010). Peripheral nerve entrapment and injury in the upper extremity. *American Family Physician, 81*, 147–155.

Page, M. J., Massy-Westropp, N., O'Connor, D., & Pitt, V. (2012). Splinting for carpal tunnel syndrome. *Cochrane Database Systematic Review,* CD010003.

Premoselli, S., Sioli, P., Grossi, A., & Cerri, C. (2006). Neutral wrist splinting in carpal tunnel syndrome: A 3- and 6-months clinical and neurophysiologic follow-up evaluation of night-only splint therapy. *Europa Medicophysica, 42*, 121.

Scanlon, A., & Maffei, J. (2009). Carpal tunnel syndrome. *Journal of Neuroscience Nursing, 41*, 140–147.

Walker, J. A. (2010). Management of patients with carpal tunnel syndrome. *Nursing Standard, 24*, 44–48.

Werner, R. A., & Andary, M. (2011). Electrodiagnostic evaluation of carpal tunnel syndrome. *Muscle Nerve, 44*, 597.

Wu, Y. T., Ho, T. Y., Chou, Y. C., Ke, M.-J., Li, T.-Y., Tsai, C.-K., & Chen, L.-C. (2017). Six-month efficacy of perineural dextrose for carpal tunnel syndrome: A prospective, randomized, double-blind, controlled trial. *Mayo Clinic Proceedings, 92*, 1179.

Case 8.14 Chronic Diarrhea

Which diagnostic studies should be considered to assist with or confirm the diagnosis?

Serologic testing is done while the patient remains on a gluten-containing diet.

tTG-IgA antibody: This is a serological test for immunoglobulin A (IgA) antibodies against tissue transglutaminase (tTG). The test has a sensitivity of more than 90% and a specificity of more than 95%. This is considered the first-line screening test for celiac disease.

EMA-IgA test: This test is moderately sensitive and highly specific for untreated celiac disease with 85–98% sensitivity and a specificity of 97–100%.

CBC: This is used to look for nutritional deficiencies. Patients with celiac disease have malabsorption, which can result in iron-deficiency anemia.

Total IgA: This would rule out IgA deficiency. IgA deficiency decreases the sensitivity of tTG-IgA, resulting in false negative serologies. Negative tTG-IgA serologies in a symptomatic patient would warrant a total IgA to help explain the negative serologies.

If there is a positive tTG–IgA, the patient should be referred to Gastroenterology for a celiac disease confirmatory small bowel biopsy.

Dermatitis herpertiformis biopsy: In patients with biopsy-proven dermatitis hepertiformis, celiac disease can be diagnosed by serology alone (Cichewicz et al., 2019; Rubio-Tapia, Hill, Kelly, Calderwood, & Murray, 2013).

It is also appropriate to order a CBC, comprehensive metabolic panel, TSH, IgA antiendomysial antibody (EMA), and IgA antitissue transglutaminase antibody (anti-tTG). It would not be appropriate to order a duodenal biopsy at this time, though it may be part of a diagnostic workup after the results of the current screening lab work are received. The CBC will show whether Amelia has iron deficiency anemia, as this would be a crucial part of the clinical picture. It will also rule out systemic illness and give a picture of general health. The CMP will show Amelia's kidney and liver function, as well as her fluid status. The TSH will show thyroid function, and the IgA studies are part of the autoimmune workup for celiac disease.

The lab results are as follows: hemoglobin: 11.7; HCT: 32; MCV: 80; ferritin: 100; LFTs: normal; TSH: 2.08. The IgA antitissue transglutaminase (anti-tTG) antibody was positive. The IgA antibody was positive. The skin biopsy was positive.

The Family Nurse Practitioner: Clinical Case Studies, Second Edition. Edited by Leslie Neal-Boylan.
© 2021 John Wiley & Sons Ltd. Published 2021 by John Wiley & Sons Ltd.

What is the most likely differential diagnosis and why?
Celiac disease:
Celiac disease is a chronic, multiorgan autoimmune disease affecting the gastrointestinal tract; it affects about 1% of the population is often underdiagnosed due to similar symptom presentation to other conditions, such as IBS and IBD. It is triggered by exposure to gluten, a storage protein found in wheat, rye, and barley (American Gastroenterological Association [AGA], 2006). Gluten triggers an autoimmune reaction that causes chronic inflammation of the intestinal mucosa, which leads to malabsorption. It is common in persons with European ancestry and in those of Middle Eastern, Indian, South American, and North African descent (Green & Cellier, 2007; Setty, Hormaza, & Guandalini, 2008). The most common symptoms are diarrhea and flatulence. Other intestinal symptoms include abdominal pain, weight loss, and poor appetite. Extraintestinal symptoms include dermatitis herpetiformis, fatigue, headaches, metabolic bone disease, and others (Pelkowski & Viera, 2014). Amelia's presentation, including diarrhea and weight loss over a long period of time, findings of rash on the elbows and extensor surface of the arms (likely dermatitis herpetiformis), and family history of Type 1 diabetes, point to celiac disease. Confirmation of the diagnosis is based on the lab results and biopsy findings.

Diagnostic criteria include a minimum of 4 out of 5 or 3 out of 4 of the following (if the HLA genotype test is not done to confirm): symptoms as described in this case, positive IgA class autoantibodies with high titer, celiac enteropathy if a biopsy is done of the small intestine, and response to a gluten-free diet. The average age of diagnosis is during one's 50s. Celiac disease is an inflammatory condition of the small bowel that manifests due to an allergy or sensitivity to foods containing gluten. Foods that contain gluten include wheat, barley, and rye. Other classic symptoms of typical celiac disease include steatorrhea and weight loss. Atypical celiac disease presents without gastrointestinal symptoms, but may present with osteoporosis, anemia, infertility, seizures, and other neurologic symptoms.

Screening for celiac disease should be done whenever an individual presents with chronic symptoms of abdominal pain and bloating, diarrhea, and weight loss. Initial screening can be done via bloodwork, and the IgA antiendomysial antibody and IgA antitissue transglutaminase antibody tests are over 95% sensitive and specific when done together. A capsule endoscopy of the small intestine is recommended initially followed by another biopsy after treatment. The biopsy can also identify small bowel lymphoma, which has a higher risk for patients with celiac disease. Celiac disease is difficult to diagnose due to its similar presentation to other gastrointestinal disorders.

What are other possible differential diagnoses?
Irritable bowel syndrome:
Irritable bowel syndrome, a functional and highly prevalent disorder, is characterized by severe disturbance in bowel functions. The Rome III diagnostic criteria describe IBS as "recurrent abdominal pain or discomfort at least 3 days per month in the last 3 months associated with 2 or more of the following: (1) improvement with defecation, (2) onset associated with a change in frequency of stool, and (3) onset associated with a change in form of stool" (Rome Foundation, 2006). It can be noted that Amelia's symptoms fall into the criteria of IBS. However, since approximately 10% of those diagnosed with IBS have celiac disease, the 2 conditions are not mutually exclusive and must both be considered in a workup.

Inflammatory bowel disease:
Another diagnosis to consider with individuals presenting with chronic loose stools is inflammatory bowel disease, which includes ulcerative colitis and Crohn's disease. IBD hallmarks include bloody diarrhea, urgency, steatorrhea, fever, abdominal pain, and weight loss. Both disease processes of IBD must be diagnosed via endoscopy. While Amelia's symptoms do not fit perfectly into this pattern, it is a differential to be considered if our initial diagnosis proves to be incorrect.

Viral gastroenteritis:
Viral gastroenteritis is not a likely diagnosis as this patient does not have nausea, vomiting, or abdominal cramps.

What is the plan of treatment?

If there is a positive tTG–IgA, the patient should be referred to Gastroenterology. Individuals with positive serology require a GI endoscopy with small bowel biopsy to confirm the diagnosis.

Treatment for celiac disease is a lifelong commitment to a gluten-free diet. Foods that contain wheat, barley, or rye must be omitted. In most individuals with gluten sensitivity, oats are well tolerated. Such a diet can be a challenge, as many foods today contain gluten derivatives. There are, however, many support networks, grocery stores, and restaurants that make a gluten-free life much easier.

* Lifelong gluten-free diet
* Referral to a dietician for education on gluten-free diet
* Treatment of nutritional deficiencies
* Referral to an advocacy group
* Nutritional supplements

(Bai & Ciacci, 2017; Rubio-Tapia et al., 2013)

What is the plan for referrals and follow-up?

Amelia will be instructed to follow a gluten-free diet and will be scheduled for an endoscopy and duodenal biopsy. After 1 month, Amelia should return to the clinic for reevaluation. A diagnosis of celiac disease involves lifelong management of one's diet, which is why routine meetings with a dietician should be strongly encouraged. If Amelia's symptoms are not alleviated by a gluten-free diet, it is appropriate to consider referral to a GI specialist. Amelia should be sent for a bone mineral density test that should then be used as a baseline. Repeat serologies (IgA-tTG) in 6–12 months to check response, then annually. Perform a follow-up CBC (Rubio-Tapia et al., 2013).

Are there standardized guidelines or resources that would help in this case?

The Celiac Disease Foundation (https://celiac.org/) is an excellent resource for both the health care professional and the consumer.

The American Gastroenterological Association (https://gastro.org) has published guidelines and position statements for many GI diseases and syndromes.

The Rome Foundation (https://theromefoundation.org/) criteria for IBS is an excellent resource.

What demographic characteristics might affect this case?

Serologic tests have decreased sensitivity in children under 2. Deamidated gliadin peptides (DGPs) have better sensitivity.

If this patient had no insurance or lived in a rural area without access to health care (difficult to get to a clinic), how would that change management, or would it change management?

If the patient lived in a rural area with few or no gastroenterologists, treatment could be started without confirmatory small bowel biopsy. A gluten-free diet would still be the mainstay of treatment.

REFERENCES AND RESOURCES

American Gastroenterological Association. (2016). AGA Institute medical position statement on the diagnosis and management of celiac disease. *Gastroenterology,131*(6), 1977–1980.

Bai, J. C., & Ciacci, C. (2017). World Gastroenterology Organisation global guidelines: Celiac disease. *Journal of Clinical Gastroenterology, 51*(9), 755–768.

Cichewicz, A. B., Mearns, E. S., Taylor, A., Boulanger, T., Gerber, M., Leffler, D. A., . . . Lebwohl, B. (2019). Diagnosis and treatment patterns in celiac disease. *Digestive Diseases and Sciences, 64,* 2095–2210. https://doi.org/10.1007/s10620-019-05528-3

Ferri, F. F. (2019). Celiac disease. *Ferri's clinical advisor 2019* (pp. 293–295). Philadelphia: Elsevier.

Green, P. H., & Cellier, C. (2007). Celiac disease. *New England Journal of Medicine, 357*(17), 1731–1743.

Pelkowski, T. D., & Viera, A. J. (2014). Celiac disease: Diagnosis and management. *American Family Physician, 89*(2), 99–105.

Rome Foundation. (2006). Guidelines—Rome III diagnostic criteria for functional gastrointestinal disorders. *Journal of Gastrointestinal & Liver Diseases, 15*(3), 307–312. Retrieved from Ovid (MEDLINE).

Rubio-Tapia, A., Hill, I. D., Kelly, C. P., Calderwood, A. H., & Murray, J. A. (2013). ACG clinical guidelines: Diagnosis and management of celiac disease. *American College of Gastroenterology, 108*(5), 656–676; quiz 677. doi:10.1038/ajg.2013.79

Simren, M., Palsson, O. S., & Whitehead, W. E. (2017). Update on Rome IV criteria for colorectal disorders: Implications for clinical practice. *Current Gastroenterology Reports, 19*(4), 15. doi: 10.1007/s11894-017-0554-0

Setty, M., Hormaza, L., & Guandalini, S. (2008). Celiac disease: Risk assessment, diagnosis, and monitoring. *Molecular Diagnosis & Therapy, 12*(5), 289–298.

NOTE: The author would like to acknowledge the contribution to this case of Geraldine F. Marrocco, EdD, APRN, CNS, ANP-BC in the first edition of this book.

Case 8.15 Intractable Pain

Which diagnostic studies should be considered to assist with or confirm the diagnosis? If you choose imaging studies, state what part of the body you will image.
No testing is needed at this time.

What is the most likely differential diagnosis and why?
Phantom limb pain (PLP):
PLP can be caused by a skin infection, pressure points, skin breakdown, ischemia in the remaining limb, a neuroma, hetereotopic ossification, or deep tissue infection. It is important to rule out medical causes of the pain and not automatically assume it is PLP. When evaluating a chief complaint of pain, it is important to look at a detailed history to identify the possible source of the pain, if there is one. Roger's trauma history points strongly to PLP, as he describes pain in the limb that is no longer present. His description of pain is congruent with PLP, which is often described as tingling, burning, or pins and needles. PLP is common in amputees and should always be part of the follow-up assessment.

Phantom pain is loosely defined as pain that is associated with nerve injury or as pain in a limb that is either no longer present due to trauma/amputation or completely numb due to major injury. The source of PLP is unknown; discussion suggests it either derives from the peripheral nervous system activity or changes in the spinal/supraspinal body surface representations. The difficulty in knowing the source of the pain results in difficulty treating it. The evidence suggests that PLP can be prevented preoperatively via regional anesthesia such as an epidural. There are several risk factors for developing PLP: stump pain, older age, repeated limb surgeries, and postoperative pain that is severe.

What is the plan of treatment?
Opioids are not recommended and have limited value. Perineural blockade via a catheter for a minimum of 80 hours following the amputation can prevent PLP. Clonidine is sometimes added in cases at risk for severe PLP. There is emerging evidence that gabapentin and pregabalin are effective in treating PLP. Ketamine given intravenously is the most frequently used treatment for severe PLP. Nonpharmacologic methods are sometimes used, such as TENS (transcutaneous electrical nerve stimulation) and biofeedback. Tricyclics are no longer recommended.

The Family Nurse Practitioner: Clinical Case Studies, Second Edition. Edited by Leslie Neal-Boylan.
© 2021 John Wiley & Sons Ltd. Published 2021 by John Wiley & Sons Ltd.

There are no definitive guidelines for the treatment of phantom limb pain; however, several sources outline the different options. The consensus seems to be to either treat with pharmacotherapy, combined with adjunct symptom management, or with the procedural options of TENS or biofeedback. If neither of those treatment modality pathways leads to alleviation of pain, specialty care should be sought out in or by a pain clinic, rehabilitation care, or an orthopedic specialist.

Several adjuvant therapy options should be considered, such as mental relaxation, wrapping, heat, massage, pressure, and mirror box therapy. One of these methods that has been studied and shows considerable promise is mirror box therapy. This technique allows the amputee to perceive the missing limb through strategically placed mirrors. Focusing on the reflection of the limb can allow reconfiguration of the sensory cortex, thus leading to a reduction in PLP (Black et al., 2009). Acupuncture and **repetitive transcranial magnetic stimulation (rTMS) may provide relief.**

Since Roger's pain is severe and untouched by over-the-counter pain medications, it is appropriate to consider a combination of medications. Roger can start taking pregabalin (Lyrica), an anti-seizure medication used often for neuropathic pain. He should receive a prescription for 100 mg in the morning, 50 mg at noon, and 50 mg at bedtime. In adjunct to pharmacotherapy, Roger can consider the adjuvant therapies listed above, including hypnotherapy, mirror box therapy, and acupuncture. In the meantime, the clinician should tell Roger to try heat, massage, and pressure on the affected limb if he finds himself in pain between now and his follow-up visit. Roger will be asked to follow up in 10 days, at which point his old records will be transferred and first assessments can be made regarding his pain control.

What is the plan for referrals and follow-up?

At this time, it is appropriate to manage Roger's phantom pain in the primary care clinic setting. If pharmacotherapy does not work, or if he is interested in specific adjuvant or procedural therapies, referrals can be made to the appropriate specialist. If the therapies tried are unsuccessful, the patient should be referred to the pain clinic, orthopedics, or rehabilitation.

Are there standardized guidelines or resources that would help in this case?

There are no universal guidelines for the treatment of phantom limb pain. However, the Department of Veterans Affairs has a published set of guidelines that are widely referenced. Particularly insightful organizations include the Amputee Coalition of America (https://www.amputee-coalition.org/) and the American Society of Regional Anesthesia and Pain Medicine (https://www.asra.com/page/44/the-specialty-of-chronic-pain-management).

REFERENCES AND RESOURCES

Baird, J. C. (2018). Pain in the residual limb. In R. S. Porter, J. L. Kaplan, R. B. Lynn, & M. T. Reddy (Eds.), The Merck manual of diagnosis and therapy (p. 3205). Kenilworth, NJ: Merck Sharp & Dohme Corp.

Black, L. M., Pearsons, R. K., & Jamieson, B. (2009). What is the best way to manage phantom limb pain? *The Journal of Family Practice, 58*(3), 155–158.

Neil, M. J. E. (2016). Pain after amputation. *BJA Education, 16*(3), 107–112, https://doi.org/10.1093/bjaed/mkv028

NOTE: The author would like to acknowledge the contribution of Geraldine F. Marrocco, EdD, APRN, CNS, ANP-BC to this case in the first edition of this book.

Case 8.16 Wrist Pain and Swelling

What is the most likely differential diagnosis and why?
Rheumatoid arthritis (RA):
The patient most likely has rheumatoid arthritis (RA). There are several findings that support this diagnosis: wrist and foot pain and swelling, more than 1 hour of morning stiffness, fatigue, and weakness. According to the American College of Rheumatology 1987 criteria for a diagnosis of rheumatoid arthritis, the patient must have 4 of the following 7 criteria for at least 6 weeks:

1. Morning stiffness lasting more than 1 hour.
2. Arthritis pain in 3 or more joints.
3. Swelling in the hand joints.
4. Symmetrical joint swelling.
5. Erosions or decalcifications on X-rays of the hands.
6. Rheumatoid nodules.
7. Abnormal rheumatoid factor.

Rosa has had the symptoms mentioned in the first 4 criteria for 3 months. Her diagnostic workup will include a rheumatoid factor and X-rays of the hands and feet.

Rosa is an unlikely candidate for osteoarthritis because of her youth. She may have systemic lupus erythematosus (SLE), as it is present in her family and the symptoms of SLE are similar to those in RA and also occur most often in young women.

Which diagnostic studies should be considered to assist with or confirm the diagnosis?
Her diagnostics should include tests for SLE, which include at this time: ANA (antinuclear antibody), C3, C4, and DS DNA (double stranded DNA). Sjögren's disease can also be ruled out—although the patient denies dry eyes or dry mouth—by testing her SS-A and SS-B levels. A rheumatoid factor, CRP (c-reactive protein), ESR, or CCP should be done to confirm inflammatory disease. In addition, a CBC can rule out anemia that often accompanies RA, and a CMP should be done to check the status of blood sugar, electrolytes, and liver function. Several treatments for RA require normal liver function. Carpal tunnel syndrome (CTS) often accompanies or follows a diagnosis of RA. In addition, the patient does perform repetitive movements in her job. Consider an

---

The Family Nurse Practitioner: Clinical Case Studies, Second Edition. Edited by Leslie Neal-Boylan.
© 2021 John Wiley & Sons Ltd. Published 2021 by John Wiley & Sons Ltd.

ultrasound of the hand because the patient has swelling. Hand and wrist X-rays will be helpful in assessing whether there are erosions in the wrists, but a nerve conduction test might be done in the future on each wrist to evaluate for the loss of nerve function. This is not urgent at this point because tests during the physical exam were negative for CTS.

What is the plan of treatment?

The lab work and imaging studies described above should be performed, and the results should be evaluated and discussed with the patient at the follow-up visit. Treatment in the meantime should consist of NSAIDs such as ibuprofen or naproxen sodium. The patient can be provided with wrist splints and be encouraged to alternate ice and heat to the painful joints.

What is the plan for referrals and follow-up?

A referral to a rheumatologist is appropriate at this time. However, if an appointment is not possible for several months, it is important to consult with the rheumatologist by phone regarding starting the patient on methotrexate. Further, it may be advisable to give the patient a short course of prednisone during this time if symptoms flare.

Would the primary diagnosis be different if the patient were 55 years old?

If the patient were 55 years old, the diagnosis of RA would still be the most likely diagnosis, given the same history and presentation.

Would there be treatment considerations if the patient had a history of tuberculosis?

If the patient had a history of tuberculosis, the treatment might differ in that the rheumatologist would be likely to steer away from the use of TNF alpha inhibitors, which are often used to treat RA if methotrexate does not work sufficiently to control symptoms.

REFERENCES AND RESOURCES

American College of Rheumatology. (2020). *Rheumatoid arthritis*. Guidelines. Retrieved from https://www.rheumatology.org/Practice-Quality/Clinical-Support/Clinical-Practice-Guidelines/Rheumatoid-Arthritis

Imboden, J., Hellman, D., & Stone, J. (2007). Current diagnosis and treatment: Rheumatology (2nd ed.). New York: McGraw-Hill Lange.

Singh, J.A., Saag, K. G., Bridges, J. R. Jr., Akl, E. A., Bannuru, R. R., Sullivan, M. C., . . . McAlindon, T. (2015). 2015 American College of Rheumatology guideline for the treatment of rheumatoid arthritis. *Arthritis Care & Research*. doi10.1002/acr.22783

Case 9.1 Sad Mood

What are the top three differential diagnoses in this case and why?

Adjustment disorder with depressed mood:
To meet the criteria for adjustment disorder with depressed mood, symptoms must emerge in response to an identifiable stressor that occurred within the prior 3 months. In Julia's case, the stressor could be her transition to college and the subsequent loss of direct family support and structure of home life.

Major depressive disorder:
Julia reports a constellation of symptoms that meet the criteria for a major depressive episode, including sad mood, low energy and motivation, difficulty concentrating, increased appetite, and hypersomnia. These symptoms have been present for more than 2 weeks and are causing impairments in academic and social functioning. Further, they cannot be attributed to substance use or an underlying medical condition.

Bipolar depression:
Bipolar depression is frequently misdiagnosed as unipolar depression due to the clinical challenge of accurately identifying a history of (hypo)mania, a criterion that must be met to fulfill the diagnostic criteria for bipolar disorder. This happens, in part, because patients are more likely to seek treatment during depressive episodes and do not necessarily view hypomanic symptoms as problematic or disruptive to functioning and, as such, they frequently go unreported.

Which diagnostic tests are required in this case and why?
Diagnostic tests, including TSH, CBC with differential, basic metabolic panel, B12 and folic acid, should be obtained to rule out any underlying medical conditions, including hypothyroidism, anemia, vitamin deficiency. The PHQ-9 should be completed to assess both the severity of depressive symptoms and their impact on daily functioning.

What are the concerns at this point?
It is important to distinguish between unipolar and bipolar depression. A thorough psychiatric history should be obtained to determine whether Julia has ever experienced a manic or hypomanic episode. Understanding the impact of depressive symptoms on Julia's functioning can serve to inform the development an appropriate and comprehensive treatment plan. The possibility that

The Family Nurse Practitioner: Clinical Case Studies, Second Edition. Edited by Leslie Neal-Boylan.
© 2021 John Wiley & Sons Ltd. Published 2021 by John Wiley & Sons Ltd.

Julia's symptoms could worsen before beneficial effects of pharmacological treatment are realized makes her vulnerable to self-neglect and/or suicidal ideation. Social support can be a protective factor in patients with depression, so encouraging social engagement should be a behavioral treatment strategy in Julia's case.

What are 3–5 case-specific questions to ask?

Is the patient experiencing suicidal ideation?

Is there a history of hypomania or mania?

Is the patient using alcohol, marijuana, or other substances?

Has the patient confided about how she is feeling to family or friends? What type of support is being provided?

What is the plan of treatment?

First, it is important to treat any underlying medical condition. In the absence of an underlying medical condition, determine the severity of depressive symptoms based on PHQ-9 score. Julia's PHQ-9 score is 19, which indicates moderately severe depression. Appropriate treatment includes medication, and SSRIs are typically the first-line pharmacological treatment. It would be helpful to know which, if any, antidepressant Julia's mother is taking for her depression. A medication that works effectively for Julia's mother may be a good first choice for Julia. In the absence of this information, fluoxetine is a good choice because of its long half-life. Most SSRIs have a half-life of approximately 24 hours and missed doses can lead to discontinuation syndrome. Fluoxetine has a half-life of 2–4 days and its active metabolite has a half-life of 7–15 days. Occasional missed doses are less likely to cause withdrawal symptoms.

It is important to review the risks, benefits, and common side effects of fluoxetine with the patient. This includes warning the patient about the link between the use of these medications and a small increased risk of suicidal thinking and behavior in adolescents and young adults. Any worsening of symptoms should be reported immediately. It is important for the patient to understand that fluoxetine needs to be taken daily and that beneficial effects may not be fully realized for 6–8 weeks. It is generally recommended that medication be continued for 6–9 months to reduce the risk of depression recurrence and discontinuing medication should be done under the supervision of the prescribing clinician.

Treatment may also include psychotherapy. Cognitive behavioral therapy (CBT) is an effective treatment for mild to moderate depression, alone or in combination with pharmacological interventions. Educate the patient on how exercise, adequate sleep, relaxation, and other behavioral strategies may also help to relieve depressive symptoms.

What are the plans for referral and follow-up care?

Julia should return for follow-up in 2 weeks to assess her depressive symptoms and how well she is tolerating the medication. Although beneficial effects may require more time, it is important to assess for any worsening of symptoms, including the presence of suicidal ideation.

A referral for cognitive behavioral therapy is indicated. Julia could benefit from engaging in this evidence-based intervention and, in doing so, be followed closely and supported by a clinician with an expertise in treating depression. Since Julia's mother has a history of depression, Julia's risk of recurrence is higher than that of the general population.

What health education should be provided to this patient?

It is important to educate Julia about what to expect of treatment, including how long it may take to feel better, and that symptom improvement will be gradual. Lifestyle strategies that can help relieve depressive symptoms, including exercise, social interaction, and stress management, as well as behaviors that may worsen symptoms, including poor sleep hygiene, social isolation, and the use of alcohol and substances, should also be shared.

What demographic characteristics might affect this case?

Men are less likely than women to seek treatment for depression and may be underdiagnosed in health care settings because they often present with anger and irritability versus sadness. In general, non-white Americans are less likely to engage in mental health treatment, so a culturally sensitive approach is critical to ensure participation.

Does the patient's psychosocial history impact how you might treat her?

Patients with few psychosocial supports may not respond as robustly to pharmacological interventions as patients with strong supports. They are also at a higher risk of depression recurrence. It is important to educate and assist patients in identifying strategies to improve functioning in this area.

What if the patient lived in a rural (or urban) setting?

If a patient lives in an area with inadequate health services, it may be more difficult to engage in treatment for depression without traveling a significant distance. The use of telemedicine is one way to address this issue. Urban settings are more likely to have adequate treatment resources; however, access to these resources may be delayed due to a scarcity of mental health clinicians.

Are there any standardized guidelines that should be used to treat this case?

The American Psychiatric Association has published guidelines for the treatment of depression in adults. UpToDate also provides treatment guidelines for depression in both adults and children.

REFERENCES AND RESOURCES

American Psychiatric Association. (2013). *Diagnostic and statistical manual of mental disorders* (5th ed.). Arlington, VA: Author.

Dixon, L. B., Holoshitz, Y., & Nossel, I. (2016). Treatment engagement of individuals experiencing mental illness: Review and update. *World Psychiatry*, 15(1), 13–20.

Kroenke, K., Spitzer, R. L., & Williams, J. B. (2001). The PHQ-9: Validity of a brief depression severity measure. *Journal of General Internal Medicine*, 16(9), 606–613.

Miller, G. E., & Noel, R. L. (2019) Unipolar vs bipolar depression: A clinician's perspective. *Current Psychiatry*, 18(6), 10–18.

National Institute for Mental Health. (2017). Men and depression. Retrieved September 9, 2019 from https://www.nimh.nih.gov/health/publications/men-and-depression/index.shtml

National Institute for Mental Health. (2018). Depression. Retrieved September 9, 2019 from https://www.nimh.nih.gov/health/topics/depression/index.shtml#part_145396

Park, L.T., & Zarate, C.A. (2019). Depression in the primary care setting. *New England Journal of Medicine*, 380(6), 559–568.

Roohafza, H. R., Afshar, H., Keshteli, A. H., Mohammadi, N., Feizi, A., Taslimi, M., & Adibi, P. (2014). What's the role of perceived social support and coping styles in depression and anxiety? *Journal of Research in Medical Sciences: The Official Journal of Isfahan University of Medical Sciences*, 19(10), 944–949.

Simon, G. (2017). Unipolar major depression in adults: Choosing initial treatment. In Roy-Byrne, P. P. (Ed.), UpToDate. Waltham, MA: UpToDate Inc. https://www.uptodate.com (accessed September 9, 2019.)

Warner, C. H., Bobo, W., Warner, C., Reid, S., & Rachal, J. (2006). Antidepressant discontinuation syndrome. *American Family Physician*, 74(3), 449–456.

Case 9.2 More Than Depression

RESOLUTION

What are the top three differential diagnoses in this case and why?

In order for a patient to meet criteria for any mental health disorder there is a diagnostic requirement that the patient be currently experiencing a significant distress in multiple domains including in their social life, work or school, or in other activities resulting in a decrease in functioning (American Psychiatric Association [APA], 2013).

The top three differential diagnoses in this case are:

Major depressive disorder (MDD):

The patient presents with symptoms congruent with depression related problems, given the normative findings on vitals and in review of symptoms (APA, 2013). Depression symptoms include lethargy, difficulty falling asleep and staying asleep, slow response and movements, difficulties feeling motivated, and reduced functioning in grades over a period of months "during this marking period," in addition to reduced work attendance. Further assessment is needed to refine a diagnosis of MDD, including the use of tools, including Patient Health Questionnaire (PHQ) 9, given that only the PHQ-2 has been administered thus far. The level of depression and potential of suicidality require additional clinical assessments, such as the Columbia Suicide Severity Rating Scale (C-SSRS) (Mundt et al., 2013). The patient meets criteria for major depressive disorder, unspecified currently.

Other specified depressive disorder:

The patient presentation includes recurrent experiences of depressed mood, over a period of months, more often than not; additionally, the frequent presence of negative affect has affected sleep, level of psychomotor and physical activity, and work/ school functioning. The patient demonstrates decreased interest in activities once found enjoyable and fulfilling, including work and school, evidenced by reduced attendance to work and slipping grades. Additionally, symptoms of lethargy, a marked decrease in energy level, also with changes in sleep with onset and intermittent insomnia, taken together with the previously mentioned presentation are indicative of a depression disorder. However, this diagnosis is less refined than major depressive disorder, and given that the MDD diagnosis is warranted, this otherspecified depressive disorder is not given, even though the criteria are met (APA, 2013).

The Family Nurse Practitioner: Clinical Case Studies, Second Edition. Edited by Leslie Neal-Boylan.
© 2021 John Wiley & Sons Ltd. Published 2021 by John Wiley & Sons Ltd.

Personal history of self-harm:
The patient presents with history of self-injurious behavior (SIB) including presence of several thin linear scars approximately 2 inches long and 2 centimeters thick that were visible. Some scars appeared white; silvery in tone; one mark was pink in tone with minimal scabbing, indicative of probable reemergence of SIB s. While it is likely given the pattern of these wounds, various degrees of healing are in fact a result of SIB, further inquiry with the patient is required prior to making the diagnosis. Assessment in accordance with psychometric tools such as the Non-Suicidal Self-Injury Assessment Tool (NSSI-AT) can aid a clinician to rule in this provisional diagnosis (Whitlock et al., under review).

Hypothyroidism:
When diagnosing depression, organic causes should also be considered in the differential. Hypothyroidism (a sluggish or underactive thyroid) is linked to depression, as a thyroid deficiency can cause fatigue, weight gain, and a lack of energy, all of which Marc is also experiencing in his presentation. Other symptoms include bloating, memory loss, and difficulty processing information. Conversely, hyperthyroidism (overactive thyroid) can cause insomnia, anxiety, elevated heart rate, high blood pressure, mood swings, and irritability. A diagnosis of hypothyroidism does not mean that Marc does not also have a mental health condition, but often when diagnosing mental health conditions, the ruling out of organic causes or contribution(s) to clinical symptoms may be inadvertently overlooked.

What diagnostic tests are required in this case and why?

Further screening questionnaires and assessment are indicated at this time. At this point, the PHQ-2 is positive and so a full Patient Health Questionnaire-9 (PHQ-9) is required and will yield further areas of potential concern related to depression and anxiety. The PHQ-9 is a specific screening tool designed to assess for symptoms of depression in teenagers. The Non-Suicidal Self-Injury Assessment Tool (NSSI-AT) is useful at this point to guide the assessment in terms of standardized self-injury questions. Further assessment for suicidality and safety is essential in any initial presentation of self-injury. The Columbia Suicide Severity Rating Scale (C-SSRS) is recommended by the American Academy of Child and Adolescent Psychiatrists for use in suicide assessment in primary care.

A blood panel that includes thyroid-stimulating hormone (TSH) and T3 and T4 hormone levels for specific indicators of a thyroid condition contributing to the patient's mood stability.

What are the concerns at this point?

It is important to assess the patient's risk for self-harm or suicide. It is necessary to obtain a Suicide Risk Assessment and a Self-Harm Risk Assessment. Is the patient motivated to engage in a safety plan to reduce the risk of self-harm and suicide? Marc is the oldest of 4 children, his father is unknown to him, and he had early childhood exposure to domestic violence. He has experienced episodes of housing insecurity and his mother works 3 jobs to provide for the family so Marc supervises his younger siblings. The psychosocial factors and family dynamics that influence this case are of concern and should be explored.

What is the plan of treatment?

- Treatment should include an immediate assessment for suicidal risk. In accordance with the Patient Health Questionnaire (PHQ) 9 (Kroenke & Spitzer, 2002) and the Columbia Suicide Severity Rating Scale (C-SSRS) (Mundt et al., 2013), assessment of suicidal risk should include the following questions stated directly in age- appropriate language:
  1. **Do you ever wish you were dead?**
  2. **Do you think about killing yourself?**
  3. Do you have a plan to kill yourself?
  4. Do you have means to carry out that plan?
  5. Do you intend to carry out the plan to kill yourself?

A **"No"** response to **Question 1** or **Question 2** means that the remaining questions are not mandatory.

A **"Yes"** response to **Question 1** or **Question 2** mandates that ALL the questions be asked (Questions 1 – 5).

■ If all subsequent answers are "No" (Question 3, 4, or 5) and an effective safety plan is not already in place, then the provider must create a safety plan with the patient (and caregiver, if applicable). An inability to execute a safety plan by the patient or caregiver requires further assessment from a mental health professional for possible hospitalization.

Example safety plan:

- List of coping skills to use to remain safe (e.g., distraction activities, deep breathing, etc.)
- List of triggers to avoid (e.g., caregiver will lock up sharp knives).
- List of supportive people to utilize when triggered (all people named must be aware they are part of the safety plan).
- Emergency contact information (e.g., suicide hotline phone number).

"Yes" responses to Question 3, 4, or 5 needs to result in an immediate assessment from a mental health professional for possible hospitalization. Calling emergency services (911) or having the patient safely transported to the Emergency Department (ED) are indicated treatment with expressed suicidality.

- Assessment for self-injurious behavior (SIB) follows a similar trajectory to suicidality assessment but with notable differences. Clinical best practices for SIB assessment falls in line with the Non-Suicidal Self-Injury Assessment Tool (NSSI-AT) (Whitlock et al., under review) and should include the following questions in age- appropriate language:

1. **Do you ever intentionally hurt yourself?**
2. When you hurt yourself, what function does it serve? (e.g., to no longer feel numb)
3. How recent/ How frequent do you hurt yourself?
4. How old were you when you first started to self-harm?
5. When you self-harm where on your body do you hurt yourself?
6. How severe are the wounds? (i.e., any wounds in need of medical care)

"Yes" to **Question 1** requires all questions for patient to respond to (Questions 2 – 6) and requires a safety plan (see the previous example safety plan).

"No" to **Question 1** results in no further questions being mandatory.

However, use good clinical judgment, a "No" with visible wounds requires additional investigation.

- Ask the patient if they have ever been to a therapist for counseling and assess where, with whom, and for long, as well as the patient's feelings about engaging in therapy. Referral for mental health care including psychotherapy and subsequent psychopharmacology are necessary given the clinical presentation. However, asking the patient's possible previous experience with therapy may help in the referral process. Evidence-based treatment interventions such as cognitive behavioral therapy (CBT) have demonstrated efficacious treatment for depression and their comorbid disorders, such as anxiety disorder (Hofmann et al., 2012).

- Further inquiry and psychoeducation on sleep hygiene are of benefit in this case, but may best be saved for a future visit. Disrupted sleep can be a symptom of a mental disorder but also can exacerbate a mental disorder. Assess inadequate levels of sleep including the quantity, quality, and satisfaction with sleep, as well as sleep hygiene (caffeine consumption later in the day, bedtime routine, etc.), and sleep schedule. Inability to sleep (as opposed to poor sleep hygiene) is more likely psychiatric in origin. If sleep is a concern, ask the patient to complete a 2-week sleep diary (see an example at www.brightfutures.org/mentalhealth/pdf/families/ec/diary. pdf). Incorporation of ongoing education on the importance of sleep as it relates to depression is appropriate for the treatment plan.

- An accurate and refined diagnosis is needed prior to advent of psychopharmacology into the treatment plan. There is no standard (specific or sensitive) way to determine if a child/adolescent will respond to medication or if a patient will experience side effects.

The *Diagnostic and Statistical Manual of Mental Disorders* (5th ed.; *DSM-5*; APA, 2013) recommends that the following is assessed first in determination of the appropriateness of psychotropic medication:

1. The patient has sufficient symptoms to support a mental health disorder;
2. Symptoms are present for a sufficient period;
3. There is significant impairment or distress from the symptoms;
4. The mental health disorder is different from normal levels of activity, worry and concern, or grief;
5. The patient has utilized evidence-based therapies (including cognitive-behavioral therapy for depression) been done sufficient in quality and duration.

The U.S. Food and Drug Administration has approved fluoxetine or escitalopram in the psychopharmacological treatment for treatment of MDD in youth and teens. Fluoxetine and escitalopram are selective serotonin reuptake inhibitors (SSRIs) and are indicated for MDD for patients 8–17 years of age (fluoxetine) and 12–17 years of age (escitalopram). The initial dose for fluoxetine in a teen is 10–20 mg with the max daily dose of 60 mg (and supplied in 10, 20, or 40 mg capsules). The initial dose for escitalopram is 10 mg with the max daily dose of 20 mg (supplied in 5, 10, and 20 mg scored tablets or 1 mg/ml oral solution). The most common adverse reactions for SSRIs include nausea, diarrhea, insomnia, somnolence, fatigue, sexual dysfunction, increased sweating, agitation, and tremors.

Safety monitoring is required with drug administration of the psychotherapeutic medications, especially in youth. Monitoring for contraindications, adverse effects, and potential drug interactions are to occur no less than every 30 days with closer monitoring on initiation of SSRI prescribing. All SSRIs have a boxed warning of suicidal thoughts and behaviors and suicidal assessment should remain a priority in follow-up care.

Beyond suicide risk, other precautions to be aware of include:

- Serotonin syndrome, which may occur with co administration of other serotonergic agents (such as triptans, tricyclic antidepressants, fentanyl, lithium, tramadol, tryptophan, buspirone, and St. John's wort).
- Activation of mania, which occurs with misdiagnosis of MDD and actual diagnosis of bipolar disorder.
- Seizures, which occur with conditions that potentially lower the seizure threshold in patients who have a history of seizures.
- Abnormal bleeding may occur with use of nonsteroidal anti-inflammatory drugs, aspirin, warfarin, or other drugs that affect coagulation.
- Hyponatremia in patients with syndrome of inappropriate antidiuretic hormone.
- Cognitive or motor impairment may occur.
- Be cautious in use with patients who have disorders that produce altered metabolism or hemodynamic reactions.
- Weight loss or gain may occur and requires close monitoring. Routine weight, height, and BMI are to be included as a part of follow-ups with medication management.
- Anxiety or insomnia may occur with fluoxetine.
- Fluoxetine has been associated with QT prolongation and is prescribed only with caution in patients with conditions that predispose to arrhythmias.

What health education should be provided to this patient?

Self-harm/risk for infection: Patients with SIB often are nonsuicidal in their injurious behavior but can end up with complications from infections, poor wound care, or unclean instruments used for self-harming. Education about wound care while the patient is seeking mental health care is helpful in reducing possible confounding medical conditions until the SIB subsides with appropriate care.

Neurobiology of depression: Psychoeducation is a well-established practice in the mental health field, often found to be the first step on a gradual exposure treatment, such as cognitive behavioral therapy (CBT), for patients with anxiety, depression, and trauma disorders, among many others (Hofmann et al., 2012). The simple learning process that their brains and bodies are functioning in a particular pattern due to neurobiology can be very anchoring to people whom often feel unsure of why they have "lost control" over their thoughts, behaviors and mood.

Sleep: The regenerative processes involved in sleep are essential for healthy functioning minds and bodies. Depression can affect sleep and vice versa. Sleep hygiene education and establishing healthy sleep habits would be essential in the holistic treatment of this patient.

Nutrition: The quality of the food ingested by each patient directly affects the ability for the brain to produce healthy thoughts. In addition, nutrition counseling about the impact food has on blood sugar and mood would aid greatly in helping to reduce the depressive symptoms, or at least not exacerbate the negative mood.

What demographic characteristics might affect this case?

Cultural considerations are important when evaluating this case. While it is essential not to stereotype, it is also important to be reflective that patients of nonmajority cultures can feel marginalized or have their symptoms inappropriately viewed through the majority culture lens. Given that this patient is Hispanic in America, it is important to acknowledge family systems of interdependence that include childcare for younger siblings is not taboo. Whereas, majority culture standards in America tend towards prioritizing individuality and independence this is not universal values across all cultures. Additionally, discussions of topics such as depression, SIB, or suicidality in medical or religious framework are more tolerable to most individuals of Hispanic culture than mental health terms (Baruth & Manning, 2002).

Does the patient's psychosocial history impact how you might treat him?

Family systems resulting in this patient being required to provide a primary caretaker role for younger siblings when not at school or work is a likely stressor, but also a potential source of pride and accomplishment for the patient, depending on his perspective. Maternal history of depression can be an indicator of a genetic predisposition toward depressive mood. Finally, if onset of depression and reduced functioning symptoms had occurred more immediately following exposure in childhood to domestic violence, then a trauma or adjustment diagnosis would also be an appropriate differential.

What if the patient were elderly or under age 13?

Should the patient's age be different, practitioners would additionally need to account for mandated reporting laws for populations at risk (elderly or under age 13). Clinicians are to review the restrictions to confidentiality with the patient while engaged in risk assessments. Additionally, given this patient's presentation of self-injurious behavior, symptoms of depression, and the need to assess for potential suicidality, it is highly likely that a patient of a more vulnerable age will require external supports, such as a caregiver, to execute any safety plan fully.

REFERENCES AND RESOURCES

American Psychiatric Association. (2013). Diagnostic and statistical manual of mental disorders (5th ed.). Arlington, VA: Author.

Baruth, L. G., & Manning, M. L. (2012). Multicultural counseling and psychotherapy: A lifespan approach (5th ed.). Boston: Pearson.

Hofmann, S. G., Asnaani, A., Vonk, I. J., Sawyer, A. T., & Fang, A. (2012). The efficacy of cognitive behavioral therapy: A review of meta-analyses. *Cognitive Therapy and Research, 36*(5), 427–440. doi:10.1007/s10608-012-9476-1.

Kroenke, K., & Spitzer, R. L. (2002). The PHQ-9: A new depression and diagnostic severity measure. *Psychiatric Annals, 32*, 509–521.

Kroenke, K., Spitzer, R. L., & Williams, J. B. (2003). The Patient Health Questionnaire-2: validity of a two-item depression screener. *Medical Care, 41*, 1284–1292.

Mundt, J. C., Greist, J. H., Jefferson, J. W., Federico, M., Mann, J. J., & Posner, K. (2013). Prediction of suicidal behavior in clinical research by lifetime suicidal ideation and behavior ascertained by the electronic Columbia-Suicide Severity Rating Scale. *The Journal of Clinical Psychiatry, 74*(9), 887–893.

Riddle, M. (2016). Pediatric psychopharmacology for primary care (2nd ed.). Itasca, IL: American Academy of Pediatrics.

Steer, R. A., & Beck, A. Use of the Beck Depression Inventory, Hopelessness Scale, Scale for Suicidal Ideation, and Suicidal Intent Scale with adolescents. (1988). *Advances in Adolescent Mental Health, 3*, 219–231.

Whitlock, J. L., Exner-Cortens, D., & Purington, A. (under review). Validity and reliability of the non-suicidal self-injury assessment test (NSSI-AT).

Case 9.3 Postpartum Depression

What is the diagnosis and its contributing factors?

For Jake

Small for gestational age (SGA), etiology unknown, requiring catch-up growth:

SGA babies are at risk for later neurodevelopmental problems due to the interuterine growth retardation implied by SGA.

For Laura

Maternal postpartum depression (PDD):

Aside from observation of the mother alternating between a flat affect and anxiety, Laura has some risk factors for developing PDD: She

- Has a previous history of depression.
- Lives in a northern climate with a winter-born baby, who requires extra care.
- Is socially isolated.
- Has a difficult baby. SGA babies typically tend to be fussy and difficult to comfort, often rejecting attempts to cuddle them, which can discourage maternal bonding. Mothers of SGA babies require a lot of support and this mother doesn't seem to have that support.
- A previous history of infertility is associated in some studies with depression in the case of marital conflict and social isolation.

There are breastfeeding concerns related to closely spaced feedings, the undersize of the infant, lack of supplemental calories for catch-up growth, lack of maternal knowledge regarding what constitutes enough milk per feeding for a small baby, and other breastfeeding concerns.

Why must concerns about Laura be addressed at this appointment?

Laura's depression can alter her interactions with the baby, thereby negatively affecting Jake's development. Depressed mothers engage less with their babies, and have trouble reading their infant's cues. Animated face-to-face engagement stimulates the growth of the brain through the release of dopamine. Dopamine serves as a growth stimulus for the orbital frontal region of the brain and is implicated in neurodevelopment. Depressed mothers' lessened engagement with their infants reduces the amount of dopamine bathing the orbital region of the infant's brain, thereby increasing the infant's risk for developmental and behavioral problems.

The Family Nurse Practitioner: Clinical Case Studies, Second Edition. Edited by Leslie Neal-Boylan.
© 2021 John Wiley & Sons Ltd. Published 2021 by John Wiley & Sons Ltd.

What additional information is needed?

- Formal depression screening for Laura. While the Edinburgh Postnatal Depression Screen (EPDS) is the most commonly used instrument to screen for PPD, the Patient Health Questionnaire (PHQ-9) also has strong reliability and validity. Both instruments are brief at 10 questions each.
- Resource for availability of mother-infant support services in Laura's area.

What are the treatment options?
For Jake

- Vitamin D supplement 600 IU by mouth daily.
- Give second dose of the Hepatitis B vaccine.
- Encourage pacifier use over prolonged pacification at the breast to give Laura's milk supply a chance to replenish for the next feeding.
- Continue with breastfeeding if Laura is amenable to this, as the research indicates that it is an effective feeding method for SGA infants. Proper nutrition for an infant with SGA with the goal of catch-up growth is one contributing factor to optimizing neurodevelopmental outcome. Encourage Laura to provide three bottle feedings a day with either pumped breast milk or formula fortified with extra calories to further encourage catch-up growth, and to allow for more options for who may feed the infant to allow Laura to attend to her own needs.
- Refer to Early Intervention Program developmental services for developmentally at-risk infants and toddlers if Jake lags in milestones or continues with hyperactive reflexes and ankle clonus.

For Laura
Consult the American Academy of Pediatrics (APA) recommended LactMed website for medication safety with the breastfed infant for consideration of starting Laura on an antidepressant.

What are the plans for referral and follow-up care? Include resources that may be needed to determine treatment options.

- Refer Laura to an International Board of Lactation Consultant (IBCLC) certified lactation consultant in her area to help with her breastfeeding goals in the context of Jake's special needs. An IBCLC consultant is the only lactation support service specifically trained in working with at-risk breastfeeding mothers and infants with special needs.
- Refer to the Visiting Nurses Association to support Laura's adjustment to caring for a challenging infant and to recommend community mother-infant support resources in the family's community. They can also monitor the baby's weight at home to reduce the number of office visits, thereby reducing Jake's exposure to illness during the flu season.
- Psychiatric referral resource for therapy as needed after medication is initiated.
- Instructions on how to access mother-baby Internet cafes for in-home support.
- Follow up with primary care clinic for weight check, immunizations, and continued developmental assessment in 4 weeks. Return sooner if weight gains level or drop off per VNA report.
- Refer Jake to Early Intervention if needed per neurodevelopmental assessment over subsequent office visits.

What demographic characteristics might affect this case?

- More affluent families may be able to pay out of pocket for cost-related services.
- The family's proximity to an urban area might give more choices for services than may be available in a more rural area.
- A person who is a fluent English speaker might also have access to a greater range of services.
- A woman who can stay at home is not faced with the concerns of returning to work that a woman who must work would have in terms of finding someone who is able and willing to continue with Jake's intensive care plan. Women returning to work have the additional concern of how to continue with breastfeeding, especially if working in an environment that does not provide time or facilities for pumping breast milk.

Are there any standardized guidelines that should be used to treat this case? If so, what are they?

The AAP, in its practice guidelines, recommends medicating depressed mothers even if breastfeeding, since the evidence of the harm to breastfeeding infants of any maternal medication that might pass into breast milk is currently much less than the evidence of the harm to the infant when the depressed mother is left unmedicated.

REFERENCES AND RESOURCES

Carducci, B., & Bhutta, Z. A. (2018). Care of the growth-restricted newborn. *Best Practice & Research in Clinical Obstetrics & Gynaecology, 49*, 103–116.

Castanys-Munoz, E., Kennedy, K., Castaneda-Gutierrez, E., Forsyth, S., Godfrey, K. M., Koletzko, B., . . . Ong, K. K.(2017). Systematic review indicates postnatal growth in term infants born small-for-gestational-age being associated with later neurocognitive and metabolic outcomes. *Acta Paediatrica, 106*(8), 1230–1238.

Edinburgh Depression Scale. (n.d.). https://www.fresno.ucsf.edu/pediatrics/downloads/edinburghscale.pdf

Falah-Hassani, K., Shiri, R., & Dennis, C. (2016). Prevalence and risk factors for comorbid postpartum depressive symptomatology and anxiety. *Journal of Affective Disorders, 198*, 142–147.

International Board of Lactation Consultant Examiners. https://iblce.org.

Kesavan, K., & Devaskar, S. U. (2019). Intrauterine growth restriction: Postnatal monitoring and outcomes. *Pediatric Clinics of North America, 66*(2), 403–423.

LactMed. https://toxnet.nlm.nih.gov/newtoxnet/lactmed.htm

Patient Health Questionnaire (PHQ-9). (n.d.). https://www.uspreventiveservicestaskforce.org/Home/GetFileByID/218

Pope, C. J., & Mazmanian, D. (2016). Breastfeeding and postpartum depression: An overview and methodical recommendations for future research. *Depression Research and Treatment, 2016*(2).

Sachs, H. C., & Committee On Drugs. (2013). The transfer of drugs and therapeutics into human breast milk: An update on selected topics. *Pediatrics, 132*(3), e796–e809.

Sethna, V., Pote, I., Wang, S., Gudbrandsen, M., Blasi, A., McCusker, C., ... McAlonan, G. M. (2017). Mother-infant interactions and regional brain volumes in infancy: An MRI study. *Brain Structure and Function, 222*(5), 2379–2388.

Smith-Nielsen, J., Tharner, A., Krogh, M. T., & Vaever, M. S. (2016). Effects of maternal postpartum depression in a well-resourced sample: Early concurrent and long-term effects on infant cognition, language, and motor development. *Scandinavian Journal of Psychology, 57*.

Case 9.4 Anxiety

What are the top three differential diagnoses in this case and why?
Generalized anxiety disorder:
Jonathan presents with symptoms consistent with generalized anxiety disorder, including excessive anxiety, irritability, sleep disturbance, and concentration difficulties.

Substance/medication-induced anxiety disorder:
Jonathan reports drinking 2–3 twelve-ounce Red Bull energy drinks per day and 2–3 beers daily in the evening. Reducing or eliminating intake of alcohol and caffeine could help to determine to what degree they are contributing to his anxiety symptoms.

Adjustment disorder with anxiety:
To meet criteria for adjustment disorder with anxiety, symptoms must emerge in response to an identifiable stressor that occurred within the prior 3 months. It is unclear if Jonathan's anxiety is a reaction to a recent increase in stress at work.

Which diagnostic tests are required in this case and why?
Diagnostic tests, including TSH, CBC with differential, basic metabolic panel, B12, and folic acid should be obtained to rule out underlying medical conditions including hyperthyroidism, B-12 deficiency, electrolyte imbalances, and infectious and malignant processes. GAD-7 should be completed to assess both the severity of Jonathan's anxiety symptoms and their impact on his daily functioning.

What are the concerns at this point?
It is important to distinguish between substance-induced anxiety disorder and generalized anxiety disorder. Reducing or eliminating caffeine and alcohol could assist in determining the extent to which they are contributing to his anxiety symptoms. Understanding the impact of anxiety symptoms on Jonathan's functioning and level of distress can serve to inform the development of an appropriate and comprehensive treatment plan. Without appropriate treatment, the severity of Jonathan's anxiety symptoms put him at risk of developing comorbid depression.

> *Ask 3–5 case-specific questions:*
> How long have anxiety symptoms been present?

The Family Nurse Practitioner: Clinical Case Studies, Second Edition. Edited by Leslie Neal-Boylan.
© 2021 John Wiley & Sons Ltd. Published 2021 by John Wiley & Sons Ltd.

Do symptoms wax and wane or are they constant throughout the day? When are symptoms at their worst?

Can the patient identify what makes anxiety worse or anything that helps to relieve symptoms?

How are symptoms impairing functioning at work, at home, and in relationships?

What is the plan of treatment?

It is critical to first treat any underlying medical condition. In the absence of an underlying medical condition, determine the severity of anxiety symptoms based on GAD-7 score. Jonathan's GAD-7 score is 14, which indicates moderate anxiety. Appropriate treatment options include cognitive behavioral therapy, medication, or a combination of the two. Patient preference should be considered. There are situations when medication can help to facilitate cognitive behavioral therapy. SSRIs are first-line pharmacological treatment for anxiety disorders. Escitalopram is a good choice. It is generally effective in treating anxiety symptoms with relatively low risk of GI distress, insomnia, and agitation in comparison to other SSRIs.

It is important to review the risks, benefits, and common side effects of escitalopram with the patient. Any worsening of symptoms should be reported immediately. It is important for the patient to understand that escitalopram needs to be taken daily and that beneficial effects may not be fully realized for 6–8 weeks. It is generally recommended that medication be continued for 6–9 months to reduce the risk of anxiety recurrence and discontinuing medication should be done under the supervision of the prescribing clinician.

Treatment may also include psychotherapy. Cognitive behavioral therapy (CBT) is an effective treatment for anxiety, alone or in combination with pharmacological interventions. Educate the patient on how exercise, adequate sleep, relaxation, and other behavioral strategies may also help to relieve anxiety symptoms.

What are the plans for referral and follow-up care?

Jonathan should return for follow-up in 2–4 weeks to assess his anxiety symptoms and how well he is tolerating the medication. Although beneficial effects may require more time, it is important to assess for any worsening of symptoms and medication tolerability.

A referral for cognitive behavioral therapy (CBT) would be beneficial. Jonathan could benefit from engaging in this evidence-based intervention and, in doing so, be followed closely and supported by a clinician with an expertise in treating anxiety disorders.

What health education should be provided to this patient?

It is important to educate Jonathan about what to expect of treatment, including how long it may take to feel better and that symptom improvement will be gradual. Lifestyle strategies that can help relieve anxiety symptoms including exercise, yoga, and stress management techniques should be emphasized. It is imperative to also advise Jonathan on behaviors that may worsen his symptoms, including poor sleep hygiene and regular use of caffeine, alcohol, and other substances.

What demographic characteristics might affect this case?

Men and non-white Americans are less likely to seek and engage in mental health treatment, so a culturally sensitive approach is critical to ensure participation.

Does the patient's psychosocial history impact how you might treat him?

Patients with few psychosocial supports may not respond as robustly to pharmacological interventions as patients with strong supports. They are also at a higher risk of developing a comorbid depression or substance use disorder. It will be necessary to educate and assist the patient in identifying ways to make improvements in this area. Urban settings are more likely to have adequate treatment resources; however, access to these resources may be delayed due to a scarcity of mental health clinicians.

What if the patient lived in a rural (or urban) setting?

If the patient lives in an area with inadequate health services, it may be more difficult to engage in treatment without traveling a significant distance. The use of telemedicine would be one way to address this issue.

Are there any standardized guidelines that should be used to treat this case? If so, what are they?

The American Academy of Family Physicians has published guidelines for the treatment of anxiety in adult patients. UpToDate provides treatment guidelines for anxiety in adults and children.

REFERENCES AND RESOURCES

American Psychiatric Association. (2013). Diagnostic and statistical manual of mental disorders (5th ed.). Arlington, VA: Author.

Craske, M., & Bystritsky, A. (2019). Approach to treating generalized anxiety disorder in adults. UpToDate. Waltham, MA: UpToDate Inc. https://www.uptodate.com (accessed September 9, 2019.)

De Sanctis, V., Soliman, N., Soliman, A. T., Elsedfy, H., Di Maio, S., El Kholy, M., & Fiscina, B. (2017). Caffeinated energy drink consumption among adolescents and potential health consequences associated with their use: A significant public health hazard. *Acta bio-medica: Atenei Parmensis*, *88*(2), 222–231.

Hentz, P. (2008, March 18). Separating anxiety from physical illness. *Clinical Advisor*.

Locke, A., Kirst, N., & Schultz, C. (2015). Diagnosis and management of generalized anxiety disorder and panic disorder in adults. *American Family Physician*, *91*(9), 617–624.

National Institute for Mental Health. (2018). Anxiety disorders. Retrieved September 9, 2019 from https://www.nimh.nih.gov/health/topics/anxiety-disorders/index.shtml#part_145338

Saeed, S., Cunningham, K., & Bloch, R. (2019). Depression and anxiety disorders: Benefits of exercise, yoga, and meditation. *American Family Physician*, *99*(10), 620–627.

RESOLUTION

What are the most likely differential diagnoses in this case and why?
Post-traumatic stress disorder (PTSD):

This diagnosis is supported by the symptomology in addition to the recent ongoing traumatic events of witnessing emotional and physical domestic violence within the home. Brittany reports difficulty sleeping, recurrent distressing dreams, markedly diminished interest/participation in significant activities, and difficulty concentrating. Furthermore, her school counselor's statements speak to feelings of detachment and estrangement from others, all of which is causing impairment in her social and academic areas of functioning. Further assessment needs to be completed to determine if the content of Brittany's nightmares relate to the traumatic events and if Brittany experiences avoidance of stimuli associated with the traumatic event(s). As both of these questions can be framed as "yes or no" questions (e.g., "*Do your bad dreams relate to what used to happen at home with Mom being hurt by Stepdad?*"), it is likely that Brittany will be more apt to answer than with an open-ended question that requires her to verbalize the trauma in detail. If these questions result in affirmative answers, Brittany meets the full criteria for a PTSD diagnosis.

Unspecified trauma- and stressor-related disorder:

Without further information about the trauma stimuli avoidance and a known link between the traumatic events and distressing dreams, Brittany will not meet the full criteria for a diagnosis of PTSD. Frequently, an adolescent will not initially disclose details of their trauma symptoms due to the distressing nature of the thoughts ("I don't want to talk about it or think about it"). For Brittany, there was an exposure to trauma with significant symptoms that are impacting her functioning across environments. Diagnosing the depressive or anxiety symptoms without taking into account the trauma experienced will not capture the likely root cause of Brittany's struggles or help assure proper management and treatment. Thus, this diagnosis can be helpful in communicating that the symptomology is related to trauma, while acknowledging that the full criteria for another disorder in this diagnostic class is not met at this time based on the information provided by the patient. If this diagnosis is needed, as soon as enough information is gathered through interviews and screening tools to allow for a more specific diagnosis (PTSD, other specified trauma- and stressor-related disorder), the diagnosis should be updated.

Major depressive disorder (MDD):

While Brittany describes several symptoms of MDD such as a diminished interest in activities and a diminished ability to think or concentrate, she does not report enough symptoms to meet the criteria

---

The Family Nurse Practitioner: Clinical Case Studies, Second Edition. Edited by Leslie Neal-Boylan.
© 2021 John Wiley & Sons Ltd. Published 2021 by John Wiley & Sons Ltd.

for this disorder, and the symptoms reported do not include enough information to indicate a depressed mood, despite the fact that a shift in Brittany's typical presentation is noted. Further assessment—with age-appropriate screening tools—is recommended to assure a full picture of Brittany's mood.

Generalized anxiety disorder (GAD):
Brittany describes several symptoms of anxiety, including worrying something bad will happen and difficulty concentrating, both of which are impacting her functioning at school. However, GAD requires at least 6 months of anxiety symptoms, and Brittany's report is that her symptoms began about 3 months ago with the move of homes. Similar to MDD, Brittany's anxiety symptoms are likely better explained as a response to her exposure to significant trauma.

Child affected by parental relationship distress:
This Z-code in the *DSM-5* (Z codes describe other areas of clinical focus that may influence a child's mental or medical well-being) allows for a descriptor of conditions that may explain the need for treatment and provide information on a patient's circumstances. Given Brittany's exposure to partner violence between her mother and stepfather, this would be an important code to utilize to allow future providers to understand Brittany's presentation and symptomology.

Which diagnostic tests required in this case and why?
Further screening questionnaires and assessment are indicated at this time. The Patient Health Questionnaire-9 (PHQ-9) and the Columbia–Suicide Severity Rating Scale (S-SSRS) are recommended for use in primary care to further screen for concerns related to depression and anxiety (PHQ-9) and suicidality (C-SSRS). The Non-Suicidal Self-Injury Assessment Tool (NSSI-AT) can be used to guide assessment in terms of standardized self-injury questions.

Because the patient is reporting extreme fatigue, as well as frequent headaches and changes in mood stability, baseline blood panels are useful to include a thyroid panel (including thyroid-stimulating hormone (TSH), T3 and T4 hormone levels) for specific indicators of a thyroid condition contributing to the patient's mood stability as well as a CBC with diff and a metabolic panel to further explore the headaches and fatigue to ensure that there is no organic contributing factor to the depressive symptoms. Hypothyroidism (from an underactive thyroid) is the most common medical condition associated with depressive symptoms; however, hyperthyroidism (from an overactive thyroid) and Cushing's disease are also associated with depression and should not be overlooked. Checking electrolytes and liver and kidney functions are also important, as medications (including SSRIs that can help with depression) are involved in the elimination of depression medications. Brittany also does not regularly follow one provider and does not routinely receive primary care, making baseline lab tests important, given her presentation.

Diagnostic Tests

Thyroid Panel	CBC and Differential	Lytes and Metabolic Panel
TSH: 1.7 miU/L	WBC: $5.9 \times 10^3/mm^3$	Na: 140 mmol/L
Total T3: .9 ng/dL	RBC: $5.0 \times 10^6/mm^3$	K: 4.1 mmol/L
Free T3: 1.0 ng/mL	Hgb: 12.0 g/dL	Glucose: 101 mg/dL
Total T4: 5.0 mg/dL	Hct: 37%	Ca: 2.0 mol/L
	MCV: 100 fL	Cl: 95 mmol/L
	RDW: 14%	Mag: 2 mEq/L
	Retics: 1%	BUN: 9 mg/dL
	Neutrophils: $3.6 \times 10^9/L$	Creatinine: 1.0 mg/dL
	Monocytes: $.3 \times 10^9/L$	Urea: 1.2 mmol/L
	Platelets: $389 \times 10^9/L$	Uric acid: 0.19 mmol/L
		Triglycerides: 100 mg/dL
		Total cholesterol: 5.0 mmol/L
		HDL: 40 mg/dL
		LDL: 85 mg/dL

What are the concerns at this point?

Brittany's diagnostic lab panel and physical assessment were normal. Her fatigue and lack of sleep, as well as frequent headaches, are still a concern. However, the immediate concerns at this visit include:

Suicide risk assessment

Self-harm risk assessment

Safety of going home

What is the plan of treatment?

Suicide risk assessment: Given the changes in Brittany's presentation and functioning, a clinical suicide risk assessment should be completed. This assessment would clarify if Brittany has ever had suicidal ideation or plans, and has the means to harm herself. Brittany should be asked if she has or has ever had (present or historical) thoughts of ending her life/killing herself (suicidal ideation). If Brittany responds affirmatively, screening would need to continue to find out if Brittany had ever thought about how she might end her life (plans), and, if so, how she would kill herself (means) (see Case 9.2, "More than Depression," for more in-depth suicidal assessment). Given that adolescents may be more likely to share information in writing than verbally, a PHQ-9 and/or a Columbia–Suicide Severity Rating Scale Screener will also offer helpful information in addition to the interview and guide the clinician in standardized questioning of statements.

Self-harm risk assessment: While Brittany has not stated self-harm, given the trauma exposure and the internalizing nature of her symptoms, a self-harm risk assessment should also be completed. Brittany should be asked if she's ever thought of or carried out harming herself (without the intentions of killing herself). If Brittany responds yes, further assessment of any physical injuries should be completed.

Safety of going home: Safety at home and Brittany's current feelings of safety in general should be discussed. Brittany should be asked about any alcohol or other substances being utilized in the home given mother's history of alcohol use, and about her plans if she at any point feels unsafe at home or with her caregivers.

Fatigue: Brittany's fatigue is most likely related to a lack of sleep and her PTSD. Thyroid concerns for fatigue have been ruled out from the labwork as well as organic causes of fatigue from a normal CBC and electrolyte panel. Brittany also describes poor sleep hygiene, which is common in adolescents regardless of mental health concerns.

Sleep hygiene: Sleep problems are symptomatic of a variety of mental health disorders and it is important to obtain more information about sleep patterns and hygiene, as lack of sleep can also exacerbate mental health concerns. Sleep hygiene can be saved for a future visit, as this is not the most pressing concern at this time. However, since Brittany is registered for SBHC use, the nurse practitioner can follow up for a sleep-related visit in the near future.

Consideration of SSRI to manage anxiety symptoms related to post-traumatic stress: Not every patient who presents with depressive symptoms, anxiety symptoms, and a history of trauma should be automatically be started on SSRIs. In some cases, specifically when a patient begins therapy (such as cognitive behavioral therapy [CBT]), a medication to manage anxiety symptoms can aid in reaching therapeutic goals. If after further assessment of Brittany medication is deemed appropriate, escitalopram (Lexapro) 10 mg QD would be a good choice related to trauma presenting with anxiolytic properties. For further determination on if psychotherapeutic medication should be used, please see Case 9.2.

Regardless of medication utilization, psychotherapy should be considered first and foremost. Cognitive behavioral therapy with a trauma-informed therapist may help for longer-term symptom reduction. A referral should be made as soon as possible and discussed with mother.

What is trauma-informed care?

The Substance Abuse and Mental Health Services Administration (SAMHSA) defines trauma-informed care as "a program, organization, or system that . . . **realizes** the widespread impact of trauma and understands potential paths for recovery; **recognizes** the signs and symptoms of trauma in clients, families, staff, and others involved with the system; and **responds** by fully integrating knowledge about trauma into policies, procedures, and practices, and seeks to actively **resist re-traumatization**." Trauma-informed frameworks also include six key principals, per SAMHSA: (1) Safety; (2) Trustworthiness and Transparency; (3) Peer Support; (4) Collaboration and Mutuality; (5) Empowerment, Voice and Choice; (6) Cultural, Historical, and Gender Issues.

Two research-supported therapy models for trauma-informed care for adolescents are trauma-focused cognitive behavioral therapy and eye movement desensitization and reprocessing (EMDR).

What are the plans for referral and follow-up care?

For the referral to behavioral health services, Brittany should be asked if she's ever attended counseling before and her willingness to try it out or return to treatment. Attending therapy should be normalized as taking care of herself and helping Brittany return to the level of functioning that she enjoyed before her symptoms began. As this visit is taking place in a school-based health center, it's likely that the provider has access to a behavioral health provider colleague to whom Brittany can be referred. A trauma-informed therapist who is familiar with trauma-informed treatment modalities would be best suited for Brittany based on her clinical presentation and history known at this point.

If an SSRI is prescribed, a follow-up visit is needed within the first 2 weeks of treatment to evaluate for effect of the medication as well as any potential side effects. SSRI black box warnings regarding worsening of suicidal ideation or intent should be considered and a follow-up suicide assessment conducted.

Basic sleep hygiene (aka good sleep habits) includes consistency at bedtime. Going to bed the same time each night and getting up at the same time each morning, including on weekends, is especially difficult for preadolescents and adolescents, but is instrumental in forming a healthy sleep pattern. Integrative sleep medicine experts also recommend that the bedroom is quiet, dark, relaxing, and at a comfortable temperature and that all electronic devices (TVs, computers, smartphones) be turned off or even removed from the bedroom. Exercising and being physically active during the day can help with fall asleep but exercising too close to bedtime can also cause difficulty falling asleep. Avoiding large meals, caffeine, and alcohol before bedtime is also important. Excessive consumption of caffeine, especially late in the day, is common in adolescents and assessment and psychoeducation should be done with Brittany related to caffeine intake. Brittany can also complete a sleep log to better track quantity and quality of sleep. There are many examples online but the American Academy of Pediatrics recommends the Bright Futures sleep log at: www. brightfutures.org/mentalhealth/pdf/families/ec/diary.pdf.

What demographic characteristics might affect this case?

Depending on Brittany's cultural background, she and her family might have questions or concerns about seeing a therapist or mental health provider of any kind, given some cultures' beliefs that the appropriate way to handle family problems is within the family system. Psychoeducation about the counseling process and benefits of therapy at this time rather than waiting until Brittany's symptoms potentially worsen may be needed. Additionally, some cultures and families from different backgrounds may be very opposed to psychotherapeutic medications, including SSRIs. Exploring the family's knowledge and possible concerns with SSRI use will be helpful and should be done as soon as possible in case SSRI is indicated once therapy begins.

Does the patient's psychosocial history impact how you might treat her?

Given Brittany's exposure to significant domestic violence and the concern that her stepfather has a no contact order with the children suggests that careful follow-up should be completed to assure Brittany's safety and care.

If this patient was male (instead of female), how might that change management and treatment?

As with other mental health disorders, trauma symptoms may include more externalizing behaviors with adolescent boys. Symptomology may include irritability and/or disruptive and defiant behaviors, which are often diagnosed as a behavioral disorder rather than a response to trauma or another mental health concern. While treatment may be the same, it is easy for providers to forget to assess for trauma or more serious underlying mental health issues when "behavioral" or "out of control" concerns seem to be the primary presenting problem.

REFERENCES AND RESOURCES

American Psychiatric Association. (2013). Diagnostic and statistical manual of mental disorders (5th ed.). Arlington, VA: Author.

Earls, M. (2018). Trauma-informed primary care: Prevention, recognition, and promoting resilience. *North Carolina Medical Journal*, 79(2), 108–112. doi:10.18043/ncm.79.2.108

Hagan, J. F. Jr., Shaw, J. S., & Duncan, P. M. (Eds.). (2017). Bright futures: Guidelines for health supervision of infants, children, and adolescents (4th ed.). Elk Grove Village, IL: American Academy of Pediatrics.

Kovachy, B., O'Hara, R., Hawkins, N., Gershon, A., Primeau, M. M., Madej, J., & Carrion, V. (2013). Sleep disturbance in pediatric PTSD: Current findings and future directions. *Journal of Clinical Sleep Medicine*, 9(5), 501–510. doi:10.5664/jcsm.2678

Kroenke, K., & Spitzer, R.L. (2002). The PHQ-9: A new depression and diagnostic severity measure. *Psychiatric Annals*, 32, 509–521.

Mundt, J. C., Greist, J. H., Jefferson, J. W., Federico, M., Mann, J. J., & Posner, K. (2013). Prediction of suicidal behavior in clinical research by lifetime suicidal ideation and behavior ascertained by the electronic Columbia–Suicide Severity Rating Scale. *The Journal of Clinical Psychiatry*, 74(9), 887–893.

Riddle, M. (2016). Pediatric psychopharmacology for primary care (2nd ed.). Elk Grove Village, IL: American Academy of Pediatrics.

Substance Abuse and Mental Health Services Administration (SAMHSA). (2014). SAMHSA's concept of trauma and guidance for a trauma-informed approach. HHS Publication No. (SMA). Rockville, MD: Author. Available at: http://www.traumainformedcareproject.org/resources/SAMHSA%20TIC.pdf

Case 10.1 Forgetfulness

What are the top three differential diagnoses in this case and why?

Major depression:
PHQ-9 indicates moderately severe depression and combined with her history and physical exam findings, Sophie's depression is not well controlled and she is experiencing an exacerbation.

Cognitive impairment:
The MoCA score reveals mild cognitive impairment (MCI). Her symptoms of forgetfulness are concerning and she has diabetes, which is associated with cognitive impairment.

Anxiety disorder:
Sophie is exhibiting increased anxiety symptoms by displaying excessive worry, accompanying sleep disturbance, and ongoing family stressors, which are contributing.

Which diagnostic tests are required in this case and why?

Brain imaging, preferably MRI to rule out an intracranial abnormality such as a stroke. The patient has demonstrated cognitive impairment on exam and several vascular risk factors, which increase the risk of a stroke.

Referral for neuropsychological testing: The patient's in-office testing indicate MCI and also major depression. In addition, she has anxiety and insomnia, which also can contribute to cognitive impairment. Neuropsychological testing can ascertain whether this patient is experiencing an emerging dementia or if her underlying psychiatric diagnoses are confounding her clinical picture.

Laboratory workup to rule out an underlying metabolic disorder, which can cause memory decline. These tests include:

a. CBC
b. TSH
c. Vitamin B12
d. CMP
e. RPR or FTA testing (if applicable)
f. HgA1C to assess the patient's overall glycemic control

The Family Nurse Practitioner: Clinical Case Studies, Second Edition. Edited by Leslie Neal-Boylan.
© 2021 John Wiley & Sons Ltd. Published 2021 by John Wiley & Sons Ltd.

What are the concerns at this point?

1. Cognitive impairment
2. Depression exacerbation
3. Anxiety exacerbation
4. Sleep disturbance
5. Breakthrough DPN pain

What are 3–5 case-specific questions to ask the patient?

- Are you experiencing any thoughts of harming yourself?
- Do you feel your anxiety and depression are currently well controlled on your prescribed medications?
- Have you forgotten names of your family, important dates, or left the oven/stovetop on?
- Is the Trazodone or Alprazolam helping you sleep?
- Do you find the gabapentin to be helpful for your DPN?

What is the plan of treatment?

Rule out an underlying intracranial abnormality and possible metabolic cause for the cognitive impairment, including brain imaging, referral to neuropsychological testing, and lab testing. Consider referral to a psychiatrist for management of anxiety and depression. This may not be feasible and wait times can be quite lengthy, so the provider should consider reducing Buproprion, as this may be contributing to anxiety. Start to address polypharmacy at this visit. The patient is on multiple central nervous system–acting medications, which all may possibly be contributing to her cognitive impairment and could increase the risk of falls. The patient is on the maximum dose of Citalopram. Consider switching to Duloxetine to treat both depression and DPN. Consider reducing gabapentin as the patient is on the maximum dose and is still experiencing breakthrough pain that is contributing to her sleep disturbance. The patient is on benzodiazepines, which has shown to be associated with cognitive impairment. It is preferable that she be weaned off this medication very slowly in the future once her depression and anxiety are under better control.

What are the plans for referral and follow-up care?

Referral to neuropsychologist
Referral to psychiatrist
Referral to counseling services; can also consider cognitive behavioral therapy, which is indicated for depression, anxiety, and sleep disturbance.
Follow-up in 2 weeks to assess response to medication changes
Possible referral for caregiving respite services if family indicates a need
Possible referral for driving evaluation to assess for any safety concerns given her cognitive impairment

What health education should be provided to this patient?

Provide written information on mild cognitive impairment. MCI increases the risk of developing dementia and the patient is already at risk, especially for vascular dementia, given her PMH of Type 2 DM, HTN, HLD. Provide medication information including the reason for prescribing, adverse effects, and how to take the medication.

What demographic characteristics might affect this case?

Age, which increases the risk of adverse drug events due to polypharmacy.

Does the patient's psychosocial history impact how you might treat her?

Yes, the provider needs to take Sophie's history of PTSD and the fact that she is a survivor of domestic abuse into consideration and be sure to establish trust and shared decision making with the patient and her family.

REFERENCES

Edlund, B. J., Lauerer, J., & Drayton, S. J. (2015). Recognizing depression in late life. *The Nurse Practitioner*, *40*(2), 37–42.

Falk, N., Cole, A., & Jason Meredith, T. (2018). Evaluation of suspected dementia. *American Academy of Family Physicians*, *97*(6), 398–405.

Harvey, P. D. (2012). Clinical applications of neuropsychological assessment. *Dialogues Clinical Neuroscience*, *14*(1), 91–99.

Kang, H., Zhao, F., You, L., Giorgetta, C., Venkatesh, D., Sarkhel, S., & Prakash, R. (2014). Pseudo-dementia: A neuropsychological review. *Annals Indian Academy of Neurology, 17*(2), 147–154. doi:10.4103/0972-2327.132613

Tobe, E. (*2012*). Pseudodementia caused by severe depression. *BMJ Case Reports, 2012*, 1–4. doi:10.1136/bcr-2012-007156

Tsoi, K. K., Chan, J., Hirai, H. W., Wong, S., & Kwok, T. (2015). Cognitive tests to detect dementia: A systematic review and meta-analysis. *JAMA Internal Medicine, 175*(9), 1450–1458.

Case 10.2 Behavior Change

RESOLUTION

Which diagnostic or imaging studies should be considered to assist with or confirm the diagnosis?

The choice of diagnostic tests should be guided by the list of likely differential diagnoses. Many factors guide the choice of diagnostics, including urgency of the clinical condition, sensitivity and specificity of the diagnostic test, availability of the test, burden to the patient (cost, invasiveness, and transportation), and, most importantly, the goals of care. The clinician should consider whether the results of the specific diagnostic test will change the treatment plan in any way. If the answer is no, the diagnostic test should be reconsidered.

In this case, laboratory and diagnostic studies should be used as part of a targeted evaluation based on clues in the history and physical (Inouye, Westendorp & Saczynski, 2014) to detect common conditions such as infection, dehydration, metabolic imbalance, or other acute illness. These typically include complete blood count with differential, serum electrolytes, glucose, calcium, measurement of renal, liver and thyroid function, drug levels (e.g., digoxin, lithium), toxicology screen, ammonia level, vitamin B12 and folate levels, cortisol level, arterial blood gas, and culture of urine, blood and sputum. EKG and CXR may be ordered in persons with cardiac or respiratory diseases or symptoms and an EEG may be useful in some patients to rule out occult seizures (Inouye et al., Oh, Fong, Hshieh, & Inouye, 2017; Westendorp & Saczynski, 2014).

Brain imaging (such as CT or MRI) is indicated in patients with focal neurological findings or those suspected of having a brain lesion (e.g., stroke, bleed, or tumor) and/or patients without other identifiable causes of delirium. Patients with delirium and recent unexplained falls or symptoms of NPH (triad of gait changes, memory disturbance, and urinary incontinence) should also be referred for brain imaging. Lumbar puncture is used for patients with meningeal signs or suspicion of encephalitis (e.g. fever with headache). Additional diagnostic tests should be based on the patient's clinical presentation (Inouye et al., 2014).

For Antonio, the studies would include an EKG because of his history of coronary artery disease with assessment findings of bradycardia and irregular rhythm. His new complaint of heartburn may also be cardiac in origin. Pulse oximetry should be done to provide a quick, noninvasive assessment of oxygen saturation. Antonio's recent fall and his gait and balance difficulties are suspicious, and a head CT should be ordered. If head trauma had been sustained, he has any localizing

The Family Nurse Practitioner: Clinical Case Studies, Second Edition. Edited by Leslie Neal-Boylan.
© 2021 John Wiley & Sons Ltd. Published 2021 by John Wiley & Sons Ltd.

neurological findings, or if he was taking warfarin (an anticoagulant), intracranial bleeding would be high on the list of differential diagnoses.

A standardized depression screen using the GDS or PHQ-9 may be useful because depression can mimic dementia, coexist with delirium and dementia, and/or mimic hypoactive delirium. Standardized screening tools identify individuals needing further assessment and provide indicators of responses to treatment over time. Depression screening may not be feasible in the acutely delirious person, due to impaired attention and/or more urgent clinical symptoms. Antonio has difficulty staying focused, so this assessment should be deferred.

Taking orthostatic vital signs (blood pressure and pulse in both lying and standing positions) is useful to obtain a baseline in all geriatric patients. Orthostatic blood pressure and pulse measurement are essential in patients with a history of falls, symptoms of lightheadedness, or weakness with position changes. Older adults are more likely to experience orthostatic drops in blood pressure due to changes in baroreceptor sensitivity in the carotid sinus. Orthostasis is more likely in patients on antihypertensives and/or diuretics and in patients who are dehydrated. Orthostatic hypotension is unlikely to be a sole cause of persistent delirium, but it may be one indicator of hypovolemia (e.g., due to dehydration and/or anemia) that may impair brain perfusion and precipitate delirium (Oh et al., 2017).

If the initial workup does not reveal a cause, physician and/or neurology consultation is recommended. Patients with fever or other features suggesting possible meningitis or encephalitis require a lumbar puncture (after brain imaging). An EEG may be ordered to rule out seizure activity in patients with altered level of consciousness (Inouye et al., 2014; Oh et al., 2017).

Which differential diagnoses should be considered at this point?

Delirium:

Antonio had an acute onset of symptoms, including inattention, disorganized thinking, and an altered level of consciousness. (Symptom fluctuation pattern is unclear and may be complicated by antipsychotic administration.) Antonio's clinical presentation is consistent with delirium.

Delirium is an acute change from baseline mental status that develops over a short period of time (usually hours to days) and tends to fluctuate over the course of the day (increasing and decreasing in severity). Key features include altered arousal (lethargic or hyperalert or alternating from one to the other), impaired attention (reduced ability to focus and/or distractibility), and disturbed cognition (a confusing flow of ideas, incomprehensible conversation, and/or unpredictable switches in topic; *Diagnostic and Statistical Manual*, 5th ed. [*DSM-5*], American Psychiatric Association [APA], 2013).

The Confusion Assessment Method (CAM) is a standardized, efficient assessment tool to assist clinicians in recognizing delirium and differentiating it from dementia or depression. It is usually completed after elements of cognitive assessment are conducted, including attentional testing (trail-making, digit span or reciting months of the year, days of the week or spelling words (such as "world" backward) (Inouye, Fearing, & Marcantonio, 2009). These tasks specifically challenge attention span and focus, and help to distinguish delirium from dementia and depression (Inouye et al., 1990; Waszynski, 2007).

Dementia is more subtle in onset (months to years) and slowly progressive, with problems in memory and executive function (planning, sequencing, and performing goal-directed activities). Attention processes are normal until later stages, and arousal is not impaired. Lewy body dementia may be difficult to distinguish from delirium since patients with this disease may experience hallucinations and/or fluctuating cognition as part of the dementia. The coexistence of Parkinson's-like features of Lewy body dementia and the less acute onset may help distinguish between the diagnoses. Persons with preexisting dementia or other types of brain disease are vulnerable to developing superimposed delirium; and therefore any sudden, significant deviations from usual cognition, behavior, or function should be assumed to be delirium until it is ruled out (Fick, Hodo, Lawrence, & Inouye, 2007).

A new onset of primary psychiatric disease is possible, but less likely in this case. Medical causes of delirium should also be ruled out prior to attributing symptoms to psychiatric disease. Antonio has no apparent symptoms of psychosis (paranoia, hallucinations, delusions, or thought disorder) and no past psychiatric history.

Depression may slow mental processing and impair cognitive performance on mental status tests. The depressed patient may make a poor effort on cognitive testing or answer questions with "I don't know" or "I can't." Antonio has recently experienced grief and associated anxiety and sleep disturbance, but he was beginning to improve in activity and social engagement. His irritability may be a sign of depression; but his distractibility, impaired attention, and acute behavior changes are classic symptoms of delirium, rather than depression or dementia. His mood and mental status should both be reassessed after infection or other acute contributors to delirium are treated.

Delirium is a syndrome or cluster of symptoms, rather than a diagnosis. It reflects a condition in which precipitants or "insults" overwhelm individual capacities due to underlying predisposing factors or "vulnerabilities" (Inouye et al., 2007). If delirium is suspected, a prompt, systematic search for reversible contributors should be conducted. The mnemonic "MIND ESCAPE" is useful in remembering potential reversible contributors to changes in mental status in the elderly (Molony, Waszynski, & Lyder, 1999, p. 78). The mnemonic and findings from Antonio's assessment that correspond to each potential contributor are listed in Table 10.2.1.

After reviewing Antonio's history and exam findings, infection, metabolic disturbance, nutritional deficiency, drug effects, and cardiac problems are identified as the most likely precipitants of delirium, with sensory deprivation (poor vision and hearing) and possibly sleep deprivation as contributing factors.

Older adults often have atypical presentations of disease (Wilbur, Gerson, & Mcquown, 2017). This is particularly true in advanced age and in persons with multiple chronic conditions or frailty. For example, older adults may have serious infections (including sepsis) with only a low-grade fever and minimal elevation in the white blood cell count. Myocardial infarctions may present

Table 10.2.1. Potential Contributors to Antonio's Delirium.

Potential Contributor to Delirium	Antonio's Risk Factors
Metabolic changes (e.g., dehydration, electrolyte imbalance, hypercalcemia, liver, kidney, or thyroid disease, hypo- or hyperglycemia, hypoxia, and hypercarbia)	Lab work pending; dry oral mucosa—possible dehydration; irregular rhythm/K+, ARB, diuretic—possible K+ imbalance
Infection (acute or chronic)/impaction/inability to void	Fever, adventitious lung sounds—possible respiratory infection; BPH—risk for urinary retention; need further assessment of bowel function
Nutrition (B12/folate, other nutritional deficiencies/neoplasm/NPH	Poor appetite, recent loss/grieving, recent 3-lb. weight loss
Drugs/drug withdrawal (including prescription and OTC or street medications)	Haldol dose; OTC medication for heartburn may be deliriogenic; beta blocker—risk for bradyarrhythmia; need further assessment re: street drugs, opioids, etc.
Environmental toxins/environmental changes	Recent move to CCRC
Sleep deprivation/sensory overload or sensory deprivation	Slight decline in visual acuity; decreased hearing related to cerumen impaction
Cardiovascular/cerebrovascular (stroke, hypoxia, shock, heart failure, myocardial infarction, arrhythmia)	History of cardiovascular disease, heart failure, bradycardia, irregular rhythm
Alcohol or alcohol withdrawal/anemia	Need additional history
Pain	Not applicable
Emotional or mental illness	Depression may be present; further assessment needed

without chest pain ("silent" or atypical symptoms such as sudden shortness of breath, hypotension, dyspnea, mental status change, or gastrointestinal symptoms). Hyperthyroidism may present with apathetic lethargy and constipation. Depression may present with irritability and feelings of worthlessness or helplessness instead of sadness. Older adults with acute intraabdominal conditions (e.g., appendicitis, ruptured diverticulum, mesenteric thrombosis) may present without severe pain, guarding, or rebound tenderness. Poor appetite, declining physical function, new urinary incontinence, falls, and mental status changes are often the heralds of geriatric clinical distress. These symptoms signal a need for skilled assessment and management.

Older adults have a lower resting body temperature at baseline as well as a lowered ability to produce a febrile response (High, 2017). Therefore, Antonio's temperature is >2.4°F above his baseline, a sensitive threshold for possible infectious disease (High et al., 2009), and his lung findings suggest a possible pneumonia. The urinalysis and chest X-ray will help to identify a source of infection and guide treatment.

Adverse drug effects are common contributors to delirium. A comprehensive medication list that includes prescription, over-the-counter (OTC), and nutritional/herbal supplements is an important part of clinical assessment in all health visits with older adults. Older adults have changes in body composition, liver enzyme systems, and renal function that affect drug distribution, activity, and clearance (Rochon, Gill, & Gurwitz, 2017). They are also more likely to experience drug-drug, drug-food, and drug-disease interactions, due to the number of medicines prescribed, the presence of multiple concurrent diagnoses, and the use of inappropriate doses (based on half-life, renal function, etc.). Older adults may also be more sensitive to drugs that cross the blood-brain barrier. While some medicines have been identified as potentially inappropriate for older adults due to risks that outweigh benefits, it is essential for the clinician to review all medicines as possible contributors to delirium (American Geriatrics Society [AGS], 2019; Molony, 2003, 2009). Pharmacist consultation is recommended, if available.

Antonio received Haldol, an antipsychotic medication with extrapyramidal side effects including dystonias (prolonged unintentional muscular contractions), Parkinson's-like symptoms (i.e., tremor, rigidity, and bradykinesia) and akathisia (restlessness, often exhibited as pacing or rocking). Akathisia is often mistaken for worsening agitation and treated with additional doses of the offending antipsychotic agent. Haldol also has anticholinergic properties (including confusion, dry mouth, urinary retention, and constipation). The higher the degree of anticholinergic burden related to medication dosing, the higher the risk for cognitive impairment. These medications are considered potentially inappropriate for older adults, based on the updated 2019 Beers criteria. Anticholinergic effects of different drugs accumulate and may contribute not only to delirium, but also to urinary retention in patients with BPH. Antonio reported using some type of OTC product for heartburn. Many proton pump inhibitors and histamine-2 receptor antagonists such as omeprazole (Prilosec®) and cimetidine (Tagamet®) are available OTC for short-term treatment of heartburn. Cimetidine worsens delirium or combines with other medications to precipitate delirium. Cimetidine, particularly in higher doses, may interact with other medicines, through effects on cytochrome P450 enzyme systems in the liver (AGS, 2019; Medical Letter, 2018).

Constipation is common in older adults if they take insufficient fluid or fiber; are inactive; are immobile; and/or take constipating medicines such as iron, calcium, and/or opioids. Prevention, assessment, and management of constipation are important aspects of geriatric care. Adequate fluid and fiber intake are important prevention strategies (Mounsey, Raleigh & Wilson, 2015). Fecal impaction or bowel obstruction may contribute to delirium, but these have been ruled out for Antonio.

Primary neurologic diseases such as Parkinson's disease (PD), normal pressure hydrocephalus (NPH), and cerebrovascular accident (CVA) are less likely diagnoses for Antonio. PD is sometimes misdiagnosed in patients with drug-induced parkinsonism. Antonio's small, shuffling steps could be consistent with parkinsonism, particularly if they appeared only after he received antipsychotic medication; but his gait may also reflect generalized imbalance, fear of falling, and chronic changes. His gait should be monitored during follow-up visits. He does not display cogwheel rigidity, resting tremor, or bradykinesia, which are the cardinal signs of PD (Kotagal & Bohnen, 2017). His slight decrease in upward gaze is consistent with normal aging. Persons with normal pressure hydrocephalus (NPH) typically have a wide-based gait with difficulty taking steps (sometimes described as a magnetic gait). In NPH, urinary incontinence and memory loss cluster together with gait changes to form a diagnostic triad typical of the disease. A cerebrovascular accident (ischemic, thrombotic, or hemorrhagic) is possible in view of Antonio's cardiovascular risk factors, but his examination revealed no focal neurological deficits. Small infarcts may still be present, and brain imaging has been ordered to rule this out. If his EKG demonstrated new-onset atrial fibrillation (a-fib), a common condition in older adults, the clinical suspicion for CVA would be much higher, since a-fib increases the risk of thrombotic stroke.

What is the treatment plan?

Antonio's chest X-ray shows left lower lobe infiltrates consistent with pneumonia and his WBC is elevated. These findings are consistent with pneumonia. His BUN is elevated and his BUN:creatinine ratio is 26:1 (usually 14:1). This suggests impaired renal perfusion, most likely due to hypovolemia/dehydration (other possible causes include acute hypotension, heart failure, or renal ischemia due to artery stenosis).

The first priority is to decide whether to treat Antonio's pneumonia in the hospital. By preventing unnecessary hospitalization, iatrogenic risks that may worsen cognitive function (e.g., changes in medication, sleep patterns, diet, sensory stimulation, and/or environment; antibiotic-resistant infections; and/or immobility) may be avoided. On the other hand, older adults are at higher risk for serious complications of pneumonia, including sepsis or respiratory failure; and hospitalization is indicated for high-risk groups and/or worrisome clinical presentations.

Otherwise-healthy older adults with community-acquired pneumonia may be treated as outpatients with appropriate followup. The decision to treat in the community relies in part on the clinician's assessment of the overall severity of illness and patient function, the patient's (or caregiver's) ability to follow through with the treatment plan, the ability to monitor clinical status, and the ability to contact the clinician if symptoms persist or worsen. The severity of the delirium, the ability to take needed fluids and medication, and the availability of around-the-clock support until mental status improves will also be factored into the decision.

Algorithms such as the Pneumonia Severity Index (PSI) and the CURB-65 are available to assist with decision-making regarding the site of care for older adults with community-acquired pneumonia (del Castillo & Sánchez, 2017). Antonio's age, BUN, and confusion place him in an intermediate to high risk category, and his pulse oximetry reading is declining. The decision to hospitalize him should be made.

Antonio's delirium should improve with appropriate diagnosis and treatment of reversible contributors and with the provision of supportive care, but some cases of delirium linger for weeks or months (Kiely et al., 2009). Skillful nursing care is needed to minimize polypharmacy and optimize nutrition and hydration, oxygenation, electrolyte balance, comfort, bowel and bladder function, sleep, and activity. Regular reassessment of function and care needs is important to prevent negative sequelae (Yevchak et al., 2017).

Are any referrals needed?

Pneumonia, dehydration, and delirium are the top three concerns, and physician involvement is advisable. Cardiology consultation is recommended due to the recent changes in Antonio's beta-blocker therapy and episode of pulmonary edema. A geriatric team consult is indicated to advise re: supportive care for delirium and to make recommendations for fall prevention.

What aspects of the health history require special emphasis in older adults?

One of the most important components of geriatric assessment is the functional assessment. It is essential to assess and document the degree to which an older adult can independently complete activities of daily living (feeding, toileting, bathing, turning in bed, moving from bed to standing or bed to chair, and walking) and the amount of supervision or assistance needed. Older adults in independent living should also be assessed for the ability to perform instrumental activities of daily living (cooking, housecleaning, laundry, managing medications, using a telephone, managing finances, shopping, and use of transportation).

When assessing the health of older adults, the clinician should recognize that many conditions and symptoms are underreported in older adults. The geriatric review of systems and physical examination should therefore specifically include assessment for the following: cognitive impairment, dental/oral health, falls, foot problems, gait or balance problems, hearing loss, vision loss, incontinence, nutrition, pressure ulcers, mental health issues (including depression, anxiety, and grief), sexual history, and sleep problems.

A careful and thorough review all medications, including oral, injectables, topical, inhalants, eye drops, over the counter, and herbal substances is necessary in the health history. It is recommended that older adults gather all medications when possible and review them with the practitioner. Assuring the safe and effective use of medications by older adults is a critical component of geriatric assessment (Steinman & Fick, 2019).

What if this patient were under age 65? Would that change the management plan?
An otherwise-healthy younger adult with community-acquired pneumonia is likely to be treated as an outpatient. Treatment of pneumonia in younger adults would include consideration of appropriate prescribing practices for possibly pregnant or breastfeeding women.

What patient, family, and/or caregiver education is important in this case?
Patient and family education should focus on prevention and early detection. If the patient is treated in the community, the importance of taking all medicine as prescribed must be emphasized. Education on prevention includes counseling to promote pneumonia and influenza vaccine, smoking cessation, and information about hand and cough hygiene. After hospital discharge, Antonio should be encouraged to continue cough and deep-breathing exercises to clear mucus and to maintain adequate fluid intake. Oxygen safety principles should be reviewed if he is discharged on oxygen. Antonio (and/or his caregivers) should be educated regarding symptoms that require a call to the clinician, such as difficulty breathing, fever, or becoming more confused or very sleepy.

It is essential that nursing assistants and personal care assistants benefit from the clinical education given to patients and family members. They are often the first ones to notice clinically important changes and are the most influential determinants in whether follow-up care or self-care strategies are maintained.

Are there any standardized guidelines that should be used to assess or treat this case?
Clinicians should be familiar with guidelines on the prevention, identification, assessment, and management of delirium (Australian Commission on Safety and Quality in Health Care, 2016); Young, Murthy, Westby, Akunne, & O'Mahony, 2010).

The 2007 Infectious Diseases Society of America/American Thoracic Society consensus guidelines on the management of community-acquired pneumonia in adults and the 2009 update are key references (Lim et al., 2009; Mandell et al., 2007).

Lower respiratory infections (LRIs) often result in avoidable hospitalizations in nursing home residents. INTERACT is a quality improvement model to reduce avoidable hospitalization due to LRI and/or other causes (Ouslander, Bonner, Herndon, & Shutes, 2014).

Follow-up:
Antonio is admitted to the hospital, started on intravenous (IV) fluids and ceftriaxone. His atenolol is switched to labetalol in response to elevated blood pressure readings. On day 3 of treatment, he develops acute pulmonary edema treated with IV diuretics followed by an increase in his oral diuretic dose.

On day 5, he develops watery diarrhea, which continues for days. Donnatal is ordered to treat the diarrhea. A *C-difficile* titer is sent, and he is started on metronidazole (which is discontinued after negative titers ×2). On day 6 of his admission, he develops acute urinary retention and a Foley catheter is inserted. He is started on tamsulosin and finasteride. The diarrhea slows and the Foley catheter is removed. Antonio's lungs are clear, but he is weak and has no appetite. He is alert and oriented, and his mental status is back to baseline. He is discharged to the rehabilitation facility for physical therapy to improve strength, balance, and endurance.

His primary care provider is asked to see him because he had a "fainting spell" the day after admission, after walking 50 feet in physical therapy. His blood pressure at the time was 80 systolic (palpable). His temperature, pulse, and respiratory rate are normal. His weight is 157 lb. His color is good, and his MoCA score is 24/30. His affect is mildly depressed. Oral mucous membranes and tongue are dry. His heart rate is 88 and regular with occasional pauses. His lungs are clear, and he has 1–2+ ankle edema (L > R). His blood pressure in both arms, while sitting, is 98/60 and drops to 84/50 upon standing. He is "woozy" after walking a few feet from the chair to the bed. His neurologic exam is unchanged from the previous exam and the remainder of the exam is unremarkable.

What are some of the possible contributors to this patient's hypotension? Are any referrals needed? What management strategies should be considered?

Age-related changes in baroreceptor function increase the risk of orthostatic hypotension in the elderly. Medications, hypovolemia, and electrolyte imbalances may contribute to orthostasis. Autonomic nervous system disease or neuropathies are other common causes. Unexplained hypotension (with or without position change) may be an early sign of shock or cardiac pathology. Antonio is dehydrated and is taking several medicines that may contribute to hypotension, including tamsulosin, labetalol, and isosorbide mononitrate. In addition to ordering elastic support stockings, teaching Antonio to perform ankle exercises before standing, and increasing his oral fluid intake, it should be recommended that he discontinue the tamsulosin with instructions to monitor for urinary retention. While liberalizing sodium is an option in some cases or orthostatic hypotension, Antonio's history of heart failure warrants caution. His recent weight loss may represent fluid and nutritional losses, and further assessment of his intake is needed.

Donnatal, a highly anticholinergic agent, is not recommended for use in older adults. Anticholinergic medications can contribute to short-term (delirium) and long-term (dementia) cognitive deficits, as well as dry mouth, blurry vision and lack of coordination, often resulting in dizziness and falls. (AGS, 2019; Gray et al., 2015).

REFERENCES AND RESOURCES

American Psychiatric Association. (2013). *Diagnostic and statistical manual of mental disorders* (5th ed.). Arlington, VA: Author.

American Geriatrics Society (AGS) Beers Criteria® Update Expert Panel. (2019). American Geriatrics Society 2019 updated AGS Beers Criteria® for potentially inappropriate medication use in older adults. *Journal of the American Geriatrics Society. 67*(4), 674–694. doi:10.1111/jgs.15767

Australian Commission on Safety and Quality in Health Care. (2016). Delirium clinical care standard. Sydney ACSQHC. Accessed at https://www.safetyandquality.gov.au/our-work/clinical-care-standards/delirium-clinical-care-standard

del Castillo, J. G., & Sanchez, F. J. M. (2017). General principles of pharmacology and appropriate prescribing. In J. B. Halter, J. G. Ouslander, S. Studenski, K. P. High, S. Asthana, M. A. Supiano, & C. Ritchie (Eds.), *Hazzard's geriatric medicine and gerontology* (7th ed., Chapter 67). McGraw-Hill.

Fick, D. M., Hodo, D. M., Lawrence, F., & Inouye, S. K. (2007). Recognizing delirium superimposed on dementia: Assessing nurses' knowledge using care vignettes. *Journal of Gerontological Nursing, 33*(2), 40–47.

Gray, S. L., Anderson, M. L., Dublin, S., Hanlon, J. T., Hubbard, R., Walker, R., . . . Larson, E. B. (2015). Cumulative use of strong anticholinergic medications and incident dementia. *Journal of the American Medical Association, 175*(3), 401–407.

High, K. P., Bradley, S. F., Gravenstein, S., Mehr, D. R., Quagliarello, V. J., Richards, C., & Yoshikawa, T. T. (2009). Clinical practice guideline for the evaluation of fever and infection in older adult residents of long-term care facilities: 2008 update by the Infectious Diseases Society of America. *Journal of the American Geriatrics Society, 57*(3), 375–394.

High, K. P. (2017). Infection: General principles. In J. B. Halter, J. G. Ouslander, S. Studenski, K. P. High, S. Asthana, M. A. Supiano, & C. Ritchie (Eds.), *Hazzard's geriatric medicine and gerontology* (7th ed., Chapter 126). McGraw-Hill.

Inouye, S. K., Fearing, M. A., & Marcantonio, E. R. (2009). Delirium. In J. B. Halter, J. G. Ouslander, M. E. Tinetti, S. Studenski, K. P. High, & S. Asthana (Eds.), *Hazzard's geriatric medicine and gerontology* (6th ed., Chapter 53). McGraw-Hill.

Inouye, S. K., Van Dyck, C. H., Alessi, C. A., Balkin, S., Siegal, A. P., & Horwitz, R. I. (1990). Clarifying confusion: The confusion assessment method: A new method for detection of delirium. *Annals of Internal Medicine, 113*(12), 941–948.

Inouye, S. K., Westendorp, R. G., & Saczynski, J. S. (2014). Delirium in elderly people. *Lancet, 383*(9920), 911–922. doi:10.1016/S0140-6736(13)60688-1

Inouye, S. K., Zhang, Y., Jones, R. N., Kiely, D. K., Yang, F., & Marcantonio, E. R. (2007). Risk factors for delirium at discharge: Development and validation of a predictive model. *Archives of Internal Medicine, 167*(13), 1406–1413.

Kiely, D. K., Marcantonio, E. R., Inouye, S. K., Shaffer, M. L., Bergmann, M. A., Yang, F. M., . . . Jones, R. N. (2009). Persistent delirium predicts greater mortality. *Journal of the American Geriatrics Society, 57*(1), 55–61.

Kotagal, V., & Bohnen, N.I. (2017). General principles of pharmacology and appropriate prescribing. In J. B. Halter, J. G. Ouslander, S. Studenski, K. P. High, S. Asthana, M. A. Supiano, & C. Ritchie (Eds.), *Hazzard's geriatric medicine and gerontology* (7th ed., Chapter 67). McGraw-Hill.

Lim, W. S., Baudouin, S. V., George, R. C., Hill, A. T., Jamieson, C., Le Jeune, I., . . . Woodhead, M. A. (2009). BTS guidelines for the management of community acquired pneumonia in adults: Update 2009. *Thorax, 64*(Suppl. 3), iii1–iii55.

Mandell, L. A., Wunderink, R. G., Anzueto, A., Bartlett, J. G., Campbell, G. D., Dean, N. C., . . . Whitney, C. G. (2007). Infectious Diseases Society of America/American Thoracic Society consensus guidelines on the management of community-acquired pneumonia in adults. *Clinical Infectious Diseases, 44* (Suppl 2):S27–S72. doi:10.1086/511159

Medical Letter. (2018, January 15). Drugs for GERD and peptic ulcer disease. *The Medical Letter on Drugs and Therapeutics, 60*(1538), 9–16.

Molony, S. L. (2003). Beers' criteria for potentially inappropriate medication use in the elderly. *Journal of Gerontological Nursing, 29*(11), 6.

Molony, S. L. (2009). How to try this: Monitoring medication use in older adults. *American Journal of Nursing, 109*(1), 68–78.

Molony, S. L., Waszynski, C. M., & Lyder, C.H. (Eds.). (1999),.Gerontological nursing: *An advanced practice approach* (p. 78). Stamford, CT: Prentice Hall.

Mounsey, A., Raleigh, M., & Wilson, A. (2015). Management of constipation in older adults. *American Family Physician, 92*(6), 500–504. doi:d12117

Oh, E. S., Fong, T. G., Hshieh, T. T., & Inouye, S. K. (2017). Delirium in older persons: Advances in diagnosis and treatment. *Jama, 318*(12), 1161–1174. doi:10.1001/jama.2017.12067

Ouslander, J. G., Bonner, A., Herndon, L., & Shutes, J. (2014). The interventions to reduce acute care transfers (INTERACT) quality improvement program: An overview for medical directors and primary care clinicians in long term care. *Journal of the American Medical Directors Association, 15*(3), 162–170. doi:S1525-8610(13)00690-7

Rochon, P. A., Gill, S. S., & Gurwitz, J. H. (2017). General principles of pharmacology and appropriate prescribing. In J. B. Halter, J. G. Ouslander, S. Studenski, K. P. High, S. Asthana, M. A. Supiano, & C. Ritchie (Eds.), *Hazzard's geriatric medicine and gerontology* (7th ed., Chapter 24). McGraw-Hill.

Steinman, M., & Fick, D. (2019). Using wisely. A reminder on how to properly use the American Geriatrics Society Beer's Criteria®. *Journal of Gerontological Nursing, 45*(3), 3–6.

Yevchak, A., Fick, D. M., Kolanowski, A. M., McDowell, J., Monroe, T., LeViere, A., & Mion, L. (2017). *Journal of Gerontological Nursing, 43*(12), 21–28.

Young, J., Murthy, L., Westby, M., Akunne, A., & O'Mahony, R. (2010). Diagnosis, prevention, and management of delirium: summary of NICE guidance. *British Medical Journal, 341.* http://dx.doi.org/10.1136/bmj.c3704

Waszynski, C. M. (2007). How to try this: Detecting delirium. *The American Journal of Nursing, 107*(12), 50–59, quiz 60.

Wilber, S. T., Gerson, L. W., & McQuown, C. (2017). Emergency department care. In J. B. Halter, J. G. Ouslander, S. Studenski, K. P. High, S. Asthana, M. A. Supiano, & C. Ritchie (Eds.), *Hazzard's geriatric medicine and gerontology* (7th ed., Chapter 17). McGraw-Hill. http://accessmedicine.mhmedical.com/content.aspx?bookid=1923&sectionid=144518612.

RESOLUTION

What are the top three differential diagnoses in this case and why?
Parkinson's disease (PD):
PD is in the differentials given his tremor history and also his PMH of anxiety, which is a common nonmotor symptom of PD.

Essential tremor (ET) (This is the diagnosis):
The patient has bilateral hand tremors that are present with action and has no other signs or symptoms on exam to suggest Parkinson's disease. His spiral drawing also reveals a tremor consistent with ET.

Anxiety:
The patient could also be experiencing enhanced physiological tremor worsened by his PMH of anxiety. However, an enhanced physiological tremor is intermittent and the patient is experiencing tremors consistently.

Which diagnostic tests are required in this case and why?
The diagnosis of essential tremor and Parkinson's disease really rests in the provider's ability to complete a thorough history and physical exam. Mr. Suarez's neurological exam does not reveal any focal neurological abnormalities with the exception of action and postural tremors, which are consistent with a diagnosis of essential tremor. Given the possibility of enhanced physiological tremor, the provider would want to rule out a metabolic cause such as a thyroid abnormality or liver toxicity. In addition it would be important for the provider to assess any heavy metal exposure (e.g., does the patient have well water?), as these can cause tremors.

- Check TSH
- Check LFTs
- Check serum lead, arsenic, mercury (if the history indicates)
- Imaging is not necessary due to the absence of focal neurological findings on exam.

What are the concerns at this point?
- How much are the tremor symptoms interfering with daily life? (ADLs, hobbies, etc.)
- How does the patient feel his anxiety is controlled at this point?

The Family Nurse Practitioner: Clinical Case Studies, Second Edition. Edited by Leslie Neal-Boylan.
© 2021 John Wiley & Sons Ltd. Published 2021 by John Wiley & Sons Ltd.

- Do any other family members have symptoms of tremors?
- What is the patient worried about most in regard to his hand tremors?
- Does alcohol improve the tremor? (Alcohol can decrease essential tremor, but it is *not* a recommended treatment!)
- Does the patient he drink alcohol to help with anxiety? This is important to assess for any emerging alcohol use disorder.

What is the plan of treatment?

- Utilizing shared decision making, the NP needs to assess how problematic these symptoms are and, given the fact that they are interfering with some of the patient's ADLs and hobbies, treatment can be discussed. It is important for the NP to understand that the mainstay of treatment in ET is symptom management.
- Utilizing the American Academy of Neurology (AAN) ET treatment guidelines, level A evidence advises starting with Propranolol or Primidone. The NP should know that Propranolol is contraindicated given the patient's pulmonary disease. Primidone should therefore be initiated as long as the patient desires treatment.
- Also, consider the dose of Fluoxetine. This medication can cause tremors as an adverse effect or exacerbate tremors.
- Occupational therapy (OT) is also highly recommended to assist the patient in utilizing techniques at home that may make it easier to complete ADLs. Also, OT can provide specific devices such as weighted utensils that make it easier for individuals with ET to consume meals.

What are the plans for referral and follow-up care?

- Start Primidone at a low dose: 50 mg at bedtime for 1 week and then increase to 50 mg bid for 1 week; then can increase to 50 mg tid until f/u.
- Referral to occupational therapy.
- Follow up in 6 weeks.
- Assess response to therapy at this time.
- Assess anxiety and consider switching to another agent.

What health education should be provided to this patient?

- Provide written information about essential tremor, including the etiology, causes, and treatment options.
- Provide written information on Primidone, including adverse effects and how to take medication.
- Provide reassurance to the patient and his daughter that at this time, his physical exam and history is consistent with a diagnosis of essential tremor and that he does not have Parkinson's disease.
- It is important to stress to the patient and his daughter that medication for essential tremor can only work to reduce the tremor and that this disorder is, unfortunately, chronic and typically does worsen over time despite medication treatment.

What demographic characteristics might affect this case?

The patient's age, widowhood, and that he lives alone.

Does the patient's psychosocial history impact how you might treat him?

Yes, the NP would want to make sure his anxiety is well-managed with not only his current regimen but also advise on nonpharmacological options such as meditation or cognitive behavioral therapy. The NP would also want to make sure that his alcohol consumption is carefully monitored for the emergence of an alcohol use disorder and also for safety reasons since he does live alone.

What if the patient lived in a rural (or urban) setting?

- Treatment and recommendations would be the same.
- However, it would be imperative that the provider assess for access to transportation to get medications and to go to occupational therapy.

Are there any standardized guidelines that you should use to treat this case? If so, what are they?

- The American Academy of Neurology treatment guidelines for essential tremor.

Are there other history questions that are pertinent when assessing a patient with tremors?

Other history questions that are pertinent when assessing a patient with tremors may include:

- o Any history of environmental or toxic exposure to chemicals or heavy metals? Ask about past military and occupational experience.
- o Does the patient's anxiety increase the tremors?
- o Is he anxious about attending social events due to his tremors?

If this patient did not have insurance, would that change the management strategy?

Primidone is a generic medication and the cost averages about $9.00 for a 1-month supply. Occupational therapy would be very expensive, so this may be prohibitive without insurance. The provider could inquire if any local schools that have OT programs offer free care to people in the community.

REFERENCES AND RESOURCES

Crawford, P., & Zimmerman, E. E. (2011). Differentiation and diagnosis of tremor. *American Family Physician*, *83*(6), 697–702.

Deuschl, G., Bain, P., Brin, M., & Ad Hoc Scientific Committee. (1998). Consensus statement of the Movement Disorder Society on Tremor. *Movement Disorders*, *13*(3), 2–23.

Jankovic, J., & Fahn, S. (1980). Physiologic and pathologic tremors: Diagnosis, mechanism, and management. *Annals of Internal Medicine*, *93*(3), 460–465.

Louis, E. D., Rohl, B., & Rice, C. (2015). Defining the treatment gap: What essential tremor patients want they are not getting. *Tremor and Other Hyperkinetic Movements*, *5*, 1–12. doi:10.7916/D87080M9

Pal, P. K. (2011). Guidelines for management of essential tremor. *Annals of Indian Academy of Neurology*, *14*, S25–S28. doi:10.4103/0972-2327.83097

Puschmann, A., & Wszolek, Z. K. (2011). Diagnosis and treatment of common forms of tremor. *Seminal Neurology*, *31*(1), 65–77. doi: 10.1055/s-0031-1271312

Shanker, V. L. (2016). Case studies in tremor. *Neurologic Clinics*, *34*, 651–655. http://dx.doi.org/10.10.1016/j.ncl.2016.04.012

Sharma, S., & Pandey, S. (2016). Approach to a tremor patient. *Annals of Indian Academy of Neurology*, *19*(4), 433–443. doi:10.4103/0972-2327.194409

Zesiewicz, T. A., Elble, R. J., Louis, E. D., Gronseth, G. S., Ondo, W. G., Dewey, R. B. Jr., . . . Weiner, W. J. (2011). Evidence-based guideline update: Treatment of essential tremor. *Neurology*, *77*(19), 1752–1755.

Case 10.4 Weight Gain and Fatigue

Which diagnostic studies should be considered to assist with or confirm the diagnosis?

The basic metabolic panel reveals the following: creatinine level: 0.89; blood urea nitrogen: 14; sodium: 137; potassium: 4.5; chloride: 104. Liver function tests are within normal limits. GFR is 85. Rapid HIV test is negative. Complete blood count—white blood count: 5.7; hemoglobin: 14.3; hematocrit: 43.2; macrocytic corpuscle volume: 84; fasting blood glucose: 168; A1C: 8.5. Testosterone is within normal limits. Erythrocyte sedimentation rate is within normal limits. Urinalysis is positive for 2+ glucose; trace protein. TSH is 4.50. Because fatigue can be a marker for cancer, a chest X-ray and investigation for other cancer markers would be appropriate.

What is the most likely differential diagnosis and why?

Diabetes mellitus Type 2:

Maxwell has had a gradual onset of fatigue over the past few months, which presents as a classic symptom of diabetes. Noted also is nocturia, which awakens him at least 2 times during the night. Polyuria and/or nocturia are also classic presenting symptoms, due to the glucose-concentrated urine creating a diuretic effect. He also has had a 15-lb weight gain over the past 2 years. His body mass index has progressed from 29 (which is the overweight category) to 31 (the obese category). Obesity is a leading cause of insulin resistance. He reports a sedentary lifestyle, which contributes to the obesity and the insulin resistance. Low libido may be related to a lack of energy in conjunction with some erectile dysfunction relevant to the hyperglycemia causing an autonomic neuropathy.

Fatigue is a major symptom reported with inadequately treated hypothyroidism, HIV, anemia, and inadequate testosterone levels. The patient does have a history of hypothyroidism and therefore may require additional levothyroxine due to a thyroid hormone deficiency. Also, the patient reported occasional constipation, some cold intolerance, and significant weight gain. Patients with hypothyroidism have a diminished red blood cell mass, which may present as a macrocytic anemia. A small percentage of patients with hypothyroidism have the occurrence of pernicious anemia. Therefore, anemia is a relevant differential diagnosis. The patient reports that he is in a monogamous homosexual relationship and denies fevers and night sweats and has had a positive weight gain; however, it would be wise to rule out the diagnosis since he is in a high-risk category. African Americans have the highest rates of HIV and AIDS in the United States. Maxwell exhibits high-risk

The Family Nurse Practitioner: Clinical Case Studies, Second Edition. Edited by Leslie Neal-Boylan.
© 2021 John Wiley & Sons Ltd. Published 2021 by John Wiley & Sons Ltd.

behavior since he is a male who is sexually active with a male. Symptoms of HIV are often nonspecific but may include fatigue. The patient has numerous risk factors for diabetes due to family history, hypertension, increased body mass index, sedentary lifestyle, and being African American. Detection of hypogonadism in males with sexual dysfunction is warranted. Male hormone deficiency can be a cause of fatigue as well as sexual dysfunction.

What is the plan of treatment?

The patient has a moderate degree of hyperglycemia ranging from 151 to 250. Therefore, diet, exercise, and 1 oral agent is appropriate therapy with which to begin. The patient's creatinine and liver function studies are within normal limits. Start with metformin 500 mg daily in the evening. Instruct the patient to take 1 tablet daily with the first bite of food in the evening. Explain the mechanism of action, contraindications, adverse effects of the metformin, and the need to remain hydrated while taking the medication to prevent lactic acidosis.

If he is unable to drink oral solutions and/or hold liquids down, then he should stop the metformin and call the office. If the metformin is well tolerated without significant gastrointestinal affects, then tell the patient to increase the dose of metformin to twice a day following the week of initiation. Provide him with basic education about diabetes signs and symptoms and potential treatment. Stress the importance of lifestyle modifications and consumption of a heart-healthy diet and routine modest aerobic exercise of 30 minutes, 5 days a week. Provide instruction in self–blood glucose monitoring and use of the glucose meter. Write prescriptions for the metformin, a glucose meter, and supplies of strips and lancets. Order routine diabetes management labwork such as fasting lipids and a urine microalbumin/creatinine ratio.

Instruct the patient to call the office in 1 week for follow-up regarding the use of the glucose meter and blood glucose readings. At that time, determine if the patient should receive another phone call or return to the clinic sooner than 1 month. Otherwise, schedule the patient to return to the clinic in a month for follow-up of self–blood glucose monitoring results and possible adjustment of medications. Repeat the HbA1C in 3 months along with fasting lipids and a urine microalbumin/creatinine ratio if any of the previous levels are abnormal. Carefully monitor this patient for changes in his cardiac and renal health.

What is the plan for referrals and follow-up?

A referral to a dietitian is appropriate for a discussion related to meal planning, cooking methods, and portion control. An ophthalmology referral for a dilated eye exam in 3 months will allow time for improved glycemia and improved vision. A referral should be made to a certified diabetes educator for further diabetes education and co-management. Offer the patient the opportunity to attend a series of diabetes education classes. Consider a cardiology referral given his risk factors and family history. Consider a podiatry referral for diabetic foot care and management. If the low libido persists following normoglycemia, then referral to a urologist would be appropriate. Follow up based on the results of the chest X-ray.

Does the patient's psychosocial history impact how you might treat him?

This patient's psychosocial history does not impact how this patient will be treated.

What if this patient were a premenopausal female?

If this were a female patient, more questioning would be necessary to assess her menstrual cycle, including the duration and the amount of flow of her menses. A ferritin level would have been included in the initial workup. Also, a pregnancy test might be indicated.

What if the patient were over the age of 80?

Metformin may not be the first drug of choice since impaired renal function and the greater potential for dehydration exists in this age group. The possibility of lactic acidosis is higher in this age group, though it rarely occurs. Patients over the age of 80 should have a normal creatinine clearance documented prior to beginning therapy. All patients on metformin should have their liver function test and creatinine checked annually.

Are there standardized guidelines that should be used to assess and treat this patient?
American Diabetes Association. (2019). Introduction: *Standards of Medical Care in Diabetes—2019, Diabetes Care, 42*(Suppl. 1), S1–S2. https://doi.org/10.2337/dc19-Sint01

REFERENCES AND RESOURCES

American Diabetes Association. (2019). Introduction: *Standards of Medical Care in Diabetes—2019, Diabetes Care, 42*(Suppl. 1), S1–S2. https://doi.org/10.2337/dc19-Sint01
Ferri, F. F. (2019). Diabetes mellitus. *Ferri's clinicial advisor 2019* (pp. 424–433). Philadelphia: Elsevier.

NOTE: The author would like to acknowledge the contribution of Vanessa Jefferson, MSN, BC-ANP, CDE to this case in the first edition of this book.

Case 10.5 Visual Changes

RESOLUTION

Which diagnostic studies should be considered to assist with or confirm the diagnosis?

The history should include the date of the last eye exam, whether a retinal exam and glaucoma assessment was done, and a family history of eye disease. Assessment of the eye begins with measuring visual acuity. Acute vision loss or unexplained low vision warrants urgent referral (to an ophthalmologist or emergency room depending upon the clinical scenario (e.g., for risk factors for ocular or neurological disease, recent ocular injury, or foreign body). If a foreign body or possible corneal scratch is suspected, fluorescein staining and Wood's lamp examination may be done.

If overall visual acuity is within the usual range, a screening test for macular degeneration should be done using an Amsler grid (Su et al., 2016). Alternatively, visual acuity can be tested using an Internet-based macular mapping test called MacuFlow™ can potentially be completed at home (Garcia-Layana, Cabrerea-Lopez, Garcia-Arumi, Arias-Barquet, L. & Ruiz-Moreno, J., 2017). Other helpful assessment tools include the National Eye Institute Visual Functioning Questionnaire 25 (NEV-VFQ-25) (Abe et al., 2016). Although vision screening in asymptomatic older adults will not result in improved clinical outcomes, these tests may help to detect hidden diseases among at-risk individuals and facilitate a tailored plan of care for older adults with visual impairment (Abe et al., 2016). Visual acuity assessment is an important consideration when devising integrated interventions designed to prevent and treat delirium, such as medication management (Carlson, Merel, &Yukawa, 2015).

Which of the symptoms or signs related to Marion's eyes or vision represent pathological changes versus normal aging?

Marion reports gradual, insidious changes in her vision. Her fear of blindness relates to her concern about having macular degeneration (like her mother). Normal aging changes in the eyes may result in an increased sensitivity to glare, difficulty with light/dark adaptation, decreased color discrimination, and loss of acuity in low-contrast and low-light conditions. Pupil size decreases. Visual processing time may also be decreased, potentially affecting reading and driving; but this may improve with training. While ectropion (outward turning of the lids) is not a normal aging change, it is a common, correctable condition (Golan, Rabina, Kurtz, & Leibovitch, 2016).

The Family Nurse Practitioner: Clinical Case Studies, Second Edition. Edited by Leslie Neal-Boylan.
© 2021 John Wiley & Sons Ltd. Published 2021 by John Wiley & Sons Ltd.

Which differential diagnoses should be considered at this point? What are the three most common diagnoses/conditions affecting vision in older adults? Are Marion's signs and symptoms similar to the clinical presentations of these conditions?

The three most common pathological conditions in older adults include cataracts (the most common cause of low vision in the elderly), glaucoma, and macular degeneration. Diabetic retinopathy is also common in diabetics and this results in visual loss that will ultimately have a negative impact on safety due to cognitive deficits, such as falls, incorrect identification of appropriate medication and dose, as well as impairment on the patient's daily routines and function (Hanna, Hepworth, & Rowe, 2016). Symptoms of cataracts include increased sensitivity to glare and/or to light, decreased contrast sensitivity, and decreased blue-yellow color vision. Although glaucoma decreases peripheral vision, the loss is gradual, painless, and rarely noticed until severe (Vujosevic et. al., 2019). Macular degeneration results in blurred or distorted central vision or central vision loss. Unless hemorrhage occurs, changes are gradual and may not be noticed until moderate or severe. A new onset of pain in the eye suggests a serious condition that must be evaluated promptly. Sudden vision loss in part or all of the visual field in one or both eyes is an emergency and may represent ocular, neural, or vascular pathology (including stroke, and retinal hemorrhage) (Abe et al., 2016). Older adults are also at higher risk for a condition known as temporal arteritis (also called "giant cell arteritis"), which may present with headache and sudden vision loss (Vujosevic et al., 2019). Immediate evaluation and treatment are necessary to prevent permanent blindness and to differentiate this condition from acute stroke (Powers et al., 2018).

Based on this exam, what is the plan of care? Would you seek any referrals from the interprofessional team?

A dilated retinal examination is needed to more thoroughly assess the health of the retina and macula. Marion should be referred to an ophthalmologist for this examination, as well as a measurement of eye pressure and peripheral vision testing (Vujosevic et al., 2019).

If Marion were under 65 years of age, would the management plan change?

These symptoms would be suspicious for ocular pathology in a younger person and comprehensive assessment and ophthalmology follow-up would be essential. Macular degeneration is almost exclusively found in persons over age 55 and cataracts in a younger person are usually secondary to other diseases/conditions, such as uncontrolled diabetes (Vujosevic et al., 2019). Giant cell arteritis (GCA) is an inflammatory disorder that occurs primarily in adults 50 years of age and older and is associated with visual disturbances, due to ischemia in the cranial vessels, which causes headache and jaw claudication (Pioro, 2018). If GCA is suspected, emergent corticosteroid treatment can prevent irreversible vision loss (Pioro, 2018). The provider should also rule out other possible conditions such as stroke, dementia, and Parkinson's disease (Miller, 2019; Powers et al., 2018).

What patient, family, and caregiver education is most important in this case?

Marion will require reinforcement regarding the importance of regular eye exams to ensure that her visual changes are consistent with her diagnosis. Marion will also benefit from learning about other potential age-related changes in vision such as presbyopia (loss of accommodation), diminished acuity, delayed dark and light adaptation, increased glare sensitivity, reduced visual field, diminished depth perception and altered color vision, and slower visual information processing (Miller, 2019). A review of medications that may impact vision (such as nonsteroidal anti-inflammatory agents, anticholinergics, phenothiazines, amiodarone, alpha blockers, diuretics, antihistamines, anticholinergics, phenothiazines, beta blockers, and anticoagulants) will be helpful (Miller, 2019). Moreover, although visual rehabilitation will not restore vision, it is helpful to ensure safety for persons with visual loss that is affecting function or quality of life (Miller, 2019).

A few weeks after the visit described above, you receive a phone call from Marion's friend, who calls the clinic with news that Marion experienced a brief episode of slurred speech and right-sided weakness that lasted a few minutes. These symptoms occurred about 30 minutes ago. What is your priority recommendation? Her friend reports that Marion is feeling fine now but she is frightened. What is your advice?

You advise Marion to seek immediate evaluation in the emergency room. Her symptoms are consistent with a transient ischemic attack (TIA) (a transient episode of neurological dysfunction caused by focal brain, spinal cord, or retinal ischemia, without acute infarction) but cannot be differentiated from a stroke without neurovascular imaging. The most common symptoms of brain ischemia include sudden weakness or numbness on one side (face, arm, or leg), trouble speaking or slurred speech, trouble walking (due to sudden unexplained dizziness, loss of coordination, or sudden "drop" attack and fall), or trouble seeing (sudden loss of visual field, sudden monocular or binocular vision loss, blurred vision, or diplopia). Headaches, tinnitus, and hearing loss may accompany vertebrobasilar insufficiency. The inherent uncertainty of classifying ischemic stroke as being distinct from a TIA is a result of the inadequacy of the diagnostic workup in some cases to visualize the occluded artery or localize the source of the embolism (Powers et al., 2018). However, due to their shared physiological mechanisms, both TIA and ischemic stroke patients should have an evaluation sufficient to exclude high-risk modifiable conditions such as carotid stenosis or AF as the cause of ischemic symptoms (Powers et al., 2018). The ABCD^2 clinical risk prediction score has been shown to predict stroke risk and should be used in the early period following stroke to determine risk (Wardlaw, 2015). However, the ABCD^2 does not reliably discriminate those at low and high risk of early recurrent stroke, identify patients with carotid stenosis or AF needing urgent intervention, or streamline clinic workload (Wardlaw, 2015).

What diagnostic evaluation should be completed?

A diagnostic evaluation will differentiate stroke mimics (SMs), which are nonvascular conditions that can produce symptoms that resemble an acute stroke (Viela, 2017) constitute a large percentage of acute stroke admissions to hospitals. The most common SMs include Bell's palsy, conversion disorders, seizures and postictal paralysis or toxic-metabolic disturbances such as brain tumors, infections, and migraine (Viela, 2017). If her symptoms included a loss of vision, visual field, or other acute vision changes, ocular neuropathy or intraocular pathology may be included in the differential diagnosis (Viela, 2017).

If Marion's clinical presentation demonstrated a score of 1 or 2 on the ABCD^2, she would be considered low risk in the initial emergency department evaluation, and subsequently she would be referred back to her primary care provider for further evaluation. A neurology consult is recommended to effectively plan and implement a comprehensive and cost-effective workup that includes appropriate neurovascular imaging. A head CT is generally performed in the emergency room, and as such an MRI of the head is recommended for outpatient diagnosis and treatment. Doppler ultrasound, transcranial ultrasound, cardiac echo, EKG, MR angiography, or CT angiography can detect carotid cardiac abnormalities or vascular pathology. If symptoms recur, a telemedicine network may be indicated to ensure a timely treatment (Powers 2018).

What education is needed?

Marion will need to learn the importance of phrases such as "Time is brain" that signify the emergent nature of accessing care because antithrombolytic agents (if indicated) must be given emergently within the first 3 to 4.5 hours after the onset of symptoms for optimal effect.

Patients and family members are taught to recognize the signs of a "brain attack" or stroke, using the mnemonic FAST.

- **F** (Face)—Ask the person to smile. Does one side of the face droop?
- **A** (Arms)—Ask the person to raise both arms. Does one arm drift downward?

- **S** (Speech)—Ask the person to repeat a simple sentence. Are the words slurred or is there difficulty repeating the sentence correctly?
- **T** (Time)—If the person has any one of these symptoms, they should activate EMS (call 911) and go to the hospital immediately. Emergency personnel will want to know the last known symptom-free time, since duration of symptoms is an important parameter in calculating the risk/benefit of various treatment options. A family member or friend should travel to the hospital, if possible, to provide information.

Other symptoms of stroke include trouble seeing in one or both eyes, trouble walking, dizziness, loss of balance or coordination, or sudden severe headache with no known cause.

What is the management plan?

Acute/initial inpatient management includes appropriate brain imaging; airway and breathing support; blood pressure, temperature, and glycemic regulation; in tandem with antithrombotic medication as indicated (Powers et al., 2018).

The nurse practitioner plays a critical role in partnering with the patient and interprofessional health care team to facilitate risk factor reduction, to reduce the likelihood of secondary strokes, and disability, as well as vascular dementia. Therefore, it will be critical to follow the latest American Heart Association guidelines and recommendations for mitigating future stroke risk, such as management of Marion's hypertension, and assessing and treating potential hyperlipidemia, diabetes mellitus, or atrial fibrillation. Antiplatelet therapy or an anticoagulant is recommended for secondary prevention of noncardioembolic, ischemic stroke, as dictated by a patient's comorbid conditions (Powers et al., 2018). Anticoagulation may be preferred for treatment in lieu of antiplatelet therapy for patients with atrial fibrillation. Older adults are at higher risk of bleeding from antiplatelet and/or anticoagulation therapy, and the risk-to-benefit ratio needs to be evaluated for each patient, guided by the latest available evidence. Physician consultation and collaboration is recommended. Age alone is not a contraindication to anticoagulant therapy, and there is evidence of undertreatment in high-risk older adults (Powers et al., 2018). If she is hospitalized, mechanical thrombectomy using a stent retriever may be selected for Marion if she meets all established criteria (Powers, 2018). Screening for dysphagia will be performed, and blood pressure, blood sugar, temperature, and nutrition will be closely monitored.

If Marion was admitted to the hospital, upon discharge, she may be transferred to a rehabilitation center following her hospital course, either for inpatient or ambulatory care treatment as indicated by her condition.

What are some of the most important domains of nursing assessment and management (physical, psychological) during these first few hours after symptoms? In the early post-stroke period?

As systems of care evolve in response to health care reform efforts, post-acute care and rehabilitation are considered a costly area of care to be trimmed, without recognition of their clinical impact and ability to reduce the risk of downstream medical morbidity resulting from immobility, depression, loss of autonomy, and reduced functional independence (Weinstein et al., 2016). Goals in the early post-stroke period are to restore maximal function and to assist with emotional and physical adjustment during the rehabilitation period. Skillful nursing assessment, care, education, and monitoring are needed in collaboration with the interdisciplinary team, the patient, and the family. The goals of care include maintaining or improving mobility and speech (if impaired), self-care, swallowing, bladder control, bowel function, sexual function, emotional adjustment, and family coping. Instructing formal and informal caregivers is an important nursing role in order to prevent injury (e.g., shoulder dislocation), avoidable complications (choking, aspiration, fecal impaction), and frustration related to unrealistic expectations and unmet needs for adaptive equipment, technologies, or assistance. The provision of comprehensive rehabilitation programs with adequate resources, dose, and duration is an essential aspect of stroke care and should be a priority in these redesign efforts (Weinstein et al., 2016).

REFERENCES AND RESOURCES

Abe, R., Diniz-Filho, A., Costa, V., Gracitelli, C., Baig, S., & Medeiros, F. (2016). The impact of location of progressive visual field loss on longitudinal changes in quality of life of patients with glaucoma. *Ophthalmology, 123*(3), 552–557.

Carlson, C., Merel, S., & Yukawa, M. (2015). Geriatric syndromes and geriatric assessment for the generalist. *Medical Clinics of North America 99*(2), 263–279.

Garcia-Layana, A., Cabrerea-Lopez, F., Garcia-Arumi, J., Arias-Barquet, L., & Ruiz-Moreno, J. (2017). Early and intermediate age-related macular degeneration: Update and clinical review, *Clinical Interventions in Aging, 12,* 1579–1587.

Golan, S., Rabina, G., Kurtz, S., & Leibovitch, I. (2016). The prevalence of glaucoma in patients undergoing surgery for eyelid entropion or ectropion. *Clinical Interventions in Aging, 11,* 1429–1432.

Hanna, K., Hepworth, L., & Rowe, R. (2016). Screening methods for post stroke visual impairment: A systematic review. *Disability Rehabilitation, 39*(25), 2531–2543.

Miller, C. (2019). *Nursing for wellness in older adults* (8th ed., pp. 337–362 & 419–434). Philadelphia: Wolters Kluwer.

Pioro, M. (2018). Primary care vasculitis, polymyalgia rheumatica and giant cell arteritis. *Primary Care: Clinics in Office Practice, 45*(2), 305–323.

Powers, W. J., Rabinstein, A. A., Ackerson, T., Adeoye, O. M., Bambakidis, N. C., Becker, K., . . . American Heart Association Stroke Council. (2018). 2018 guidelines for the early management of patients with acute ischemic stroke: A guideline for healthcare professionals from the American Heart Association/American Stroke Association. *Stroke, 49*(3), e46–e110. doi:10.1161/STR.0000000000000158

Revicki, D. A., Rentz, A. M., Harnam, N., Thomas, V. S., & Lanzetta, P. (2010). Reliability and validity of the National Eye Institute Visual Function Questionnaire-25 in patients with age-related macular degeneration. *Investigative Ophthalmology & Visual Science, 51*(2), 712–717.

Su, D., Greenberg, A., Simonson, J., Teng, C., Liebmann, J., Ritch, R., & Park, S. (2016). Efficacy of the Amsler Grid Test in evaluating glaucomatous central visual field Defects. *Ophthalmology, 123*(4), 737–743.

Viela, P. (2017). Acute stroke differential diagnosis: Stroke mimics. *European Journal of Radiology, 96,* 133–144.

Vujosevic, S., Toma, C., Villani, E., Gatti, V., Brambilla, M., Muraca, A., . . . De Cilla, S. (2019). Early detection of microvascular changes in patients with diabetes mellitus without and with diabetic retinopathy: Comparison between different swept-source OCT-A instruments. *Journal of Diabetes Research, 19.* https://doi.org/10.1155/2019/2547216

Wardlaw, J. M., Brazzelli, M., Chappell, F. M., Miranda, H., Shuler, K., Sanderock, P. A. G., & Dennis, M. S. (2015). ABCD^2 score and secondary stroke prevention. *Neurology, 85*(4). https://doi.org/10.1212/WNL.0000000000001780

Weinstein, C. J., Stein, J., Arena, R., Bates, B., Cherney, L. R., Cramer, S. C., . . . Zorowitz, R. D. (2016). Guidelines for adult stroke rehabilitation and recovery: A guideline for healthcare professionals from the American Heart Association/American Stroke Association, *Stroke, 47*(6), e98–e169.

Case 10.6 Back Pain

RESOLUTION

What are the most likely differential diagnoses in this case and why?
Vertebral compression fracture (VCF):

A late midlife woman who presents with a chief complaint of acute onset of upper midback pain that limits active range of motion and deep breathing and radiates to her lower chest and abdomen prompts the clinician to consider several differential diagnoses. The most common differential that accounts for this constellation of symptoms is vertebral compression fracture (VCF) due to osteoporosis (OP). This is a common presentation of OP as bone loss does not cause any pain or symptoms until a fracture occurs (Bethel, 2019; Camachoet al., 2016; Cosman et al., 2014). However, several other differentials may mimic some symptoms of VCFs or exacerbate these symptoms and must be carefully explored; these include back strain, atypical angina, and costochondritis. Less common differentials that the clinician will consider given Mary's history include an RA flare and extra-articular pulmonary RA manifestations.

VCFs commonly occur with usual activities when the spine is hyperextended or flexed as the vertebral bones are weakened due to bone loss and the anterior or posterior edges of the bones are crushed with the pressure of the flexion or extension of the spinal column. About two-thirds of patients who experience VCFs do not have significant pain. These patients may present with height loss or kyphosis. VCFs change the vertebral bone to a wedge shape instead of a square shape and lead to the classic forward-bent posture seen in patients with kyphosis of the spine. OP often presents with a fracture because there are no symptoms associated with bone loss until an actual fracture occurs. This is why early screening is advocated (Bethel, 2019; Camacho et al., 2016; Cosman et al., 2014).

OP is diagnosed with a comprehensive history and physical exam, selected laboratory testing, and central bone density measurement such as dual-energy absorptiometry (DXA). Mary's DXA revealed a T-score of −2.6 at her lower spine, −2.0 at her hip, and −1.7 for her combined hip. Her FRAX® 10-year fracture risk at the hip was reported as 3.0%; and for any major OP fracture, it was reported as 22.0%. Her physical examination findings are consistent with thoracic VCFs. Her laboratory testing revealed a normal fasting serum calcium and 24-hour urinary calcium and a serum 25-OH-D of 20 ng/mL, suggesting nutritional insufficiency. Finally, her spine films revealed stage 1 VCFs at T7 and T8 (20–25% deformity).

The Family Nurse Practitioner: Clinical Case Studies, Second Edition. Edited by Leslie Neal-Boylan.
© 2021 John Wiley & Sons Ltd. Published 2021 by John Wiley & Sons Ltd.

The history and physical examination and laboratory tests are done to evaluate the possible presence of secondary OP. Secondary OP is present when a disease process or medication causes bone loss that results in OP. Mary is at risk for secondary OP because she has a high-risk disease (RA) and has needed to take high-risk medications (oral steroids) for many years (Bethel, 2019; Camacho et al., 2016; Cosman et al., 2014). Since her need for daily steroids continued for many years, it is highly likely that her OP is secondary, at least in part, due to steroid use. The rate of bone loss also normally increases significantly in women during the early postmenopausal years (bone loss of up to 5% per year can occur); thus it is likely that Mary's OP is also partly primary and due to her postmenopausal status.

Other musculoskeletal causes:
Musculoskeletal causes of back or chest-wall pain that are unrelated to OP must also be considered. Such differentials would include back strain and costochondritis. Mary's physical examination findings of pain upon movement and tenderness with chest-wall compression support each of these differentials. Back strain is the more likely of these differentials because of the history of physical activity that precipitated the onset of Mary's pain. Costochondritis is less likely as it tends to develop over time with overuse and inflammation as opposed to acute injury. However, neither of these differentials is supported by the physical examination finding of vertebral tenderness; this finding is more indicative of VCF.

Angina:
Angina is an important differential that Mary's clinician cannot afford to miss. Mary is at increased risk for cardiovascular disease due both to her RA and to her age. Although cardiac manifestations of RA can occur; they are not common. RA is, however, associated with an increased risk for cardiovascular disease (Jagpal & Navarro-Millan, 2018). Women are more likely to develop cardiovascular disease as they age, with postmenopausal women having an equal or greater risk for cardiovascular disease than men of the same age cohort (Jagpal & Navarro-Millan, 2018). While women do experience typical angina symptoms, angina often presents atypically among women with fatigue, neck pain, nausea, and shortness of breath. Women are less likely than men to present with acute infarction; rather, they have symptoms over a longer period of time and at rest. As women age, the likelihood that they will present with more typical angina symptoms increases (Maas, 2017). In Mary's case, she has not described symptoms of atypical angina such as nausea or prolonged fatigue; rather, she stated that she usually awakes refreshed and well rested. Additionally, her pain is the posterior chest rather than the anterior chest, an acute onset related to a specific activity, radiates to her lower chest and abdomen, and is exacerbated with chest-wall palpation—all findings that suggest VCF more strongly than angina-related chest pain.

RA Flare:
Given Mary's history of RA, her clinician would also likely consider an RA flare and extra-articular pulmonary RA manifestations as possible, yet less likely, causes of her pain. RA flares tend to present with increased symptoms in previously affected joints such as the metacarpal phalangeal (MCP) and proximal interphalangeal (PIP) joints in the hands. As the disease progresses, other joints may be affected such as the elbows or wrists; ankles, knees, or hips; shoulders; and cervical spine (such as C1 and C2) (Smith, 2018). In Mary's presentation, she describes this pain as distinct from her usual morning stiffness associated with RA and does not associate it with the many RA flares that she has experienced in the past. Additionally, RA is not likely to affect other areas of the spine (Smith, 2018), and Mary's symptoms are specifically centered in the T7–T8 region by both her history and her physical examination. Extra-articular pulmonary RA manifestations are even less likely. Pericardial effusions related to RA are normally asymptomatic. Pulmonary manifestations may include asymptomatic pleural effusions and are more commonly seen among men (Smith, 2018). Similarly, lung nodules caused by RA are also more common in men. These pulmonary manifestations do not present with acute onset upper back pain.

Which diagnostic tests are required in this case and why?

Diagnostic testing is needed to diagnose both osteoporosis (OP) and vertebral compression fractures (VCFs).

1. EKG: Obtaining an EKG would be prudent for a 63-year-old woman who presented with either typical or atypical angina symptoms. However, an EKG is not useful in verifying OP or VCFs, and may not accurately identify myocardial distress.
2. CPKs: Obtaining CPKs would be prudent for a 63-year-old woman who presented with typical or atypical angina symptoms or who presented with myalgias such as are sometimes seen with statins. However, CPKs are not used to verify OP or VCFs.
3. Fasting lipid panel, fasting blood glucose, and hemoglobin A1C (HgA1c) level: While these tests would be useful to determine cardiovascular disease and diabetes risk profiles and might be appropriate if Mary has not been screened recently, these tests will not assist with verifying OP or VCFs.
4. CBC, ESR, and CRP: A CBC is drawn to evaluate the number and types of cells present in a serum sample. Anemia of chronic disease is a common finding with RA. A CBC is also useful to assess in patients suspected of having OP to rule out secondary causes of bone loss and to determine overall health status (Bethel, 2019; Camacho et al., 2016; Cosman et al., 2014). ESR and CRP are nonspecific markers for inflammation and are indicative of disease activity with RA; however, they are not highly specific and will be elevated with other inflammatory processes as well (Smith, 2018).
5. LFTs, BUN/creatinine, eGFR, phosphorous: These tests are often measured to assess general health and are appropriate to test in Mary to evaluate for secondary causes of OP. Knowing her liver and kidney function status may be important when determining whether to use pharmacotherapeutics to manage her OP and VCFs.
6. TSH: Obtaining a TSH level is appropriate to evaluate for secondary causes of OP despite the fact that Mary does not describe symptoms consistent with thyroid abnormality.
7. Fasting serum calcium, 24-hour urinary calcium, and serum 25-OH-D (vitamin D): These tests are done to identify calcium and vitamin D levels. This data is important for any patient suspected of OP, as low calcium levels may suggest underlying pathology or secondary OP and must be rectified prior to starting any antiresorptive medication (Bethel, 2019; Camachoet al., 2016; Cosman et al., 2014). Similarly, low vitamin D levels (below 30 ng/mL) need to be corrected (Bethel, 2019; Camacho et al., 2016; Cosman et al., 2014). Adequate vitamin D is needed both for normal bone resorption processes and for calcium absorption.
8. Spine films: Spine films can be used to diagnose VCFs. In patients with greater than 30% bone loss, OP can be seen on radiological examination. However, X-ray is not used to diagnose OP. Patients with bone loss identified on X-ray are referred for DXA.
9. DXA with FRAX®: DXA is considered the gold standard for the diagnosis of OP (Bethel, 2019; Camacho et al., 2016; Cosman et al., 2014). Results are provided that include both T-scores and Z-scores; and, since early 2009, most reports also include the 10-year risk probability for hip and major OP fractures identified by the FRAX® algorithm. T-scores identify how the patient's bone density compares to that of a normal young adult of the same gender. The Z-score identifies how the patient's bone density compares to others of the same age and gender. Both T-scores and Z-scores are reported as standard deviations, with 0 indicating an exact match. Since they are standard deviations, a normal T-score is −1 to +1. Low bone mass, or osteopenia, is identified with T-scores of −1 to −2.5; and osteoporosis is identified with T-scores below −2.5. Severe OP is identified with T-scores below −2.5 in the presence of fragility fracture(s) (World Health Organization [WHO], 1994). Low trauma fractures (formerly called fragility fractures) are those that occur with low trauma or a fall from standing height or less (Bethel, 2019; Camacho et al., 2016; Cosman et al., 2014). FRAX® is an individualized algorithm that identifies the probability of fracture over the next 10 years based on the patient's height, weight, and bone density raw score and the presence or absence of 11 additional risk factors such as smoking, history of RA,

steroid use, and parental history of hip fracture (WHO, 2007a, 2007b). FRAX® is used to assist with determining whether a specific patient would benefit from the use of pharmacotherapeutics to prevent fracture and thus is used for patients who have not previously been treated with medication. Analyses were done on the U.S. population to evaluate the cost of fracture and pharmacotherapy. These analyses revealed that it is cost effective to treat those with a 10-year risk of hip fracture of above 3% or a 10-year risk of major OP fracture of above 20% (Bethel, 2019; Camacho et al., 2016; Cosman et al., 2014). It is important to note that a diagnosis of OP is not made based on DXA results alone. All patients, even those with a T-score of below −2.5, require a detailed history and physical examination with selected laboratory evaluations to identify any secondary causes of OP that can be treated and to determine safety in using possible pharmacotherapeutic agents (Bethel, 2019; Camacho et al., 2016; Cosman et al., 2014).

What is the plan of treatment?

Mary and her clinician need to address both of her diagnoses. She has documented VCFs identified by X-ray as well as OP identified by DXA. The plan for her pain management for the VCFs will be of a more short-term nature, while OP management will be long term.

Self-management lifestyle changes:

Mary will initially need to avoid activities that increase her pain. She needs to understand that it may take 3 months before she is fully healed and that a return to activity as soon as possible is important. It will be important for her to see the physical therapist for pain modalities early on, as well as for strengthening exercises for her upper midback and body mechanics retraining later to prevent further injury.

For OP management, she will need to adjust her activity and intake of vitamin D and calcium. Mary needs to increase her activity and ensure that it includes both resistance and weight-bearing activities each day. These activities will serve to increase osteoblast activity and thus strengthen bone. Mary also needs to assure daily intake of vitamin D of 800–1000 IU and calcium of 1200 mg (Bethel, 2019; Camacho et al., 2016; Cosman et al., 2014). This level of vitamin D intake is enough to rectify her vitamin D deficiency within about a 3-month period. Since most people cannot achieve the recommended daily intake of vitamin D and calcium through diet alone, it is likely that Mary will require ongoing calcium and vitamin D supplementation, even after her vitamin D levels are normalized. Many different supplement brands and types are available. Calcium citrate is less constipating than calcium carbonate and can be taken with or without meals. Calcium carbonate must be taken with meals, as an acid environment is needed for it to be absorbed. Calcium carbonate would not be an appropriate option for Mary if she uses antacids of any kind. Both calcium carbonate and calcium citrate are also available as a combination tablet with vitamin D.

Mary also needs to implement a fall prevention program (Bethel, 2019; Camacho et al., 2016; Cosman et al., 2014). This is not because she is at an increased risk for falls simply due to her OP; it is more that the likelihood of fracture caused by a fall is increased significantly due to her OP. Mary's clinician will advise her to look around at home and remove any loose rugs or cords that she might fall or trip on. She will need to assure adequate lighting in case she needs to get up at night, again to lessen the risk of a fall. Similarly, she will need to ensure removal of snow, ice, or wet leaves and uncluttered walkways around her home to reduce the risk of a fall.

Complementary and alternative medicine therapies:

Mary may be interested in light massage therapy or acupuncture for pain management. While neither of these therapies will increase bone strength, each may help to reduce her pain while the VCFs are healing. Continuing with these therapies may increase her tolerance for exercise later as well. Other relaxation therapies that may be beneficial include yoga, aromatherapy, and meditation. Yoga should not be initiated until the VCFs have healed and will need to be modified to avoid any forward bending (flexion) of the spine.

Research results evaluating the use of soy to improve bone strength have been contradictory; some demonstrate a benefit, while others show none. A meta-analysis that reviewed randomized, controlled trials did not find overall support for the use of soy to prevent bone loss (Zheng, Lee, & Chun, 2018).

Pharmacotherapeutics:

Pharmacotherapeutic agents for both Mary's VCF pain and management of her OP are reasonable. Her pain may be adequately managed by consistent use of acetaminophen, dosed at 1000 mg by mouth every 6 hours, or in combination with a nonsteroidal anti-inflammatory drug (NSAID). If an NSAID is used, she must be cautioned to take it with food to reduce the likelihood of developing gastrointestinal irritation as a side effect, especially if she is prescribed a bisphosphonate for her OP. If acetaminophen or a combination of acetaminophen and NSAIDs is ineffective, then acetaminophen combined with a narcotic analgesic, such as acetaminophen with codeine, may be tried. A return to usual activity as soon as possible is the goal.

Mary meets the criteria established by both the National Osteoporosis Foundation (NOF) and the American Association of Clinical Endocrinologists (AACE) for pharmacotherapeutic treatment of her OP (Camacho et al., 2016; Cosmanet al., 2014). Both organizations recommend initiating medication therapy in individuals with documented OP, which Mary has. In fact, Mary meets the diagnostic criteria established by the WHO for severe osteoporosis, because she has a spine T-score of −2.5 on DXA plus fragility or low-trauma fractures (VCFs) (WHO, 1994). Even if Mary's DXA scores had not indicated OP and she did not have VCFs, her clinician would still consider pharmacotherapeutic therapy for her, as her FRAX® 10-year risk for major OP fracture was above the cutoff of 20.0%. This suggests that it would be cost effective, based on U.S. population calculations, to treat Mary with medications for OP (Bethel, 2019; Camacho et al., 2016; Cosman et al., 2014).

The purpose of pharmacotherapy for OP is to reduce fracture incidence and its related sequelae. Several different effective medications for OP management are currently available in the United States and approved by the FDA, including bisphosphonates, calcitonin, estrogen agonist/antagonists, hormone therapy (estrogen or estrogen-progestin therapy), a RANK-ligand inhibitor, and parathyroid hormone (see Table 10.6.1). These medications can be categorized into two groups: antiresorptive or anabolic. Antiresorptive agents increase bone strength by inhibiting the function of the osteoclasts and include bisphosphonates, calcitonin, estrogen agonist/antagonists (which were previously known as selective estrogen receptor modulators [SERMs]), and hormone therapy (HT, estrogen or estrogen-progestin therapy). Denosumab is also in this category and increases bone density by binding with RANK-ligand, which ultimately inhibits osteoclast formation and function. Anabolic agents stimulate bone formation by increasing osteoblast activity and include one agent—teriparatide.

For Mary, selecting an agent will focus on identifying an effective therapy that is acceptable to her, does not interfere with her current medications, and has a reasonable side-effect profile. Because she has established OP, she needs a medication that is approved for OP treatment. This means that hormone therapy is not an appropriate option. If Mary had osteopenia and was also experiencing significant menopause-related symptoms, then HT or estrogen + bazedoxifene (Duavee®) might be a good option (ePocrates, updated daily; North American Menopause Society, 2014). Bisphosphonates are frequently identified as first-line options for OP. Several different medications are now available in this class with varied frequency of dosing and varied routes of administration. Some are also available in generic formulation, which can significantly reduce cost. A precise procedure for taking oral bisphosphonates must be followed to reduce the risk of esophageal irritation. Other rare side effects are also possible (see Table 10.6.1). If Mary starts with a bisphosphonate and is unable to follow the oral medication regimen or has a low bone-density response, she might have better adherence with an injectable bisphosphonate or denosumab. Denosumab is also identified as a first-line option. If Mary was at high risk for breast cancer, raloxifene might be a better option for her. Calcitonin is sometimes used for the pain associated with VCFs and might be considered for Mary. However, other OP medications have better fracture prevention data and Mary's pain will likely be well managed with analgesics instead. Teriparatide or abaloparatide are unlikely options for Mary as these are generally reserved for use in patients who do not respond to first-line medication options. Poor adherence to OP medication is a significant problem. Therefore, it is important that Mary is an active participant in deciding which medication to use. She is much more likely to continue with the medication if it is taken on a schedule that

Table 10.6.1. Prescription Agents for Osteoporosis Management.

Medication	FDA-Approved Use and Dose	Considerations
Alendronate (Fosamax)	PMO prevention—5 mg by mouth daily or 35 mg by mouth weekly. SIO—5 mg by mouth daily or 10 mg by mouth daily if postmenopausal and off estrogen PMO and MOP treatment—10 mg by mouth daily or 70 mg by mouth weekly.	Take oral doses first thing in the morning on an empty stomach with 8-oz glass of plain water; remain upright and take no other food or drink for at least 30 minutes. Take oral doses 2 hours before antacids/calcium. Caution with oral forms if upper gastrointestinal disease, clinical association with dysphagia, esophagitis, or ulceration. Beneficial effects may last for years after medication is discontinued.
Alendronate + cholecalciferol (Fosamax plus D)	PMO and MOP treatment—70 mg plus 2800 IU Vitamin D_3 or 70 mg plus 5600 IU vitamin D_3 in combined tablet by mouth weekly.	Fosamax plus D—combined bisphosphonate and vitamin D_3 in a single tablet taken weekly. Actonel with calcium—blister pack for 28-day use, provides Actonel in 1 tablet taken on day 1 and calcium in other 6 tablets taken days 2–7, repeated sequence over 4 weeks.
Risedronate (Actonel)	PMO prevention or treatment— 5 mg by mouth daily, 35 mg by mouth weekly, 75 mg by mouth 2 consecutive days each month, or 150 mg by mouth monthly. SIO—5 mg by mouth daily. MOP—35 mg by mouth weekly.	IV ibandronate and zoledronic acid are not associated with gastrointestinal side effects or limitations on timing dose around food, water, calcium, or medication intake. Hypocalcemia must be corrected prior to use.
Ibandronate (Boniva)	PMO prevention or treatment— 2.5 mg by mouth daily or 150 mg by mouth monthly. PMO treatment—3 mg IV every 3 months.	Subtrochanteric fracture is an extremely rare event that has been associated with bisphosphonate use. Advise patients that the risk of this extremely rare event is far less than the risks associated with hip fracture and encourage them to take their prescribed bisphosphonates consistently.
Zoledronic acid (Reclast)	PMO prevention—5 mg IV every 2 years. PMO, MOP, and SIO treatment— 5 mg IV yearly.	
Calcitonin (Miacalcin, generic nasal spray)	PMO treatment—200 IU intranasal spray daily (generic) or 100 IU subcutaneously 3 times each week (Miacalcin).	Usually administered as nasal spray. Alternate nares for nasal spray. Most often used for analgesic effect on acute pain due to vertebral compression fractures.
Denosumab (Prolia, Xgeva)	PMO treatment—60 mg injection (subcutaneous) every 6 months.	Denosumab is for those with multiple risks for fracture, with osteoporotic fracture history, and who have not responded to other treatments. Requires administration by a health care professional. Use may be associated with ONJ, oversuppression of bone turnover, skin infections, and dermatologic conditions. Individuals with a latex allergy should not handle gray needle cover. Hypocalcemia must be corrected prior to use.
Estrogen (e.g., Alora, Climara, Estrace, Menest, Menostar, Premarin, Vivelle Dot)	PMO prevention—doses and routes vary.	Also effective in alleviating most symptoms related to menopause (even Menostar, which has a very low dose and was shown to effectively reduce severity and frequency of hot flashes).
Estrogen + Bazedoxifene (Duavee)	PMO prevention	Also effective in alleviating most symptoms related to menopause.

Table 10.6.1. (Continued)

Medication	FDA-Approved Use and Dose	Considerations
Estrogen-Progestin combination products (e.g., Activella, Climara, Climara Pro, Femhrt, Prefest, Premphase, Prempro)	PMO prevention—doses and routes vary.	Available in several forms (e.g., pills, patch, ring, cream, gel). Use for 2–3 years immediately following menopause may provide some beneficial effects on bone health after discontinuation.
Raloxifene (Evista)	PMO prevention or treatment— 60 mg by mouth daily.	May cause hot flashes. Not recommended if taking ET or EPT. Also approved for prevention of breast cancer in women at high risk for invasive breast cancer.
Teriparatide [recombinant human PTH 1–34] (Forteo) Abaloparatide (Tymlos)	PMO, MOP, and SIO treatment (high fracture risk)—20 mcg subcutaneously daily. (A teriparatide patch for osteoporosis is under investigation.)	Reserved for use after failure of first-line agents. Most effective when used sequentially following bisphosphonate.

PMO = postmenopausal osteoporosis; SIO = steroid-induced osteoporosis; MOP = male osteoporosis.
Source: ePocrates (updated daily); Bethel (2019); Camacho et al. (2016); Cosman et al. (2014).

works for her life. This may mean daily or nondaily oral medications, or possibly infrequent office visits for injectable medications. Ensuring insurance coverage of her selection is also crucial.

What are the plans for referral and follow-up care?

Referral to physical therapy initially for pain modalities and later for strengthening exercises and body mechanics training is appropriate. If Mary does not respond to routine pain management strategies or if her DXA T-scores continue to fall, then referral to a specialist may be indicated. Consultation with an OP specialist may be warranted if she is not responding to therapy. A pain specialist or ongoing physical therapy may help to alleviate her pain. Some patients with VCFs require referral for surgical intervention, such as kyphoplasty or vertebroplasty, to relieve pain and preserve function. Kyphoplasty (a balloon is inserted into the vertebral space, is inflated to straighten the vertebral bones, and is then replaced with a cement-like substance) is performed under local anesthesia so pain and function can be monitored throughout the procedure. Vertebroplasty is similar and was the precursor to kyphoplasty. Vertebroplasty is usually performed by interventional radiologists and involves injection of a cement-like substance into the fractured vertebrae. If effective, pain relief is almost immediate after either procedure.

In addition to reevaluating Mary's ability to follow the management plan including both medications and self-management strategies at every visit, a follow-up DXA scan will be ordered for about 1–2 years to evaluate the efficacy of Mary's management strategies (Bethel, 2019; Camacho et al., 2016; Cosman et al., 2014). It will be repeated every 1–2 years until her results are stable. If her T-scores do not improve after a few years, her clinician might consider changing the pharmacotherapeutic agent to an alternate class or consider referral to an OP specialist.

What health education should be provided for this patient?

While OP is not wholly reversible, slowing bone loss with the described self-management strategies is crucial to reducing the impact of the disease and preventing future fractures. It is important for Mary to understand that she has a lifelong challenge ahead of her to retain her current bone strength and hopefully build upon it. This can only be successful with a combined management plan that includes self-management lifestyle strategies—such as regular exercise, adequate calcium and vitamin D intake, and careful monitoring of her RA—and consistent use of her OP medications.

What demographic characteristics might affect this case?

Several of the medications available for OP treatment and prevention only carry FDA approval for use in postmenopausal women, so agent selection options would be narrowed (see Table 10.6.1).

Does the patient's psychosocial history impact how you might treat her?

If Mary were under 40, a more aggressive search for other secondary causes of OP would be appropriate. Any conditions identified would then need to be managed to reduce bone loss. Additionally, most of the medications available for OP treatment and prevention do not carry FDA approval for use in premenopausal women, so agent selection options would be narrowed (see Table 10.6.1).

Consideration of Mary's psychosocial history is important when developing a management plan with her. Consideration of Mary's health care insurance coverage of medications, physical therapy, and DXA evaluations is important. Many insurance companies dictate which pharmacotherapeutic agents are covered. Similarly, most companies have rules governing the frequency of covered DXA testing and the length of physical therapy treatments. These issues are taken into account when deciding on a management plan with Mary so that financial barriers to the cost of medications, follow-up DXA testing, or PT do not become barriers to her ability to follow the agreed upon plan.

Are there any standardized guidelines that should be used to treat this case? If so, what are they?

Both the National Osteoporosis Foundation and the American Association of Clinical Endocrinologists have published guidelines for osteoporosis prevention, identification, and management (Camacho et al., 2016; Cosman et al., 2014).

REFERENCES

Bethel, M. (2019). Osteoporosis. *eMedicine, MedScape*. Accessed September 27, 2019. Available at: https://emedicine.medscape.com/article/330598-overview.

Camacho, P. M., Petak, S. M., Binkley, N., Clarke, B. L., Harris, S. T., Hurley, D. L., . . . Watts, N. B. (2016). American Association of Clinical Endocrinologists and American College of Endocrinology clinical practice guidelines for the diagnosis and treatment of postmenopausal osteoporosis—2016. *Endocrine Practice*, 22(Suppl. 4), 1–42. https://journals.aace.com/doi/pdf/10.4158/EP161435.GL

Cosman, F., de Beur, S. J., LeBoff, M. S., Lewiecki, E. M., Tanner, B., Randall, S., & Lindsay, R. (2014). Clinician's guide to prevention and treatment of osteoporosis. *Osteoporosis International, Online* (August 2014), 1–25. file:///C:/Users/ima00001/Downloads/Clinicians-Guide.pdf

ePocrates. (Updated daily). Computerized pharmacology and prescribing reference [Mobile application software]. Retrieved from http://www.epocrates.com

Jagpal, A., & Navarro-Millan, I. (2018). Cardiovascular co-morbidity in patients with rheumatoid arthritis: A narrative review of risk factors, cardiovascular risk assessment and treatment. *BMC Rheumatology*, 2, article no. 10. https://bmcrheumatol.biomedcentral.com/articles/10.1186/s41927-018-0014-y

Maas, A. H. E. M. (2017). The clinical presentation of "angina pectoris" in women. *E-Journal of Cardiology Practice*, *15*(3). https://www.escardio.org/Journals/E-Journal-of-Cardiology-Practice/Volume-15/The-clinical-presentation-of-angina-pectoris-in-women.

North American Menopause Society (NAMS). (2014). *Menopause practice*: A clinician's guide (5th ed.). Mayfield Heights, OH: Author.

Smith, H. R. (2018). Rheumatoid arthritis. *eMedicine. Medscape*. Accessed July 30, 2019. Available at: https://emedicine.medscape.com/article/331715-overview

World Health Organization. (1994). *Assessment of fracture risk and its application to screening for postmenopausal osteoporosis. Technical report series*. Geneva: Author.

World Health Organization. (2007a). WHO FRAX Technical Report. Retrieved June 6, 2008, from http://www.shef.ac.uk/FRAX/

World Health Organization. (2007b). *WHO scientific group on the assessment of osteoporosis at the primary health care level: Summary meeting report*. Geneva, Switzerland: Author.

Zheng, X., Lee, S-K., & Chun, O. K. (2018). Soy isoflavones and osteoporotic bone loss: A review with an emphasis on modulation of bone remodeling. *Journal of Medical Food*, *191*(1), 1–14. doi:10.1089/jmf.2015.0045.https://www.ncbi.nlm.nih.gov/pmc/articles/PMC4717511/pdf/jmf.2015.0045.pdf

Case 10.7 Acute Joint Pain

What is the most likely diagnosis and why?

Acute gouty arthritis:

The location of the joint pain in the first metatarsophalangeal (MTP) joint, redness, swelling, warmth, and tenderness to light touch are all consistent with an acute gout flare. Other factors that make this the most likely diagnosis include Rami's male sex, history of hypertension, lack of known injury, unilateral presentation, and absence of fevers/chills.

What are possible differential diagnoses?

See Table 10.7.1.

Which diagnostic or imaging studies should be considered to assist with or confirm the diagnosis?

When suspecting gout the most important diagnosis to rule out is septic arthritis, as they have similar presentations. If there is concern for septic arthritis a joint aspiration with synovial fluid analysis should be performed. The presence of monosodium urate (MSU) crystals in the joint fluid confirms the presence of gout; the presence of bacteria and white blood cells in the joint fluid confirms septic arthritis. If the risk for septic arthritis is low and a joint aspiration cannot be easily obtained other diagnostics including joint X-ray, CBC and serum uric acid levels can help to make the diagnosis. Of note, an elevated serum uric acid level lends support to the diagnosis of gout but is not diagnostic. Interestingly, serum uric acid levels can be normal during acute gout flares. Renal function should be checked to help guide treatment choice as several of the treatment options for gout are contraindicated in renal insufficiency.

What is the plan of treatment?

There are several options to consider when treating an acute gout flare. The need to start treatment as soon as possible after a flare occurs should be discussed. The choice of pharmacologic agent is mostly dependent on the patient's other comorbidities as one is not superior to the other in clinical trials. Options include:

- NSAIDs: High-dose NSAIDs, such as naproxen or indomethacin, are effective in the management of gout. Common contraindications to NSAID use include renal insufficiency,

The Family Nurse Practitioner: Clinical Case Studies, Second Edition. Edited by Leslie Neal-Boylan.
© 2021 John Wiley & Sons Ltd. Published 2021 by John Wiley & Sons Ltd.

Table 10.7.1. Differential Diagnoses.

Condition	Signs and Symptoms
Sprain/strain	Acute pain and swelling following an injury. Decreased range of motion, possibly with ecchymosis. Pertinent negatives: redness, fever, warmth.
Septic arthritis	Acute monoarticular joint pain with associated redness, swelling, and warmth; Significantly decreased range of motion; often accompanied by fever, chills. Hip and knee joints are the most commonly affected.
Osteoarthritis	Insidious, progressive joint pain and stiffness; worse upon first arising and after significant activity; generally relieved by rest; welling and crepitus may be present; generally not symmetrical.
Rheumatoid arthritis	Insidious onset over weeks or months; often bilateral, symmetrical joint pain with associated swelling, aching, and morning stiffness lasting over an hour; associated systemic symptoms such as weakness, weight loss, malaise, fatigue, and loss of appetite are often present.

history of gastrointestinal bleeding/peptic ulcer disease, and prior bariatric surgery. The concomitant use of a proton pump inhibitor (PPI) with an NSAID could be considered to help minimize the risk of stomach upset and perforation. Given that Rami has stomach upset with ibuprofen, other treatment options should be considered.

- Colchicine: This medication is most effective if started within 24 hours of an acute gout flare. Some patients may be on colchicine for prevention of acute gout episodes. Patients with renal or hepatic dysfunction should not use colchicine. A common side effect is diarrhea.
- Oral corticosteroids: Oral steroids are recommended for patients with contraindications to NSAIDs and/or colchicine; however, they should be used with caution in patients with a concurrent infection or history of diabetes mellitus. Corticosteroids can also be administered intraarticularly after a joint aspiration.

In addition to pharmacotherapy, icing and elevation may help relieve symptoms.

Are there any modifiable risk factors or medications Rami is taking that could contribute to this diagnosis?

Alcohol use is a risk factor for the development of gout. Discussing with Rami the reduction of his nightly alcohol intake would be recommended. Thiazide diuretics are also associated with an increased risk of gout. Consider changing Rami's chlorthalidone to an alternate blood pressure medication. There is some evidence that use of the angiotensin receptor blocker losartan can help decrease uric acid levels.

What are the plans for referral and follow-up care?

Should Rami require a joint aspiration, referral to a provider able to perform this procedure and analyze the joint fluid is appropriate. In cases of refractory gout symptoms, referral to rheumatology may be appropriate. Follow-up within 1–2 days is recommended if there is no improvement in symptoms.

What health education should be provided to Rami at this visit?

Several lifestyle changes can be made for Rami. Consumption of meat, seafood, alcohol, and sugar-sweetened beverages and foods containing high-fructose corn syrup can contribute to the development of gout and the incidence of acute attacks. Education around limiting these foods and beverages is recommended. Weight loss can also be beneficial for preventing future attacks. Reiterating the importance of starting treatment as soon as possible in future attacks would also be beneficial.

What if Rami had uncontrolled diabetes mellitus? How would this affect the treatment plan?

It would be important to avoid the use of oral corticosteroid if possible in patients with diabetes.

Rami recovers from his current symptoms but comes in again in 4 months with a similar problem. What should be done for him at this visit?

Rami would require treatment for his acute gout attack; however, he now meets criteria for initiation of urate-lowering therapy (ULT). ULT is not recommended after the first gout attack or in patients with infrequent attacks. In patients with more frequent attacks or evidence of tophaceous deposits on exam or X-ray, the initiation of ULT is recommended. The most common medication used for ULT is allopurinol 100–300 mg daily. When starting ULT, patients may experience an increased number of gout flares. In order to prevent this, prophylaxis with either NSAIDs or colchicine is recommended along with ULT for the first 6 months, assuming no contraindications. The goal for ULT is to titrate the serum uric acid level to <6 mg/dL.

REFERENCES AND RESOURCES

Qaseem, A., McLean, R. M., Starkey, M., & Forciea, M. A. (2017). Diagnosis of acute gout: A clinical practice guideline from the American College of Physicians. *Annals of Internal Medicine, 166*(1), 52–57.

Qaseem, A., Harris, R. P., & Forciea, M. A. (2017). Management of acute and recurrent gout: A clinical practice guideline from the American College of Physicians. *Annals of Internal Medicine, 166*(1), 58–68.

Schlesinger, N. (2017). Gout. In T. M. Buttaro, J. Trybulski, P. Polgar-Bailey, & J. Sandberg-Cook (Eds.), *Primary care: A collaborative practice* (5th ed., pp. 928–932). St. Louis: Elsevier.

Case 10.8 Itching and Soreness

RESOLUTION

What is the most likely differential diagnosis and why?

Aside from cherry angiomas and seborrheic keratoses, Rosa has no visible entry wound or lesions. She has no papules, vesicles, urticaria, redness, or swelling in the affected area. The absence of a rash, lesion, inflammation, or visible insect bite makes bug bites, contact dermatitis, and seborrheic dermatitis unlikely. The initial small, red papule associated with scabies may be difficult to see, but it is often accompanied by small linear burrows that assist in diagnosis. Scabies often appears in areas such as the finger webs, axillary or subgluteal folds, and/or flexor (wrists) or extensor (elbows and knees) surfaces of the joints. This condition is intensely pruritic, especially at night (Raffi, Suresh, & Butler, 2019). Rosa's irritation and tenderness are not consistent with scabies. Xerosis and systemic diseases may contribute to pruritus (as described earlier), but they do not explain the localized sensory symptoms.

Medication side effects should always be considered in the differential diagnosis of new symptoms in the elderly. Medications may precipitate changes in mental status, falls, or functional decline. Older adults experience adverse drug effects more often due to polypharmacy, drug interactions, and age-related changes in pharmacokinetics and pharmacodynamics. Dermatologic side effects of medicines may result in maculopapular rashes, photosensitivity, or desquamation. Toxic epidermal necrosis (TEN) and Stevens–Johnson Syndrome (SJS) are rare, life-threatening conditions that may appear within weeks to months of starting a new medicine. (There are also non-medication-related causes.) These syndromes may present with skin pain and other systemic symptoms prior to evolution of the characteristic skin lesions (Schneider & Cohen, 2017). Allopurinol is one of the medicines that may precipitate this reaction, but Rosa has been taking this medicine for some time. She has no suspicious eye or mucous-membrane findings and has not had any prodromal flu-like symptoms.

Musculoskeletal pain may also be associated with medications. Rosa is taking alendronate; cases of serious bone, joint, or muscle pain have been reported with the use of bisphosphonates (U.S. Food and Drug Administration, 2018). Pain begins days to months after beginning therapy and typically begins locally but spreads and may become severe, interfering with daily activities. Rosa's pattern of symptoms and her findings on examination suggest a distinctly different etiology for her discomfort, but it would not be unreasonable for the clinician to hold the next dose of alendronate pending confirmation of the diagnosis.

The Family Nurse Practitioner: Clinical Case Studies, Second Edition. Edited by Leslie Neal-Boylan.
© 2021 John Wiley & Sons Ltd. Published 2021 by John Wiley & Sons Ltd.

Rosa's history of osteoporosis suggests an increased risk of fracture. The nurse practitioner would know that thoracic discomfort and tenderness may be consistent with a rib fracture, which can occur with little or no trauma in older adults with osteoporosis. Fracture would be suspected if Rosa's pain was aggravated by inspiration or if point tenderness was found on palpation when she took a deep breath. Rosa's corticosteroid therapy increases her risk for osteoporosis, skin changes (thinning and easier bruising), high blood sugar, and other effects.

Rosa's history of polymyalgia rheumatica (PMR) may result in symptoms such as aching, stiffness (worse in the morning and late at night), and weakness in the upper arms, thighs, neck, or lower back, but PMR is *not* associated with itching or significant tenderness on palpation. *Note:* Older adults with PMR should be educated to notify their clinician immediately if they have vision changes or headache, since PMR can be associated with a serious condition in the elderly called giant cell arteritis (GCA), also known as temporal arteritis. Early recognition and treatment of GCA may prevent permanent blindness and other serious sequelae (Resnick & Gershowitz, 2019).

Nostalgia paresthetica is an underdiagnosed condition characterized by pruritis in the mid-scapular region associated with pain or sensory symptoms. It may or may not include a hypo- or hyperpigmented macule. It may be associated with intervertebral disc or nerve impingement and is more common in women; mean age of onset is 50–60 years. Symptoms may last 2–3 years (Howard, Sahhar, Andrews, Bergman, & Gin, 2018).

Rosa has no prior history of a similar rash. She did have chickenpox in childhood and has no history of receiving the herpes zoster vaccine. Risk factors for varicella zoster virus (VZV) reactivation include older age and immunosuppression (Schmader, 2016). You suspect shingles based on the acute onset and neurosensory symptoms in a dermatomal pattern. Your suspicions are confirmed when Rosa returns several days later with a weeping rash along the T5 dermatome associated with a sharp stinging sensation. You find a mixture of erythematous papules and vesicles.

Which diagnostic or imaging studies should be considered to assist with or confirm the diagnosis?

Herpes zoster is a clinical diagnosis based on dermatomal-pattern vesicular rash with neurosensory symptoms. Diagnostic tests are not needed unless there is diagnostic uncertainty or possible disseminated disease in an immunocompromised individual. Viral identification by PCR or fluorescent antibody testing may be helpful in those cases (Saguil, Kane & Mercado, 2017). An ESR may be used to assess inflammation related to PMR, but it is not as useful in the context of an acute dermatologic condition. Chemistry profiles may identify systemic disease but are not warranted by dermatologic symptoms alone. Skin scrapings and microscopy are useful for scabies identification.

What is the management plan?

The management plan has three main goals: to treat the presenting disease or condition, to prevent negative sequelae and excess disability, and to promote comfort. Antiviral therapy is recommended within the first 72 hours after onset of rash to lessen acute discomfort and reduce symptom duration (O'Connor & Paauw, 2013; Schmader, 2016). While there is insufficient evidence to support benefit after 72 hours, this may still be considered if new lesions are still emerging or in cases of ophthalmic involvement. Research is mixed on whether antiviral therapy reduces the risk of postherpetic neuralgia (PHN), a painful complication of shingles. The two greatest risk factors for PHN are older age and severity of acute symptoms (i.e., pain and rash). Acyclovir, famciclovir, and varaciclovir are the currently available antiviral agents. They differ in cost, dosing frequency, and efficacy in treating acute and postherpetic neuralgia. The most common side effects of these agents are nausea, vomiting, diarrhea, and headache.

Patients with disseminated lesions and/or impaired immune competence (e.g., patients with HIV, and malignancies) should be referred to a specialist. Facial lesions or paralysis should prompt an assessment of the ear canals for involvement. If the VZV affects the facial nerve (Ramsay Hunt syndrome), it may cause facial paralysis, intense ear pain, hearing loss, dizziness, tinnitus, or loss of balance. Patients with facial or trigeminal nerve involvement or lesions in the ears or near the eyes should be referred. Ocular zoster is an emergency that may result in permanent vision loss, and patients should be immediately referred to an ophthalmologist.

The American Dermatology Association recommends using cool wet cloths, cool baths, or ice packs for comfort (American Association of Dermatology, 2019). When not using these, the area should be kept clean and dry, covered with nonstick, sterile bandages. Calamine lotion may be applied to the rash and blisters to reduce itching. Colloidal oatmeal baths are also used for symptomatic relief and loose, cotton clothing may improve comfort.

The varicella zoster virus (VZV) can spread from a person with active shingles and cause chickenpox in someone who is not immune to the disease. Contact with fluids from the rash blisters poses risk of transmission. Until all lesions are crusted over, the individual should avoid contact with pregnant women and persons who are not immune to chickenpox. Airborne precautions are recommended in cases of disseminated zoster (Centers for Disease Control, 2018).

Pain management is a key component of care. Corticosteroids do not prevent or shorten PHN but may be used to reduce acute pain. Acetaminophen and nonsteroidal anti-inflammatory drugs (NSAIDS) are used for generalized pain relief in acute zoster. NSAIDs pose greater risks for older adults (Wehling, 2014) and, if prescribed, should be used in the lowest dosage and for the shortest time necessary. Tricyclic antidepressants (TCAs) and anticonvulsants such as gabapentin and pregabalin are used to treat the neuropathic pain of PHN (John & Canaday, 2017). Topical lidocaine is a well-tolerated option for PHN and some patients may also receive benefit from capsaicin, but the burning sensation may not be tolerable, and some patients are adverse to touch and all topical therapies.

Nonpharmacologic strategies for pain management and/or stress reduction include progressive muscle relaxation, meditation, guided imagery, deep breathing, physical exercise, and distraction. Nutritional assessment and counseling are key strategies to support immunologic competence.

Frequent follow-up and evaluation of pain relief and psychosocial well-being are essential. Stress management techniques and psychosocial interventions may be indicated. PHN-related pain may decrease quality of life and may result in depression, decreased activity level, decreased appetite, impaired sleep, decreased function, and social isolation. Some older adults may use alcohol or other substances to obtain symptom relief.

Are any referrals appropriate at this time?

Referral to an ophthalmologist is essential to prevent vision loss related to herpes zoster opthalmica (HZO), a prodrome of headache, malaise, and fever followed by unilateral pain in the eye, forehead, or top of head and conjunctivitis (Conceicao, 2018; John & Canaday, 2017).

Referral to a pain specialist is indicated for severe or persistent pain. Cognitive-behavior modification, biofeedback, and relaxation training may be used, as well as nerve blocks. Referral to a mental health professional for assessment and counseling may also be indicated.

Which of the clinical findings are consistent with normal aging changes?

Aging is associated with changes in cellular structure and function resulting in changes in skin dryness, fragility, atrophy, and decreased elasticity (Resnick & Gershowitz, 2019). Aging skin is more susceptible to wrinkling, uneven tearing, and purpura (purplish discolorations caused by extravasation of blood into the tissues after minor trauma).

Benign lesions such as seborrheic keratoses (yellow, light tan, brown, or brown-black scaly or waxy growths) and cherry angiomas (tiny, bright-red papules) are more common in older adults. Many skin changes are related to environmental factors including air quality and chronic sun exposure over the life course, contributing to accelerated skin aging, dryness, and increased risk for premalignant (e.g., actinic keratoses) or malignant skin growths (including basal cell and squamous cell carcinomas and malignant melanomas). Genetic factors and lifestyle habits contribute to heterogeneity in dermatologic changes in older adults.

Some of Rosa's dermatologic findings may be attributed to normal, age-related interactions with genetic factors (e.g., the cherry angiomas and seborrheic keratoses); and her new complaint of pruritus (itching) may stem in part from xerosis (dry, cracked, or rough skin, which occurs more commonly in cold, low-humidity environments and in older age); but neither aging nor xerosis provides a sufficient explanation for her sensory symptoms and tenderness to touch. The nurse practitioner needs to pursue a more comprehensive assessment and diagnostic approach.

What are the most common causes of pruritus (itching) in older adults? What are the risks and benefits of antihistamine therapy for pruritus, such as diphenhydramine (Benadryl©)?

Itching may be associated with dermatologic conditions (xerosis, scabies, urticaria insect bites), neuropathic conditions (herpes zoster or postherpetic neuralgia, neuropathic syndromes), systemic disease (cholestasis, kidney disease, malignancies, thyroid disease), and psychiatric conditions (obsessive-compulsive disorders, somatization disorders) (Nowak & Yeung, 2017). Dry, rough skin (xerosis), especially over the lower legs, is a common skin finding in older adults, occurring in more than 50% of elderly patients (Berger, Shive & Harper, 2013). Medication side effects are another common cause of pruritis, particularly with thiazide diuretics and calcium channel blockers, as well as photosensitizing medications (Berger et al., 2013).

Older adults with contact dermatitis, eczema, psoriasis, folliculitis, and infestation may also present with itching as the primary complaint. In scabies, the severity of the itching is usually out of proportion to the skin appearance. If these dermatoses have been ruled out and pruritis persists, metabolic and systemic causes must be considered.

Pruritis is a common symptom associated with pre- and postherpetic disease in shingles (Valdes-Rodriguez, Stull & Yosipovitch, 2015). Systemic conditions associated with pruritus include renal disease, liver disease, thyroid disease, endocrine disease, hematologic disease, infectious disease, autoimmune disease, and cancer (Chinniah & Gupta, 2014; Fazio & Yosipovitch, 2019). These conditions typically cause generalized, rather than limited, pruritis. Moses (2003) provides a diagnostically useful pictorial chart, organizing likely causes of pruritis by body location.

Dry skin is treated by avoiding or reducing exposure to aggravating agents (e.g., harsh detergents and alkaline soaps; chemicals including chlorine; and long, hot baths or soaks) and treating liberally with emollients applied to moist skin, immediately after bathing, to seal in moisture (Kirkland-Kyhn, Zaratkiewicz, Teleten & Young, 2018). Urea-based products, glycerin, and petrolatum products are often used to maintain moisture and scaling may be treated with keratolytics that contain alpha hydroxy or lactic acid (Fazio & Yosipovitch, 2019; Kirkland-Kyhn et al., 2018). Humidification of dry environments may be helpful.

Diphenhydramine is appropriate for emergency allergic reactions, but is not recommended for routine use in older adults as a hypnotic or antipruritic, due to the risk of confusion and sedation. Diphenhydramine is one of the medications listed in the American Geriatrics Society 2015 Updated Beers Criteria for Potentially Inappropriate Medication Use in Older Adults (American Geriatrics Society 2019 Criteria Update Expert Panel, 2019). The published Beers criteria include an explicit list of medications that are best avoided in older adults or must be used with caution due to increased risk for delirium, falls, or increased mortality.

If new lesions continue to appear after 1 week, what additional considerations should be addressed?

Patients with new lesions appearing after 1 week may have underlying conditions that impair immune function and should be referred for more extensive evaluation.

Which specific vaccines' dates of administration should be included in immunization documentation for older adults?

In addition to the standard recommendations for all adults, the Centers for Disease Control (CDC, 2018) recommends the following vaccines for adults age 65 and older: influenza (inactivated or recombinant), tetanus and diphtheria booster, zoster recombinant (2 doses) or zoster live (1 dose), pneumococcal conjugate (PCV13), and pneumococcal polysaccharide (PPSV23). The recombinant zoster vaccine (Shingrix) is recommended by the Advisory Committee on Immunization Practices (ACIP) as the preferred vaccine because it is more than 90% effective at preventing shingles and PHN, but Zostavax® may be used if the patient is allergic to Shingrix. Shingrix should be given even if the older adult has had shingles, received Zostavax in the past or is not certain whether they have had chickenpox (CDC, 2018).

> *When an older adult presents with new symptoms, accurate diagnosis facilitates appropriate treatment to prevent further health and functional decline. List two additional questions the practitioner should consider to guide clinical care.*

How can excess disability be prevented?

While early and recognition and treatment with antivirals may prevent or mitigate the severity of PHN, these strategies are not always effective. The best opportunity to prevent pain and disability is vaccination with Shingrix. Education in primary care and community health settings is critical to make older adults aware of the need for prompt evaluation and treatment.

How can comfort (physical, psychosocial, and spiritual) be enhanced, beginning immediately? How can suffering be reduced?

By correcting any myths or unfounded fears, alleviating uncertainty, enhancing a sense of control and participation in self-care, and providing reassurance, as well as using nonpharmacologic and pharmacologic comfort measures.

REFERENCES AND RESOURCES

American Association of Dermatology. (2015). Tips for treating shingles. Available at: https://www.aad.org/media/news-releases/dermatologists-share-tips-for-treating-shingles

American Geriatrics Society 2019 Beers Criteria Update Expert Panel. (2019). American Geriatrics Society 2019 Updated AGS Beers Criteria® for Potentially Inappropriate Medication Use in Older Adults. *Journal of the American Geriatrics Society, 67*(4), 674–694. doi:10.1111/jgs.15767.

Berger, T. G., Shive, M., & Harper, G. M. (2013). Pruritus in the older patient: A clinical review. *JAMA, 310*(22), 2443–2450. doi:10.1001/jama.2013.282023

Centers for Disease Control. (2018). *What everyone should know about shingles vaccine* (Shingrix). Available at: https://www.cdc.gov/vaccines/vpd/shingles/public/shingrix/index.html

Chinniah, N., & Gupta, M. (2014). Pruritus in the elderly: A guide to assessment and management. *Australian Family Physician, 43*(10), 710–713. Retrieved from https://search-ebscohost-com.libraryproxy.quinnipiac.edu/login.aspx?direct=true&db=ccm&AN=109680891&site=ehost-live&scope=site

Conceicao, V. (2018). Prevention and management of shingles and associated complications. *Journal of Community Nursing, 32*(6), 40–43.

Dodiuk-Gad, R. P., Chung, W. H., Valeyrie-Allanore, L., & Shear, N. H. (2015). Stevens–Johnson syndrome and toxic epidermal necrolysis: An update. *American Journal of Clinical Dermatology, 16*, 475–493. https://doi.org/10.1007/s40257-015-0158-0

Fazio, S., & Yosipovitch, G. (2019). Pruritus: Etiology and patient evaluation. In R. P. Dellavalle & J. Callen (Eds)., *UpToDate*. Waltham, MA: UpToDate Inc. https://www.uptodate.com (Accessed October 6, 2019).

Howard, M., Sahhar, L., Andrews, F., Bergman, R., & Gin, D. (2018). Notalgia paresthetica: A review for dermatologists. *International Journal of Dermatology, 57*(4), 388–392. doi:10.1111/ijd.13853

John, A. R., & Canaday, D. H. (2017). Herpes zoster in the older adult. *Infectious Disease Clinics of North America, 31*(4), 811–826. doi:S0891-5520(17)30070-3 [pii]

Kirkland-Kyhn, H., Zaratkiewicz, S., Teleten, O., & Young, H. M. (2018). Caring for aging skin: Preventing and managing skin problems in older adults. *American Journal of Nursing, 118*(2), 60–63. doi: 10.1097/01.NAJ.0000530249.91452.4e.

Moses S. (2003). Pruritus. *American Family Physician, 68*(6), 1135–1012. Retrieved from https://search-ebscohost-com.libraryproxy.quinnipiac.edu/login.aspx?direct=true&db=ccm&AN=106707867&site=ehost-live&scope=site

Nowak, D. A., & Yeung, J. (2017). Diagnosis and treatment of pruritus. *Canadian Family Physician Medecin De Famille Canadien, 63*(12), 918–924. doi:63/12/918 [pii]

O'Connor, K. M., & Paauw, D. S. (2013). Herpes zoster. *Medical Clinics of North America, 97*(4), 503–522. https://doi-org.libraryproxy.quinnipiac.edu/10.1016/j.mcna.2013.02.002

Raffi, J., Suresh, R., & Butler, D. C. (2019). Review of scabies in the elderly. *Dermatology and Therapy, 9*, 623–630. https://doi.org/10.1007/s13555-019-00325-2

Resnick, B., & Gershowitz (Eds.). (2019). *Geriatric nursing review syllabus* (6th ed.). American Geriatric Society.

Saguil, A., Kane, S., Mercado, M., & Lauters, R. (2017). Herpes zoster and postherpetic neuralgia: Prevention and management. *American Family Physician, 96*(10), 656–663

Schneider, J. A., & Cohen, P. R. (2017). Stevens–Johnson syndrome and toxic epidermal necrolysis: A concise review with a comprehensive summary of therapeutic interventions emphasizing supportive measures. *Advances in Therapy, 34*(6), 1235–1244. doi:10.1007/s12325-017-0530-y

Schmader, K. (2016). Herpes zoster. *Clinics in Geriatric Medicine, 32*(3), 539–553. https://doi-org.libraryproxy.quinnipiac.edu/10.1016/j.cger.2016.02.011

U.S. Food and Drug Administration. (2018). FDA drug safety communication: Safety update for osteoporosis drugs, bisphosphonates, and atypical fractures. Available at: https://www.fda.gov/drugs/drug-safety-and-availability/fda-drug-safety-communication-safety-update-osteoporosis-drugs-bisphosphonates-and-atypical

Valdes-Rodriguez, R., Stull, C., & Yosipovitch, G. (2015). Chronic pruritus in the elderly: Pathophysiology, Diagnosis and Management. *Drugs & Aging, 32*(3), 201–215. doi:10.1007/s40266-015-0246-0.

Wehling, M. (2014). Non-steroidal anti-inflammatory drug use in chronic pain conditions with special emphasis on the elderly and patients with relevant comorbidities: Management and mitigation of risks and adverse effects. *European Journal of Clinical Pharmacology, 70*(10), 1159–1172. doi:10.1007/s00228-014-1734-6

What is the most likely differential diagnosis and why?

Osteoarthritis (OA):

Obesity, age, and a previous history of an active lifestyle can contribute to OA. People with OA usually have symptoms that occur with activity or shortly after embarking on activity. Stairs can present a particular problem. OA is most often unilateral but can be polyarticular and symmetric. Sharon did not experience any popping, twisting, clicking, or giving way, so ligamental strains and tears are less likely. She denies experiencing a tick bite, but it is important to remember that one does not always remember a bite or being outdoors and may still have Lyme disease. However, Lyme disease typically presents with unilateral knee pain and swelling. A Lyme titer might be a good test to include in the diagnostics for this case just to rule out the possibility. Gout and pseudo-gout typically include acute onset of severe pain accompanied by erythema and warmth. They are most often unilateral.

Patellofemoral syndrome is most common in teens and young adults. Anterior knee pain is the most common complaint. Difficulty with stairs is a symptom with difficulty going down stairs typically more severe than going up stairs. Sitting for prolonged periods causes pain that is relieved with walking, and a sense of joint locking instability is common. Rheumatoid arthritis (RA) is typically symmetric and may appear in later life, so Sharon should be questioned regarding morning stiffness, other joint pain and swelling, and fatigue, especially since she has a positive family history for RA. If Sharon experienced unilateral knee pain with an acute onset specific to the area just inferior and medial to the patella (classic location), she would most likely have anserine bursitis.

Which diagnostic studies should be considered to assist with or confirm the diagnosis?

It is important to determine whether the pain is acute or chronic and whether the patient's activity level or ability to move or function has changed because of the pain. Ask the patient to point to the part of the knee causing her pain. Knee pain can be a sign of systemic disease so a thorough history and diagnostic testing are necessary depending on presentation.

A rheumatoid factor, Lyme titer, and a CCP as well as an ESR should be included in the lab work for Sharon. Further, Sharon may be osteoporotic and should therefore receive a DEXA scan if she

The Family Nurse Practitioner: Clinical Case Studies, Second Edition. Edited by Leslie Neal-Boylan.
© 2021 John Wiley & Sons Ltd. Published 2021 by John Wiley & Sons Ltd.

hasn't had one in the past year or 2. Sharon should have X-rays of the knees if these have not previously been done or if they have not been done for a long time. An ultrasound is necessary if an effusion is suspected. An MRI is appropriate if a soft tissue injury is suspected. In addition to labwork this visit (Lyme titer, rheumatoid factor, CCP, ESR, vitamin D), Sharon should have a CBC, CMP, and TSH, as her blood pressure is elevated and she is fatigued. These tests could be delayed, for insurance reimbursement purposes, until she returns to the office for a complete physical. At that time, the clinician should order a mammogram, colonoscopy, and DEXA scan, and also should include a pelvic exam.

What should be the plan of treatment?

Clearly, Sharon needs a physical to determine her overall health status and to evaluate her health maintenance. She should be advised to lose weight, exercise, and begin taking calcium and vitamin D, if deficient. Sharon's blood pressure is elevated during this visit. She should be encouraged to check her blood pressure at home every day for 3 weeks and return for a follow-up visit. She should be educated about symptoms of hypertension and red flags associated with potential complications and when to report them. She should be counseled to eat a low-sodium diet.

In addition, Sharon should decrease weight bearing while her knees are causing her pain. Swimming in a heated pool is a good alternative. She should avoid kneeling and try to do less housework, if possible. Plan to see Sharon back to discuss the imaging and lab results and to perform her physical and pelvic exams.

Lifestyle changes are the first-line treatment. However, oral and topical NSAIDs, intra-articular steroid injections, capsaicin, and braces may be helpful. Surgery is a final option. Acetaminophen is not recommended.

What should be the plan for health maintenance testing for this patient?

Sharon should see the dermatologist annually to assess and treat any suspicious skin lesions. If the primary care clinician observes any suspicious lesions between these annual visits, the patient should see the dermatologist sooner. Sharon should also have a colonoscopy if she has not had one or if the last one was 5 or more years ago depending on the findings at that time. She should also have annual mammograms. Sharon should have a DEXA scan to look for osteoporosis or osteopenia. In addition, she should have basic laboratory screening including CBC, LFTs, CMP, and a lipid panel.

Does this patient need gynecological care and treatment at this time?

Sharon is a widow and is not engaged in sexual activity; however, she and her nurse practitioner should jointly discuss the advisability of a pelvic exam to check for abnormalities. The vaginal dryness is probably due to atrophy and should be examined. Sharon may want and/or require treatment. The American Cancer Society recommends Pap test screening until age 65 years for a healthy patient who has not had an abnormal test fort 10 years (https://www.cancer.org/cancer/cervical-cancer/prevention-and-early-detection/cervical-cancer-screening-guidelines.html).

What is the plan for referrals and follow-up?

No referrals are needed at this time. However, if treatment fails, then an orthopedic and/or a rheumatologic referral should be considered. Sharon can be treated with NSAIDs to begin with, and diclofenac gel can be used to rub into her knees. Alternation of ice and heat may also help. If swelling increases and limits her mobility, corticoid injections into the knee should be considered. Synvisc injections are also possible treatments. Finally, total knee replacements may need to be considered in the future if her symptoms worsen.

REFERENCES AND RESOURCES

American Cancer Society. (2018, May 30). *American Cancer Society guideline for colorectal cancer screening*. https://www.cancer.org/cancer/colon-rectal-cancer/detection-diagnosis-staging/acs-recommendations.html

Cameron, D. J., Johnson, L. B., & Maloney, E. L. (2014). Evidence assessments and guideline recommendations in Lyme disease: The clinical management of known tick bytes, erythema migrans rashes and persistent disease. *Expert Review of Anti-Infective Therapy, 12*(9), 1103–1135. https://www.ilads.org/patient-care/ilads-treatment-guidelines

Deveza, L. A., Bennell, K., Hunter, D., & Curtis, M. R. (2019). Osteoarthritis. *UpToDdate*.

Mayo Clinic. (2018, April 21). *Pseudogout*. https://www.mayoclinic.org/diseases-conditions/pseudogout/symptoms-causes/syc-20376983

National Osteoporosis Foundation. (n.d.). https://www.nof.org

O'Dell, J. R. (2007). Rheumatoid arthritis: The disease—diagnosis and clinical features. In J. Imboden, D. Hellmann, & J. Stone (Eds.), *Current diagnosis & treatment: Rheumatology* (2nd ed., pp. 161–169). New York: McGraw Hill-Lange.

What are the top three differential diagnoses in this case and why?

1. Heat-related illness (classic heat stroke vs. heat exhaustion)
2. Neurological condition (e.g., stroke, meningitis, encephalitis)
3. Infection (systemic or central nervous system)

Which diagnostic tests are required in this case and why?

1. MRI or CT to assess for central nervous system causes of altered mental status
2. Blood and urine cultures with urinalysis to rule out systemic and urinary tract infection
3. Laboratory studies:
   - CBC to assess for increased WBC
   - Serum electrolytes to assess for abnormalities, particularly sodium
   - BUN, creatinine to assess for acute kidney injury
   - Liver enzymes to assess for heat-induced liver injury
   - Coagulation panel (PT, PTT, INR) to assess for heat-induced liver injury and disseminated intravascular coagulation

What are the concerns at this point?

Given Judith's risk factors and her current neurological and cardiovascular status, the etiology of hyperthermia is unclear. However, heat stroke, which is a medical emergency that can lead to multisystem organ failure and death, cannot be ruled out. It is important to note that the temperature reported by the EMTs at the scene was an oral temperature and therefore corresponds to a higher core temperature. Efforts to decrease her core temperature should be the priority to prevent further deterioration while other diagnoses are investigated.

The elderly are particularly vulnerable to heat-related illnesses (HRIs), such as heat exhaustion and heat stroke. List the symptoms and treatment associated with each condition.

Heat-related illnesses (HRIs) are the most common cause of weather-related deaths in the United States. Older adults, those living with chronic illness, pregnant women, and prepubertal children

The Family Nurse Practitioner: Clinical Case Studies, Second Edition. Edited by Leslie Neal-Boylan.
© 2021 John Wiley & Sons Ltd. Published 2021 by John Wiley & Sons Ltd.

are particularly at risk for developing an HRI. These are classified as mild (heat edema, heat rash, and muscle cramping), moderate (syncope, heat exhaustion), and severe (heat stroke). There are two types of heat stroke—exertional hyperthermia and nonexertional (classic heat stroke) hyperthermia, both of which are life-threatening, medical emergencies.

1. Heat exhaustion
   - Symptoms: Thirst (late sign in the elderly), headache, fatigue, tachycardia, weakness, ataxia, syncope, nausea, vomiting, diarrhea, cold/clammy skin, core temperature 101–104°F
   - Treatment: Remove from heat, rest in supine position, evaporative cooling, oral/IV rehydration.
2. Heat stroke
   - Symptoms: Altered mental status (confusion, delirium, seizures, coma, tachycardia, tachypnea, hypotension, pulmonary crackles, oliguria, core temperature 104°F or greater.
   - Treatment: Rapid cooling to below 102°F, using conductive or evaporative cooling techniques (infusion of cool fluids, application of ice packs or wet gauze with fanning). These are better tolerated in the elderly as compared to cold water immersion.

NOTE: Antipyretics should *not* be used to treat heatstroke.

Identify six risk factors that Judith has for developing heatstroke.

1. Age
2. Gender
3. Socioeconomic status
4. Chronic medical condition (cardiovascular disease)
5. Social isolation
6. Medications
   a. Lasix: Dehydration
   b. Beta-blockers: Reduced cardiac output decreases blood flow to skin, limiting the shunting of warm blood to periphery, which impairs cooling

Identify three physical assessment findings from the case that support a diagnosis of heatstroke.

It should be noted that heatstroke is diagnosed clinically, and there is no diagnostic test that can confirm it. However, in the face of hyperthermia, neurological symptoms, and recent exposure to hot weather, heatstroke should be considered. In this case, Judith presented with:

1. Hyperthermia
2. Confusion and restlessness
3. Hemodynamic indicators (tachycardia, tachypnea, hypotension)

Identify and explain three elements from the patient's history that support a diagnosis of heat stroke.

1. No air conditioning in the home in the context of a heatwave.
2. EMT's report of neurological status upon arrival to the home.
3. Documented oral temperature in the home. Of note, a PO temperature of 103.3°F is particularly concerning because it correlates with a core temperature greater than 104°F.

What is the differential diagnosis for heatstroke?

Meningitis, encephalitis, epilepsy, drug intoxication, severe dehydration, and metabolic syndromes such as neuroleptic malignant syndrome and thyroid storm. Alternative diagnoses should be considered only after ruling out heatstroke since a delay in treatment increases morbidity and mortality.

What is the plan of treatment?
<u>*Send Judith to the emergency room by ambulance.*</u>

1. *Rapid cooling* in the emergency room to below 102°F, using convective or evaporative cooling techniques (infusion of cool fluids, application of ice packs or wet gauze with fanning). These are better tolerated in the elderly as compared to cold water immersion. The longer hyperthermia persists, the greater chance of complications related to the underlying systemic inflammatory response triggered.
2. Hospital admission for supportive care and continued monitoring for prompt recognition of complications including: acute respiratory distress syndrome, rhabdomyolysis, compartment syndrome, liver dysfunction, acute renal failure, disseminated intravascular coagulopathy, and electrolyte abnormalities

NOTE: Antipyretics should *not* be used to treat heatstroke.

What are the plans for referral and follow-up care?

- Home health care services:
  - Nursing to continue patient education and to provide care as required based on her clinical status at the time of discharge.
  - Occupational therapy (OT) to assess Judith's home environment for safety.
  - Physical therapy as needed.
- Referral to local community agency to determine if local cooling centers are available during periods of heat wave and to determine process for accessing (i.e., transportation).

What health education should be provided to this patient?

- Education about heat and health and home environment
- Heat-related prevention measures
  - Stay indoors during between 10 a.m. and 4 p.m. when it is the hottest.
  - Ensure that shades are on windows and draw during periods when sun is most intense.
  - Wear a hat and light clothing when going outside.
  - Take cool showers.
  - Drink plenty of cool liquids before you feel thirsty (check with your doctor to see what amount is appropriate).
  - Do not use the oven to cook on very hot days.
  - *Note:* The research on the use of fans for cooling in the elderly, while limited, is equivocal. Some studies suggest that the use of electric fans impedes heat loss at high ambient temperatures while others suggest fans contribute to heat loss. If the ambient temperature is hotter than the core temperature of an individual, the use of a fan can lead to an increase in core temperature, particularly on hot, dry days above 95°F.
- Worrisome signs and symptoms
  - Dizziness or fainting
  - Nausea or vomiting
  - Headache
  - Rapid breathing
  - Rapid heart rate
  - Extreme thirst
  - Decreased urination and dark urine
- What to do if you experience symptoms
  - If outside, move to a cool place immediately and drink cool liquids.
  - If inside, call 911.

What demographic characteristics might affect this case?

- Age
- Gender
- Social isolation/lives alone
- Low socioeconomic status

Does the patient's psychosocial history impact how you might treat her?

The patient's psychosocial history is important in the treatment plan since social isolation is a concern for Judith. Addressing the need for social services with additional services such as social work involvement are important considerations.

How does Judith's living in an urban area impact her risk for heatstroke?

Living in an urban area is an additional risk for heatstroke, particularly for vulnerable populations. Urban heat islands are a risk for heatstroke, particularly for the elderly. The urban heat island refers to a city or metropolitan area that experiences significantly higher temperatures than rural areas. Because urban areas have areas with asphalt and concrete, temperatures are significantly higher than rural areas with greenspace. Asphalt absorbs the sun's rays because of its dark color and both asphalt and concrete retain heat at higher temperatures than green areas. Buildings also reflect heat, which then leads to higher temperatures.

Are there any standardized guidelines that should be used to treat this case? If so, what are they?

Canadian Guidelines on Heat Stress and Health: Retrieved from https://www.canada.ca/en/health-canada/services/environmental-workplace-health/reports-publications/climate-change-health/extreme-heat-events-guidelines-technical-guide-health-care-workers.html

REFERENCES AND RESOURCES

Epstein, Y., & Yanovich, R. (2019). Heatstroke. *New England Journal of Medicine, 380*(25), 2449–2459. doi:10.1056/NEJMra1810762

Gaudio, F. G., & Grissom, C. K. (2016). Cooling methods in heat stroke. *Journal of Emergency Medicine, 50*(4), 607–616. doi:10.1016/j.jemermed.2015.09.014

Gauer, R., & Meyers, B.K. (2019). Heat-related illnesses. *American Family Physician, 99*(8), 482–489.

Gupta, S., Carmichael, C., Simpson, C., Clarke, M. J., Allen, C., Gao, Y., . . . Murray, V. (2012). Electric fans for reducing adverse health impacts in heatwaves. *Cochrane Database of Systematic Reviews, 7*, CD009888. doi:10.1002/14651858.CD009888.pub2

Lemery, J., & Auerbach, P. (2017). *Enviromedics: The impact on climate change on human health.* London: Rowman & Littlefield.

Luber, G., & McGeehin, M. (2008). Climate change and extreme heat events. *American Journal of Preventative Medicine, 35*(5), 429–435. doi:10.1016/j.amepre.2008.08.021

Mechem, C. C. (2019). Severe nonexertional hyperthermia (classic heat stroke) in adults. *UpToDate.* Retrieved from: www.uptodate.com

Wald, A. (2019). Emergency department visits and costs for heat-related illness due to extreme heat or heat waves in the United States: An integrated review. *Nursing Economic$, 37*(1), 35–48.

Water, Air, and Climate Change Bureau, Health Environments and Consumer Safety Branch. (2011). *Extreme heat events guidelines: Technical guide for health care workers.* Retrieved from: www.healthcanada.gc.ca

Index

The Family Nurse Practitioner: Clinical Case Studies, Second Edition. Edited by Leslie Neal-Boylan.
© 2021 John Wiley & Sons Ltd. Published 2021 by John Wiley & Sons Ltd.